PROPERTY OF RIVERWOOD CENTER

PROPERTY OF
RIVERWOOD COMMUNITY MENTAL HEALTH

Edited by
ALAN KERR
PHILIP SNAITH

With the assistance of
STANLEY THORLEY (Indexing)
ALISON CAMPBELL

Contemporary Issues in Schizophrenia

For all the physicians and authors in the world could not give a clear account of his madness. He is mad in patches, full of lucid intervals.

CERVANTES   *Don Quixote*

GASKELL

© The Royal College of Psychiatrists 1986

ISBN 0 902241 13 3
ISBN 0 902241 14 1 (*Pbk*)

Gaskell is an imprint of the Royal College of
Psychiatrists, 17 Belgrave Square, London SW1

Printed in Great Britain at The Bath Press, Avon

Distributed in North America by
American Psychiatric Press, Inc.

ISBN 0-88048-228-1

Contents

*Articles commissioned for this publication

Part III   Organic aspects

Part IV   Genetic aspects

List of Contributors

David Abrahamson, Consultant Psychiatrist, Goodmayes Hospital, Essex

G. W. Ashcroft, Professor of Psychiatry, Department of Mental Health, University of Aberdeen, University Medical Buildings, Foresterhill, Aberdeen

Roger Baker, Research Principal Psychologist, Royal Cornhill Hospital, Aberdeen

Manfred Bleuler, Professor of Psychiatry, University of Zurich, Bahnhofstrasse 49, CH-8702 Zollikon, Switzerland

Luc Ciompi, Specialist FMH for Psychiatry and Psychotherapy, Director of the Sociopsychiatric University Clinic, Murtenstrasse 21, CH-3010 Berne, Switzerland

John Cooper, Professor of Psychiatry, University Department of Psychiatry, Mapperley Hospital, Porchester Road, Nottingham

Timothy J. Crow, Head of Division and Honorary Consultant Psychiatrist, Division of Psychiatry, Clinical Research Centre, Northwick Park Hospital, Harrow, Middlesex

Raymond R. Crowe, Associate Professor of Psychiatry, Department of Psychiatry, University of Iowa College of Medicine, Iowa City, Iowa 52242, USA

John Cutting, Consultant Psychiatrist, Bethlem Royal Hospital, Monks Orchard Road, Beckenham, Kent

N. J. Delva, Assistant Professor, Department of Psychiatry, Queen's University, Kingston, Ontario, Canada

Kenneth Dewhurst, late Professor of Psychiatry, University of the West Indies, Mona, Kingston, Jamaica

Donald Eccleston, Professor of Psychiatry, Royal Victoria Infirmary, Newcastle upon Tyne

Herbert Fox, Clinical Director, Grace Square Hospital, 420 East 76 Street, New York, USA

Hugh Freeman, Consultant Psychiatrist, Hope Hospital, Salford, Manchester

Joe Galdi, Behavioral Neurology Program, New Hampshire Hospital, Concord, New Hampshire 03301, USA

John Hall, District Psychologist, Department of Psychology, Warneford Hospital, Headington, Oxford

Edward Hare, Emeritus Physician, Maudsley Hospital, Denmark Hill, London SE5

George G. Hay, Consultant Psychiatrist, Department of Psychiatry, University Hospital of South Manchester, West Didsbury, Manchester

Steven R. Hirsch, Professor of Psychiatry, Charing Cross Hospital Medical School, Fulham Palace Road, London W6

J. Hoenig, Professor of Psychiatry, Clarke Institute, 250 College Street, Toronto, Ontario, Canada

D. A. W. Johnson, Consultant Psychiatrist, Withington Hospital, West Didsbury, Manchester

Eve Johnstone, Honorary Consultant Psychiatrist, Division of Psychiatry, Clinical Research Centre, Northwick Park Hospital, Harrow, Middlesex

Jon Karlsson, Institute of Genetics, Hraunteig 16, Reykjavick, Iceland

David W. K. Kay, Emeritus Professor of Psychiatry, University of Tasmania

R. E. Kendell, Professor of Psychiatry, University Department of Psychiatry, Royal Edinburgh Hospital, Morningside Park, Edinburgh

Seymour Kety, Professor of Psychiatry and Associate Director for Basic Research, Laboratory of Clinical Science, National Institute for Mental Health, Bethesda, Maryland 20205, USA

Karl Koehler, Universitäts-Nervenklinik-Psychiatrie, Sigmund Freud Str. 25, 5300 Bonn 1, West Germany

Julian Leff, Consultant Psychiatrist, MRC Social Psychiatry Unit, Friern Hospital, Friern Barnet Road, London N11

F. J. J. Letemendia, Professor, Department of Psychiatry, Queen's University, Kingston, Ontario, Canada

Hamish A. McClelland, Consultant Psychiatrist, St Nicholas Hospital, Gosforth, Newcastle upon Tyne

Robin G. McCreadie, Director of Clinical Research and Consultant Psychiatrist, Crichton Royal Hospital, Dumfries, Scotland

R. A. Machón, Department of Psychology and Social Science Research Institute, University of Southern California, Los Angeles, California 90089-111, USA

Angus V. P. Mackay, Physician Superintendent, Argyll and Bute Hospital, Lochgilphead, Argyll, Scotland

S. A. Mednick, Director, Psykologisk Institut, Kommunehospitet, 1399 Copenhagen, Denmark

C. S. Mellor, Department of Psychiatry, Memorial University, St John's, Newfoundland, Canada

Sukdeb Mukherjee, Assistant Clinical Professor of Psychiatry, College of Physicians and Surgeons of Columbia University, Department of Biological Psychiatry, New York State Psychiatric Institute, New York, USA

Alistair Munro, Head, Department of Psychiatry, Dalhousie University, Halifax, Nova Scotia, Canada

Robin M. Murray, Dean, Institute of Psychiatry, De Crespigny Park, London SE5

Adrianne M. Reveley, Senior Lecturer, Institute of Psychiatry, De Crespigny Park, London SE5

Michael A. Reveley, Senior Lecturer and Honorary Consultant, Institute of Psychiatry, De Crespigny Park, London SE5

Sir Martin Roth, Professor of Psychiatry, Department of Psychiatry, University of Cambridge Clinical School, Addenbrooke's Hospital, Cambridge

Norman Sartorius, Chief, Office of Mental Health, World Health Organization, Geneva, Switzerland

Fini Schulsinger, Professor and Chairman, Department of Psychiatry, Kommunehospitalet, 1399 Copenhagen, Denmark

Andrew Scull, Professor of Sociology, University of California, San Diego, California, 92093, USA

Graham P. Sheppard, Consultant Psychiatrist, Hayes Priory Hospital, Prestons Road, Hayes, Kent

Andrew Sims, Professor of Psychiatry, Department of Psychiatry, St James's University Hospital, Leeds

Andrew C. Smith, Consultant Psychiatrist, Greenwich District Hospital, London SE10

Thomas Szasz, Professor of Psychiatry, State University of New York, Upstate Medical Center, Syracuse, New York, USA

John Todd, formerly Consultant Psychiatrist, High Royds Hospital, Menston, W. Yorkshire

Ming T. Tsuang, Professor of Psychiatry, Department of Psychiatry, University of Iowa College of Medicine, Iowa City, Iowa 52242, USA

H. M. van Praag, Professor and Chair, Department of Psychiatry, Albert Einstein College of Medicine, Montefiore Hospital, Bronx, New York 10461, USA

Geoffrey Wallis, formerly Consultant Psychiatrist, High Royds Hospital, Menston, W. Yorkshire

David C. Watt, Consultant Psychiatrist, St John's Hospital, Stone, Aylesbury, Buckinghamshire

George Winokur, Professor and Head, Department of Psychiatry, University of Iowa College of Medicine, Iowa City, Iowa 52242, USA

Foreword

The first Special Publication of the *British Journal of Psychiatry* appeared in 1967. The topic was 'Recent Developments in Schizophrenia' with reports on ten lectures on the broad range of themes related to schizophrenia. After a decade and a half, interest in the disorder has not slackened and the Editorial Board of the *Journal* considered that an update would be helpful to students, researchers and clinicians. The *British Journal of Psychiatry* has published the reports of some of the outstanding papers of the period and we decided that a reprinting of these would form the basis of the present book. Space has imposed rather rigid criteria and many interesting scientific papers have not been included, preference being given to papers presenting broad reviews. The papers we have reprinted are not in precisely the same format as the originals and abbreviations by the removal of tabulated data and summaries have taken place. At times we have asked researchers, prominent in a particular field, to provide a new review of their field of interest and we have invited distinguished psychiatrists to present a series of Overviews of the present status of knowledge.

Furtherance of knowledge is impossible without definition, and schizophrenia is notoriously resistant to definition. A major endeavour in the past fifteen years has been concerned with the delineation of the disorder. The urgent need for this effort was underlined by the recognition that in at least two countries, the UK and the USA, the concept of schizophrenia was very different; this discovery also posed the question whether a disorder discernable as schizophrenia occurred in all parts of the world or whether it had a more limited geographical and racial distribution. These questions were addressed by the most thorough and searching investigation ever undertaken in the area of psychiatry. Specially trained psychiatrists from nine cities in nine countries (Denmark, India, Columbia, Nigeria, Great Britain, USSR, Taiwan, USA and Czechoslovakia) constituted the group for the International Pilot Study of Schizophrenia. Their findings were published in 1973 and the most important of the conclusions was that a central syndrome recognizable as schizophrenia occurred in all parts of the world where the study was undertaken.

The period has seen the development of aetiological theory and speculation. The previous emphasis on interpersonal and social causation has to some extent lost ground to biological factors but there is an increasing recognition of the multi-dimensional nature of this complex disorder. Work on biochemical abnormalities has supported the hypothesis of abnormal dopamine transmission and provides some part of the explanation for the effectiveness of certain drugs in the treatment of schizophrenia. A wealth of other possible aetiological factors are being proposed, all or any of which may eventually throw some light on the conundrum.

The relationship of disorders of mood to schizophrenia is now under closer scrutiny than at any time since rigid categorical distinctions in the psychotic illnesses were proposed. This inter-relationship will inevitably cause research findings to be more difficult to interpret but, in clinical practice, recognition and appropriate management may lead to improved outcome of the schizophrenic disorders. The link between schizophrenia and the paranoid disorders, especially the intriguing forms of monodelusional psychoses, is an area which has received insufficient attention in the period. Interest in the recognition of schizophrenia, or at least schizophreniform disorders, in the setting of mental handicap has been promoted by some excellent studies and more are required.

The decade and a half has been a period of further criticism of psychiatric practice and the reporting of major hospital scandals added fuel to the flames. Stances have been adopted which have not necessarily lead to the better care of the patient, and discharge policies of long-stay patients, adumbrated in the Hospital Plan of 1962, have proceeded before alternative care has been established. Often the burden of care is placed on the family, untrained and sometimes unsupported in the task, and the President of the National Schizophrenia Fellowship has spoken of the family life being laid in ruins. Adequate community care is still lacking but one hopeful development in the period is the establishment of the grade of psychiatric community nurse who establishes links with the discharged patient and family.

We have aimed to draw attention to the present broad range of comment and research in schizophrenia. Research and practice should be intimately linked and we look forward to the state of knowledge and of care for the individual in another fifteen years, the year 2001 AD.

THE EDITORS

I. General and historical concepts

1   General and historical concepts in schizophrenia: Overview

ANDREW C. SMITH

To psychiatrists, schizophrenia remains the classical severe and disabling mental illness. Lives are ruined by neurosis and personality disorder, early promise unfulfilled because of manic-depressive psychosis, and epidemiological studies show that 95 per cent of psychiatric disorder is seen and treated (if at all) in general practice, but the greatest affliction is schizophrenia. It baffles us, and disables the patients, justifiably counting as the paradigm of mental illnesses, worthy subject of our attention as psychiatric physicians. Yet if we raise our eyes from the task in hand, we find very different views expressed by those in other fields of endeavour. They seem to see our schizophrenia as a horse of entirely different colour, if not as no horse but of a different species, or even a ghost of an animal. Although the views often come from those who never meet schizophrenics, and may thus be regarded as underqualified to express wisdom on the nature of the disorder, I believe that rival views give us perspective and provoke thought.

For this reason I shall mention anti-psychiatric views first, before moving to the familiar field of discussions of the definitions of illness that have been proposed by doctors. Keeping a distant point of view a little longer, I touch on schizophrenia in past ages before our own and in other places than our familiar base, before shortening the length of focus and examining more closely, as psychiatrists are accustomed to doing, some aspects of research on causes, and discussions of diagnosis. Finally I try to collect the many theories into four groups, and tentatively offer the outline of a widely based theory of the disorder.

Does the illness exist?

The high point of anti-psychiatric writing occurred in the 1960s—the age of Laing's *The Divided Self* (1965) and Szasz's *The Myth of Mental Illness* (1962) and *The Manufacture of Madness* (1971). Little explicit criticism of the concept of schizophrenia has been heard from Laing in recent years, and Szasz's continuing attacks contain no new ideas: he is resting on the earlier ones (**Szasz, 1976***). He chooses clear-cut cases to ease his argument—the medical model is represented by an infectious disease of single aetiology and clear-cut pathology—syphilis, and he finds it easy to argue that psychiatrists by contrast

---

References given in **bold denote those papers reprinted in this publication.*

with other doctors are dealing only with behaviour. These psychiatric doctors are then alleged to call eccentric behaviour diseased, which exercise is a disgraceful abrogation of human freedom and responsibility. A sociological argument is pursued according to which the nineteenth century psychiatrists (Kraepelin, castigated again for debasing his patients, in the same role as he appears in Laing's famous passage in *The Divided Self*, 1965), under pressure from society, re-defined awkward deviants as diseased people suitable to be coerced by doctors. The criticism, written as it is with reckless gusto, touches a raw nerve in psychiatrists, as witness the angry riposte by **Roth (1976)**.

A later classic in this area, *de rigueur* on sociological reading lists, is the Rosenhan experiment (1973) in which normal volunteers had themselves admitted incognito to American mental hospitals after claiming to hear monosyllabic hallucinated voices. They were diagnosed as schizophrenic by the staff, and thereafter behaved normally, but were still described as abnormal, presumably because of the effect of the stigma of being mentally ill. The experiment is said to show the drastic effects of labelling and the hopeless subjectivity of psychiatric diagnosis. It does indeed need some explaining, although pilloried psychiatrists have put forward many defences: the experiment needs replication, it could not happen in good mental hospitals here, the procedure of deceiving the staff is unfair, and Wing (1978) on each occasion when he refers to the experiment mentions the investigators' 'lies'.

The anti-psychiatric case, that psychiatrists 'medicalize deviance' as a profession and that there is literally no such thing as mental illness, became the received wisdom among radical critics outside psychiatry, so perhaps no further texts were needed for some time. The mantle of critic of the psychiatrists has now, however, fallen on Scull (1979), who, although not a maverick member of the psychiatric ranks but a sociologist, has been well-informed on the nineteenth century history of the asylums, the inmates and the doctors.

Wing is one of those psychiatrists who have recently defended the psychiatric enterprise and its involvement with the condition and illness of schizophrenia, by writing detailed expositions of the state of knowledge: four examples are his own *Reasoning about Madness* (1978), Clare's *Psychiatry in Dissent* (1976), Tsuang's *Schizophrenia: the Facts* (1982) and Smith's *Schizophrenia and Madness* (1982b). They have explained the broad base of the models of illness used in psychiatry, and shown how the crude 'medical model' allegedly used is an Aunt Sally set up by the critics for ease of being knocked down again. Attention to definitions of illness or disease (unfortunately the two are rarely distinguished) has come from Kräupl Taylor (1979), and from **Kendell (1975)**, who mentions Szasz in his second sentence. Kendell rejects definitions of disease as syndromes of complaints of feeling ill, or as consisting of those needing to be under medical care, or Taylor's suggestion of those awaking therapeutic concern in self or others, as being vague or circular. If there is no objective criterion then doctors or society could call deviants ill (as Szasz claims they do). Basing the definition of disease on physical lesions is objective, but there are still problems with functional syndromes such as migraine or trigeminal neuralgia. In the end he adapts Scadding's (1967) definition, that the criterion is that the abnormality is a biological disadvantage, applying it to psychiatry by pointing out the low fertility of schizophrenics.

Kendell insists on individual biological disadvantage in fertility and procreation as the criterion of disease (but will get into difficulty, as the theory seems then to require homosexuality to be a disease, an awkward conclusion). The conclusion is that some psychiatric disorders fulfil the same criteria as those of physical illness (even ignoring for the moment the partial genetic transmission, and therefore physical basis, of schizophrenia). And he concludes: 'By all means let us insist that schizophrenia is an illness [it was "disease" in the title of the paper] and that we are better equipped to understand and treat it than anyone else. But let us not try to do the same for all the woes of mankind'. So that is the position: schizophrenia is in the medical heartland of psychiatry, and the critics' discussion of medical empire-building concerns other conditions.

Other times

Was the modern illness, schizophrenia, found in past times? **Hare (1983)**, in his survey of the figures on the rapidly increasing numbers of asylum patients in England in the nineteenth century, comes to the conclusion that the numbers of first-ever admissions (the figures we need, which are not given in the official statistics) can be deduced, and rise between 1859 and 1900, denoting an actual increase in insanity, and not merely an artefact of recognition of milder cases, better ascertainment and longer survival of patients (see also **Scull, 1984**). The cases were probably not of general paralysis of the insane, but functional psychosis, i.e. the patients subsequently regarded as schizophrenic. Hare is impressed, as have been others such as Torrey (1980), by the rarity of descriptions of typical schizophrenia before the nineteenth century, and suspects an epidemic of a new illness, the evidence being 'certainly compatible with a somatic cause'—he favours an infective one.

Yet Scull (1979), also studying the history of the asylums and 'the social organization of insanity in nineteenth century England', comes to very different conclusions. He believes that the medical profession helped society to send awkward people to the asylums, and it was because they were doctors that the alienists believed that insanity was based on brain disease, which would be found one day. There was no new illness, but a new 'confinement' (discussed also in Foucault, 1967) of the deviant. 'In fact', according to Scull, 'by sustaining the illusion that asylums were medical institutions, they placed a humanitarian and scientific gloss on the community's behaviour, legitimizing the removal of difficult and troublesome people whose confinement would have been awkward to justify on other grounds.' Contrast the usual view as in Kendell's (1975) aside: 'The asylums of the nineteenth century were after all built primarily for the protection of the insane and only secondarily for the protection of society.'

Historians of ideas, too, have watched the doctors and what they do, and interpreted medical practice in terms of changing societies and how they function, without requiring the concept of named illnesses. Thus MacDonald (1981a) suggests that the history of insanity in early modern England 'was profoundly influenced by a growing divergence between the mental worlds of the upper and lower orders of society. During the sixteenth century, most people shared a common assessment of what the most destructive kinds of insanity were, and they often employed traditional religious and demonological symbolism to describe abnormal thoughts and actions ... Because competing religious beliefs became matters of political controversy during the late sixteenth and seventeenth centuries, the governing élite rejected those aspects of popular religion and demonology which had become politically charged.' Religious theories and therapies became politically dangerous, and were slowly discredited by the advance of science and the growth in size and respectability of the medical profession. By the eighteenth century insanity was a medical and social problem, he claims (1981b), and the madhouses and asylums were needed. Thus, in our terms, schizophrenia could be a modern disease because modern society has modern insanity. But we can still look ourselves for schizophrenia in the records of past ages.

Historical studies in the last few years have been more sophisticated than when Zilboorg and Henry (1941) diagnosed Socrates as schizophrenic because he was guided by inspiring voices at times, and stood immobile in the freezing cold lost in thought for hours. We can now read descriptions of patients in Simon (1978) on ancient Greece, Rosen (1968) on *Madness in Society* for the Old Testament and the ancient world, Clarke (1975) on *Mental Disorder in Earlier Britain*, Leigh (1961) on the eighteenth and nineteenth centuries, and Hunter and MacAlpine's (1964) *Three Hundred Years of Psychiatry, 1535–1860*, as well as Allderidge (1979) and Jones (1972) on the history of the organization of services. Torrey (1980) collected evidence that schizophrenia is a 'disease of civilization', and, like **Hare (1983)**, pointed out that there is always madness in the records of past ages, but typical schizophrenia, with onset in early adulthood and progressive deterioration, is very rarely described before the late eighteenth century (and he ascribes the rare cases to organic syndromes mimicking true schizophrenia). Hare adds that even the first edition of Haslam's book in 1798 has no account of what we would recognize as acute schizophrenia.

In the Bible Ezekiel is described as having a sudden experience of a message and visions of God, followed by years of prophesying in communications full of symbolic meaning. He lay on his left side for 390 days and then on his right side for 40 days to represent the years of iniquity of the peoples; he cut off his hair and divided it into three portions, burning one, chopping one with a knife and scattering one to the wind, to symbolize death from pestilence, death by the sword, and the scattering of the tribes of Israel. Are these actions of a great prophet different from the delusional mood and symbolic acting of modern schizophrenics? In Greece there are descriptions of individuals with delusions of persecution and being plotted against, and delusions of grandeur. One believed that all the shipping in and out of Piraeus belonged to him—and he recovered later.

Most of the patients described in mediaeval records, for example when visiting shrines, are impossible to diagnose as schizophrenic, but Clarke's (1975) account of Henry VI's illness has been discussed by Smith (1982b) in his survey of the retrospective search for schizophrenic cases as being a reasonably convincing example. At the age of 31 he suddenly became severely withdrawn, inaccessible to conversation, silent, and slumped in posture, a condition which continued for a year and a half. Delegations came repeatedly to beg for attention to business, but he 'gave no answer, word or sign'. He afterwards had no memory of what had occurred during the time, including the birth of a son. The treatment was designed to be medical, by a commission of three physicians, entrusted by the Council to treat him according to the best textbooks and 'according to the advice of experienced doctors who have written on this type of case.' In subsequent years his earlier religious eccentricities and remoteness were more marked, with awkward silences during ceremonies and during a battle 'the king was placed under a tree a mile away, where he laughed and sang.'

In Renaissance and seventeenth century Britain, there are more abundant descriptions of the insane, in fact and fiction. Denials that schizophrenia is described in Shakespeare (Torrey, 1980) must disqualify the madness portrayed in Hamlet, Macbeth, Othello and King Lear, but Bark (1985) argues that Edgar, when masquerading as a Tom o' Bedlam in *King Lear*, displays in his speech typical thought disorder with loosening of associations, neologisms and imaginary persecuting voices. The seventeenth century has stories of grandiose Messiahs in plenty, Hunter and Macalpine's George Trosse with voices of many fairies talking to him in the walls of his room, and Alexander Cruden the eccentric and zealot who proclaimed himself Alexander the Great, 'Corrector of the Morals of the Nation', whose friends had him confined as insane to a private madhouse for three periods.

By 1801 Pinel (1806; Smith, 1967), in the Bicêtre, had a patient who believed he was Mahomet; many patients had grandiose delusions of being kings and even deities, and had vivid hallucinations; one wandered about the institution muttering and smiling to himself but answered questions correctly; one was normal to talk to and in most of his behaviour, but always signed himself 'Christ'. There may have been some doubt in earlier times, but here at last are some of the institutionalized chronic schizophrenics of yesteryear. In 1810 Haslam's patient (Leigh, 1961) was tortured by 'bomb-bursting, lobster-cracking and lengthening the brain', by means of an 'air loom', a picture of which the patient supplied. Of further typical modern-seeming patients I need only mention Daniel McNaughton, tried for murder in 1843, who believed he was watched and followed everywhere by spies and signals that brought on a 'grinding of the mind' (West and Walk, 1977), and Daniel Schreber, the judge with an extremely complicated and bizarre system, including God turning him into a woman by miracles and rays, female orgasms induced by remote control, talking scorpions inserted into his head, and friendly souls migrating into the sexual organs whereas unfriendly souls lodged on his left ear to disturb him (Schreber, 1955).

It is true that cases of insanity that resemble the modern syndrome of schizophrenia are rare before the end of the eighteenth century, but this does not confirm that there must be a new disease from that time onwards. That culture influences content is a commonplace, but it must influence form too. As we come nearer to modern times and modern society, modern attitudes and demands, tolerance and rejection, modern conceptions of charisma and stigma, and modern institutions (in every sense of the word), the plastic effect of culture on all human life will ensure that insanity too takes on ever more modern forms. In the speculations of **Cooper and Sartorius (1977)**, social and family structures found in pre-industrial societies exert a benign effect upon patients with schizophrenia, these effects being lost during and after industrialization. Thus the severe and chronic forms of the disease become prominent and recognized in the asylums. They say that they are speculating not necessarily about the aetiology of schizophrenia—not suggesting it is a condition caused by industrialization—but rather about variations in the outcome of an ancient and widespread condition.

Withdrawal, unusual and idiosyncratic styles of thinking, and concern for hidden meanings, will be differently regarded in different ages. Ezekiel was honoured. Now there is little of Plato's divine madness, and mysticism is not understood in the suburbs. We live in secular times.

Other places

'In what sense can it be said that schizophrenic disorders exist in different parts of the world?' was the question addressed by the International Pilot Study of Schizophrenia (WHO, 1973). The attempt to answer it was made by studying young patients with onset of illness within the previous five years in Aarhus, Agra, Cali in Colombia, Ibadan in Nigeria, London, Taiwan, Prague, Washington and Moscow. The research showed that typical cases of severe schizophrenia, as described in European textbooks of psychiatry, and centring on delusions, hallucinations, flattening of affect and lack of insight, occurred in all nine places. The boundaries set for the syndrome were remarkably similar in seven of the nine countries, whereas a wider and different concept of schizophrenia was found in Washington (as had been fully studied in the separate US–UK diagnostic project (Cooper *et al*, 1972) and Moscow. (The findings in Moscow obscured the protests by many psychiatrists, notably in the Royal College of Psychiatrists and in America, against the incarceration of political dissidents in forensic mental hospitals in the Soviet Union on apparently flimsy evidence of their suffering from the more vague forms of schizophrenic poor adjustment to society, as described in Soviet textbooks. This is discussed cautiously in Wing (1978) and passionately in Bloch and Reddaway (1984).) In China too, the symptoms of psychotic patients include 'hearing voices that criticize, abuse, threaten them or give them orders, or they see strange things, smell strange smells. Some are full of suspicion and feel persecuted ... some are still as statues, they neither eat nor drink and are unable to relieve themselves' (Brown, 1980). So all these centres have typical schizophrenic patients, but are of course sufficiently sophisticated to have teams of research psychiatrists affiliated to the WHO and studying diagnostic techniques. What of more isolated peoples?

In India Neki (1973) found patients with various schizophrenic syndromes, some partially accepted as religious mendicants, and in Africa German (1972) noted that chronic schizophrenia occurred in all classes, and was the predominant condition in the mental hospital in Kampala. From Central Australia Cawte and Kidson (1965) described mentally ill aborigines of whom at least one (*Tjapaltjari*) sounds schizophrenic in our terms.

Sociologists, anthropologists and other critics of psychiatry continue to aver that 'anthropology shows that each society has its own "correct way of going mad", and that this model is furnished by the myths or customs of the people ... the sick person, to be recognized as sick, has to make his behaviour conform to the behaviour traditionally expected of the madman. Psychotics tend to develop the symptomatology that will enable the psychiatrist to classify their disturbances according to socially defined criteria. A Chippewa Indian tends to develop a *windigo* syndrome, a Malayan a *latah* psychosis. Fundamentally speaking, all madness is a *folie à deux* involving the psychiatrist and the patient, in which the psychiatrist represents the public (the collective conceptions of madness) and the patient endeavours to help him make his diagnosis by taking the opposite course to the behaviour of normal people by making his disturbances into a ritual of rebellion' (Bastide, 1972). This is similar to the position of Laing (1965; and see Smith, 1982a) when he says, more succinctly: 'sanity or psychosis is tested by the degree of conjunction or disjunction between two persons where the one is sane by common consent'; and (1967) 'the "cause" of schizophrenia is to be found by the examination, not of the prospective diagnosee alone, but of the whole social context in which the psychiatric ceremonial is being conducted.'

There is, as we have seen, evidence that this is incomplete if not wrong, and the studies in the field tend to support Murphy's conclusion (1976) after her work with the Eskimos and Yorubas, and contrary to her initial expectations:

It appears that (i) phenomenal processes of disturbed thought and behaviour are found in most cultures; (ii) they are sufficiently distinctive and noticeable that almost everywhere a name has been created for them; (iii) over and above similarity in processes, there is variability in content which in a general way is coloured by culture; and (iv) the role of social fictions [i.e. labelling the disturbed people as suffering from a metaphorical mental illness] in perceiving and defining the phenomenon seems to have been very slight ... Patterns such as schizophrenia, *were* [in the Yoruba] and *nuthkavihak* [in the Eskimos] appear to be relatively rare in any one human group but are broadly distributed among human groups. Rather than being simply violations of the social norms of particular groups, symptoms of mental illness are manifestations of a type of affliction shared by virtually all mankind.

Causes

In genetic research family studies were long ago replaced by the now classical studies of series of twins up to the 1960s and 1970s, and the Genain quadruplets (identical, all schizophrenic: Rosenthal (1963)). By 1968 'it was definitely and openly agreed by our foremost students of family interaction that heredity is implicated in the development of schizophrenia' and the problem had become 'how the implicated hereditary and environmental variables interact or coact to make for various kinds of schizophrenic and non-schizophrenic outcomes' (Rosenthal and Kety, 1968). The adoption and cross-fostering studies in Denmark and America followed (Heston, 1966; Wender *et al*, 1974; and see especially Gottesman and Shields, 1982), confirming that the raised familial incidence of schizophrenia follows genetic links rather than upbringing.

So the genetic evidence for much of the aetiology, but not all, is strong, despite the absence of an agreed genetic theory (see the discussion later in this volume), and some tantalizing puzzles that seem never to be cleared up. I give three examples from Gottesman and Shields (1982). The Danish long-term twin study allowed the examination of the adult offspring of discordant monozygotic twins. Did the schizophrenic twin pass on the illness and the normal twin have normal progeny? The results are: three schizophrenics out of 31, and three out of 23—i.e. small numbers, but looking like similar rates, as if the predisposition is inherited genetically and is passing on through the phenotypically normal twin to his descendants. The detailed study of discordant twin pairs might reveal enlightening environmental factors making the sick twin vulnerable or the healthy twin robust. But despite fascinating published case histories the results are disappointing, and it is not possible to see why the outcome was as it was. The collected results on the crucial case of monozygotic twins reared apart are 12 or 14 pairs (eight Western and either four or six Japanese, depending on one's confidence in the judgement of zygosity), of whom seven or nine are concordant for schizophrenia.

One of Wender's careful comments on the state of knowledge comes in his paper on cross-fostering (1974): 'What the data from this study do suggest is that those personality types seen commonly in the biological and rearing parents of schizophrenics do not produce schizophrenia when the offspring have biological parents who are not schizophrenic.'

Research on other physical causes of schizophrenia continues vigorously and optimistically, although a historical perspective shows that past optimism has not always been lasting, for many once new theories are later discarded. **Kety**'s article (**1980**) is a masterly review of the state and possibilities of the art, encompassing biochemical and neurological theories, and touching upon other possibilities such as birth injury and the wonderful enigma of the slight skew in the distribution of the season of birth of schizophrenics. He regards acute illnesses as being probably different and therefore well worth separating in research projects. He finds it 'difficult to avoid the conclusion that in a substantial fraction of typical chronic schizophrenics there is an underlying neurological disturbance.'

This is the promising part of what **Szasz** (**1976**) calls the search for the crooked molecule (because doctors wish to repeat the success of discovering the crooked spirochaete of syphilis). A few years later Kety would have been describing the findings of computerized axial tomography of the brain in finding enlarged cerebral ventricles in schizophrenia (Weinberger *et al*, 1980), the theory of a disorder of lateralization between the two cerebral hemispheres and discussion whether schizophrenics have an abnormal corpus callosum, and virus theories (mentioned by **Hare** (**1983**) and developed by **Crow** (1983; **1984**)). The field contains many other theories, however, as it has always done, varying from the popular (food allergy—Mackarness, 1976); through the scientifically sophisticated (immunogenetics—Roberts and Kinnell, 1981); the pineal (Mullen and Silman, 1977); and cytomegalovirus (Torrey, 1983), to the more obscure (hyperformaldehydism—Barker *et al*, 1980). Some, such as perinatal hypoxaemia and abnormal lymphocytes, are being discarded (Stevens, 1984). The virus theory appeared to be disproved when 'analysis of age of onset in pairs of siblings ruled out horizontal transmission', but the theory was reborn in more complicated form: 'Some characteristics of schizophrenic illness, particularly their selectivity for the dominant hemisphere, can be understood on the assumption that the virus (perhaps a retrovirus) responsible for the disease interacts with a proto-oncogene, which induces the asymmetrical brain growth responsible for laterality and cerebral dominance'

(**Crow, 1984**). Is the theory of viruses now so elaborate that it can provide an explanation for nearly all data (as did incomplete penetrance in genetics), with consequent weakening of its refutability?

Theories that schizophrenia is traceable to abnormal communications in the family have been much espoused, especially in America, where they go back at least to the tradition of Adolf Meyer's psychobiological theories that psychiatric illnesses are forms of adaptation of the developing individual to abnormal situations. In Bateson *et al*'s theory (1956) the schizophrenic phenomena were understandable as responses to 'double-binds', and it was implicit that the patient was young and the double-binds came from a parent. From 1948 onwards (Fromm-Reichmann) the parent was more commonly thought of as a 'schizophrenogenic mother' than father—and there has always been a deafening silence from family theorists about the development of schizophrenia in middle age, in people living alone, in married people, and in the elderly and hard of hearing. In Laing's speculations (Laing and Esterson, 1964) it always seems to be parents who are confusing the patients and undermining them ontologically, in fact, driving them mad.

Specific theories that have been influential include those of Lidz (1975) (parents' marriages 'skewed' or 'schismatic': 'the schizophrenic patient escapes from irreconcilable dilemmas and unbearable hopelessness by breaking through these confines [i.e. the meanings and logic of his culture] to find some living space by using his own idiosyncratic meanings and reasoning, but in so doing impairs his ego functioning and ability to collaborate with others'); and Wynne and his collaborators (1978) ('pseudomutuality' in the family, which while appearing harmonious to those outside, in fact harbours deep gulfs between members, and irrational distorted modes of communication that fragment the thinking of that member of the family who becomes schizophrenic). These authors claimed to be able to detect these forms of communication 'blind', an exciting finding. Hirsch and Leff (1975), after a thorough review of the evidence for abnormalities in the parents of schizophrenics (and finding it scanty: e.g. '. . . the concept of the cold, aloof hostile schizophrenogenic mother, for which, surprisingly in view of its popularity, we could not find any reliable supporting evidence'), described their very careful attempted replication of Wynne and Singer's work, with largely negative results. The observed abnormalities doubtless occur, but in many unhappy families.

In the last few years there have been no major advances in these theories, and some earlier excesses have been retracted. Arieti (1974) said that psychotherapists had 'made an unwarranted generalization that includes all the mothers of schizophrenics', and Lidz (1975) stated that he did not believe that 'such torsions exerted upon the patient's rationality have the purposeful malevolence that these investigators seem to imply.'

Hirsch and Leff (1975) stated that 'it seems likely that the popular theorists are describing ways of behaving that generate high emotion or over-involvement. This is a form of stress which, according to the recent environment model, is likely to precipitate florid schizophrenia in the vulnerable individual.' The recent environment model to which they refer is that developed in the research at the Institute of Psychiatry on relapses in schizophrenics and the family factors involved. This work, justifiably highly regarded and influential, is described fully later in this volume.

Concept and diagnosis

In the absence of knowledge of the causes, discussion of concept and diagnosis continues much as it always has, with description of typical syndromes, appeal to the original authorities, and minute examination of history.

So **Hoenig** (**1983**) in his review of the concept of schizophrenia quotes widely from classical authors from Kraepelin onwards. We hear how Kraepelin had to rely on the overall syndrome, and as Hoenig says: 'nowhere do we find any precise demarcation of the illness, but are always referred to the overall picture.' There are no pathognomonic symptoms. We hear again how Kraepelin thought the illness was nearly always irreversible, but that there might be some full recoveries. E. Bleuler is quoted also, as so often before, on 'a group of psychoses whose cause can at times be chronic, at times run in intermittent thrusts, and which can become arrested at any stage or show improvement, but will probably not permit full *restitutio ad integrum*.' **Kety** (**1980**) refers to the same definition. He also criticizes Schneider severely, saying that he defines schizophrenia by E. Bleuler's accessory symptoms, which are more easily recognized than the primary symptoms. Thus, Kety avers of Schneider's schizophrenia, 'that syndrome may be more prevalent, have a more favourable outcome, and be more responsive to a wide variety of treatments, but it is not schizophrenia.' This is not good news for those many who have looked to Schneider's first-rank symptoms as to a beacon in a fog, although they can take some comfort by finding Hoenig criticizing Kety and praising Schneider's approach as being particularly appropriate in its use of course and description to delimit the boundary of schizophrenia for working purposes. The use of Schneider's first-rank symptoms is noted as being devoid of theory, and useful purely for pragmatic purposes, so that we all can be agreed on what we are saying when we diagnose the condition.

General agreement to use working definitions has marked the last decades—the years of Feighner *et al* (1972), Spitzer *et al*'s Research Diagnostic Criteria (1978), the Catego programme for computerized diagnosis, and the phenomenal success of the DSM-III (American Psychiatric Association, 1980). This subject is discussed more fully below and was studied by Kendell *et al* (1979).

Four theories

Four principal groups of theories of schizophrenia are current: neurological, psychiatric, sociological and prophetic.

According to the *neurological* theories, schizophrenia is a brain disease. This is the point of view of many psychiatrists, including most in the 19th century and many at the present time. It is the theory of the researchers in genetics, biochemistry, and cerebral lateralization and pathology, and the theory of Hunter (1973) in his neurological variant of 'the myth of mental illness'—e.g. after discussing subtle neurological signs he says 'the concept of psychosis or schizophrenia is a historical accident. The abnormal mental state is not the illness, nor even its essence or determinant, but an epiphenomenon. Had the epidemic of encephalitis broken out only ten years earlier, or had its manifestations in endemic form been recognized for what they were, psychiatry would look very different today.' It is the theory of Slater and Roth (1977) in the most influential textbook of the 1960s and 1970s, in which after stating that schizophrenia comprises a group of mental illnesses characterized by specific psychological symptoms, they continue: 'If these primary symptoms are present, then they are features which refute any purely psychogenic theory.'

According to the *psychiatric* theories, schizophrenia is indeed a mental disorder, a malfunction of the life of the mind, but a psychosis, because it is ultimately a disorganization, a breakdown, if not incomprehensible. It is neither brain disease nor straightforward reaction to stress, but in a mysterious category of its own. This is the metaphorical illness on the analogy of physical illness, so often criticized, especially by Szasz in *The Myth of Mental Illness* (1962). This is the theory of Murphy (1976) when she says it is visionary thinking gone out of control; of **Ciompi** (**1980**)—'it more closely resembles a life process than an illness with a given course'; and of Lidz (1972), who regards it as a desperate and handicapping withdrawal 'in the nature of illusion and delusion, with very little to do with anything real or practical ... it tends to be a self-perpetuating condition in which people give up validating their experience.'

In particular, the psychiatric theory is espoused by M..Bleuler (1978) and Lewis (1973), in one of the greatest studies of recent years, based on long-term personal follow-up of 208 patients. His summary must be given in full: '(1) The patients are not physically ill; (2) The state is experienced subjectively as a problem between the patients' own being and their experience of life; (3) This agrees with our own observations of their difficulties; (4) There are no environmental stresses in the past lives of schizophrenics which are specific ones for the development of this condition; (5) There are hereditary factors, but we do not understand how they work; (6) The (frequently co-existing) schizoid personality itself represents a lack of harmony between the person and the events of his life; (7) Schizophrenic ways of experiencing and thinking occur in a hidden form in the mentally healthy, and similarly healthy ways of experiencing and thinking remain in a hidden way preserved in schizophrenia; (8) The schizophrenic patient does not dement (i.e. undergo depletion of mental functions through deterioration of the cerebral processes)—a rich inner life remains; (9) Afer some five years on the average, there is no further deterioration, and more often some improvement takes place; (10) All the methods of treatment help by reaching the healthy parts of the personality.' And in addition 'the schizophrenic loses himself in the discord between the disharmony of his own personality and the disharmony of his environment ... the schizophrenic happening takes place in the realms of the mind and the emotions, that is, in mental spheres that exist only in man.'

According to the *sociological* theories, madness is a social role, a form of deviance, probably with functions in society, and only to be understood in social terms. The psychiatric profession is regarded, as we have seen, as 'medicalizing' deviance by saying it is a form of illness, a (mythical) mental illness. Versions have been stated by Becker (1963: 'social groups create deviance by making rules whose infraction constitutes deviance'); Lemert (1951; 1967), in his analysis of labelling; Scheff (1966); Szasz (1962; 1971), and by Laing when he discusses labelling (1967). It is in fact the usual view of sociologists and social anthropologists, and akin to the stance of historians (MacDonald,

1981a; 1981b). Bastide (1972) says that 'the isolation which for some psychiatrists characterizes the world of the mentally ill is merely the translation, in morphological terms, of the marginality of values that have been rejected or repressed by the rest of society ... clearly one is insane only in relation to a particular society.'

A fourth group of theories sees madness, as it would be termed, as at least sometimes *akin to prophecy*, offering comments and occasionally the most profound insight into society and the human condition. This is an offshoot of the sociological theory, for there is no illness, and prophecy is a social institution. Madness is seen as incomprehensible only to the benighted or unimaginative; but psychiatrists unfortunately are usually among the insensitive who miss the message. The tradition of this kind of madness goes back to Plato, and is found widely in literature since, down to our own time when the patient in Doris Lessing's *Briefing for a Descent into Hell* (1971) is cured by ECT, but the author makes the reader regret the return to normality. This is the theory of Bateson (1962), and of Laing in *The Politics of Experience* (1967).

A disorder of development?

It may be that the different viewpoints are not so incompatible as appears at first sight. My own dark horse for promising progress in future would be a complex developmental psychiatric theory, concerning long periods of the patient's life and many different factors bearing upon it. It would include genetic transmission of a vulnerability to the condition, and possibily future research on the effect of family environments. It would include Watt's research (1978) on the school records of subsequent schizophrenics, which shows that, more than controls, the boys were negativistic and unstable, the girls passive and immature. The theory would make allowance for the mystifying and stressful effect on parents of bringing up such a child, envisaging vicious circles in which the physically and emotionally immature child of schizoid unhappy parents called forth natural protective responses seen by researchers, and possibly felt by the child, as cold intrusion, causing withdrawal, alienation, more strangeness, more labelling as strange, and further protectiveness.

The theory might describe preschizophrenic children, as does Crider (1979), as seeing themselves 'as driven by uncontrollable impulses and urges, as friendless in a rejecting and hostile world, as increasingly retarded *vis-à-vis* peers in social-emotional development. Low self-esteem begins to merge with the harbingers of psychotic breakdown: hallucinatory experience, depersonalization, delusions of control by others, and experiences of derealization.'

At the onset of psychosis new processes will be involved, or older ones gather fresh momentum. Physical, biochemical factors may be present, and an increase in adverse life events. Then the responses of family, workmates and society at large to the oddity, outrageous rule-breaking and handicaps of the schizophrenic will be seen to have many of the effects postulated by sociologists, anthropologists, historians, and **Cooper and Sartorius** (**1977**). What happens next is sure to be affected by society's tolerance of peculiar behaviour, whether it has a role for prophets, what it expects the insane to do, and what kind of institutions, including the psychiatric profession and mental hospitals, are available. In this reaction of society, at least as plausibly as in the search for the schizococcus, may lie the key to the extent to which schizophrenia is a 'disease of modern civilization'.

In this theory, the illness would be the pathological end of a long process of human maladaptation. The genetic vulnerability would have to arise by mutation or have some procreative advantage for the individual or his group in some circumstances. (Theories here have been tentative and need development: could mild degrees of the genetic specification result in thoughtful, detached and original individuals, not handicapped in marrying and reproducing?) Cerebral, familial and social processes would contribute pressure to retreat from outer world to inner, from reason to unreason, from normality to psychosis.

References

ALLDERIDGE, P. (1979) Hospitals, madhouses and asylums: cycles in the care of the insane. *British Journal of Psychiatry*, **134**, 321–334.

AMERICAN PSYCHIATRIC ASSOCIATION (1980) *Diagnostic and Statistical Manual of Mental Disorders*, 3rd Ed. (DSM-III). Washington, DC.: APA.

ARIETI, S. (1974) *Interpretation of Schizophrenia* (2nd Ed). London: Crosby Lockwood Staples.

BARK, N. M. (1985) Did Shakespeare know schizophrenia? The case of Poor Mad Tom in *King Lear*. *British Journal of Psychiatry*, **146**, 436–438.

BARKER, S. A., CARL, G. F. & MONTI, J. A. (1980) Hyperformaldehydism: a unifying hypothesis for the major biochemical theories of schizophrenia. *Medical Hypotheses*, **6**, 671–686.

BASTIDE, R. (1972) *The Sociology of Mental Disorder*. (Translated by J. McNeil.) London: Routledge and Kegan Paul.

BATESON, G. (ed.) (1962) *Perceval's Narrative: A Patient's Account of his Psychosis 1830–1832*. London: Hogarth Press.

—— JACKSON, D., HALEY, J. & WEAKLAND, J. (1956) Towards a theory of schizophrenia. *Behavioural Science*, **1**, 251–264.

BECKER, H. S. (1963) *Outsiders: Studies in the Sociology of Deviance*. New York: Free Press.

BLEULER, M. (1978) *The Schizophrenic Disorders: Long-Term Patient and Family Studies*. (Translated by S. M. Clemens from German edition of 1972.) New Haven: Yale University Press.

BLOCH, S. & REDDAWAY, P. (1984) *Soviet Psychiatric Abuse*. London: Gollancz.

BROWN, L. B. (1980) A psychologist's perspective on psychiatry in China. *Australian and New Zealand Journal of Psychiatry*, **14**, 21–35.

CAWTE, J. E. & KIDSON, M. A. (1965) Ethnopsychiatry in Central Australia—II: The evolution of illness in a Walbiri lineage. *British Journal of Psychiatry*, **111**, 1079–1085.

CIOMPI, L. (1980) The natural history of schizophrenia in the long term. *British Journal of Psychiatry*, **136**, 413–420.

CLARE, A. (1976) *Psychiatry in Dissent*. London: Tavistock.

CLARKE, B. (1975) *Mental Disorder in Earlier Britain*. Cardiff: University of Wales Press.

COOPER, J. & SARTORIUS, N. (1977) Cultural and temporal variations in schizophrenia: a speculation on the importance of industrialization. *British Journal of Psychiatry*, **130**, 50–55.

COOPER, J. E., KENDELL, R. E., GURLAND, B. J. et al (1972) *Psychiatric Diagnosis in New York and London*. Oxford University Press.

CRIDER, A. (1979) *Schizophrenia: A Biopsychological Perspective*. Chichester: John Wiley.

CROW, T. J. (1983) Is schizophrenia an infectious disease? *Lancet*, i, 173–175.

—— (1984) A re-evaluation of the viral hypothesis: Is psychosis the result of retroviral integration at a site close to the cerebral dominance gene? *British Journal of Psychiatry*, **145**, 243–253.

EZEKIEL. Passim, especially chapters 1–5, and 14, (i)–(ii).

FEIGHNER, J. P., ROBINS, E., GUZE, S. B., WOODRUFF, R. A., WINOKUR, G. & MUNOZ, R. (1972) Diagnostic criteria for use in psychiatric research. *Archives of General Psychiatry*, **26**, 57–63.

FOUCAULT, M. (1967) *Madness and Civilisation*. (Translated by Richard Howard from the French edition of 1961.) London: Tavistock.

FROMM-REICHMAN, F. (1948) Notes on the development of treatment of schizophrenia by psychoanalytic psychotherapy. *Psychiatry*, **11**, 263–273.

GERMAN, G. A. (1972) Aspects of clinical psychiatry in sub-Saharan Africa. *British Journal of Psychiatry*, **121**, 461–479.

GOTTESMAN, I. I. & SHIELDS, J. (1982) *Schizophrenia, the Epigenetic Puzzle*. Cambridge University Press.

HARE, E. (1983) Was insanity on the increase? *British Journal of Psychiatry*, **142**, 439–455.

HESTON, L. L. (1966) Psychiatric disorders in foster home reared children of schizophrenic mothers. *British Journal of Psychiatry*, **112**, 819–825.

HIRSCH, S. R. & LEFF, J. P. (1975) *Abnormalities in Parents of Schizophrenics*. Oxford University Press.

HOENIG, J. (1983) The concept of schizophrenia: Kraepelin–Bleuler–Schneider. *British Journal of Psychiatry*, **142**, 547–556.

HUNTER, R. (1973) Psychiatry and neurology: psychosyndrome or brain disease. *Proceedings of the Royal Society of Medicine*, **66**, 359–364.

—— & MACALPINE, I. (1964) *Three Hundred Years of Psychiatry 1535–1860*. Oxford University Press.

JONES, K. (1972) *A History of the Mental Health Services*. London: Routledge and Kegan Paul.

KENDELL, R. E. (1975) The concept of disease and its implications for psychiatry. *British Journal of Psychiatry*, **127**, 305–315.

—— BROCKINGTON, I. F. & LEFF, J. P. (1979) Prognostic implications of six alternative definitions of schizophrenia. *Archives of General Psychiatry*, **36**, 25–31.

KETY, S. S. (1980) The syndrome of schizophrenia: unresolved questions and opportunities for research. *British Journal of Psychiatry*, **136**, 421–436.

LAING, R. D. (1965) *The Divided Self*. London: Penguin. (Originally published in 1960; Chicago: Quadrangle Books.)

—— (1967) *The Politics of Experience*. London: Penguin.

—— & ESTERSON, A. (1964) *Sanity, Madness and the Family*. London: Tavistock.

LEIGH, D. (1961) *The Historical Development of British Psychiatry, Volume 1, 18th & 19th century*. Oxford: Pergamon.

LEMERT, E. (1951) *Social Pathology*. New York: McGraw-Hill.

—— (1967) *Human Deviance, Social Problems and Social Control*. Englewood Cliffs, N.J.: Prentice-Hall.

LESSING, D. (1971) *Briefing for a Descent into Hell*. London: Jonathan Cape.

LEWIS, A. (1973) Manfred Bleuler's *The Schizophrenic Mental Disorders*: an exposition and a review. *Psychological Medicine*, **3**, 385–392.

LIDZ, T. (1972) Schizophrenia, R. D. Laing and the contemporary treatment of psychosis. In *Laing and Antipsychiatry* (eds. R. Boyers and R. Orrill). London: Penguin.

—— (1975) *The Origin and Treatment of Schizophrenic Disorders*. London: Hutchinson.

MACDONALD, M. (1981a) Insanity and the realities of history in early modern England. *Psychological Medicine*, **11**, 11–25.

—— (1981b) *Mystical Bedlam: Madness, Anxiety, and Healing in Seventeenth Century England*. Cambridge University Press.

MACKARNESS, R. (1976) *Not All in the Mind*. London: Pan.

MULLEN, P. E. & SILMAN, R. E. (1977) The pineal and psychiatry: a review. *Psychological Medicine*, **7**, 407–417.

MURPHY, J. M. (1976) Psychiatric labelling in cross-cultural perspective. *Science*, **191**, 1019–1028.

NEKI, J. S. (1973) Psychiatry in South-East Asia. *British Journal of Psychiatry*, **123**, 257–269.

PINEL, P. (1806) *A Treatise on Insanity*. (Translated in 1962 by D. D. Davis). New York: Hafner.

ROBERTS, D. F. & KINNELL, H. G. (1981) Immunogenetics and schizophrenia. *Psychological Medicine*, **11**, 441–447.

ROSEN, G. (1968) *Madness in Society*. London: Routledge and Kegan Paul.

ROSENHAN, D. (1973) On being sane in insane places. *Science*, **179**, 250–258.

ROSENTHAL, D. (1963) *The Genain Quadruplets*. New York: Basic Books.

—— & KETY, S. S. (eds.) (1968) *The Transmission of Schizophrenia*. New York: Pergamon.

ROTH, M. (1976) Schizophrenia and the theories of Thomas Szasz. *British Journal of Psychiatry*, **129**, 317–326.

SCADDING, J. G. (1967) Diagnosis: the clinician and the computer. *Lancet*, ii, 877–882.

SCHEFF, T. J. (1966) *Being Mentally Ill—a Sociological Theory*. London: Weidenfeld and Nicholson.

SCHREBER, D. P. (1955) *Memoirs of My Nervous Illness*. (Translated and edited by I. Macalpine and R. Hunter.) London: Dawson.

SCULL, A. (1979) *Museums of Madness*. London: Allen Lane.

—— (1984) Was insanity increasing? A response to Edware Hare. *British Journal of Psychiatry*, **144**, 432–436.

SIMON, B. (1978) *Mind and Madness in Ancient Greece*. Ithaca: Cornell University Press.

SLATER, E. & ROTH, M. (1977) *Clinical Psychiatry* (3rd Ed.). London: Baillière Tindall.

SMITH, A. C. (1967) Clinical notes on Pinel's *Treatise of Insanity. British Journal of Medical Psychology*, **41**, 255–259.

—— (1982a) R. D. Laing's *The Divided Self. British Journal of Psychiatry*, **140**, 637–642.

—— (1982b) *Schizophrenia and Madness.* London: George Allen & Unwin.

SPITZER, R. L., ENDICOTT, J. & ROBINS, E. (1978) Research diagnostic criteria: rationale and reliability. *Archives of General Psychiatry*, **35**, 773–782.

STEVENS, J. R. (1984) Schizophrenia and the brain at the 1984 winter workshop at Davos, Switzerland. *Archives of General Psychiatry*, **41**, 816–817.

SZASZ, T. S. (1962) *The Myth of Mental Illness.* London: Secker & Warburg.

—— (1971) *The Manufacture of Madness.* London: Routledge and Kegan Paul.

—— (1976) Schizophrenia: the sacred symbol of psychiatry. *British Journal of Psychiatry*, **129**, 308–316.

TAYLOR, F. K. (1979) *The Concepts of Illness, Disease and Morbus.* Cambridge University Press.

TORREY, E. F. (1980) *Schizophrenia and Civilization.* New York: Jason Aronson.

TORREY, E. F., YOLKEN, R. H. & ALBRECHT, P. (1983) Cytomegalovirus: a possible etiological agent in schizophrenia. In *Research on the Viral Hypothesis of Mental Disorders* (ed. P. V. Morozov). Basel: Karger.

TSUANG, M. T. (1982) *Schizophrenia: the Facts.* Oxford University Press.

WATT, N. F. (1978) Patterns of childhood social development in adult schizophrenia. *Archives of General Psychiatry*, **35**, 160–170.

WEINBERGER, D. R., BIGELOW, L., KLEINMAN, J., KLEIN, S., ROSENBLATT, J. & WYATT, J. (1980) Cerebral ventricular enlargement in chornic schizophrenia. *Archives of General Psychiatry*, **37**, 11–13.

WENDER, P. H. ROSENTHAL, D., KETY, S. S. & WELNER, J. (1974) Cross-fostering. *Archives of General Psychiatry*, **30**, 121–128.

WEST, D. J. & WALK, A. (1977) *Daniel McNaughton: His Trial and the Aftermath.* London: Royal College of Psychiatrists.

WING, J. K. (1978) *Reasoning about Madness.* Oxford University Press.

WORLD HEALTH ORGANIZATION (1973) *Report of the International Pilot Study of Schizophrenia: Vol. 1.* Geneva: WHO

WYNNE, L. C., CROMWELL, R. L. & MATTYHYSSE, S. (1978) *The Nature of Schizophrenia: New Approaches to Research and Treatment.* New York: John Wiley.

ZILBOORG, G. & HENRY, G. W. (1941) *A History of Medical Psychology.* London: George Allen & Unwin.

2 The concept of disease and its implications for psychiatry

R. E. KENDELL

It has often been suggested in recent years that there is no such thing as mental illness; that the conditions psychiatrists spend their time trying to treat ought not, properly speaking, to be regarded as illness at all, or even to be the concern of physicians. Szasz is the best-known exponent of this viewpoint, and the core of his argument is essentially this: that as prolonged search has never demonstrated any consistent physical abnormality in those regarded as mentally ill, and as their 'illness' consists simply in behaving in ways that alarm or affront other people, or in believing things which other people do not believe, there is no justification for labelling them as ill, and to do so is to use the word illness in a purely metaphorical sense (Szasz, 1960). Schneider had previously been led by the same reasoning to the conclusion that neurotic illness and personality disorders were 'abnormal varieties of sane mental life' rather than disease, but he took care to exempt schizophrenia and cyclothymia by assuming that both would in time prove to possess an organic basis (Schneider, 1950). The argument Eysenck puts forward in the first edition of his textbook, though written from the quite different standpoint of academic psychology, is a similar one. After observing that 'the term psychiatry does not denote any meaningful grouping of problems or subjects of study' he went on to suggest that the traditional subject-matter of psychiatry should be divided into a small medical part 'dealing with the effects of tumours, lesions, infections and other physical conditions' and a much larger behavioural part 'dealing with disorders of behaviour acquired through the ordinary processes of learning', thereby implying that most of what doctors regarded as mental illness was really learnt behaviour rather than disease, and therefore much better understood, and dealt with, by psychologists than by physicians (Eysenck, 1960). A third line of attack is provided by R. D. Laing, and a fourth is exemplified by the sociologist Scheff. Laing argues that schizophrenia, far from being a disease or a form of insanity, is really the only sane or rational way adolescents have of coping with the intolerable emotional pressures placed on them by society and their families (Laing, 1967). Scheff has developed the somewhat similar argument that what psychiatrists call mental illness is largely a response to the shock of being labelled and treated as insane and the expectations this produces; in other words that schizophrenia is created by the people and institutions that purport to treat it (Scheff, 1963).

Psychiatrists have generally reacted to these various assaults with indignation or disdain. They have either ignored their critics, or told them, with varying degrees of candour, that they do not know what they are talking about, or suggested, with varying degrees of subtlety, that they are motivated by professional jealousy, a taste for publicity, or emotional difficulties of their own. Perhaps there is some truth in these retaliatory jibes. But what matters is the strength of the critics' arguments, not their motives. They come from a variety of backgrounds—psychology, sociology and psychiatry itself—and although they disagree with one another almost as vehemently as they do with orthodox psychiatry, they have one central argument in common—that what psychiatrists regard as mental illnesses are not illnesses at all. The purpose of this essay is to examine this proposition.

The need for a definition of illness

To question the existence of mental illness, or to assert that the word illness in such a context is no more than a misleading metaphor, assumes that one already has a clear idea of what illness is. It is equally meaningless to assert either that something is, or that it is not, illness unless one has a clearly defined concept of illness to start with. Unfortunately, although medicine has adequate working definitions for most individual illnesses, it does not possess an agreed definition or an explicit concept of illness in general (Engle and Davis, 1963). So before we can begin to decide whether mental illnesses are legitimately so called we have first to agree on an adequate definition of illness to decide if we like what is the defining characteristic or the hallmark of disease.

Most doctors never give a moment's thought to the precise meaning of terms like illness and disease, nor do they need to. They simply treat the patients who consult them as best they can, diagnose individual diseases whenever they can, and try to relieve their patients' suffering even if they cannot. At times they are well aware that they are dealing with matters other than illness—childbirth and the circumcision of infants are traditional examples, and family planning a more recent innovation—but rarely do they pause to consider what is the essential difference between the two. The practical nature of medicine is not conducive to theorizing. But there are some situations in which this unthinking empiricism is inadequate. Psychiatrists are only too well aware of this, since they are often required to express opinions about the presence or absence of illness in the courts, and to defend these opinions to hard-headed lawyers, but they have not been conspicuously successful in finding a solution.

An American writer has recently pointed out that when doctors disagree whether a particular condition is a disease or not it is almost invariably the case that those who regard the subject of the condition as ill also regard some medical procedure—either treatment or investigation—as necessary, while those who do not regard the subject as ill do not regard either as warranted. This gives rise to the suspicion that, whether or not they realize it, doctors do not have a clearly formulated concept of illness, and that the answer they give to the question 'Is this a disease?' is really a covert answer to the quite different question 'Should this person be under medical care?' (Linder, 1965). This rather cynical judgement is not entirely justified, if only because doctors do perceive that some of their activities, such as the delivery of babies and the circumcision of infants, are not the treatment of illness, despite the fact that the technology and expertise involved are the same in both. But it is undoubtedly extremely difficult to pin down the essential element distinguishing illness from non-illness, or, to put it another way, to produce a definition of disease which neatly covers all the individual diseases we currently recognize, and excludes other phenomena.

Changing concepts of disease

The main reason why this is so is that, for historical reasons, the defining characteristics of individual diseases are very diverse. To most of the schools of medicine of the ancient world symptoms and signs were themselves diseases. Fever, joint pains and skin rashes were all separate diseases to be studied individually. The idea of disease as a syndrome, a constellation of related symptoms with a characteristic prognosis, originated with Sydenham in the seventeenth century, though the Hippocratic school had had the germ of the idea long before. However, the popularization of post-mortem dissection of the body in the latter half of the eighteenth century by Morgagni and Bichat slowly converted disease from a syndrome observed at the bedside to a characteristic morbid anatomy observed in the cadaver, and thereafter new concepts followed one another in rapid succession, mainly in response to the introduction of new types of observational technology. The development of powerful microscopes in the middle of the nineteenth century enabled individual cells to be examined for the first time, and the consequent detection of cellular pathology led Virchow and his contemporaries to assume that cellular derangements were the basis of all disease. This concept was in turn displaced by the discovery of bacteria by Koch and Pasteur, and currently new techniques like electrophoresis, chromosome analysis and electron microscopy are producing further concepts of disease expressed in terms of deranged biophysical structures, genes and molecules.

Each of these waves of technology has added new diseases, and from each stage some have survived. A few, like senile pruritus and proctalgia fugax, are still individual symptoms. Others, like migraine and most psychiatric diseases, are clinical syndromes—Sydenham's constellation of symptoms. Mitral stenosis and hydronephrosis are based on morbid anatomy, and tumours of all kinds on histopathology. Tuberculosis and syphilis are based on bacteriology and the concept of the aetiological agent, porphyria on biochemistry, myasthenia gravis on physiological dysfunction, Down's syndrome on chromosomal architecture, and so on. In fact the diseases we currently recognize are rather like the furniture in an old house, in which each generation has acquired a few new pieces of its own but has never disposed of those it inherited from its predecessors, so that amongst the inflatable plastic settees and glass coffee tables are still scattered a few old Tudor stools, Jacobean dressers and Regency commodes, and a great deal of Victoriana.

A logician would have started by defining what he meant by disease as a whole and then produced individual diseases by sub-dividing the territory whose boundaries he had thus defined. Medicine, being essentially practical and opportunist, proceeded the other way and started with individual diseases.

As a result, many of these overlap with one another, and the outer perimeter between disease and health is based on different criteria in different places. Hence the difficulty in producing a satisfactory definition.

Historically it seems likely that the concept of disease originated as an explanation for the onset of suffering and incapacity in the absence of obvious injury, and that the concept of health was a later development, implying the absence of disease. Naturally enough, therefore, attempts have often been made to define illness in terms of suffering and incapacity, or at least in terms of a complaint of some sort. But this immediately leads to difficulties. Many people whom we regard as ill neither complain nor suffer, either because they experience no symptoms, or because they ignore what in others would be cause for complaint, or simply because they drop dead without warning. A man with a cancer growing silently in his lung, or someone with anginal pain which he dismisses as a touch of wind, would be regarded by both doctors and laymen as ill and urgently in need of treatment, yet neither complains, or even suffers to any significant extent. The same is true of the typhoid carrier harbouring salmonellae in his gall bladder. Other people, whom we call hypochondriacs or hysterics, complain incessantly, and insist that they suffer, without either their doctors or anyone else being convinced that they are genuinely ill.

Partly because of such problems, attempts have sometimes been made to define illness in terms of the need for treatment rather than the presence of a complaint; in other words to make the situation to which Linder was drawing attention overt rather than covert. Kräupl Taylor, for instance, recently suggested that disease, or patienthood, should have 'as its sufficient and necessary condition the experience of therapeutic concern by a person for himself and/or the arousal of therapeutic concern for him in his social environment' (Kräupl Taylor, 1971). A criterion of this kind is certainly capable of embracing people whom doctors, or society as a whole, regard as in need of treatment as well as those who complain or suffer personally, but in doing so it creates worse problems than it solves. Equating illness with a complaint allows the individual to be sole arbiter of whether he is ill or not, and is unsatisfactory because some people who should be complaining do not do so, and others who complain repeatedly do not seem to have adequate reasons for doing so. Equating illness with 'therapeutic concern' implies that no one can be ill until he has been recognized as such, and also gives doctors, and society, free rein to label all deviants as ill, thus opening the door to all the inconsistencies and abuses that Szasz has so vividly conjured up.

The fact is that any definition of disease which boils down to 'what people complain of', or 'what doctors treat', or some combination of the two, is almost worse than no definition at all. It is free to expand or contract with changes in social attitudes and therapeutic optimism and is at the mercy of idiosyncratic decisions by doctors or patients. If one wished to compare the incidence of disease in two different cultures, or in a single population at two different times, whose criteria of suffering or therapeutic concern would one use? And if the incidence of disease turned out to be different in the two, would this be because one was healthier than the other, or simply because their attitudes to illness were different?

Disease as a lesion

During the last century the development first of morbid anatomy and then of histology produced widespread evidence that illness was accompanied by structural damage to the body, at either a gross or a microscopic level. It was only a short step from this observation to the assumption that these lesions constituted the illness, and that illness always involved structural damage. Subsequently, as knowledge of physiology and biochemistry grew in the first half of this century, this concept was expanded to include biochemical and physiological abnormalities, without relinquishing the basic assumption that illness necessarily involved a demonstrable physical abnormality of some sort.

In this milieu it was almost inevitable that the presence of an identifiable lesion should come to be regarded as the essential attribute of disease, and this concept of illness held sway for over a hundred years. Such a standpoint certainly has many advantages. It provides an objective and usually reliable criterion which is not at the mercy of changing social attitudes and therapeutic fashions, and also embodies at least a partial explanation of the patient's symptoms or disabilities. On close examination, however, it has several shortcomings. In the first place, conditions whose physical basis is still unknown cannot legitimately be regarded as diseases. Trigeminal neuralgia, senile pruritus and dystonia musculorum deformans must all be discarded. Twenty years ago the same would have been true of migraine and narcolepsy, and sixty years ago most forms of epilepsy, Parkinson's disease, chorea, Bornholm disease and pellagra would all have failed to qualify. Indeed, to insist on the presence of a demonstrable lesion implies that most of the great scourges of mankind have only become diseases during the last hundred and fifty years. A further difficulty is that no distinction is drawn between what is trivial and what is crippling. A child with spina bifida and an oligophrenic imbecile both suffer from congenital diseases—the first by virtue of an anatomical defect acquired early in embyronic development, the second because of the absence of the enzyme needed to convert phenylalanine to tyrosine. But children with fused second and third toes have a similar congenital defect to those with spina bifida, and those with albinism also lack an enzyme involved in tyrosine metabolism, yet despite the presence of these lesions we do not normally wish to regard them as ill.

There is a third problem as well. The concept of an abnormality or a lesion is quite straightforward so long as one is concerned with deviation from a standard pattern. But as soon as we begin to recognize that there is no single set pattern of either structure or function, that even in health human beings and their constituent tissues and organs vary considerably in size, shape, chemical composition and functional efficiency, it becomes much less obvious what constitutes a lesion; where normal variation ends and abnormality begins. Is, for instance, hypertension a disease, and if so what is the level beyond which the blood pressure is abnormal? And at what point does a raised blood sugar level, or a prolonged response to a carbohydrate load, become the disease diabetes?

It was in fact the example of hypertension which finally discredited the nineteenth-century assumption that there was always a qualitative distinction between sickness and health (Oldham *et al*, 1960). The demonstration by

Pickering and his colleagues twenty years ago that such a major cause of death and disability as this was a graded characteristic, dependent, like height and intelligence, on polygenic inheritance and shading insensibly into normality, was greeted with shock and disbelief by most of their contemporaries, and the prolonged resistance to their findings showed how deeply rooted the assumptions of Koch and Virchow had become.

The resistance finally crumbled not only because Pickering's evidence was strong but because at the same time advances in other fields were also discrediting another of the major assumptions of the old concept—the assumption that every illness had a single cause, both necessary and sufficient. As the focus of medical research widened from an exclusive concern with individual patients to embrace the study of disease in populations, it slowly became apparent that a host of interacting factors, both internal and environmental, all contributed to the development of disease; and as knowledge increased the decision to regard one of these as 'the cause' and the rest merely as 'precipitating or exacerbating factors' appeared increasingly arbitrary. This was true not only of degenerative diseases like arteriosclerosis but even of classical illnesses like tuberculosis. Although tuberculosis cannot develop in the absence of the *Mycobacterium tuberculi*, the presence of the organism is insufficient to produce the illness. It is ubiquitous in many populations, yet only a minority develop the disease. Genetic studies reveal differences in concordance between MZ and DZ twins, and epidemiological studies show that these constitutional differences are matched by a host of environmental factors—dietary, climatic, occupational and social—all exerting a powerful influence on the liability of individuals exposed to the tubercle bacillus to develop the disease.

A statistical concept of disease

By 1960 the 'lesion' concept of disease, and its associated assumptions of a single cause and a qualitative difference between sickness and health had been discredited beyond redemption, but nothing had yet been put in its place. It was clear, though, that its successor would have to be based on a statistical model of the relationship between normality and abnormality. Lord Cohen (1943) had anticipated this in an essay in which he defined illness simply as 'deviation from the normal ... by way of excess or defect', and indeed Broussais and Magendie had had the germ of a quantitative concept of disease a hundred years before. But Cohen never developed his suggestion any further, and as it stands his definition is inadequate because it fails to distinguish between deviations from the norm which are harmful, like hypertension, those which are neutral, like great height, and those which are positively beneficial, like superior intelligence. Scadding was the first to recognize the need for a criterion distinguishing between disease and other deviations from the norm that were not matters for medical concern, and suggested that the crucial issue was whether or not the abnormality placed the individual at a 'biological disadvantage' (Scadding, 1967). Although he was primarily concerned with defining individual diseases, his definition of *a* disease has clear implications for the corresponding global concept. He defines illness not by its antecedents— the aetiological agent or the lesion producing the overt manifestations—but by its consequences. In itself this is not new; previous attempts to define illness as a condition producing suffering or as meriting medical intervention had done the same but, as we have seen, had proved inadequate. The concept of 'biological disadvantage' differs from these, however, in being more fundamental and less obviously an epiphenomenon, and in being immune to the idiosyncratic personal judgements of patients or doctors which had proved the undoing of its predecessors.

I should like to examine Scadding's definition in detail. He defines a disease as 'the sum of the abnormal phenomena displayed by a group of living organisms in association with a specified common characteristic or set of characteristics by which they differ from the norm for their species in such a way as to place them at a biological disadvantage'. Differing from the norm for the species is Cohen's 'excess or defect' set out in more explicitly statistical terms and carrying with it several fundamental implications—that deviation in either direction, too much or too little, is equally capable of producing disease; that the boundary between health and disease may need to be an arbitrary one, like the boundary between mental subnormality and normal intelligence; and that the majority are debarred from being regarded as ill. The 'specified common characteristic or set of characteristics' is the defining characteristic of the disease in question. Its presence is essential for establishing the presence of that disease, and it is worth noting that the wording allows it to be either monothetic (a single trait) or polythetic (a set of traits no one of which is mandatory).

The 'biological disadvantage' criterion

Scadding avoided elaborating on what he meant by 'biological disadvantage'. Presumably, though, it must embrace both increased mortality and reduced fertility. Whether it should embrace other impairments as well is less obvious, and the consequences need considering carefully before deciding.

Despite this uncertainty, Scadding's definition does not founder on the shoals which were the undoing of its predecessors. Diseases like hypertension and diabetes which are or may be purely quantitative deviations from normality present no problem. Nor do conditions like dystonia musculorum deformans in which no consistent lesion has yet been identified and whose aetiology remains unknown. Provided that it can be established that a biological disadvantage is involved, their status as diseases is secure. The definition is also independent of whether the affected individual complains or suffers; and it provides a clear indication of which conditions should and which should not merit medical attention, without being influenced by whether or not they currently do so. It also successfully discards lesions, like congenitally fused toes, whose ill-effects are trivial, and provides a clear cut answer to the problem posed by conditions like the sickle cell trait which are disadvantageous in some environments but harmless, or positively beneficial, in others. Despite the presence of a qualitative deviation—an abnormal haemoglobin molecule—it is only to be regarded as a disease in environments in which its presence is a real disadvantage. By the same token, albinism would rank as a disease in Delhi or Khartoum, but probably not in Newfoundland. The 'lesion' concept of disease ignored the environment, except as a source of pathogens, but the biological disadvantage criterion gives environmental influences a powerful role, rightly so in an age in which all disease is increasingly seen as the result of a complex interaction between the individual and his environment, rather than as arising *de novo* within him, or attacking him from without.

My interpretation of 'biological disadvantage'—restricting it to conditions which reduce fertility or shorten life—means that some conditions, like post-herpetic neuralgia and psoriasis, fail to qualify as illnesses despite the fact that they cause considerable suffering, are accompanied by well-defined lesions, and are capable of being relieved by medical means, and on all these counts it seems unreasonable not to regard them as diseases. This is admittedly rather disconcerting, but the problem is that if the meaning of the phrase is broadened to take account of conditions of this kind there is a danger that it will lose all sharpness of meaning, and that as a result anyone with a complaint, or whom doctors think they can treat, will once more be accepted uncritically as ill. (It is also advisable, if one is trying to show that mental illnesses fulfil the same criteria as other illnesses and finds onself presented with a choice of criteria, to use the stricter of the two.)

Despite these doubts about precisely how to define 'biological disadvantage', Scadding's definition is better matched to the ethos of contemporary medicine and to current attitudes to the nature of disease than any of its predecessors, and also more successful in embracing conditions that by common consent are diseases and excluding those that are not. It could still be argued that it and all the other definitions I have discussed are equally inadequate, in which case assertions about the existence or non-existence of mental illness would remain untestable. But if any definition is to be accepted it must surely be this one, or some modification of it.

Having reached this decision I can now come back to my starting point and pose my original question once more. Do mental illnesses possess the essential attributes of illness or not? Do they, by reducing either fertility or life expectancy, produce a significant biological disadvantage?

The fertility of the mentally ill

In purely biological terms fertility is all-important. It is this that determines which species flourish and expand and which die out, and which genotypes within a species become dominant and which remain rare. The fertility of the mentally ill has been the subject of over a dozen studies in the last fifty years, and these indicate that psychotics as a whole marry less often than other people, remain childless more often even when they do marry, and have fewer children than other people in or out of wedlock. To some extent these findings are an artificial consequence of confining the mentally ill in asylums, but this is only a partial explanation. Dahlberg (1933) found that the fertility of psychotic women was less than that of other women of the same age even before admission to hospital, and the studies of Macsorley (1964) and Stevens (1969), carried out since the introduction of 'open door' policies, confirm that despite their increased opportunities for marrying and reproducing those with psychotic illnesses still have fewer children than other people. As Sir Aubrey

Lewis concluded in his Galton Lecture seventeen years ago, the evidence 'points towards the personal characteristics of the patients rather than their enforced residence in a mental hospital as the main reason for their low marriage rate and low fertility' (Lewis, 1958). This reduction in the fertility of psychotics as a whole is largely due to the low fertility of schizophrenics; it is open to doubt whether the fertility of manic-depressives is significantly below that of the general population. Although six studies in the last forty years have all suggested that it is reduced, Essen-Möller's classical study in Munich did not (Essen-Möller, 1935), nor did the more recent investigations by Hopkinson (1963) and Stevens (1969).

The condition which stands out above all others in its implications for fertility is homosexuality. Although there have been few formal studies of the fertility of male or female homosexuals, it can hardly be doubted that it is drastically reduced in both. In simple biological terms their lack of interest in forms of sexual activity capable of resulting in conception puts homosexuals, and other sexual deviants like transsexuals, at a quite daunting negative selection advantage. Whether neurotic illnesses and personality disorders are associated with any significant reduction in fertility is still uncertain, mainly because the question has rarely been considered. There are suggestions that the fertility of criminal psychopaths is below that of the general population (Rosenthal, 1970). There is also some evidence that the sexual activity of neurotics is reduced (Slater, 1945; Eysenck, 1971), and one might expect this to result in a reduction in fertility.

Rosenthal was recently driven to the unwelcome conclusion that fertility is reduced 'in at least four major types of disorders—schizophrenia, manic-depressive psychosis, psychopathy and homosexuality'. (The conclusion is unwelcome because it forces geneticists to postulate either a very high spontaneous mutation rate or else some compensatory advantage in gene-carrying relatives in order to explain the high incidence of these conditions.) Some might wish to dispute the evidence relating to manic-depressive illness and psychopathy, but it would be hard to do so in the case of schizophrenia or homosexuality.

The mortality of the mentally ill

Although fertility may be all-important biologically, death is a more obvious, and to the individual a more important consequence of disease. It also has a greater biological significance in social animals like man, whose off-spring are dependent on their parents for a high proportion of their life span, than in species whose young can fend for themselves from birth. The studies of Alström (1942), Ødegård (1951) and Malzberg (1953) indicate that the risk of death for patients newly admitted to public mental hospitals is, or was until recently, between four and ten times that of the general population, but this high mortality might well be due in part to physical ill-health contributing to the decision to seek hospital admission, or even to infections or other harmful influences encountered in hospital. Larsson and Sjögren (1954), in a meticulous study of the population of two Swedish islands, showed that over a 45-year period schizophrenics, and to a lesser extent manic-depressives also, had a mortality considerably higher than that of the general Swedish population, but they were unable to match the two for the many variables liable to influence mortality.

More recently, studies have been done of the mortality of patients reported to psychiatric case registers. These provide data on out-patient populations with neurotic illnesses and personality disorders, and also allow accurate matching of observed mortality rates with those of the catchment area population. Innes and Millar (1970) studied the mortality over a five-year period of a cohort of 2,000 patients reported to the N.E. Scotland Psychiatric Case Register. Even though they assumed that all untraced patients were still alive, they found that the overall mortality of their cohort was twice the expected rate. Organic psychoses accounted for much of this increase, but all age groups and all diagnostic groups except male character disorders had a mortality above expectation. Even in neurotic illness the mortality was twice the expected rate. A similar study based on the Monroe County register in the United States produced almost identical findings (Babigian and Odoroff, 1969). Even after careful matching for age, sex and marital and socio-economic status, the mortality of the patient group was three times that of the general population, and all diagnostic groups, including neurotic illnesses and character disorders, shared this increased risk. Although the suicide rate was increased tenfold in the register population, suicide was not an important cause of this increased mortality. Indeed, there was no single cause; instead there was a fairly uniform increase in mortality from all major causes of death, including neoplasms, cerebrovascular disease and coronary artery disease. It is possible that this increased mortality is due to intercurrent physical illness increasing the likelihood of psychiatric referral, or even to psychiatric symptoms developing secondarily in the presence of physical illness, but these findings do suggest that a wide range of mental illness may be associated with a significantly increased risk of death.

There have been surprisingly few studies of the mortality associated with individual conditions. Rosenthal quotes three studies of manic-depressive illness all indicating that after the onset of the illness mortality is increased about 1½-fold and life expectancy decreased by about 15 per cent. There is also evidence from numerous sources that at least 15 per cent of manic-depressives die prematurely by suicide (Sainsbury, 1968), and without treatment the mortality would be considerably higher—from exhaustion and accidents of diverse kinds in mania, and from inanition and suicide in depression. The picture is less clear where schizophrenia is concerned, mainly because of the distorting effects of prolonged institutional care. The schizophrenic inmates of the great asylums certainly died prematurely, mainly from tuberculosis and other infections, but the institutions themselves may have been partly responsible for this rather than the disease. However, if schizophrenics were simply to be ignored and provided neither with sanctuaries where they could be fed and clothed nor with modern chemotherapy there is little doubt that comparatively few would survive to old age. Many would die of exposure, the indirect effects of malnutrition, or plain starvation, and others would die in accidents of various kinds, or by suicide. The asylums of the nineteenth century were, after all, built primarily for the protection of the insane and only secondarily for the protection of society. Finally, there is the evidence that several types of drug dependence, including alcohol and heroin—and also nicotine dependence in its common form, cigarette smoking—are all associated with a well-documented increase in mortality.

There is evidence, therefore, that schizophrenia and manic-depressive illness, together with some sexual disorders and various kinds of drug dependence, are associated with either a reduction in fertility or a reduction in life expectancy, or both, and for that reason are justifiably regarded as illnesses. The same may eventually prove to be true of some neurotic states and some types of personality disorder, but at present the evidence is not strong enough to justify firm conclusions in these areas.

At this point it will be worthwhile to recall the arguments of our critics. The various assertions that what psychiatrists regard as mental illnesses are nothing of the kind have all been based on the argument that no physical lesion has ever been demonstrated in these conditions, and that some kind of lesion is essential to establish the presence of disease. This argument is quite explicit in Szasz's case, and implicit in the reasoning of Eysenck, Laing and Scheff also. The arguments of these writers are therefore all based, wittingly or unwittingly, on a concept of disease which has been abandoned not just by psychiatry but by medicine as a whole. The position they are in is like that of Ishmael in *Moby Dick*, arguing that whales must be fish because they have fins and swim under water, unaware that the defining characteristics of fishes had been revised some time before.

Biological and social disadvantages

There are other arguments, however, which do require an answer. I have argued that mental illnesses are justifiably so-called because they are associated with reduced fertility and life expectancy, and that these two constitute a biological disadvantage. Scheff and other sociologists would argue that these handicaps may exist but are secondary consequences of the individual having been labelled as ill rather than being innate and inevitable. They might argue, for example, that the main reason people labelled as schizophrenics have relatively few children is because they are regarded, both by others and by themselves, as lunatics and are less likely to marry and have children for this reason; and they die at an early age because we either lock them up in institutions where they catch tuberculosis, or shun them so that they eventually die of neglect or are driven to suicide.

Essentially the problem is to distinguish between a biological and a purely social disadvantage, and this is difficult because man is necessarily a social animal. His long post-natal immaturity and his use of language are both intimately linked to this fact, and our species has only achieved its present ascendency over others because of the ability of its members to assist one another to overcome both competing species and the physical hazards of the environment. If, therefore, an individual is discriminated against and shunned by his fellows, it could well be argued that that in itself places him at a substantial biological disadvantage, and not merely a social one. The argument could be buttressed by the evidence that other social species, like the rat and the chimpanzee, have also been observed to discriminate against deformed or diseased individuals, excluding them from the group and sharply reducing their chances of survival by doing so. The situation is further complicated by the fact that over the last two hundred years our dominance over our physical and biological environment has become so complete that cultural rather than purely biological forces are increasingly becoming the main determinants of natural selection. Which human genotypes become dominant, and how severe the negative selection pressures on others, are increasingly determined not so much by their inherent hardiness and adaptability as by cultural attitudes towards them. The increased survival chances of diabetics in the twentieth century and the reduced survival chances of Huguenots in the seventeenth century are both examples of this. There is another issue as well. It could legitimately be argued that because man is a social species what matters is the contribution the individual makes to the survival chances of the group rather than his own personal survival, and that a trait which is, biologically speaking, a disadvantage to him personally may be advantageous to his social group, or *vice versa*. If, for example, homosexuality could be shown to be associated with valuable aptitudes which others lacked, it might be positively advantageous to a community to have a proportion of homosexual members. Indeed, in an era of explosive population growth it might be beneficial to a community to have its fertility reduced. Clearly the complexities of the situation created by man's distortion of his original biological environment are almost endless. Yet somehow we have still to find a way of distinguishing between innate biological disadvantages and others attributable to cultural and social determinants of varying kinds.

The answer, I suggest, is that we must ignore the increasing importance of purely cultural factors in determining who lives and who dies; ignore the existence and fatal effects of social discrimination in other species, and also ignore the argument that it is the survival of the group rather than of the individual that matters. Despite all these complications we must still insist that for a characteristic to qualify as a biological disadvantage it must be shown to be harmful to the individual possessing it, and also to be innate and not simply one that leads to rejection by others. The criterion must be, would this individual still be at a disadvantage if his fellows did not recognize his distinguishing features but treated him as they treat one another? In the case of schizophrenia the argument hinges on whether the high mortality and low fertility associated with this condition are innate, or whether they would melt away if those whom we call schizophrenics were not merely treated like other people but not even recognized as deviant. Although the proponents of the labelling theory have demonstrated that recognition of deviance may often increase rather than reduce the handicaps associated with it, they are far from establishing that labelling is the primary problem. Indeed, the evidence from both twin and adoption studies for the genetic transmission of schizophrenia establishes beyond doubt that it is not.

Comments

I think, therefore, that my earlier conclusion is still justified: we have adequate evidence that schizophrenia and manic-depressive illness, and also some sexual disorders and some forms of drug dependence, carry with them an intrinsic biological disadvantage, and on these grounds are justifiably regarded as illness; but it is not yet clear whether the same is true of neurotic illness and the ill-defined territory of personality disorder.

What is the significance of this conclusion? First, it is an answer to the argument that there is no such thing as mental illness. At least part of the territory regarded by psychiatrists as mental illness fulfils the same criteria as those required for physical illness. But only part of it does so. Many of the conditions which psychiatrists have come to regard as illness, and hence as requiring treatment, do not qualify, or rather there is little evidence at present that they do. This does not necessarily mean that psychiatrists have no right to meddle in these areas, or that people who are anxious or depressed should be dissuaded from visiting their doctors. For one thing, childbirth and family planning provide precedents for the involvement of medicine beyond the boundaries of disease.

Even so, psychiatrists might be well advised to reconsider where their sphere of responsibility should end. A century ago they were concerned only with madness. But from that time onwards their concept of their proper role expanded steadily until the stage was reached, particularly in North America, at which some were claiming a mandate—and the ability—to treat anyone who was unhappy for whatever reason, and anyone whose behaviour was annoying or alarming to other people. It is worth reflecting whether the many attempts we have recently witnessed to discredit the concept of mental illness might not be a reaction to the equally absurd claims we have made that all unhappiness and all undesirable behaviour are manifestations of mental illness.

The attempt to relieve suffering is medicine's oldest and noblest tradition, and I am not suggesting that psychiatrists should stop trying to help husbands and wives to live together in harmony, or aimless adolescents to find their feet. But if we are to venture into such areas let it be in full recognition of the fact that in doing so we may be straying outside our proper boundary, and that in the end it may turn out that other people can deal with such problems as well as or better than we can, and that in these areas their training and their concepts are more appropriate than ours. By all means let us insist that schizophrenia is an illness and that we are better equipped to understand and treat it than anyone else. But let us not try to do the same for all the woes of mankind.

References

ALSTRÖM, C. H. (1942) Mortality in mental hospitals. *Acta Psychiatrica et Neurologica Scandinavica*, Suppl. 24.

BABIGIAN, H. M. & ODOROFF, C. L. (1969) The mortality experience of a population with psychiatric illness. *American Journal of Psychiatry*, **126,** 470–480.

COHEN, H. (1943) *The Nature, Method and Purpose of Diagnosis*. Cambridge University Press.

DAHLBERG, G. (1933) Die Fruchtbarkeit der Geisteskranken. *Zeitschrift für die gesante Neurologie und Psychiatrie*, **144,** 427.

ENGLE, R. L. & DAVIS, B. J. (1963) Medical diagnosis: past, present and future. I. Present concepts of the meaning and limitations of medical diagnosis. *Archives of Internal Medicine*, **112,** 512–519.

Essen-Möller, E. (1935) Untersuchungen über die Fruchtbarkeit gewisser Gruppen von Geisteskranken. *Acta Psychiatrica et Neurologica Scandinavica*, Suppl. 8.

Eysenck, H. J. (1960) Classification and the problem of diagnosis. In *Handbook of Abnormal Psychology* (ed. H. J. Eysenck). London: Pitman.

—— (1971) Personality and sexual adjustment. *British Journal of Psychiatry*, **118**, 593–608.

Hopkinson, G. (1963) Celibacy and marital fertility in manic-depressive patients. *Acta Psychiatrica Scandinavica*, **39**, 473–476.

Innes, G. & Millar, W. M. (1970) Mortality among psychiatric patients. *Scottish Medical Journal*, **15**, 143–148.

Kräupl Taylor, F. (1971) A logical analysis of the medico-psychological concept of disease. *Psychological Medicine*, **1**, 356–364.

Laing, R. D. (1967) *The Politics of Experience*. Penguin Books.

Larsson, T. & Sjögren, T. (1954) A methodological, psychiatric and statistical study of a large Swedish rural population. *Acta Psychiatrica et Neurologica Scandinavica*, Suppl. 89.

Lewis, A. (1958) Fertility and mental illness. *Eugenics Review*, **50**, 91–106.

Linder, R. (1965) Diagnosis: description or prescription? A case study in the psychology of diagnosis. *Perceptual and Motor Skills*, **20**, 1081–1092.

Macsorley, K. (1964) An investigation into the fertility rates of mentally ill patients. *Annals of Human Genetics*, **27**, 247–256.

Malzberg, B. (1953) Rates of discharge and rates of mortality among first admissions to the New York civil state hospitals. *Mental Hygiene*, **37**, 619–654.

Ødegård, Ø. (1951) Mortality in Norwegian mental hospitals, 1926–41. *Acta Genetica*, **2**, 141–173.

Oldham, P. D., Pickering, G., Fraser Roberts, J. A. & Sowry, G. S. C. (1960) The nature of essential hypertension. *Lancet*, i, 1085–1093.

Rosenthal, D. (1970) *Genetic Theory and Abnormal Behavior*. New York: McGraw.

Sainsbury, P. (1968) Suicide and depression. In *Recent Developments in Affective Disorders* (ed. Coppen and Walk). London.

Scadding, J. G. (1967) Diagnosis: the clinician and the computer. *Lancet*, ii, 877–882.

Scheff, T. J. (1963) The role of the mentally ill and the dynamics of mental disorder: a research framework. *Sociometry*, **26**, 436–453.

Schneider, K. (1950) Systematic psychiatry. *American Journal of Psychiatry*, **107**, 334–335.

Slater, E. (1945) Neurosis and sexuality. *Journal of Neurology and Psychiatry*, **8**, 12–14.

Stevens, B. C. (1969) *Marriage and Fertility of Women Suffering from Schizophrenia or Affective Disorders* (Maudsley Monograph No. 19.) London.

Szasz, T. S. (1960) The myth of mental illness. *American Psychologist*, **15**, 113–118; or book of same title. London: Secker and Warburg, 1961.

3   The syndrome of schizophrenia: Unresolved questions and opportunities for research

SEYMOUR S. KETY

The nosology of schizophrenia

Eugen Bleuler, who devised the term 'schizophrenia' for Kraepelin's 'dementia praecox', was careful to point out that he was not revising Kraepelin's description of the syndrome, but merely its name:

The whole idea of dementia praecox originates with Kraepelin. Almost exclusively to his work we also owe the grouping and description of the separate symptoms [p. 1].... Unfortunately we could not shirk the uncomfortable duty of coining a new name for this disease... the present one seems to be awkward. It only designates the disease, not the diseased; moreover it is impossible to derive from it an adjective denoting the characteristics of this illness, although an exasperated colleague has used 'praecox symptom'. Without such a new term, a thorough work on differential diagnosis would be hard to write and even harder to read. [Bleuler, 1911]

Others, since that time, have taken greater liberties with the syndrome, altering its essential features but retaining the name and introducing thereby considerable confusion. Justification for these changes has often been based upon the claim that the original syndrome had not been well characterized. It is true that Kraepelin insisted that no single symptom was pathognomonic, but neither he nor Bleuler left any doubt regarding the features that were essential to their concept:

By the term 'dementia praecox' or 'schizophrenia' we designate a group of psychoses whose course is at times chronic, at times marked by intermittent attacks, and which can stop or retrograde at any stage, but does not permit a full *restitutio ad integrum*. The disease is characterized by a specific type of alteration of thinking, feeling, and relation to the external world which appears nowhere else in this particular fashion [p. 9] ... The fundamental symptoms consist of disturbances of association and affectivity, the predilection for fantasy as against reality and the inclination to divorce oneself from reality (autism). Furthermore, we can add the absence of those very symptoms which play such a great role in certain other diseases such as primary disturbances of perception, orientation and memory, etc. [p. 14]

Kraepelin, who agreed with Bleuler's distinction between the fundamental disorders and accompanying phenomena of the disease, goes on to state:

The former constitute the real characteristic of the clinical state and can be demonstrated in each individual case more or less distinctly; the latter may be present but may also be absent; they are not caused by the character of the morbid process but by circumstances which are in loose connection with it... from this point of view the weakening of judgement, of mental activity and of creative ability, the dulling of emotional interest and the loss of energy, lastly, the loosening of the inner unity of the psychic life would have to be reckoned among the fundamental disorders of dementia praecox, while all the remaining morbid symptoms, especially hallucinations and delusions, . . . would be regarded more as secondary accompanying phenomena. [Kraepelin, 1913]

By the 'loosening of the inner unity of psychic life' Kraepelin included several other characteristics:

... it consists in the loss of the inner unity of the activities of intellect, emotion and volition in themselves and among one another . . . in the disorders of association, described by Bleuler, incoherence in the train of thought, in the sharp change of moods as well as in desultoriness and derailments in practical work . . . emotions do not correspond to ideas, the patients laugh and weep without recognizeable cause, without any relation to their circumstances and their experiences . . . [p. 75]

Besides these characteristic symptoms, an insidious onset in a premorbid personality with certain common features and a chronic course were also included by both. Each also included a subgroup which they termed 'dementia praecox simplex' or 'simple schizophrenia' which manifested the fundamental features but without hallucinations or delusions:

... the only possibility of acquainting physicians with this type of individual rests in giving it a distinct name. This distinction also possesses a minor theoretical value inasmuch as it demonstrates the difference between the essential and accessory symptoms: the latter are absent in simple schizophrenia. [Bleuler, 1911]

Bleuler saw simple schizophrenia tapering off into a broader and milder syndrome which he termed 'latent schizophrenia'. Kraepelin agreed that such a latent form of illness could be seen in the relatives of typical schizophrenics but was concerned about stretching the boundaries too far:

There is also a latent schizophrenia, and I am convinced that this is the most frequent form, although admittedly these people hardly ever come for treatment. It is not necessary to give a detailed description of the various manifestations of latent schizophrenia. In this form, we can see *in nuce* all the symptoms and combinations of symptoms which are present in the manifest types of the disease. [Bleuler, p. 238]

Bleuler is inclined to stretch the limits of such a 'latent schizophrenia' to an extraordinary extent and to interpret all possible psychopathic personalities in this set. How far that is justified in fact can scarcely be decided at present. [Kraepelin, p. 240]

Studies of the families and of the co-twins of schizophrenics have found a consistently high prevalence of individuals with uncertain schizophrenia and schizoid characteristics (Shields *et al*, 1975), which would support Bleuler's thesis. To what extent these, like Bleuler's observations, might have been affected by association with or mimicry of the overtly schizophrenic relative is difficult to say.

The studies on adopted schizophrenics that have been conducted with David Rosenthal, Paul Wender and Fini Schulsinger, over the past 16 years have provided an opportunity to observe the operation of genetic factors in schizophrenia, but also to examine the hypothesized relationship of a syndrome such as latent schizophrenia or schizoid personality to classical schizophrenia (Kety *et al*, 1978). In the Copenhagen sample of adoptees, 17 had been identified by four raters who agreed on a diagnosis of 'chronic schizophrenia' in accordance with the criteria of Kraepelin and Bleuler. The biological relatives of these adoptees, in contrast to the biological relatives of control adoptees, showed a significant prevalence of schizophrenia-like conditions which we had called 'latent or borderline schizophrenia', 'uncertain schizophrenia', or 'schizoid or inadequate personality'. Since the biological relatives grew up apart from the adoptee and, in most cases, unaware of his mental status, and our diagnoses were made without that knowledge, these findings provided support less open to bias for the existence of Bleuler's 'latent schizophrenia'. We now felt justified in attempting to arrive at a better characterization of these conditions than our global judgements had provided. The material on which we had based our diagnoses—comprehensive psychiatric interviews or detailed abstracts of hospital records—were submitted to Robert Spitzer and Jean Endicott for an independent evaluation, which supported our diagnosis of chronic schizophrenia in 16 of the 17 adoptees and in each of our five diagnoses of chronic schizophrenia among the biological relatives. Among those we had diagnosed as latent or uncertain schizophrenia, schizoid or inadequate personality, they found eight characteristics on which they have based a new diagnostic category of 'schizotypal personality'. From questionnaires distributed randomly to 4,000 American psychiatrists, Spitzer and his associates (Spitzer *et al*, 1979) found that these characteristics also occurred with a satisfactorily high frequency in 222 patients who had been given a clinical diagnosis of borderline schizophrenia. More important than that, however, in respect of the validity of the syndrome and its relationship to schizophrenia, is the fact that it occurred with a significantly high prevalence in the biological relatives of adoptees who had developed classical schizophrenia.

Our studies have been less successful in the case of 'acute schizophrenic reaction', another accretion to schizophrenia which Bleuler did not originate and which he specifically repudiated. We have not found a greater than chance prevalence of acute, remitting psychosis in the biological relatives of chronic schizophrenics, but the numbers involved are too small to permit a conclusion. There are, however, many other reasons for challenging that diagnostic concept.

Schizophrenia and manic-depressive disorder did not suffice to describe all psychotic patients in whom an organic basis was not apparent, and other designations were developed for these atypical psychoses. 'Schizophreniform psychosis', 'schizoaffective disorder', 'atypical schizophrenia', described illnesses with acute onset, many of the accessory symptoms, but fewer of the fundamental features of schizophrenia, and in the majority of which complete remission was to be expected (Langfeldt, 1939; Strömgren, 1965; Mitsuda, 1965). These gave way, in the United States particularly, to less precise terms like 'confusional insanity', 'good-prognosis schizophrenia' or 'acute schizophrenic reaction', often on the explicit assumption that these were indeed forms of schizophrenia. Knapp (1908) put it this way: 'If we accept... the probable identity of confusional insanity (amentia) and dementia praecox, we can extend a larger hope to the patient and his friends by recognizing that complete recovery is often possible and that the patient is not inevitably doomed to "dementia praecox"'. Of course the same salutary effect could have been accomplished by continuing clearly to separate that syndrome from dementia praecox.

Schneider, 50 years later (1959), gave renewed support to those who preferred to think of schizophrenia as a benign process by simply redefining schizophrenia to make it so. Features regarded by both Kraepelin and Bleuler as fundamental and characteristic (impoverishment of affect, disturbances in personal contact and rapport, ambivalence, lack of motivation, depersonalization, and stereotypes) were specifically rejected and the new criteria were restricted to particular types of hallucinations and delusions which Bleuler had regarded as accessory symptoms. Schneider established a new syndrome with features that are more easily perceived and described, and which therefore show a higher degree of inter-rater reliability, features which are economically put into checklists and fed into computers. That syndrome may be more prevalent, have a more favourable outcome, and be more responsive to a wide variety of treatments, but it is not schizophrenia. I suspect that Bleuler would have criticized it today as he did earlier attempts to confound the original concept: 'Naturally, nothing is gained thereby except another symptomatological picture which is then called a disease and which, moreover, is misleadingly defined by the same terms as the qualitatively and quantitatively quite different Kraepelinian concept' (p. 278).

Schneider's statement—'When any of these modes of experience is undeniably present and no basic somatic illness can be found, we may make the decisive clinical diagnosis of schizophrenia'—stands in sharp contrast to that of Bleuler: 'Hallucinations and delusions, are partial phenomena of the most varied diseases. Their presence is often helpful in making the diagnosis of a psychosis, but not in diagnosing the presence of schizophrenia' (p. 204).

Nomenclature is one of the very few areas in science where reference to authority may be decisive. The properties of a category, be it of plants or illnesses, are established by the one who named it and become characteristic of that category by definition. If different characteristics are to be adopted for schizophrenia, their validity and pertinence to it should be established, and that will require new knowledge, not simply a high inter-rater reliability. It is possible that future knowledge will provide truly pathognomic features of schizophrenia generally or, more likely, of homogeneous subgroups which can then be given more informative names. That process has been going on effectively in the case of another phenomenological syndrome, mental retardation.

The present confusion in respect of the characteristics of schizophrenia will persist until it is required that suggested redefinitions of schizophrenia should show that they accurately describe the original syndrome and more parsimoniously or reliably differentiate it from other syndromes. That was not done for the first rank symptoms of Schneider originally, and where they have been tested more recently, they have been shown to be neither characteristic nor discriminating (Mellor, 1970; Carpenter *et al*, 1973; Koehler *et al*, 1977). The acute psychoses in which they are often found do not have the type of onset or course, the family history, the fundamental symptoms, prognosis or response to treatment that are associated with schizophrenia (Pope and Lipinski, 1978).

It is true that a small fraction (approximately 10 per cent) of classical schizophrenics experience an acute psychotic episode with a relatively long-lasting remission before the chronic disorder appears. It is also evident that at the time of the initial break such patients cannot be distinguished by most competent clinicians from acute psychotic patients who will later show a permanent remission (Welner and Strömgren, 1958; Vaillant, 1978). That, however, could hardly justify labelling as schizophrenia all acute psychoses not obviously organic. In all likelihood the majority will turn out to have been manic (Tsuang *et al*, 1976), which would not permit using that term to describe them all. The group of acute functional psychoses differs so much from classical schizophrenia that it is difficult to see what advantage inheres in our continuing to confound them. It is easy to point out the disadvantages. Not only does it attach an inappropriately pessimistic diagnosis to patients with a self-limiting illness and needlessly expose them to long-term treatment with potent drugs, it also raises false hopes in those who suffer from classical schizophrenia by lending an unwarranted credibility to claims that schizophrenia can be effectively treated with large doses of vitamins, with other novel treatments enthusiastically advocated, or with no drugs at all. In fact, Laennec's familiar dictum might well be paraphrased: 'If you discover a new treatment for schizophrenia, make sure you use it on acute schizophrenic patients, for they will surely improve under it.'

Until we have new and better knowledge of the nature of the disorders which make up the syndromes, it is possible that much of the confusion and dissatisfaction may be relieved by utilizing the knowledge we already have. We would define syndromes more homogeneous in symptomatology, and more useful predictors of outcome and response to therapy for clinical practice and research, were we to restrict the term schizophrenia to its original concept of a chronic disorder of thought and feeling, in which an insidious onset, the premorbid personality qualities, and the fundamental features described by Kraepelin and Bleuler were the defining characteristics, permitting the accessory symptoms to differentiate simple schizophrenia from the rest of the syndrome. For the broader group with similar but less intense and handicapping manifestations, found to occur in the biological families of classical schizophrenics, Bleuler's 'latent schizophrenia' seems justified, although 'schizotypal personality, may be more appropriate, until the genetically related group can be differentiated. The third syndrome would include what remained of 'acute schizophrenia' after mania had been excluded by careful diagnosis, and could be called 'schizoaffective psychoses' if that term merely implied the combination of symptoms, although the designation 'acute undifferentiated psychosis' seems preferable.

I propose to limit the rest of my discussion to the classical syndrome of schizophrenia, of which, unfortunately, there are still too many examples.

The pathology of schizophrenia

Both Kraepelin and Bleuler assumed that a 'common morbid process' in the brain accounted for the common features of the syndrome and Kraepelin included the lesions described by Alzheimer in his later descriptions of dementia praecox. Those lesions and numerous others reported by many observers were not substantiated and probably represented post-mortem artefacts of non-specific changes which more rigorous controls would have obviated. Maudsley (1872) had put it succinctly: 'The morbid anatomy of insanity would take little room were speculation rigidly excluded and limited to what is actually seen and known.'

Kraepelin based his assumption of a common morbid process, not on Alzheimer's findings which were made later, but on the resemblance of many of the psychological symptoms which he observed in dementia praecox to those which were known to occur in other disorders with a clear organic basis, particularly general paresis, encephalitis and epilepsy. In addition many of the behavioural disturbances, pupillary responses, altered reflexes, tics, ataxias, fits and absences which both he and Bleuler described in these patients pointed to neurological disturbances.

Since their time both types of observation have been considerably enlarged through new knowledge in neuropathology, the application of more sophisticated technology and more rigorously controlled conditions. An increasing number of neurological and metabolic disorders have been described in which some or many of the psychological and behavioural characteristics of schizophrenia are seen and can be attributed to pathological biological processes (Davison and Bagley, 1969). In many of these the resemblance to schizophrenia is sufficiently great in some stages or throughout the course of the illness that competent clinicians have made the diagnosis of schizophrenia, to be challenged only at autopsy. Various psychotomimetic drugs produce symptoms that are observed in schizophrenia; in the case of amphetamines the resemblance is often real enough to justify a diagnosis of schizophrenia. There are a number of disorders such as Huntington's chorea, Wilson's disease, temporal lobe epilepsy, or the adult form of metachromatic leukodystrophy, which quite regularly present as schizophrenia in their early phases, and later progress to the different manifestations which are their individual characteristics. This raises the possibility that these disturbances, early in their course, share with the syndrome of schizophrenia which they resemble a common morbid process of diverse aetiology, which in the case of schizophrenia, remains limited in its distribution and unrecognized by conventional pathological techniques. A parsimonious hypothesis would be that there exists a system or systems in the brain which, when their normal functions are disturbed by one or more of a variety of aetiological factors, produce the characteristic psychological and behavioural symptoms of schizophrenia. The differences we see in the symptoms of schizophrenia may well be due to differences in the extent or severity of the disturbance, while the variations in course and outcome may be more related to the nature and persistence of the aetiological factors.

Our ability to demonstrate and elucidate pathological disturbances is limited by the state of the art, and to assume their absence because they have not been demonstrated is a *non sequitur*. Maudsley refuted Szasz and Laing long before those men were born:

> ... at present we know nothing whatever of the intimate constitution of nerve element and of the mode of its functional action, and it is beyond doubt that important molecular or chemical changes may take place in those inner recesses to which we have not gained access. Where the subtlety of nature so far exceeds the subtlety of human investigation, to conclude from the non-appearance of change to the non-existence thereof could be just as if the blind man were to maintain there were no colours or the deaf to assert that there is no sound. [p. 367]

The disturbance may be in the coarse structure or in finer details perceptible by classical staining techniques, which has been the case for most of the nervous diseases already identified. On the other hand it may reveal itself in a morphology not yet explored, in enzymatic, biochemical, or immunological processes, or in molecular, membrane or receptor mechanisms, many of which can now be examined by techniques only recently developed and which constitute a new discipline of neuropathology (Matthysse and Pope, 1975). The post-mortem examination of the brain, which for several decades has languished because of the unlikelihood of finding anything new with old techniques, may again occupy an important place in the study of mental illness (Bird *et al*, 1977).

Are there more compelling reasons than plausible hypotheses and compatible observations for believing that neurological changes underlie a major segment of the classical schizophrenia syndrome? The neurological signs found in their patients by Kraepelin and Bleuler have been repeatedly confirmed and extended by numerous authors and have been reviewed by Stevens (1973) and many others. Rochford and associates (1970), in a well controlled study, found various types of neurologic abnormality in two-thirds of the schizophrenics they studied and none among patients with affective disorder. Mosher *et al* (1971) noted that 73 per cent of the schizophrenic monozygotic twins they examined had one or more signs of neurologic defect contrasted with their virtual absence in the non-schizophrenic co-twins. Tucker and his co-workers (1975), using a 'neurological impairment index' based on several measures of psychomotor control and co-ordination, found it to be significantly elevated in schizophrenic as opposed to non-schizophrenic patients and well correlated with measures of cognitive dysfunction. The eye-tracking dysfunction found in a high proportion of schizophrenics and their non-schizophrenic relatives (Holzman *et al*, 1974) appears to be more than an attentional deficit.

Observations suggesting cortical atrophy or ventricular dilatation in the brains of chronic schizophrenics at autopsy or from pneumo-encephalographic studies have been made repeatedly and just as often criticized for deficiencies in design. The introduction of the new technique of computerized tomography has made possible a re-examination of the question during life with an objective and non-invasive technique. Johnstone and associates (1978), in an examination of 18 chronically hospitalized schizophrenics and 10 age-matched institutionalized controls, found a significantly increased ventricular size in the schizophrenic patients (particularly those with intellectual and affective dulling) and practically no overlap with the controls. They suggest the existence of a subgroup in the syndrome. Weinberger *et al* (1979) confirmed this finding in 58 chronic schizophrenic patients all under the age of 50, 40 per cent of whom showed ventricular size outside the normal range. Rieder and associates (1979) confining their sample entirely to patients between 20 and 35 years of age, in partial remission and living in the community found 4 out of 17 with widened sulci (11.5 ± 4.1 per cent of total brain area in those as opposed to 1.9 ± 1.3 per cent in the remainder of the sample).

There have been numerous studies of the electroencephalogram in schizophrenia which have found a greater percentage of abnormality than would be expected in a normal population (Kennard and Levy, 1952). Some studies (Hill, 1957; Abenson, 1970) exercising great care to avoid artefacts and employing appropriate controls have confirmed this, finding obvious abnormalities largely in the temporal region in 16 to 24 per cent of schizophrenics as opposed to 9 per cent of controls.

The possibility that neurological damage is the result of the presence of schizophrenia by virtue of increased exposure to trauma or somatic therapies can be examined by prospective studies of individuals in the course of their development. Fish (1975) has conducted such studies extending over 20 years on a total of 213 children of whom 89 eventually became schizophrenic, reporting disturbances in the timing and integration of neurological maturation in infancy and disorders of arousal, vestibular and autonomic functioning and somatic growth preceding or accompanying the first appearance of the psychological manifestations of schizophrenia.

In a careful prospective study of the birth records of 54 process schizophrenics and 46 'schizophrenia-like' disorders, which included schizophreniform, schizoaffective, confusional and reactive psychoses, McNeil and Kaij (1978) found a significantly elevated incidence of obstetrical complications in the group which eventually became typically schizophrenic, whereas the atypical group did not differ significantly from controls.

I find it difficult to avoid the conclusion that in a substantial fraction of typical chronic schizophrenics there is an underlying neurological disturbance. That fraction has not diminished with increasingly rigorous observations and it is augmented by each new technique as it is applied. It is not unlikely that the actual fraction so affected is considerably larger than has thus far been demonstrated. Whether such a process is present in all schizophrenics, I cannot say, and the ability of a hysterical psychosis to mimic some of the features of schizophrenia leaves open the possibility of forms of schizophrenia with disturbed psychological processes in a neurologically normal brain. In any case, one can keep open that undemonstrated possibility without ignoring the clear indications of neurological derangements that have been found.

Genetic factors in schizophrenia

Evidence that genetic factors play an important role in schizophrenia further support the significance of biological processes as a substrate for the symptoms and as primary aetiological factors.

The process of adoption appears to offer a means of separating the confounding genetic and environmental variables and minimizing many of the sources of error. Both Karlsson (1966) and Heston (1966) have traced individuals born of a schizophrenic parent but reared in another environment and found that the same percentage developed schizophrenia as is usually found in the offspring of schizophrenics. Attempting to minimize ascertainment and subjective bias, my colleagues and I began, in 1962, to compile a total national sample of adults in Denmark who were legally adopted by individuals not biologically related to them, and have used this population as the basis for several adoption studies on schizophrenia (Kety *et al*, 1968, 1975; Rosenthal *et al*, 1968; Wender *et al*, 1974). The prevalence of schizophrenia comparable to that found in non-adoptive samples in parents, offspring, siblings and half siblings of schizophrenic probands, reared apart from them and in most cases ignorant of their status or existence, indicates the importance of genetic factors in the aetiology of the syndrome.

The three types of disorder included in our initial selection of 34 index adoptees (chronic, latent and acute schizophrenia) were apparently not part of a homogeneous syndrome. There was considerably more schizophrenia and schizophrenia-like illness in the biological relatives of the adoptees with chronic schizophrenia than of those with the other types of illness. Furthermore, typical chronic schizophrenia appeared to occur only in the biological relatives of adoptees with the same syndrome. But these probands also had biological relatives with milder forms of illness described by 'latent' or 'uncertain' schizophrenia. Although schizophrenia was not limited to only a few of the biological families, neither was it uniformly distributed among them. In fact, only half of the schizophrenic adoptees had chronic schizophrenia or schizophrenia-like disorders in their biological relatives. Of course, many of the biological families were too small to rule out a genetic contribution to the proband's illness, but others were sufficiently large for the genetic risk in the proband to be said to be low. The unexpectedly high frequency of chronic, latent or uncertain schizophrenia in the biological half siblings of schizophrenic adoptees whose shared parent had one of those diagnoses suggested a form of schizophrenia with monogenic transmission. Consequently the 34 pedigrees were analysed from the point of view of permissible models of genetic transmission, but allowing for the presence of non-genetic phenocopies (Morton *et al*, 1979). Although the small size of sample permits a compatibility with a wide range of hypotheses, the model which gives the best fit is a single major locus of intermediate dominance, reminiscent of an earlier suggestion of Slater (1958), with 15 per cent of schizophrenics as phenocopies, 1–2 per cent as homozygotes, 84 per cent as heterozygotes, and a penetrance of 46 per cent in homozygotes and 23 per cent in heterozygotes. Böök and his associates (1978) report new evidence compatible with genetic dominance in the schizophrenia occurring in an isolate population in Sweden.

The findings of the adoption studies lend additional credibility to the aetiologic diversity of schizophrenia which has been suggested by numerous authors (Matthysse, 1978; Richter, 1976; Kety, 1959). Both Kraepelin and Bleuler, while assuming a common morbid process in the syndrome of schizophrenia, recognized a number of different possible aetiologies. The belief that the syndrome represents a single disease with a single aetiology is supported by neither authority nor empirical evidence, and much of the latter argues against it. That assumption, however, has been responsible for much of the controversy and confusion in the interpretation or acceptance of the results of research. Although hypotheses have been formulated to explain schizophrenia on the basis of some unitary process, experimental support has not been forthcoming. More modest hypotheses formulated to account for a segment of a heterogeneous syndrome, might well fare better. In addition, such hypotheses would not be mutually exclusive and results which appear to support one or the other would not imply a rejection of all others.

The assumption of heterogeneous aetiology has been employed in an ingenious search for environmental variables important in schizophrenia (Kinney and Jacobsen, 1978). On the premise that the environmental contribution would be greater in those probands with low genetic risk, they have examined a number of environmental influences, comparing their incidence in schizophrenic adoptees with a high and low genetic background. The findings to date are interesting. Those probands with a low genetic risk have more evidence of birth injury than those who became schizophrenic with a strong genetic background. The probands with a low genetic risk were born predominantly in the first four months of the year. A number of epidemiological studies employing large samples have indicated a small excess of births in the first third of the year for schizophrenics compared with the rest of the population. A recent study of more than 5,000 schizophrenics found a 7 per cent excess (Hare *et al*, 1974), but a striking difference found among only 34 probands is remarkable and likely to reflect an important variable. Although the risk of birth trauma is higher in the cold winter months, it is equally possible that some virus may have a peak incidence in that season. In addition to these environmental influences of a biological nature, some personality characteristics have also been found which appear to be more common in the adoptive parents of probands with a low genetic risk, which this technique is especially suitable for pursuing. Since all of the adoptive parents in the sample have reared a schizophrenic individual, the possibility of feedback from the child to parental personality is controlled.

Biochemical factors

In a remarkable insight which anticipated developments that have come about only in the past decade or two, Maudsley (1872) wrote:

... it is clear that we cannot at present penetrate those intimate special differences in constitution which the variety (of functions of the neurons of the brain) implies. These essential differences are not such, indeed, as the microscope is ever likely to reveal; for they probably depend on the intimate chemical composition and are not likely ... to be disclosed until chemistry has arrived at a microscopial application ... [p. 57]

Even Thudichum (1884), who established the modern science of neurochemistry, did not perceive as clearly as did Maudsley the progress that was to take place in microanalysis and histochemistry, and the implications that these would have for the understanding of the major psychoses.

In recent years, ultramicrochemistry, fluorescence- and immuno-histology, enzymatic assays, labelled amino acids, and radioactive ligands have all been brought to bear on the complexity of the brain, identifying systems of neurons which share a common transmitter, delineating their pathways, measuring the number or sensitivity of receptors to them on the postsynaptic membranes of responding cells, learning the various times at which they emerge in the developing brain, studying their growth, observing the effects on behaviour of alterations in their disposition or functional integrity.

The most obvious progress which this has made possible is in elucidating the action of numerous psychotropic drugs, which, in the case of schizophrenia has meant the antipsychotic neuroleptics. The affinity which all of these display for dopamine receptors which is, moreover, highly correlated with their therapeutic potency can hardly be a coincidence and the conclusion that these drugs achieve their therapeutic effects by reducing the efficacy of dopaminergic transmission is widely accepted. The pertinence of this to chemical disturbances that may have an aetiological role in schizophrenia or underlie some of its symptoms is at present far from clear. The simplest hypothesis, that schizo-phrenia is associated with an increased concentration of dopamine at certain of its synapses, has not been supported, although an adequate test may require a more precise knowledge of the connections of the mesolimbic dopamine system which can now be acquired (Nauta *et al*, 1978). The increase in dopa-mine receptor sensitivity that some have found in the brains of schizophrenic patients' post-mortem is confirmed by others, but the effect of chronic neuro-leptic blockade of such receptors is difficult to rule out.

There have been other hypotheses and some provocative observations sug-gesting disturbances in other neurotransmitters like noradrenalin, acetylcho-line, serotonin, or GABA, which interact or maintain a balance with dopamine, (Roberts, 1972; Kety, 1972; Iversen and Rose, 1973; Matthysse and Pope, 1975). It is becoming clear that the earlier notion that each neurotransmitter regulated a particular function or mental state was far too simple. It is more appropriate now to regard them not as solo instruments but as playing in concert. Moreover, the orchestra of transmitters and modulators is one in which the strings cannot merely complement or override the woodwinds, they may suppress them entirely, accentuate them, speed their tempo or slow them down. A single transmitter may be involved in a wide variety of neuropsycholo-gical functions, its role in each being largely determined by the state of the system and the action of other neurotransmitters. The more complex picture suggests that an understanding of the biochemical substrates that underlie the symptoms of schizophrenia will not quickly or easily be discovered, but there can be little doubt that a further understanding of these transmitters and others that remain to be characterized is an area of fundamental research of great relevance to these clinical problems. It is also significant that there is a cohort of psychiatrists and psychologists, skilled in modern techniques of neurochemistry, who are well aware of this, and that nearly ten years ago a distinguished committee of the Medical Research Council (1970) reported on the opportunities which lie in this field.

Psychosocial factors

The psychosocial milieu of the nuclear family, which twenty years ago occupied a dominant position among aetiological theories regarding schizophrenia, still represents an influence of obvious importance in acculturation and personality development, although its role in the genesis of schizophrenia remains to be unequivocally demonstrated. The observations which contributed to its early prominence consisted of various indications of severe psychopathology in the parents of schizophrenic individuals. More compelling, however, was a study which avoided subjective bias and the impact of the schizophrenic upon his family by evaluating records and psychiatric interviews from parents of pro-blem children or adolescents seen in out-patient clinics. Significantly more psychopathology, communication deviance and marital stress was found in those whose children were to become schizophrenic some years later (Waring and Ricks, 1965). This approach, as the authors recognized, was unable to rule out genetic factors, shared between parents and offspring. In an effort to correct that deficit, studies of adoptive parents of schizophrenics have been conducted which have revealed no gross pathology in them comparable to that which is found in the biological parents of schizophrenics (Wender *et al*, 1968; Kety *et al*, 1975).

In blind evaluations of the Rorschach protocols of adoptive and biological parents of schizophrenics, however, Margaret Singer has found comparable degrees of communication deviance in parents who have reared a schizophrenic individual whether or not they were genetically related to the patient (Wynne *et al*, 1976). Another study employing a similar strategy found different results, with more Rorschach pathology in the biological parents of schizophrenics than in their adoptive parents who, in turn, showed no more than the parents of a comparison group of non-genetic mentally retarded (Wender *et al*, 1977). It is still necessary, however, to explain the striking results of Dr Singer who with unerring accuracy could discern, from the Rorschach alone, individuals who had reared a schizophrenic. If it were possible to rule out the effects of such an experience on the parents' personalities and responses to psychological tests (Schopler and Loftin, 1969; Liem, 1974; Hirsch and Leff, 1975) the aetiologic significance of parental communication deviance or other characteristics identifiable in the Rorschach response would be enhanced. This could be accomplished by applying the design of Waring and Ricks to adopted children or by utilizing the strategy of Kinney and Jacobsen to control the effects of having reared a schizophrenic individual.

The ability of Harlow and his collaborators to produce extremes of autistic and bizarre behaviour in monkeys by complete maternal and peer deprivation may indicate the possibility of a causal relationship of rearing deficits to psychotic behaviour, although there is no interval in Harlow's monkeys corresponding to the period of 15 years or longer which usually precedes the onset of schizophrenia. The number of schizophrenics who have experienced so deviant a rearing milieu must be very small indeed, in fact most have not been deprived of meaningful relationship (Kohn and Clausen, 1955). While human infants exposed to severe maternal deprivation show considerable emotional impoverishment at the time, they appear to grow up quite normally (Kagan and Klein, 1973) as do Harlow's autistic monkeys if they are permitted to interact with other young monkeys (Suomi and Harlow, 1972).

Although it is difficult to believe that the deviances that have been found in the rearing parents of schizophrenics could produce in a normal child anything more than a pallid suggestion of the severe cognitive and behavioural disturbances that are seen in chronic schizophrenia, more plausible hypotheses can be developed that are based upon an interaction between a deviant parental milieu and an infant or child made vulnerable by a genetic or other constitutional deficiency (Garmezy, 1975; Watt, 1974). However, a global assessment of parent-child relationships was found to be very weakly associated with psychopathological disorders in the child (Rosenthal *et al*, 1975). The risk for schizophrenia in genetically vulnerable children, moreover, is remarkably insensitive to quite drastic extremes of rearing milieu. Heston and Denney (1968) found no significant difference in the prevalence of schizophrenia or other psychopathology between children at high genetic risk for schizophrenia reared by foster families or in foundling institutions. Higgins (1966) studied 50 young adults, all born of schizophrenic mothers, half of whom had been reared by their mothers, the other half separated from their mothers early in life and reared by agents without history of psychiatric illness. Four chronic schizophrenics were found in each group and other types of psychopathology were no higher in the group reared by their schizophrenic mothers. Individuals born of normal biological parents but reared by adoptive parents with severe psychopathology of psychosis did not show an increased risk for schizophrenia spectrum disorders (Wender *et al*, 1974).

The biological and adoptive siblings of schizophrenic adoptees offer a valuable means of examining the relative influence of genetic and rearing factors on the risk for schizophrenia. If rearing factors were significant influences, one would expect the adoptive siblings reared by the same parents to show some increase in risk, whereas the biological siblings reared in a different family should show a diminished risk. This prediction is not borne out in the two studies of which I am aware. Karlsson (1966) in his extensive study in Iceland found eight schizophrenics reared in foster families. These had 29 biological full siblings reared apart from them of which six became schizophrenic, and 28 foster siblings reared with them of whom none became schizophrenic. Our study of the national sample of adult adoptees in Denmark has identified 12 who became schizophrenic and had both biological and adoptive full siblings. Again, the biological siblings showed a high risk for schizophrenia whereas the adoptive siblings showed none.

Although there are plausible hypotheses to explain how parental influences may enhance or attenuate the expression of a genetic vulnerability, and there is no doubt that the parents of schizophrenics show a high prevalence of psychopathology and disturbance in communication, those disturbances have not yet been shown to play an aetiological role in schizophrenia.

Sociological factors

A higher prevalence of schizophrenia in the lower socio-economic classes has been a consistent finding in studies conducted in England, the Continent and North America, and several hypotheses have been developed to explain this phenomenon. Assuming that the difference is real and not an artefact of sampling or ascertainment, it could be accounted for by a greater genetic of vulnerability or of schizophrenic environmental influences or of both at the lower socio-economic levels of the population. Several recent studies in England have emphasized the important effects of social conditions and attitudes on course and rate of relapse in schizophrenia rather than on aetiology (Brown *et al*, 1972). Some have discussed the operation of particular environmental stresses known to be associated with lower social classes in conjunction with genetic vulnerability (Dohrenwend, 1975; Kohn, 1976). The factors which have been emphasized are largely psychological and pertain to role perceptions, status, value orientations, reality testing, child rearing practices, and stressful life events, but certain biological hazards associated with lower social class should also be considered. As Kohn (1968) has pointed out, the correlation between prevalence of schizophrenia and lower class status is strongest for cities of large size and not discernible in cities with a population below 100,000, where the contrasts in living conditions between social classes are not as sharp. In large cities also, as Maudsley recognized in his time and with little change in the situation since, the poor live in slums in which are found extremes of crowding, poor sanitation and diet, and inadequate medical care such as their counterparts in small cities and in the countryside do not experience. To the extent that birth injury, malnutrition and infection may play a role in the aetiology of schizophrenia, their impact would be exaggerated on the lower socio-economic class in large cities.

Several infectious diseases, especially those of viral origin, occur significantly more frequently in lower socio-economic classes (Fenner, 1971). Some of these, like cytomegalovirus, are now known to be congenitally transmitted and to lie latent in the central nervous system, eventually producing deafness or mental retardation at a rate which is considerably higher in populations of low income (Hanshaw *et al*, 1976).

Menninger (1928) cited several reports in the literature of post-influenzal psychosis and presented his own study at the Boston Psychiatric Hospital of 175 cases of acute mental disease admitted during or after the great influenza epidemic of 1918 where that infection was thought to be involved. Sixty-seven of these presented an acute syndrome which was diagnosed 'dementia praecox' by the staff. On follow-up 70 per cent had shown a good remission and 20 per cent had become chronic. In Menninger's words: 'Whatever term the nosologic categories ultimately utilized, the acute picture presented the unmistakeable schizophrenic stigmas, including intrapsychic ataxia, emotional-ideational splitting, incoherence, stereotypies, and other bizarre expressions, and were not conspicuously different from the usual types of schizophrenia.' This suggests the hypothesis that there are viral strains which show a predilection for the neural systems involved in schizophrenia and a course dependent on particular viral-host interactions. Where the response is optimal the infection and the psychosis would be short-lived; an infection which became latent or which elicited an abnormal immune response could be involved in a recurrent or chronic disorder. The types of interaction possible between virus and neuron are legion and not all need have precedents in our present knowledge of pathology (Matthysse and Matthysse, 1978). Torrey and Peterson (1976) have adduced evidence from the literature compatible with the hypothesis that some forms of schizophrenia may be of viral origin. In several studies a consistent pattern of HLA antigens in schizophrenics as a whole has not been found, which does not exclude it in a particular subgroup.

The increased prevalence of schizophrenia in lower socio-economic classes deserves more study, and it is possible that further light could be shed by twin, family or adoption studies to permit the estimation and comparison of genetic risk for schizophrenia between high and low social class or urban and rural populations. If valid estimates could thus be made, as free as possible from ascertainment and diagnostic bias, it should be possible to infer the extent to which the augmented prevalence of schizophrenia in lower class or urban populations is a reflection of genetic or environmental factors.

References

ABENSON, M. H. (1970) EEGs in chronic schizophrenia. *British Journal of Psychiatry*, **116**, 117–189.

BIRD, E. D., BARNES, J., IVERSEN, L. L., SPOKES, E. G., MACKAY, A. V. P. & SHEPHERD, M. (1977) Increased brain dopamine and reduced glutamic acid decarboxylase and choline acetyl transferase activity in schizophrenia and related psychoses. *Lancet*, *ii*, 1157–1159.

BLEULER, E. (1911) *Dementia Praecox or the Group of Schizophrenias.* Translated by H. Zinkin, 1950. New York: International Universities Press.

BÖÖK, J. A., WETTERBERG, L. & MODRZEWSKA, K. (1978) Schizophrenia in a north Swedish geographical isolate 1900–1977. *Clinical Genetics*, **14**, 373–394.

BROWN, G. W., BIRLEY, J. L. T. & WING, J. K. (1972) Influence of family life on the course of schizophrenic disorders: A replication. *British Journal of Psychiatry*, **121**, 241–258.

CARPENTER, W. T., Jr., STRAUSS, J. S. & MULEH, S. (1973) Are there pathognomonic symptoms in schizophrenia: An empiric investigation of Kurt Schneider's first-rank symptoms. *Archives of General Psychiatry*, **28**, 847–852.

DAVISON, K. & BAGLEY, C. R. (1969) Schizophrenia-like psychoses associated with organic disorders of the central nervous system: A review of the literature. In *British Journal of Psychiatry*, Special Publication No. 4: *Current Problems in Neuropsychiatry* (ed. R. N. Herrington). London: Royal College of Psychiatrists.

DOHRENWEND, B. P. (1975) Sociocultural and sociopsychological factors in the genesis of mental disorders. *Journal of Health and Social Behavior*, **16**, 365–392.

FENNER, F. (1971) Infectious disease and social change. *Medical Journal of Australia*, **2**, 1099–1102.

FISH, B. (1975) Biologic antecedents of psychosis in children. In *Biology of the Major Psychoses* (ed. D. X. Freedman). Research Publications, Association for Research in Nervous and Mental Disease, **54**, 44–83.

GARMEZY, N. (1975) The experimental study of children vulnerable to psychopathology. In *Child Personality and Psychopathology: Current Topics*. New York: Wiley.

HANSHAW, J. B., SCHEINER, A. P., MOXLEY, A. W., GAEV, L., ABEL, V. & SCHEINER, B. (1976) School failure and deafness after 'silent' congenital cytomegalovirus infection. *New England Journal of Medicine*, **295**, 468–470.

HARE, E. H., PRICE, J. S. & SLATER, E. (1974) Mental disorder and season of birth: a national sample compared with the general population. *British Journal of Psychiatry*, **124**, 81–86.

HAWK, A. B., CARPENTER, W. T., Jr. & STRAUSS, J. S. (1975) Diagnostic criteria and five-year outcome in schizophrenia. *Archives of General Psychiatry*, **32**, 343–347.

HESTON, L. L. (1966) Psychiatric disorders in foster home reared children of schizophrenic mothers. *British Journal of Psychiatry*, **112**, 819–825.

—— & DENNEY, D. (1968) Interactions between early life experience and biological factors in schizophrenia. In *The Transmission of Schizophrenia* (eds. D. Rosenthal and S. S. Kety). Oxford: Pergamon Press.

HIGGINS, J. (1966) Effect of child rearing by schizophrenic mothers. *Journal of Psychiatric Research*, **4**, 153–167.

HILL, D. (1957) The encephalogram in schizophrenia. In *Schizophrenia: Somatic Aspects* (ed. D. Richter). London: Butterworths.

HIRSCH, S. R. & LEFF, J. P. (1975) *Abnormalities in Parents of Schizophrenics*. Maudsley Monograph No. 22. London: Oxford University Press.

HOLZMAN, P. S., PROCTOR, L. R., LEVY, D. L., YASILLO, N. J., MELTZER, H. Y. & HURT, S. W. (1974) Eye-tracking dysfunctions in schizophrenic patients and their relatives. *Archives of General Psychiatry*, **31**, 143–151.

IVERSEN, L. L. & ROSE, S. P. R. (eds.) (1973) *Biochemistry and Mental Illness*. Biochemical Society Special Publication No. 1. London: Biochemical Society.

JOHNSTONE, E. C., CROW, T. J., FRITH, C. D., STEVENS, M., KREEL, L. & LE HUSTARD, J. (1978) The dementia of dementia praecox. *Acta Psychiatrica Scandinavica*, **57**, 305–324.

KAGAN, J. & KLEIN, R. E. (1973) Cross-cultural perspectives on early development. *American Psychologist*, **28**, 947–961.

KARLSSON, J. L. (1966) *The Biologic Basis of Schizophrenia*. Springfield, Ill.: C. C. Thomas.

KENNARD, M. A. & LEVY, S. (1952) The meaning of the abnormal encephalogram in schizophrenia. *Journal of Nervous and Mental Disease*, **116**, 413–418.

KETY, S. S. (1959) Biochemical theories of schizophrenia. *Science*, **129**, 1528–1532; 1590–1596.

—— (1972) Toward hypotheses for a biochemical component in the vulnerability to schizophrenia. *Seminars in Psychiatry*, **4**, 233–238.

—— ROSENTHAL, D., WENDER, P. H. & SCHULSINGER, F. (1968) The types and prevalence of mental illness in the biological and adoptive families of adopted schizophrenics. In *The Transmission of Schizophrenia* (eds. D. Rosenthal and S. S. Kety). Oxford: Pergamon Press.

—— —— —— & JACOBSEN, B. (1975) Mental illness in the biological and adoptive families of adoptive individuals who have become schizophrenic: A preliminary report based on psychiatric interviews. In *Genetic Research in Psychiatry* (eds. R. R. Fieve, D. Rosenthal and H. Brill). Baltimore: The Johns Hopkins University Press.

—— —— —— (1978) Genetic relationships within the schizophrenia spectrum: evidence from adoption studies. In *Critical Issues in Psychiatric Diagnoses* (eds. R. L. Spitzer and D. F. Klein). New York: Raven Press.

KINNEY, D. K. & JACOBSEN, B. (1978) Environmental factors in schizophrenia: new adoption study evidence and its implications for genetic and environmental research. In *The Nature of Schizophrenia* (eds. L. C. Wynne, R. L. Cromwell and S. Matthysse). New York: Wiley.

—— & MATTHYSSE, S. (1978) Genetic transmission of schizophrenia. *Annual Reviews of Medicine*, **29,** 454–473.

KNAPP, P. C. (1908) Confusional insanity and dementia praecox. *Journal of Nervous and Mental Disease*, **35,** 609–614.

KOEHLER, K., GUTH, W. & GRIMM, G. (1977) First rank symptoms of schizophrenia in Schneider-oriented German centres. *Archives of General Psychiatry*, **34,** 810–813.

KOHN, M. L. (1968) Social class and schizophrenia: a critical review. In *The Transmission of Schizophrenia* (eds. D. Rosenthal and S. S. Kety). Oxford: Pergamon Press.

—— (1976) The interaction of social class and other factors in the etiology of schizophrenia. *American Journal of Psychiatry*, **133,** 177–180.

—— & CLAUSEN, J. A. (1955) Social isolation and schizophrenia. *American Sociological Review*, **20,** 265–273.

KRAEPELIN, E. (1913) *Dementia Praecox and Paraphrenia*. Translated by R. M. Barclay from the 8th German Edition of the 'Text-book of Psychiatry. Vol. III part 2, on Endogenous Dementias', 1919. Edinburgh: E. & S. Livingstone.

LANGFELDT, G. (1939) *The Schizophreniform States*. Copenhagen: Munksgaard.

LIEM, J. H. (1974) Effects of verbal communications of parents and children: a comparison of normal and schizophrenic families. *Journal of Consulting Clinical Psychology*, **42,** 438–450.

MATTHYSSE, A. G. & MATTHYSSE, S. (1978) Bacteriophage models of neurotopic virus specificity. In *Neurochemical and Immunologic Components in Schizophrenia* (eds. D. Bergma and A. L. Goldstein). New York: A. R. Liss.

MATTHYSSE, S. (1978) Etiological diversity in the psychoses. In *Genetic Epidemiology* (eds. C. S. Chung and N. E. Morton). New York: Academic Press.

—— & POPE, A. (1975) The approach to schizophrenia through molecular pathology. In *Molecular Pathology* (eds. R. A. Good, S. D. Day and J. J. Yunis). New York: C. C. Thomas.

MAUDSLEY, H. (1872) *The Physiology and Pathology of Mind*. New York: Appleton & Co.

McNEIL, T. F. & KAIJ, L. (1978) Obstetric factors in the development of schizophrenia: Complications in the births of preschizophrenics and in reproduction by schizophrenic parents. In *The Nature of Schizophrenia* (eds. L. C. Wynne, R. L. Cromwell and S. Matthysse). New York: Wiley & Sons.

MEDICAL RESEARCH COUNCIL (1970) *Biochemical Research in Psychiatry: Survey and Proposals*. London: H.M. Stationery Office.

MELLOR, C. S. (1970) First rank symptoms of schizophrenia. *British Journal of Psychiatry*, **117,** 15–23.

MENNINGER, K. (1928) The schizophrenic syndrome as a product of acute infectious disease. *Archives of Neurology and Psychiatry*, **20,** 464–481.

MITSUDA, H. (1965) The concept of 'atypical psychoses' from the aspect of clinical genetics. *Acta Psychiatrica Scandinavica*, **41,** 372–377.

MORTON, L. A., KIDD, K. K., MATTHYSSE, S. & RICHARDS, R. (1979) Recurrence risks in schizophrenia: Are they model dependent? *Behavior Genetics*, **9,** 389–406.

MOSHER, L. R., POLLIN, W. & STABENAU, J. R. (1971) Identical twins discordant for schizophrenia: Neurologic findings. *Archives of General Psychiatry*, **24,** 422–430.

NAUTA, W. J. H., SMITH, G. P., FAULL, R. L. M. & DOMESICK, V. B. (1978) Efferent connections and nigral afferents of the nucleus accumbens septi in the rat. *Neuroscience*, **3,** 385–401.

POPE, H. & LIPINSKI, J. (1978) Differential diagnosis of schizophrenic and manic-depressive illness. *Archives of General Psychiatry*, **35,** 811–836.

RICHTER, D. (1976) The impact of biochemistry on the problem of schizophrenia. In *Schizophrenia Today* (eds. D. Kemali, G. Bartholini and D. Richter). Oxford: Pergamon Press.

RIEDER, R. O., DONNELLY, E. F., HERDT, J. R. & WALDMAN, I. N. (1979) Sulcal prominence in young chronic schizophrenic patients: CT scan findings associated with impairment on neuropsychological tests. *Psychiatry Research*, **1,** 1–9.

ROBERTS, E. (1972) An hypothesis suggesting that there is a defect in the GABA system in schizophrenia. In *Prospects for Research on Schizophrenia* (eds. S. S. Kety and S. Matthysse). *Neurosciences Research Program Bulletin*, **10** (4), 468–482.

ROCHFORD, J., DETRE, T., TUCKER, G. J. & HARROW, M. (1970) Neuropsychological impairments in functional psychiatric disease. *Archives of General Psychiatry*, **22**, 114–119.

ROSENTHAL, D.. WENDER, P. H., KETY, S. S., SCHULSINGER, F., WELNER, J. & ØSTERGAARD, L. (1968) Schizophrenics' offspring reared in adoptive homes. In *The Transmission of Schizophrenia* (eds. D. Rosenthal and S. S. Kety). Oxford: Pergamon Press.

—— —— —— —— & RIEDER, R. O. (1975) Parent-child relationships and psychopathologic disorder in the child. *Archives of General Psychiatry*, **32**, 466–476.

SCHNEIDER, K. (1959) *Clinical Psychopathology*. Translated by M. W. Hamilton. New York: Grune & Stratton.

SCHOPLER, E. & LOFTIN, J. (1969) Thought disorders in parents of psychotic children. *Archives of General Psychiatry*, **20**, 174–181.

SHIELDS, J., HESTON, L. L. & GOTTESMAN, I. I. (1975) Schizophrenia and the schizoid: The problem for genetic analysis. In *Genetic Research in Psychiatry* (eds. R. R. Fieve, D. Rosenthal and H. Brill). Baltimore: Johns Hopkins University Press.

SLATER, E. (1958) The monogenic theory of schizophrenia. *Acta Genetica et Statistica Medica*, **8**, 50–56.

SPITZER, R. L., ENDICOTT, J. & GIBBON, M. (1979) Crossing the border into borderline personality and borderline schizophrenia: The development of criteria. *Archives of General Psychiatry*, **36**, 17–24.

STEVENS, J. R. (1973) An anatomy of schizophrenia? *Archives of General Psychiatry*, **29**, 177–189.

STRÖMGREN, E. (1965) Schizophreniform psychoses. *Acta Psychiatrica Scandinavica*, **41**, 483–489.

SUOMI, S. J. & HARLOW, H. F. (1972) Social rehabilitation of isolate reared monkeys. *Developmental Psychology*, **6**, 487–496.

THUDICHUM (1884) *A Treatise on the Chemical Constitution of the Brain*. London: Ballière, Tindall & Cox.

TORREY, E. F. & PETERSON, M. R. (1976) The viral hypothesis of schizophrenia. *Schizophrenia Bulletin*, **2**, 136–146.

TSUANG, M. T., DEMPSEY, G. M. & RAUSCHER, F. (1976) A study of 'atypical schizophrenia'. *Archives of General Psychiatry*, **33**, 1157–1160.

TUCKER, G. J., CAMPION, E. W. & SILBERFARB, P. M. (1975) Sensorimotor functions and cognitive disturbance in psychiatric patients. *American Journal of Psychiatry*, **132**, 17–21.

VAILLANT, G. E. (1978) A 10-year follow-up of remitting schizophrenics. *Schizophrenia Bulletin*, **4**, 78–85.

WARING, M. & RICKS, D. F. (1965) Family patterns of children who become adult schizophrenics. *Journal of Nervous and Mental Disease*, **140**, 351–364.

WATT, N. F. (1974) Childhood and adolescent routes to schizophrenia. In *Life History Research in Psychopathology*, vol. 3 (eds. D. R. Ricks, A. Thomas and M. Roff). Minneapolis: University of Minnesota Press.

WEINBERGER, D. R., TORREY, E. F., NEOPHYTIDES, A. N. & WYATT, R. J. (1979) Lateral cerebral ventricular enlargement in chronic schizophrenia. *Archives of General Psychiatry*, **36**, 735–739.

WELNER, J. & STRÖMGREN, E. (1958) Clinical and genetic studies on benign schizophreniform psychoses based on a follow-up. *Acta Psychiatrica et Scandinavica*, **33**, 377–399.

WENDER, P. H., ROSENTHAL, D. & KETY, S. S. (1968) A psychiatric assessment of the adoptive parents of schizophrenics. In *The Transmission of Schizophrenia* (eds. D. Rosenthal and S. S. Kety). Oxford: Pergamon Press.

—— —— SCHULSINGER, F. & WELNER, J. (1974) Cross-fostering: A research strategy for clarifying the role of genetic and experiential factors in the etiology of schizophrenia. *Archives of General Psychiatry*, **30**, 121–128.

—— —— RAINER, J. D., GREENHILL, L. & SARLIN, B. (1977) Schizophrenics' adopting parents: Psychiatric status. *Archives of General Psychiatry*, **34**, 777–784.

WYNNE, L. C., SINGER, M. T. & TOOHEY, M. L. (1976) In *Schizophrenia 75: Psychotherapy, Family Studies, Research* (eds. J. Jorstad and E. Ugelstad). University of Oslo Press.

4 The concept of schizophrenia: Kraepelin–Bleuler–Schneider

J. HOENIG

In 1978 in the 52nd Maudsley Lecture, **Seymour S. Kety** (**1980**) made the following statement:

Schneider, 50 years later (1959), [after Bleuler] gave renewed support to those who preferred to think of schizophrenia as a benign process by simply redefining schizophrenia to make it so. Features regarded by both Kraepelin and Bleuler as fundamental and characteristic (impoverishment of affect, disturbances in personal contact and rapport, ambivalence, lack of motivation, depersonalisation, and stereotypes) were specifically rejected and the new criteria were restricted to particular types of hallucinations and delusions which Bleuler had regarded as accessory symptoms. Schneider established a new syndrome with features that are more easily perceived and described, and which therefore show a higher degree of inter-rater reliability, features which are economically put into check lists and fed into computers. That syndrome may be more prevalent, have a more favorable outcome, and be more responsive to a wide variety of treatments, but it is not schizophrenia.

Kety here sketches a section of the history of the concept of schizophrenia. The history of psychiatry is not always a popular subject. It belongs, so it is held, to the fringe of our discipline, and is too remote from the field of action, the clinic, the courtroom or the research work to warrant much attention. It is best left to the older psychiatrist, or the egghead blowing the dust off old books in secluded corners of libraries. But Seymour Kety is a very active researcher, as eminent as he is practical. And yet it appears that his concern with history is a necessity arising directly out of his practical research work. What do we call schizophrenia? What are the diagnostic criteria? And as the answers to these questions proffered by various authorities are by no means all the same it becomes necessary to go to the roots of these views in the history of the subject. Kety asks: what exactly was Kraepelin's concept of schizophrenia (or dementia praecox as he first called it); how does it differ from Bleuler's and how are Kraepelin's and Bleuler's views different from Schneider's. Clarity demands that we say exactly what we ourselves mean when we say 'schizophrenia'.

Emil Kraepelin 1856–1926

When Kraepelin began his work there was already a voluminous psychiatric literature. Kraepelin (1962) surveyed this field which included German and Austrian, French, Italian, English and Russian authors, in a little book called

100 years of Psychiatry. In the 4th edition of his textbook in 1893, dementia praecox first appeared as an entity under the heading of 'Psychic Degenerative Processes'. In later editions dementia praecox begins to appear as an entity of its own. Jaspers (1959, 1963), in the historical section of *General Psychopathology*, describes Kraepelin's place in the history of psychiatry as follows:

Half a century ago Emminghaus had given a comprehensive and conciliatory up to date summary of the observed facts and views presented by the several psychiatric schools ... The new ideas started from Wernicke and from Kraepelin. When they appeared the traditional world of psychiatry closed ranks against them ... They used to say: what is new in them is wrong, and what is right is not new. The productive achievement which consisted in seeing what was already known from fresh points of view in greater depth and more coherently, was seen as a reshuffling of already established knowledge. But subsequent developments have reversed this situation. The old is passed on only in as far as it was taken over by Wernicke and by Kraepelin ... Kraepelin's textbook has become the most widely read of all psychiatric books. These concepts have for the first time created a common ground for psychiatric thought. [p. 710].

What precisely was Kraepelin's creative contribution to dementia praecox? Kraepelin deprecated the widespread overvaluation of auxiliary disciplines like anatomy, physiology, etc. and the neglect of the straight forward clinical psychiatric approach. He saw the central task of psychiatry, 'analogous to our experience in general medicine', to be an open-minded detailed study and unrelenting follow through of individual cases of illness, which after separating out the accidental and unessential will lead us to a practical delineation of particular disease forms. Having failed to establish such disease entities on purely anatomical, purely aetiological or purely symptomatological criteria he nevertheless expressed his firm belief in the interdependence of these criteria.

If we had in our possession an exhaustive knowledge of every single detail in any of these three areas, it would not only be possible to come to a comprehensive and fundamental classification of the psychoses with any one of them as the starting point, but each of these three classifications—and this is the fundamental task of our scientific endeavour—would largely coincide with the other two. [In his text book, 2nd edition 1887].

To this basic idea he added later two more 'areas', namely course and treatment response. Jaspers (1959, 1963) characterizes this work as follows.

Kraepelin has taken Kahlbaum's idea of disease entities and defended it with uncommon vigor, and for a time has achieved general recognition for it. One of the most fruitful research approaches, namely the study of the entire life history of psychiatric patients, was founded by him ... Kraepelin's basic orientation remained somatic, which together with the majority of physicians he held to be the only one appropriate to medicine; not only the preferred one but absolutely the only one. [p. 711].

Kraepelin was guided by the idea of dementia praecox as a disease entity, which if 'every detail' were known would turn out to have a specific anatomical pathology, with a specific aetiology, but we are hardly any nearer to its discovery than he was. How far did he succeed in his characterization of the clinical picture, and in determining the exact circumference of the illness, i.e. the means of deciding if a particular case falls within its boundaries? This is after all Kety's concern in the paper quoted above. Kraepelin (1909–13) emphasizes the great variability of the clinical picture, but says:

Everywhere the same basic disturbances recur again and again, the loss of the inner unity of thought, feeling and acting, the blunting of higher feelings, the manifold and peculiar disorders of the will with their associated delusions of the loss of psychic freedom and of influences, finally the disintegration of the personality while the acquired knowledge and the simple skills remain relatively undamaged. To be sure not all of these characteristics can be clearly demonstrated in each and every case. Nevertheless the survey of a large number of complete observations teaches us that we never find a picture which does not show a link by very gradual transitions with all the others. [Vol. II, p. 943].

Unfortunately in the field of psychic disturbances there is not a single symptom which is pathognomonic for any particular illness. On the other hand we can expect that the composition of the individual characteristics which form the total picture, and in particular the changes which develop in the course of the illness, will not be produced in exactly the same way by any of the other diseases; [Vol. II, p. 945].

Nowhere do we find any precise demarcation of the illness but are always referred to the overall picture. Thus Gruhle (1932) notices the 'methodologically unique state of affairs' that Kraepelin had created the disease entity of dementia praecox without being able to name a single unequivocal symptom of it.

The least defined border is in the area of dementia simplex, a concept introduced by Diem, and later made much of by Bleuler, and even more so in the area of Bleuler's 'latent schizophrenia'. Kraepelin (1909–13) always had difficulties accepting the latter concept. 'This interpretation of morbid states which consist of fearfulness and lack of self confidence (as belonging to schizophrenia) will for the vast majority have to be rejected.' (Vol. II, p. 947).

As regards the outcome of the illness, Kraepelin has often been misunderstood. In general the illness is thought to be irreversible and to lead to a state of general deterioration. However, the course was found to show great variability in the speed of the decline, its extent, its consistency, i.e. the frequency, extent and quality of remissions, etc. Out of 127 cases he found 16 (12.5 per cent) where 'it was unreservedly stated, that the patients were fully recovered' (Vol. II, p. 865). This did not lead Kraepelin to revise the diagnosis.

All this was achieved to a large extent already in 1893 in the 4th edition of the text book. Kraepelin himself evolved and changed his work with every new edition of his textbook, dealing with all the new contributions, sometimes incorporating or modifying them, sometimes rejecting them. Kolle (1957) by bringing together the tables of content of all the eight editions has clearly shown these changes and unremitting efforts of their author.

What were the main edges of further growth? We turn to Mayer-Gross (1929) for an answer. In a lecture on 'The Development of Kraepelin's Clinical Views' he describes the enormous achievement of Kraepelin, but also examines its limits.

We wish to know without any preconceptions, 'phenomenologically'—as Pick and Jaspers called it—exactly what the elements are which make up the actual individual symptom and its diagnostically characteristic background which provides the context of its manifestation; . . . we no longer regard all the unusual features the patient presents as a direct expression of the illness itself . . . The studies of these features lead us to the psychological field in the narrower sense; which has found its way into the medicine of our day through Freud, the field called by Jaspers 'the psychology of meaning'. We have already seen how little in that area struck Kraepelin as being worthy of systematic study, not just because he was estranged by Freud's controversial methods, but because he was lacking a sense for this entire area of psychopathology, what L. Binswanger called 'the inner life history'.

Jaspers (1959) had earlier noticed this lack when he wrote: 'The sometimes excellent psychological passages in his (Kraepelin's) textbook succeeded as it were against his intention: he considers them temporary stopgaps until experiment, microscope or test tube will have made everything accessible to objective investigation' (p. 711).

What was felt to be lacking in Kraepelin's description of the clinical picture was 'the psyche'. The symptoms were symptoms of the underlying disease process. The patient's life history, his premorbid personality, even his own experience of the illness had no assigned place in the scheme of things. They were an irrelevancy.

Eugen Bleuler 1857–1939

One of the first to try to retrieve the 'psyche' in dementia praecox was Bleuler and his young assistant, C. G. Jung. Freud in his own work had not tackled dementia praecox, but his psychology of the neuroses influenced all these endeavours by others, particularly those by Jung and by Bleuler.

In the introduction to his monograph *Dementia Praecox or the Group of Schizophrenias*, Bleuler (1911, 1950) stresses what his work has in common with that of Kraepelin.

The whole idea of dementia praecox originates with Kraepelin; also the grouping and description of the individual symptoms we also owe almost entirely to him [p. vii] ... Kraepelin's concept however continues to be opposed by many, who because of the wide diversity of the clinical pictures, cannot accept it as a single entity, which originally appeared to be based on the uniform course of the illness, and yet could include cases with a good as well as a bad outcome [p. i] ... The circumference of the concept of dementia praecox has (since Kraepelin's final version) remained essentially the same [p. 4] ... with the term dementia praecox or schizophrenia we designate a group of psychoses whose course can at times be chronic, at times run in intermittent thrusts, and which can become arrested at any stage or show improvement, but will probably not permit full *restitutio ad integrum* [p. 6].

One almost gets the impression that the only noticeable intention with the monograph was to replace the name dementia praecox by that of schizophrenia, and that mostly for grammatical reasons: 'The name (dementia praecox) can only be used to refer to the illness not the patient, and it does not permit the formation of an adjective which could characterize the properties of the illness' (p. 4). He complains that many critics of Kraepelin have dismissed the entire concept of dementia praecox on semantic objections alone.

The worst situation in that regard exists in England where as far as I am aware the majority of psychiatrists simply cling to be word while remaining completely ignorant of the concept or disregarding it ... I call dementia praecox schizophrenia because I hope to show that the split of the several psychic functions is one of its most important characteristics [p. 5].

Bleuler also states, however, that he is going beyond Kraepelin and tries to extend the psychopathology by applying the ideas of Freud. His ideas were clearly expressed in a paper co-signed with Jung (Bleuler and Jung, 1908). The paper has two sections, each by one of the authors, indicating that they shared certain views, but not all. Bleuler explains his new views:

We differentiate sharply between the physical illness and its symptoms, the latter in dementia praecox being almost exclusively psychic ... The illness itself, the disease process, is still completely unknown. It can be an anatomical cerebral disease, or an autointoxication, or an infection, or something entirely different ... The disease itself, even when far advanced, need not produce any of the symptoms commonly considered as typical. The most prominent symptoms of dementia praecox like delusions, thought blocking, hallucinations of words, sentences and figures, negativism, can surely never correspond to cerebral processes in the way diffuse manifestations could, like general thought inhibition (*Denkhemmung*), general—as yet unidentified—disorders of the intellectual elementary functions, melancholic and manic dysphorias, subjective noise or light manifestations. The earlier class of symptoms, which as we know appear most frequently, must be determined by an additional—psychic—cause. If such a cause is in abeyance, the illness though really existing, will simply remain latent. It will become manifest when amongst other things an affect-laden complex begins to be activated. In the abnormally functioning psyche the affects have more far reaching impacts than in the normal psyche (although basically they are not different). In this way, as Jung has demonstrated, most or possibly all the known psychic symptoms come about. The complex thus is not the cause of the illness, but the cause of its symptoms or of their manifestation.

It is important that we postulate the existence of *primary* psychic symptoms, even though we do not know exactly what they are, and that the symptomatology of dementia praecox so far described consists to a large extent of secondary symptoms, which are brought about by the reaction of the sick psyche to the complexes (i.e. the affects). We thus differentiate not only between the disease process and its symptoms, but amongst the latter between primary, directly caused by the disease process, and secondary symptoms brought about by certain psychic mechanisms.

Bleuler goes further than simply giving an explanation of the content of these secondary symptoms, but explains their entire existence as a product of the complexes: 'If a woman hallucinates that she is pregnant, the complex causes not only the content of the hallucinations (that she is pregnant) but also that the patient actually has an hallucination.'

Jung, in his section, takes this beyond where even Bleuler dared to venture. He says:

An affect, just as any psychic cause, can set in motion the organic process of dementia praecox (by forming a toxin?) analogous to the manifestation of tuberculosis in a contused joint. If there were no complex the actual illness would not come about at that point in time, not on that location and not in that particular way. In such cases, therefore, the complex would have significance not merely for the determination of the content, but for the origin of the organic disease process itself.

Jaspers welcomes the reintroduction of 'the psyche' into the concept of schizophrenia—'At last there is psychological thinking'. Kraepelin (1913) himself acknowledges that Bleuler's schizophrenia includes all the forms originally described by him. However, he totally rejects the views about the complexes.

Jung moves closely to the toxin theory by pointing to the possibility that an emotional upheaval could produce a 'toxin', which would then bring about the disease. (The toxin can also at times arise spontaneously). In that case however it would be really difficult to understand why the manic-depressive patients with their stormy affective upsets, would not produce these harmful toxins which lead to deterioration in much greater quantitities. [Vol. III, p. 937].

Bleuler's distinction into primary and secondary symptoms he considers 'purely contrived'. He does concede the differentiation into basic and accessary symptoms. However, he understands these terms to mean obligatory and facultative, thus giving them a different meaning from Bleuler:

The former are the real characteristics of the clinical picture and can be demonstrated more or less clearly in every case; the latter may, but need not, be present; they are not brought about by what is essential in the disease process but by circumstances which are only loosely associated with it. [Vol. III, p. 936].

He has certain reservations about Bleuler's symptom classification:

Bleuler includes 'ambivalence' and 'autism' among the basic symptoms without, I feel full justification, as there are endstates of dementia praecox which do not show these symptoms, whereas the others are present. [Vol. III, p. 936].

Bleuler considers the accessory symptoms to be psychogenically determined by the complexes, but Kraepelin accepts none of this.

It is clear also to Bleuler that the obligatory symptoms are not very helpful when it comes to diagnosis in an individual case, particularly when there is no time for prolonged observation stretching over years to reveal in time the steady characteristic deterioration. Bleuler had never intended to create a new diagnostic approach—he was quite satisfied in that respect with Kraepelin's work—but he presented a new theory of the disease.

All the same, Bleuler's (1911) attempt had diagnostic consequences of considerable magnitude:

... in schizophrenia, ... there are a number of symptoms which fall within the wide frame of what one calls, if not exactly 'healthy', nevertheless not 'mentally ill'. Personality anomalies, indifference, anergia, querulousness, obstinancy, moodiness, and what Goethe could describe only with the English *whimsicality*, hypochondriasis, etc. need not be symptoms of a mental disease; but only too often they are the only visible signs of schizophrenia. Because of this, the diagnostic threshold is in no other illness as low, and the latent cases so common. [p. 239].

To base the diagnosis on such non-specific symptoms all of which lie on the borderline of normality, eccentricity, or personality variants, and not on easily identifiable symptoms like hallucinations, delusions, passivity experiences, etc. because the latter may not be found in every case at all times is like diagnosing idiopathic epilepsy not on the recognition of seizures but on interictal abnormalities, which would be equally difficult to recognize clearly or have the same lack of specificity.

Kraepelin agrees that among the personality disorders there may be a group of not fully developed cases of schizophrenia: 'But for the vast majority of such disorders which present with anxiety and a lack of self-confidence, such an interpretation must be rejected' (Vol. III, p. 947).

Bleuler's over-extension of the diagnosis into that group of patients, however, gained influence, particularly in Switzerland. Wyrsch (1966), a former student of Bleuler, gives an account of the extent of this usage and of its medico-legal consequences.

Around 1920 and even during the subsequent decade, we in Switzerland had a rather wide concept of schizophrenia, much wider than Kraepelin in Germany, where I understand people mocked that Bleuler just shakes schizophrenia out of his sleeve ... Bleuler never held the view like Freud and some of his followers that schizophrenia was only a special kind of a neurosis, an 'introversion neurosis', as in those days it was wont to be called. Something else carried a larger blame: we believed we could glean the diagnosis before manifest unequivocal psychic symptoms were there, and when we thought we found the poor rapport, the often misunderstood autism and the ununderstandable behavior in life, we spoke then of simple or, rather more cautiously, of latent schizophrenia ... When certain delinquents in our large cities—mostly youths around 20 years, usually with minor but repeated thefts, break-ins, frauds—stood arraigned in court, and were referred for assessment to our university clinics, the assessor often concluded that there was a latent schizophrenia, and that the accused was mentally incompetent. Consequently, he was committed to the mental hospital in his home Canton.

He then describes in a charming and witty way how as they got to know those youngsters better, the diagnosis at first was often qualified with a question mark, and later was dropped altogether and replaced by 'personality disorder'. All this led amongst Swiss psychiatrists to a soul-searching reappraisal of the entire concept of schizophrenia.

At a congress in Basel in 1929 the south-west German psychiatrists with their speaker Mayer-Gross on the one side, and the Swiss psychiatrists with their leader Eugen Bleuler on the other, gave each other a two-day battle which however ended undecided, as is proper for such struggles because scientific congresses are of course not parliamentary sessions or church councils.

The academic discussion of these issues continued for a time in the literature, and various names for all those marginal cases were invented such as symptomatic schizophrenia, schizoid-psychosis, schizophreniform, etc., 'until genetic research with its disastrous law of 1933 made it advisable to drop the word schizophrenia in such cases altogether, which I hasten to add was done not just for that reason, but for the sake of keeping the disease concept pure.'

The law had been introduced by the new German Reich and stipulated compulsory sterilization of all cases of schizophrenia as well as other hereditary mental illnesses. Gaupp (1939) in an oration, like Wyrsch, also refers to the notorious German law of 1933, but unlike Wyrsch, welcomes it, and calls for a precise diagnosis on Kraepelian lines, the better to serve its intent.

Bleuler's did not remain the only attempt to introduce psychic aspects into the understanding of the illness. One of the best known attempts is that by Kretschmer (1967) who laid great stress on the premorbid, constitutionally determined, personality and its influence on the clinical picture of the illness, and in his 'sensitive delusions of reference' had attempted actually to show a psychogenic development from personality to psychosis.

Bleuler's colleague from the Burghölzli hospital, Adolf Meyer (1948) (they were both assistants of August Forel), attempted to show schizophrenia to be altogether the result of a faulty habit formation. Less radical attempts were made in Scandinavia where the concept of 'psychogenic psychosis' is still used and treasured as a national heritage (Faergeman, 1963; Strömgren, 1974).

Even among Kraepelin's closest circle such moves were made. Gaupp (1920) tried to separate paranoia from dementia praecox by showing in the case of the schoolmaster Wagner, a psychogenic development leading from a characterological disposition via closely linked experiences to a delusional system without deterioration.

Later came other attempts by using philosophical ideas of the existential schools to understand psychologically much of the clinical picture of schizophrenia, such as that by Zutt (1956), Binswanger (1957) or Blankenburg (1958), or by using sociological and anthropological ideas which were more common in the United States.

No matter how diverse the attempt, Kraepelin's influence is still recognizable in all of them. Schneider (1956), at the centenary celebration of Kraepelin's birthday, puts it as follows:

We have to make it clear that in our descriptive psychopathology, Kraepelin's (diagnostic) forms of illness are still valid. This also applies to Kretschmer ... He extends Kraepelin's two endogenous forms to a universal anthropology ... Nothing of all that has become established. Kleist too tried in vain to shake off Kraepelin's shackles ... Even closer to Kraepelin is Leonhard with some 10 categories ... What is important is: here too Kraepelin's forms are the fundament ... The epoch of Kraepelin is far from over.

Kurt Schneider 1887–1967

Schneider, who at the end of World War II was appointed to the Chair of Psychiatry at the University of Heidelberg, continued the scientific tradition of a group of workers under Nissl who had developed a new *Forschungsrichtung*, a research approach. That group had included Gruhle, Wilmanns, Homburger, Ranke, Mayer-Gross and Jaspers. Their overriding concern here, as in Zurich, was to overcome the limitations of the Kraepelinian exclusively somatic psychiatry. Jaspers (1967a; b) writes:

Freud's influence was limited to small circles. Psychological approaches were regarded to be subjective and futile, not scientific. ... The cause for the confusion appeared to lie in the nature of the subject itself. The subject of psychiatry was man, not just his body; his body even least of all, but rather his psyche, his personality, man himself.

In that situation in 1911 I was invited by Wilmanns and the publisher Ferdinand Springer to write a general psychopathology ... I was alarmed but gripped by the spirit and exuberance of the enterprise, and so I decided to try at least to bring some order into the existing factual knowledge, and to foster as much as I could methodological awareness.

The *General Psychopathology* (Jaspers, 1963) appeared in 1913 and grew in subsequent years in size and depth until the final years of the war. Subsequent editions remained unchanged. The basic ideas however had already been presented in a number of earlier papers; the ideas in relation to schizophrenia in a paper on *Eifersuchtswahn* (delusion of jealousy) (Jaspers, 1910). The task in hand for the *General Psychopathology* appeared to be one of methodological aspects of psychiatric studies. Kräupl Taylor (1967) has succinctly summarized the essence of these efforts and described their historical context. Let us hear Jaspers (1910) himself:

For the study of psychic life we have two approaches available; we either put ourselves in the other person's place, empathise with him, 'understand' him, or we observe particular elements or phenomena (which as they too are psychological in nature, are therefore also seen 'from the inside' as it were) in their context and their sequence as something given, without 'understanding' them by empathy with the other person. Here we only 'comprehend', as we comprehend the contexts of the physical world, by presupposing an underlying objective process, be that a 'physical' or an 'unconscious' one, the nature of which does not permit empathy ... The first approach will lead us to the concept of personality development, the latter to that of the process.

Having described several cases with delusions of jealousy, he applies these methods in his analysis of their histories and mental state:

It thus would seem that in the delusions of jealousy the criteria of the 'personality development' and those of a 'process' are mixed together, with a preponderance of the latter. This need not really surprise us. We have seen that in life every development is a process in which empathically understandable and rational connections are as it were embedded. The 'process' however of normal life can be conceived as a 'development' in so far as one sees in it intuitively the total of the personality. We have seen the extreme subjectivity of that intuition, and have to concede that there is room for transitions between the 'new' which appears at certain stages of life as part of the total personality, and the 'new' which contrasts to it as something heterogeneous. Therefore we find gradual transitions between the psychic effects of processes and psychological developments, corresponding to the fact that in the field of psychology sharp lines of demarcation as they are certainly possible in certain areas of physical processes are impossible to draw. (This is the reason for ever recurring revivals of the theory of the unitary psychosis).

Jaspers thus skirts the dilemma of *a priori* deciding which features of a clinical picture are 'process determined' and which belong to the psychogenic super-structure—a decision which cannot be made empirically, and which still fails to see the patient as a whole—by showing how any given aspect of the clinical picture can be studied by several differing methods. Each method has its specific working rules and produces its own kind of knowledge. The knowledge obtained by objective scientific methods is of a different order from that obtained by subjective empathic methods. It is not permissible to take the one for the other. This methodological error, i.e. of mistaking meaning in the symptoms for objective, as it were neurophysiological events, flaws in Jasper's view some of the work of Freud. Jaspers (1913, 1974) explains:

Connections by meaning are something entirely different from causal connections. For example we *understand* or see meaning in motivated behavior; a movement brought about by nerve stimulation, on the other hand, we *explain* causally. We 'understand' how affects arise out of certain moods, out of moods certain hopes, phantasies and fears; but the presence or loss of memory performance, of fatigue, recovery etc. we 'explain' ... In research on humans the analysis of meaningful and of causal connections subtly interact in a complex way but with methodological reflection can be clearly distinguished and disentangled.

Methodological reflection also shows that in our present nosology the psychoses are psychological entities. The assumption that the psychosyndromes form a unity with a somatic disease was a postulate, a hope still unfulfilled. The new psychiatry was facing this fact squarely, and also the need to explore the patient psychologically, that is, apperceive him as a person with motives, aims, reflections, feelings—feelings also about the illness.

Bleuler had done a great deal already in that latter respect and had drawn practical conclusions, such as recommending early discharge from hospital to restore the patient to his normal environment. Because however of the deficiencies in methodological clarity, Bleuler's diagnostic approach brought about an enormous expansion of the concept of the illness.

Schneider (1925) did more than anyone else to apply these new approaches to the bedside diagnosis of the endogenous psychoses. He did not abandon the Kraepelinian landmarks, nor the Kraepelinian postulate of a somatosis; he did however underline the fact that since we do not know the somatosis, we must accept these clinical entities for what they are, namely psychopathological syndromes.

In the rich variety of the possible clinical pictures schizophrenia and cyclothymia are types. This introduces a greater relativity into the classification of the endogenous psychoses. In this way the question of 'right or wrong diagnosis' loses in severity, the arguments between schools their sharpness; it no longer makes sense to fight e.g. over such questions of whether involutional melancholia 'belongs' to the manic-depressive illness or not, but only whether it would be more practical to count it in, or more expedient not to do so. The same applies to the relationship between schizophrenia and dementia paranoides, the paraphrenias, the presenile delusions of encroachment (*Beeinträchtigung*) described by Kraepelin, the involutional paranoia of Kleist, or the sensitive delusions of reference by Kretschmer ... By and large I feel the use of such new creations to be preferable to a gradual return to a unitary psychosis ...

As regards the final biological 'right or wrongness' of such separations or fusions of various psychotic pictures (that) will one day, so we hope, be decided by somatic research ... Thus unless one wishes to abandon clinical psychiatry altogether, the task of finding psychological groupings will persist. This however is a classification by useful types: Clinical psychiatry is a pragmatic science.

Schneider was equally undogmatic about the way schizophrenia should be defined, whether by the unrelenting course to final dementia or by the symptoms in cross section. Here he entirely follows Jaspers (1959):

The causes of manic-depressive illness and dementia praecox are entirely unknown. Their definition is guided sometimes more by their essential psychological form and sometimes more by their course (recoverable or not) depending on a change in emphasis. If the first aspect is placed into the foreground (Bleuler) the group of schizophrenias becomes vastly over-extended, which is refuted by the other side which for its own part puts more weight on the course of the illness (recovery with insight or not) which in turn unduly narrows the illness (Willmanns); ... In this way the border between manic-depressive illness and dementia praecox shifts widely to and fro, and has done so for many years, like a pendulum, without achieving in the various definitions any kind of advance.

Schneider (1925), the clinician, goes on:

We shall use both; as the course itself consists of a sequence and developments of clinical states, their description will always have to precede the former. From this follows unavoidably the task so important for clinical and social psychiatry, to search them for symptoms, which from experience will permit predictions regarding the future course and outcome. This will after all be the question asked of us.

Methodologically this obliges us to be precise in our description of the symptoms, which are mostly abnormal inner experiences, phenomena, which must be elicited through skilled questioning from the patient himself. Schneider (1938) explains:

While psychiatrists before Jaspers often spoke a language which confused anatomical, physiological and psychological concepts one with the others ... Jaspers taught us the simple self-evident truth that psychopathology must speak the language of normal psychology. If Jasper's contribution is to be assessed ... we begin with the phenomenological investigations, descriptions derived from introspection (by the patient), a method in its own right, introduced and elaborated by Jaspers.

The paper which elaborates the 25th birthday of the *General Psychopathology* by Jaspers is remarkable in itself, appearing as it did in 1938, at a time when the German government of the day had forbidden Jaspers to teach or to publish, and testifies to the courage and integrity of Kurt Schneider.

Schneider, as did Jaspers, explicitly avoids any kind of preconception about the nature of these psychopathological symptoms, unlike Bleuler with his speculative classification into primary, i.e. process-bound, and secondary, i.e. complex-bound symptoms. As we do not know the somatosis such differentiations would be entirely hypothetical. In a paper on primary and secondary symptoms in schizophrenia, Schneider (1957, 1974) subjects these concepts, not only as found in Bleuler's work but also in Griesinger's and Birnbaum's, to a critical analysis, and he explains the difference of his own 'first' rank and 'second' rank symptom classification from the 'structural analytical' approach of the earlier workers:

These schizophrenic symptoms (divided into those of 1st or 2nd rank) are entirely devoid of any theory and are intended purely pragmatically-diagnostically. When we say for instance that thought withdrawal is a 1st rank symptom this means, if this symptom is present in a psychosis in the absence of an organic pathology we call it schizophrenia, as opposed to a cyclothymic psychosis, a personality abnormality or a psychogenic reaction (*Erlebnisreaktion*). These 1st rank symptoms thus only have a purely diagnostic preference over the 2nd rank symptoms which can also be found in the other psychoses and at times in non-psychotic conditions. This however does not say that we speak of schizophrenia only if 1st rank symptoms are found. 2nd rank symptoms and behavioral abnormalities very often permit such a diagnosis if present in certain combinations and numbers.

As can be seen from this Schneider is not concerned with a fresh definition of the circumference of the illness. He does not give 'renewed support to those who preferred to think of schizophrenia as a benign process by simply redefining schizophrenia to make it so' (**Kety, 1980**). Schneider emphasizes that recovery with full insight can occur, though only exceptionally so. With that he says no more than Kraepelin. Compared to Bleuler he greatly narrows the circumference by avoiding an overreliance on the recognition of Bleuler's primary or basic symptoms (the four A's as they are called) which are far too nonspecific. Schneider described 'features that are more easily perceived and described, and which therefore show a higher degree of interrater reliability, features which are economically put into check lists and fed into computers' (**Kety, 1980**), but these enormous advantages are dismissed by Kety because he feels they describe a different syndrome. This, as has been shown, has not been the intention of Schneider nor is it an unintended but somehow inevitable result of his work. Schneider's starting point was Kraepelin's dementia praecox. He never doubted the validity of that concept, but stripped it of the positivist theories and inappropriate clinical characterizations, which represented the impact on Kraepelin's thinking of his contemporary Zeitgeist.

The advantages mentioned by Kety are no mean achievement, but they do not close all the gaps in a precise and comprehensive diagnostic concept of the syndrome. Firstly it remains a syndromatic psychopathological type only, with occasional transitional forms being possible; secondly the cases go beyond the presence of first rank symptoms and so include some where the diagnosis is on less firm ground; and finally in the absence of an established somatosis any firm and dogmatic notion as to its nature as a disease with a single pathology would be rash. We have no way of proving that what Bleuler included, or what Schneider defined as schizophrenia is the same disease or is not, only whether it better serves the purposes of our work. Greater reliability and greater pragmatism as opposed to speculation are not to be despised by a practical clinician or researcher. In each of these fields it will be expedient for instance to keep separate the group with first rank symptoms from the others (without necessarily excluding them) when reporting the findings of genetic, epidemiological, prognostic or therapeutic research. This will render such work more reliably repeatable, and will make scientific communication more precise. More cannot be achieved but this would by no means be an overly modest advance.

Janzarik (1978), the present occupant of the Chair in Heidelberg, held in days gone by both Kraepelin and Schneider, sums up as follows:

At the present state of knowledge what matters is not deciding for the one or the other commonly used schizophrenia-definition, but the clear understanding that the concept of schizophrenia as such and its particular definition are based on convention ... International research must work for a unification of these conventions. The agreements reached from time to time however must not be turned into absolutes and rigidly laid down for always. Research is not impaired if for instance an investigation in Vienna or Zurich is based on a narrow concept of schizophrenia, while one in Lubeck or Heidelberg on a wider one. The only important matter is that the researcher is aware of the relativity of his premises, and that he never loses sight of the relativity of his own particular concept of schizophrenia.

Comment

We have seen the epochal achievement of Kraepelin and its impact on world psychiatry. We have also seen the subsequent attempts of clarification which all continue to build on Kraepelin, but which have in common the attempt to overcome his essentially non-psychological approach. Kraepelin saw only the illness, not the person, the patient. We saw that the impetus for these attempts to overcome this came from Freud, and that his psychology is somehow to a greater or lesser extent present in these attempts. We also saw that these efforts were often lacking in methodological clarity and consequently led into distortions of one kind or another.

In the case of Bleuler an artificial, surely speculative, division of symptoms into directly process-related and secondary complex-related, weakened the diagnostic grip. In the case of Kretschmer or Gaupp it led to an anthropological or entirely psychological apprehension of at least certain subgroups. In the case of Meyer and Sullivan the disease dissolved into a set of acquired faulty habits or interpersonal relationships. To some workers the psychological approach became the exclusive one. Understanding the psychogenic connections of the symptoms, often with the help of hypothetical underlying constructs like the unconscious, was seen as exhaustive, revealing all there is to schizophrenia.

Kubie (1971) writes 'at last a rebellion against the concept of schizophrenia is in full swing.' He quotes various participants in that revolt such as Karl Menninger, Cancro, and Altschule. He writes:

... within the general concept of progressive psychotic disorganisation there is no need (or justification) for a separate sub-category among psychotic disturbances to be called 'schizophrenia' or 'schizoid'. I am more convinced of this today than ever, and I challenge my colleagues to prove its necessity or its usefulness, and to demonstrate that it does not add to the confusions of our clinical descriptions and of our research.

This revolt is not universal and the concept has been retained in American and International classifications, but what had already struck Bleuler as a limitation is still seen as such by many and is still giving rise to 'revolts'.

Jaspers' clarification in psychopathological methodology appears to overcome this perceived gap, by allowing the exploration of each case both by a clear description of the phenomena, the symptoms, while at the same time allowing a psychological understanding of the personality and the life of the patient, and how the change brought by the process on one hand and the life and personality on the other interact. It makes possible a comprehension of the patient without sacrificing diagnosis. Schneider (1956) applies this:

Diagnostics looks at the 'How?' (the form) not at the 'What?' (the theme or content). If I find thought-withdrawal this is important to me as a certain mode of experience and as a diagnostic hint; I am not interested diagnostically whether it is the devil, the mistress or a political leader who withdraws the thoughts. Where one looks at such contents diagnostics recedes. In that case one sees only the biographical or the understandable existence. This is the case in psychoanalysis and in the new extreme types of existential analysis. There, it is true, diagnosis comes to an end and with that also the heritage of Kraepelin.

In phenomenology and the psychology of meaning, as explained by Jaspers, subjective psychology is brought back into the study of schizophrenia, not at the expense of diagnosis, but in its service.

References

BINSWANGER, L. (1957) *Schizophrenie*. Pfullingen: Neske.
BLANKENBURG, W. (1958) Daseinsanalytische Studie über einen Fall paranoider Schizophrenie. *Schweizer Archiv für Neurologie u. Psychiatrie*, **81,** 9–105.
BLEULER, E. (1911) *Dementia Praecox oder Gruppe der Schizophrenien*. Leipzig: F. Deuticke.
—— (1950) Dementia praecox or the group of schizophrenias (Transl. J. Zenkin). New York International University Press.
—— & JUNG, C. G. (1908) Komplexe und Krankheitsursachen bei Dementia praecox. *Zentralblatt für Psychiatrie u. Nervenheilkunde*, **3,** 220–227.
FAERGEMAN, P. M. (1963) *Psychogenic Psychoses: A Description and Follow-Up of Psychoses Following Psychological Stress*. London: Butterworths.
GAUPP, R. (1920) Der Fall Wagner. *Zeitschrift für die gesamte Neurologie u. Psychiatrie*, **60,** 312–327.
—— (1939) Die Lehren Kraepelins in ihrer Bedeutung für die heutige Psychiatrie. *Zeitschrift für die gesamte Neurologie u. Psychiatrie*, **165,** 47–75.
GRUHLE, H. W. (1932) Geschichtliches. In *Handbuch der Geisteskrankheiten* (ed. O. Bumke). Berlin: Springer.
JANZARIK, W. (1978) Wandlungen des Schizophrenie-begriffes. *Nervenarzt*, **49,** 133–139.

JASPERS, K. (1910) Eifersuchtswahn. *Zeitschrift für die gesamte Neurologie u. Psychiatrie*, **1**, 567–637.
—— (1913) Kausale und 'verständliche' Zusammenhänge zwischen Schicksal und Psychose bei der Dementia praecox. *Zeitschrift für die gesamte Neurologie u. Psychiatrie*, **14**, 158–263.
—— (1957a) Philosophische autobiographie. In *Karl Jaspers* (ed. P. A. Schlipp). Stuttgart: Kohlhammer.
—— (1957b) Philosophical autobiography. In *The Philosophy of Karl Jaspers* (ed. P. A. Schlipp). La Salle, Ill: Open Court.
—— (1959) *Allgemeine Psychopathologie*. Heidelberg: Springer.
—— (1963) *General Psychopathology*. (Transl. by J. Hoenig and M. W. Hamilton). Manchester University Press.
—— (1974) Causal and 'meaningful' connections between life history and psychosis. In *Themes and Variations in European Psychiatry* (eds. S. R. Hirsch and M. Shepherd). Bristol: J. Wright.
KETY, S. (1980) The syndrome of schizophrenia: Unresolved questions of opportunities for research. *British Journal of Psychiatry*, **136**, 421–436.
KOLLE, K. (1957) *Kraepelin und Freud*. Stuttgart: Thieme.
KRAEPELIN, E. (1893) *Psychiatrie*, 4th ed. Leipzig: J. A. Barth.
—— (1909–13) *Psychiatrie*, 8th ed. Leipzig: J. A. Barth.
—— (1962) *100 Years of Psychiatry*. New York: Philosophical Library.
KRÄUPL TAYLOR, F. (1967) The role of phenomenology in psychiatry. *British Journal of Psychiatry*, **113**, 765–770.
KRETSCHMER, E. (1967) *Körperbau und Charakter*. Berlin: Springer.
KUBIE, L. S. (1971) Multiple fallacies in the concept of schizophrenia. *Journal of Nervous and Mental Disease*, **153**, 331–342.
MAYER-GROSS, W. (1929) Die Entwicklung der Klinischen Anschauungen Kraepelins. *Archive für Psychiatrie*, **87**, 30–42.
MEYER, A. (1948) The dynamic interpretation of dementia praecox. In *The Common Sense Psychiatry* (ed. A. Lief). New York: McGraw Hill.
SCHNEIDER, K. (1925) Wesen und Erfassung des Schizophrenen. *Zeitschrift f.d. gesamte Neurologie u. Psychiatrie*, **99**, 542–547.
—— (1938) 25 Jahre Allgemeine Psychopathologie von Karl Jaspers. *Nervenartz*, **11**, 281–283.
—— (1956) Kraepelin und die gegenwärtige Psychiatrie. *Fortschritte der Neurologie Psychiatrie*, **24**, 1–7.
—— (1957) Primäre und sekundäre Symptome bei der Schizophrenie. *Fortschritte der Neurologie Psychiatrie*, **25**, 487–490.
—— (1974) Primary and secondary symptoms in schizophrenia. In *Themes and Variations in European Psychiatry* (eds. S. R. Hirsch and M. Shepherd). Bristol: J. Wright.
STRÖMGREN, E. (1974) Psychogenic psychoses. In *Themes and Variations of European Psychiatry* (eds. S. R. Hirsch and M. Shepherd). Bristol: J. Wright.
WYRSCH, J. (1966) Das Problem der schizophrenen Person. *Psychiatria Neurologia (Basel)*, **151**, 129–149.
ZUTT, J. (1956) Das Schizophrenie-problem. Nosologische Hypothesen. *Klinische Wochenschrift*, **34**, 679–684.

5 Was insanity on the increase?

EDWARD HARE

At the autumn meeting of the Medico-Psychological Association in 1871, Maudsley—at that time President of the Association—read a paper entitled 'Is Insanity on the Increase?'. The question was then one of profound concern both to the British public and to psychiatrists. Not only had there been for years a constant need to build new asylums—a cause 'of terrible discouragement and complaint with the ratepayers' (Arlidge, 1859)—but also, as was clearly apparent in the publications of the Poor Law Office and the Annual Reports of the Commissioners in Lunacy, the number of the registered insane was increasing every year, far out of proportion to the increase in the population. This circumstance, it was said, 'might well give rise to alarming apprehension of a mental degeneracy' in the country (Arlidge, 1862).

The increase was occurring not only in England and Wales, but in Scotland and Ireland too. 'There can be no question', said Maudsley in his paper of 1872, 'that there are a great many more insane persons shut up in asylums in this country now than there ever were at any other period of its history, or, perhaps, in any country at any period of the world's history.' But the explanation of this increase was 'more easily disputed than decided'.

Among medical men, the dispute was long and bitter. In one camp were those who believed that the incidence of insanity was increasing at an alarming rate and that the same was happening in Europe and in the USA: in the other camp were those who believed that the undoubted increase in the *numbers* of the recognized insane did not necessarily imply an increase in *incidence* and could be accounted for in other ways—ways which we might nowadays call 'nosocomial'. The term 'nosocomial' means 'of hospitals' (*OED*); but it has been usefully used in the special sense of embracing all those factors, other than the disease itself, which determine whether a person with the disease comes to be included in a register of hospital cases.

This sharp difference of opinion—between the alarmists who thought insanity was increasing and the nosocomialists who thought it was not—continued throughout the nineteenth century. In the early twentieth century, determined efforts were made by a specially appointed Statistical Committee of the Medico-Psychological Association to devise ways in which the issue might be finally decided (*Journal of Mental Science*, 1904; 1905). But their efforts were interrupted by the Great War of 1914; and soon after that war, it became apparent that the question had lost its urgency. In his Maudsley Lecture of 1926, George Robertson discussed the statistics of insanity in Scotland for the years

1910–1924, and showed that the evidence indicated a decrease rather than an increase in rate during that period. He concluded that 'in these statistics there is no cause whatever for alarm'. The old bogey, of insanity in Britain being 'fearfully on the increase', seemed at last to have been laid to rest; and I cannot find that there was any further discussion of the matter during the next 50 years.

So the question raised by Maudsley, at this autumn meeting of ours one hundred and eleven years ago, was never resolved; and indeed, it has been said that it never could have been resolved because the appropriate data were not collected, or were not collected for a sufficient period of time. Yet it is my impression that during at least the last 30 or 40 years there has existed a silent presumption that the nosocomialists were right and that the incidence of mental disorder in Britain during the nineteenth century did not increase to any significant extent. Such a presumption would be in line with the widely accepted conclusion reached by Goldhamer and Marshall in their book *Psychosis and Civilization* (published in 1953) that, except for the psychoses of old age, there was no change in the incidence of psychotic illness in the USA between the 1840s and 1940. It would also be in line with a general opinion (as expressed, for example, by Dunham in 1971) that the incidence of schizophrenia is probably about the same in all parts of the world.

These views have recently been challenged. In particular, the work of Goldhamer and Marshall has been criticized in the United States by the sociologist William Eaton (1980) and by the psychiatrist Fuller Torrey (1980). Reading their criticisms, it occurred to me that it might be of interest to re-examine, from a historical point of view, the nineteenth-century controversy over the increase of insanity in Britain. Such a study would be more than mere antiquarianism. The incidence of a disease, and its possible variations in time, are of basic importance in epidemiology; and although no decisive answer might be found, the probabilities could be re-assessed, and these might then be relevant for present hypotheses of the aetiology of the functional psychoses.

The case for the nosocomialists

The Lunacy Act of 1845 not only obliged counties to build asylums for the care of their insane poor, but placed on the Commissioners in Lunacy the power and the duty to inspect asylums and to make returns of the numbers of persons brought to their notice as 'insane' (the term was used to include lunatics and idiots). From 1846 until 1914 (when they were succeeded by the Board of Control), the Commissioners produced Annual Reports—the so-called 'lunacy Blue Books'—which gave statistics of insane persons in public and in private asylums, in workhouses (under the Poor Law Acts) and in home care. The collection of such nationwide figures on what might be considered essentially a medical condition was something quite new, and it needed a few years before the system was considered to be satisfactory. But the establishment of this system, and the fact that it then continued almost unchanged for 60 years, is a remarkable tribute to the determination and efficiency of the Commissioners.

From their Annual Reports, and from the continually increasing demand for asylum accommodation, it appeared incontrovertible that, in one sense at least, insanity was on the increase. Thus it was upon those who held that this increase was not a real one—i.e. was *not* due to an increasing incidence—that the burden of proof lay. I shall therefore present first the case for the nosocomialists.

The 1850s

In their earliest Reports, the increasing numbers of registered insane were attributed by the Lunacy Commissioners to the incompleteness of previous records. However, the increases continued even when the system of recording seemed to be adequate. In their Ninth Report (Bucknill, 1855) the Commissioners, noting that during the past eight years the numbers of pauper lunatics in asylums had increased from about 10,000 to about 16,000 (i.e. by 64 per cent), observed that this increase 'may appear at first sight startling' and might lead to the 'painful and disheartening' inference that the incidence of insanity was increasing. But, they said, the increase in numbers could be explained in other ways. These were: *first*, that asylum care caused the insane to live longer there than they would have done outside, so that long-stay cases were accumulating; *second*, that the effect of various Acts of Parliament had been to increase both the numbers of persons ascertained as insane and the numbers admitted to asylums who might previously have been cared for at home or in workhouses; and *third*, that 'the far more comprehensive as well as scientific view of insanity' had led to the recognition of cases which 'from not exhibiting any strongly developed symptoms, were in former times, wholly overlooked'. They concluded that the increase of insanity was more apparent than real.

These three reasons, lower death rate, more complete registration, and more accurate detection, which the Commissioners first put forward in the early 1850s, appear to have been generally accepted for a number of years. In 1866, for example, the *Lancet*, while observing that 'the three large asylums for the county of Middlesex are full' and that 'extended accommodation for the insane poor is urgently required all over England', could add 'It must not be thought that insanity is increasing because more asylums are required'. Likewise the Pall Mall Gazette, in an article of 1869 'on the alleged increase of insanity', was still able to find in the arguments of the Lunacy Commissioners a satisfactory explanation for the evidence that the number of insane paupers in proportion to the population of England and Wales had more than doubled between 1836 and 1868 (*Journal of Mental Science*, 1869).

The 1860s and '70s

As time went on, however, and the pressure for asylum places continued, the matter came to be studied more closely. Lockhart Robertson (1869) dealt with the problem in his presidential address of 1867, and he added something to the arguments of the commissioners. The Lunacy Act of 1845, he said 'forms a new era in the history of lunacy, and it cannot be wondered that the greater care bestowed upon the insane should lead to a larger knowledge of their numbers as well as their conditions'. Moreover, the Lunacy Registration

Act of 1853 required the medical officers of (pauper) Unions to make quarterly
returns of the numbers of pauper lunatics *not* in asylums; this added to the
accuracy of the total numbers. Similarly, the Irremovable Poor Act of 1861,
by which a pauper lunatic became chargeable to the common fund of the
Union instead of to his own parish, led to increasing numbers (especially
of idiots) being sent to asylums because, whereas parishes had tended to maintain their insane poor at home in order to keep down the local rates, this
inducement was now removed. The effect of these measures, it was argued,
could account for the increase in asylum numbers; and the time would come
when all lunatics had been ascertained and transferred, and there would be
no further increase. Indeed, this seemed already to be happening, because
the *rate* of increase of the numbers in asylums was falling, as was the rate
of increase of admissions (see Table I). 'I think I am justified in saying',

TABLE I
Yearly rate of increase in asylum population, 1844–1868
(Robertson, 1869, Table IX)

Period	Mean yearly rate of increase
1844–49	5.64%
1849–54	6.09%
1854–59	3.41%
1859–64	4.83%
1864–68	3.82%

Robertson concludes, 'that we see the limits of our labours in providing for
the care and treatment of the insane poor; and further, that we have nearly
gained the desired end. It is allowing a wide margin in our calculations for
the future if we place the possible total number of lunatics and idiots at one
in 400 of the population ... We should thus require, with a population of
22 million, 33,000 beds in public asylums. Of these, 26,000 are already provided.' (Table II).

TABLE II
Ratio of insane to total population of England and Wales
(Robertson, 1869, Table I)

Year	Total insane	Proportion of population
1844	20,611	1 in 802
1852	26,352	1 in 691
1858	35,347	1 in 544
1868	50,118	1 in 432

Maudsley, in the paper of 1872 which I have mentioned, took a similar
view: most of the increase was due to better recognition; part of it to a wider
range of conditions being included (though this might be simply the result
of administrative factors); and part of it to a diminishing recovery rate (though
he implies that the asylum system itself might be partly to blame for this).
As to the admission rate, he accepted that it had been increasing, but was

this increase (he asked) greater than might be accounted for by the causes he had enumerated? He thought not; and 'for my part', he concluded, 'I think that one might fairly venture a prophecy that, 12 years hence, the ratio of admissions to the population will not be greater, if it be not less, than it is now.'

We might notice here another paper of Maudsley's, published five years later, in which he refers to this prophecy of 1871, a prophecy which, he admits, 'does not seem at all likely to be fulfilled in regard of pauper patients.' But the fact that the admission rate was continuing to increase could *now* be attributed, he said, to the so-called 'Four Shilling' Act of 1874, whereby the Government granted four shillings towards the local authority cost of maintaining each asylum patient—or, as Maudsley put it, 'an Act whereby the Government said, in effect, to parish officials, "We will pay you a premium of four shillings a head on every pauper whom you can by hook or crook make out to be a lunatic and send into an asylum".' As to the likely collapse of his former prophecy, 'how was it possible (he asks) to foresee in 1871 that a Conservative Government would come into power and forthwith put a direct premium on the manufacture of lunacy? It was impossible' (Maudsley, 1877).

The 1880s and '90s

The question of increasing insanity was debated as vigorously during the 1880s and 1890s as it had been during the '60s and '70s. From 1880 until his death in 1895 at the age of 67, Daniel Hack Tuke was the editor of the *Journal of Mental Science*, and his position as editor, we may presume, added to the influence of his strongly-held opinion that insanity was not on the increase. In an article of 1886, he re-emphasized that the only sound test of increasing insanity was the proportion of 'occurring cases'—what we would now call the incidence rate. An increase in the number of existing cases in asylums (i.e. an increase in prevalence) was not a sound test, as this could be due to an accumulation of cases from falling rates of death or discharge. He gave figures to show a recent fall in asylum death rates, and a calculation to show that this fall would imply 3,000 fewer deaths and therefore 3,000 more patients in asylums. He noted, as Lockhart Robertson had done 20 years before, that the rate of increase in the numbers of insane had been falling, and also that the rates for first admissions (i.e. total number of admissions less transfers and re-admissions) had actually shown a decrease. Finally, he gave a graph of admission rates for 'first attacks', returns for which had been available in the lunacy Blue Books since 1876. He concluded: 'these figures are very satisfactory so far as they exhibit no increase in the amount of *occurring* insanity since the year 1878.' (Table III).

We should notice here some of the technical difficulties which Tuke had to contend with. At no time during the nineteenth century does there seem to have been any clear understanding, in the statistical study of insanity, of the need for what we would now call the definition of a case. The idea of a 'first-ever admission to an asylum' being a good working definition of a case of insanity and a basis on which a study of changes in incidence rate could usefully be made was never fully reached. Tuke did not consider 'first admission' a satisfactory index, partly because it was not necessarily a *first-ever*

TABLE III

'First' admission rates to asylums in England and Wales,
1871–1885 (adapted from Table E in Tuke, 1886)

Period	Admission rate (per million population)	Change in rate
1871–75	429	+7.4%
1876–80	461	
		−1.9%
1881–85	452	

admission (the patient might have been previously admitted to some other asylum) but more because, as Tuke rather cumbrously put it, 'first admissions ... are not identical with first attacks, for obviously a patient may be admitted for the first time into an asylum and yet not be labouring under his first attack.' He evidently believed that a true index of occurring insanity should refer only to recent cases, and that cases of insidious onset and cases where there had been earlier attacks not needing admission should be excluded. But his usage of 'first attack' was criticized, particularly from America, and Tuke himself (1894) was later ready to accept that the returns for first attacks were untrustworthy.

Another major contribution to the debate came from a statistician, Noel Humphreys. His article 'Statistics of insanity in England, with special reference to its alleged increasing prevalence' was published in the *Journal of the Royal Statistical Society* in 1890. He observed—what everyone accepted—that the available statistics did not allow of a 'sound and trustworthy' answer, but he introduced a new argument. He compared the numbers of registered insane, as found by the Lunacy Commissioners, with the numbers enumerated at the censuses of 1871 and 1881 (Table IV): these censuses had included a

TABLE IV

Numbers of insane found at census and by the Lunacy
Commisioners in 1871 and 1881
(Humphreys 1890, from Table A)

Year	Census enumeration	Number ascertained by Lunacy Commisioners	Deficit in ascertainment
1871	69,019	56,755	18%
1881	84,503	73,113	14%

question on the number of residents in each household who were 'imbecile or idiot, or lunatic'. The differences between the census numbers and the registered numbers, he said, must indicate the numbers of the unregistered insane; and the fact that the proportion of unregistered insanity was lower at the later census was an indication of 'the increasing accuracy of registration'. Thus the ever-increasing number of the insane, as shown in the Reports of the Lunacy Commissioners, was to be accounted for by a gradual mopping-up of the pool of unregistered cases. Humphreys does not mention—nor indeed does Hack Tuke, who uses this argument in his last paper of 1894—that the

Census returns, completed (we must presume) by householders of widely varying knowledge, opinion and responsibility in these matters, might not constitute
a very reliable source of data on so emotional a topic. Another comment which
might be made in retrospect is that many, perhaps most, of the non-registered
insane reported in the censuses would have been idiot children, the group
most likely to remain at home; and that the decrease in the size of the non-
registered pool might in part reflect a decreasing proportion of mentally
retarded children in the community because of the fall in birth-rate dating
from the 1870s, which implies a fall in family size and in the number of children
born to older women.

Better recognition and registration was one reason, Humphreys said, for
the increasing numbers of the 'existing cases' of insanity. Another reason for
the accumulation of patients in asylums was the diminishing death rate there:
'It is beyond question that the rate of mortality in asylums has declined' he
said, and he gave figures to show that this was so both in lunatic asylums
(Table V) and in the metropolitan asylums for imbeciles and idiots. Concerning

TABLE V
Annual asylum death rates in England and Wales, 1859–1888
(from, Humphreys, 1890, Table D, p. 228)

Period	Death rate
1859–68	10.31%
1869–78	10.17%
1879–88	9.55%

the use of 'first admissions' as an index of incidence, Humphreys had the
same doubts as Tuke; there was no way, he said, of determining what proportion of first admissions were 'really new cases' and how many were previously
existing in the reserve of cases in workhouses or with relatives. For what they
were worth, the figures showed no increase in rate during the previous ten
years, and indeed a decline during the latest quinquennium. Humphreys's
final cautious conclusion was that 'without venturing to say there has been
no increase of insanity in England in recent years, many reasons have been
pointed out for refusing to accept any insanity statistics that we at present
possess as conclusive evidence for a real increase in the rate of occurring
insanity'.

The last study to support the nosocomialist view that there was no need
to suppose any increase in the *incidence* of insanity in England and Wales was
the special report of the Commissioners in Lunacy on the alleged increase
of insanity (1897). Essentially a summary of previous arguments, it also provided one new one, based on the age distribution of asylum patients. One
of the major deficiencies of the statistics collected by the Lunacy Commissioners
was, as Humphreys had observed, the absence of any routine data on age
at admission to asylums or age at death there. The importance of age-specific
rates only gradually became recognized during the latter half of the nineteenth
century, and although Maudsley had remarked on it in his 1872 paper, no
routine data became available. However, the censuses of 1881 and 1891, which
had enumerated the insane in asylums, provided data on their ages. In the

Commissioners' Special Report a table shows that for insane persons in the age group 20–45—the period of greatest liability to insanity—the proportion relative to the population was no greater in 1891 than it had been in 1881. The 'obvious inference', says the Report, was that 'accumulation and not fresh production had been the most influential factor' in the increased numbers of asylum patients. This, together with the weight of previous arguments, led the Commissioners to the following conclusion: 'We have thus, we think, demonstrated at least the probability that much of the apparent increase of insanity has been due, not to an increase in the incidence of that disorder, but to the aggregation of persons affected by it and to their re-distribution'. These are words which, we might now be tempted to think, reflect the uneasy compromise of a committee divided in its opinions; but this was to be the last authoritative statement on the subject until George Robertson's Maudsley Lecture of 1926.

The case for increasing incidence

Those nineteenth-century psychiatrists who believed that the incidence of insanity *was* increasing had, on the face of it, a much easier case to make. They did not deny that some of the undoubted increase in prevalence was to be explained in the way the nosocomialists claimed, i.e. by increased recognition of cases and by patients staying longer in asylums, but they argued that such effects could only be temporary, whereas the increase in numbers of the insane had been continuous from the time of the earliest statistics. If Acts of Parliament or better diagnosis drew attention to cases previously unrecognized, the time should come when the pool of undiagnosed cases had been mopped up; and if patients lived longer in asylums than they would have done outside—and there was no proof of this—then after 20 years or so these patients would have reached the natural limit of their lives and so there should be no more accumulation from that cause. In any case, the admission rate to asylums showed a generally increasing trend; and even though there was considerable year-to-year fluctuation in this rate and the statistics of first admissions were somewhat unsatisfactory, the reasonable conclusion was of a real increase in the number of new patients being admitted.

The number of insane in Britain

Harrington Tuke, in his presidential address of 1873, observed that Dr Lockhart Robertson had 'adduced all that can be brought forward in advocacy of the hopeful view that the statistical returns lead to a fallacious conclusion ... I regret to say that the elaborate Annual Reports of the Commissioners in Lunacy, and the inference to be drawn from them, seem to me unanswerably to demonstrate the reverse.' These statistics, together with a table divided into age-groups, prepared for him by William Farr, 'appear to prove', said Tuke, 'that a great wave of insanity is slowly advancing.' The discussion which followed his address, and which was reported in the *Journal of Mental Science*, clearly shows the conflict of expert opinion at this time.

Much of the evidence for increase came not from the lunacy statistics but from medical men with long and close experience of particular districts. In

1869, Dr MacCabe, Superintendent of the Waterford District Asylum, contended that there were 'tolerably accurate returns' of the numbers of the insane in all parts of Ireland. Between 1851 and 1861 these numbers had increased by 6 per cent, while the population had fallen 12 per cent. In his own district during this time, the proportion of persons found to be insane had almost doubled, from one in every 690 to one in 350.

The increase in lunacy in Ireland, he believed, was 'a well-established fact'. This opinion continued to be expressed by Irish physicians. In his paper of 1894, Thomas Drapes, Superintendent of Enniscorthy Asylum, compared statistics for first admissions to asylums in Ireland with those in England and Wales. For Ireland, the first admission figures were derived from those of all admissions, less transfers and re-admissions; but they included admissions from workhouses, a group which had been omitted from Hack Tuke's tables on the ground that such cases were not 'first attacks'. It is clear now that, in so far as a first admission to an asylum would have been the best definition of a case of insanity, Drapes' procedure was right here and Tuke's was wrong. Drapes concluded that the increasing first admission rate in Ireland 'must be regarded as indicating a decided increase in occurring insanity'. As regards the cause of the increase, he noted that there was no good evidence for an increase in the part played by heredity or consanguineous marriage, and that the effects of emigration had probably been over-estimated, though he rather spoils these sensible observations, we might now think, by attributing the increase to the Celtic temperament: 'the quick-witted, passionate, versatile and vivacious Celt has, for those qualities which make him so charming, too often to pay the price of instability'.

Like Ireland, Scotland was for the most part a thinly populated country where a man might acquire close knowledge of a local community. Jamieson was physician at the Royal Aberdeen Hospital, and in 1876 he expressed his opinion, based on 35 years' professional experience, that 'the most remarkable phenomenon of our time has been the alarming increase of insanity'. Whereas in 1840 there had been seven asylums in Scotland, in 1876 there were 24; and whereas in 1844 the asylum in Aberdeen had held 150 patients, now it had 480, and in addition there were three new asylums, each with 100 patients in them.

The number of insane abroad

The question of an increase in insanity was also being debated in other countries, but I will here refer only to such observations as were noted in the *Journal of Mental Science*.

In France, the asylum population increased rapidly between 1838 and 1862 (Lunier, 1870; Robertson, 1871); but Lunier, observing that the *rate* of increase had then begun to fall off slightly, attributed most of this increase to an increased public confidence in the use of asylums, adding that any increase in incidence was 'une proportion insignificante le chiffre total des entrées'. Yet a few years later, at the discussion of Harrington Tuke's presidential address, a Parisian physician said that the intermarriage of families where insanity prevailed was one cause of the continued increase in the numbers of the insane in France (Tuke, 1873, p. 479); and in the discussion of Humphreys's paper

(1890), it was remarked that 'the increase in the number of lunatics in France had gone on in recent years at a more rapid rate than in England'.

In the United States, the increase in the number of the insane had caused concern since at least the early 1850s, when Jarvis (1852) concluded that 'insanity is an increasing disease'. From a study of the statistics of insanity in Massachusetts, which showed an 80 per cent increase in the number of first admissions between 1868 and 1886, Pliny Earle (1887) concluded that the figures 'appear to show that there has been a considerable increase, even in recent insanity, out of proportion to the gain in population'. His opinion was reinforced in a later paper by Sanborn (1894) entitled 'Is American insanity increasing?'. Sanborn accepted that the three factors of better care, better registration and a wider definition of insanity could have accounted for some of the earlier increase in the number of insane. Yet, 'still we find this insane accumulation going on as fast as 50 years ago, and in the face of influences that ought to yield just the contrary result'. For this reason—and because, as he indicated, the statistics of insanity in Massachusetts had been particularly reliable over the preceding 15 years—he believed that there must have been a 'very substantial' increase in the incidence of insanity there and, I doubt not, in most of the United States ... If any other interpretation can be put upon the figures given, nobody will be more pleased than myself; but that seems to me hardly possible.'

An assessment of the evidence

I shall now attempt to assess the evidence for and against the view that insanity was increasing in Britain during the second half of the nineteenth century. Contemporary authors could of course consider only the statistics available to them at the time, whereas we can now take a longer view. To an epidemiologist, the main deficiency of the Lunacy Commissioners' statistics is that they were designed to serve administrative rather than medical ends; but we have also to remember that epidemiology was then an undeveloped science and that the need for case definition and for age-specific rates of first-ever admissions was not recognized, or was recognized too late to be useful. In addition, of course, 'insanity' was a legal rather than a medical concept, and embraced not only all varieties of mental illness ('lunacy') but all varieties of retardation ('idiocy') as well.

Prevalence statistics

I will first consider the arguments used by the nosocomialists to support their view that the obvious increase in the numbers of ascertained insane did not necessarily imply an increase in the incidence of insanity. There were three types of argument.

Previously unrecognized insanity

The first was there had been a large number of cases of unrecognized insanity in the population, and that these were gradually being recognized as a result of various Acts of Parliament, greater medical knowledge, and increased public confidence in asylums. It was argued that although this recognition had been the cause of the increasing numbers of insane under care, the pool of unrecognized cases was being emptied and the time would come when the numbers of recognized insane would no longer continue to increase. Lockhart Robertson, in 1869, believed this desired end had almost been achieved, and he predicted that the proportion of the insane in the general population would never fall below 1 in 400, and that the limit of the need for asylums would be 1500 beds per million population. Yet his prediction of the maximum prevalence rate was overtaken within five years, and by the year 1914 the proportion of the insane to the population was 1 in 266, and the proportionate number of asylum beds was more than twice his maximum (3,100 beds per million). We have already noted Maudsley's prophecy of 1871, that in 12 years' time the admission rate would show no further increase. In fact, by that time the rate had increased by nearly 15 per cent, and in another 12 years was to be increased by 50 per cent. Hack Tuke in 1886, and Humphreys in 1890, also argued that the admission rates were levelling off, and indeed that the last quinquennial average had actually shown a fall. This was true, but the effect was only temporary and the rate rose as steeply as ever during the next three quinquennia.

Accumulation of patients

The second explanation for the increase in the number of the recognized insane was that chronic cases *accumulated* in asylums. Accumulation occurs whenever the number of admissions exceeds the combined numbers of discharges and deaths. Unfortunately, the lunacy statistics were not always such as to enable a simple calculation to be made, and arguments had to be based on a consideration of rates of recovery and of deaths. Clearly, if either of these rates were falling, there would be more patients remaining in asylums. The best statistic for recovery rate was based on the number per 100 admissions who were 'discharged as recovered'. Tuke, in 1866, noted that this rate had shown little change since 1870, when the data first became available, and concluded that recovery rate did not appear to be 'a disturbing element'. Humphreys (in 1890) found the statistics of recovery to be 'so vitiated by the disturbing element of relapses' that no useful conclusion could be drawn from them. On the other hand, the evidence for a *decrease* in recovery rate was used by the Lunacy Commissioners in their Special Report of 1897 as an argument *for* accumulation. The actual numbers point to a clear fall in recovery rates from about 1890, though we might think that when the Special Report was being written, the trend towards a fall was not then clear enough for the Commissioners' case to be very sound.

Death rates in asylums (expressed as the number of deaths divided by the daily average resident number) were more clear-cut than recovery rates, though the absence of any break-down by age at death much decreased their value. Humphreys took the evidence for decreasing death rates as supporting the case for accumulation, though he accepted that the interpretation was uncertain because the death rate would increase if the average age of patients increased and would decrease if ('as is probably the case') the proportion of acute cases diminished. Hack Tuke, in 1894, used the same argument, saying that the mortality rate in asylums 'is distinctly lower than it was 20 years ago', and the Commissioners followed suit (1897). However, the figures collected in the Board of Control's Report (1914) show there was a decline in the death rate between 1870 and 1885, but no such trend thereafter. Thus once again the nosocomialists were using evidence which supported their view when taken over a relatively short preceding period, but which was uncharacteristic of a longer period. A further difficulty in the use of death rate is that, when considered by sex, the male rate shows a general decrease and the female rate an increase.

Private patients

The third argument—and to my mind much the weakest—for the increase in the insane being due to nosocomial factors was that the increase had been mainly in pauper patients and had been relatively small in the private class. The argument was used by the Commissioners as far back as 1855, when they noted that the increase in the number of lunatics over the preceding eight years had been 64 per cent for paupers, and only 15 per cent for private patients. Forty years later, an editorial review in the *Journal of Mental Science* (1895) drew attention to the fact that the number of private patients in Scotland had not been increasing and commented that this was 'one of the strongest indicators that there is no real increase in the amount of mental disorder in the country' because if the alleged increase were due to the strain of modern life then 'it ought to show itself especially in the classes above the ranks of manual labour'. The same argument was urged in the Special Report of the Commissioners in 1897. The lunacy statistics do indeed show a fall in the ratio of private patients to the population between 1880 and 1895, but thereafter a fairly rapid increase. In any case, a separate consideration of private cases seems, from the medical point of view, to be unsatisfactory. Not only does private care reflect the varying play of market forces but, as Maudsley pointed out in 1872, insanity was a pauperizing disease, so that many once well-to-do patients had come down in the world by the time institutional care was needed.

Conclusion

There is no doubt that *some* of the increase in the numbers of insane was due to nosocomial factors—increased recognition (in the statutory sense) and increased length of asylum stay. The question is: how much? In the absence of hard data, there could only be, and still can only be, opinions. But from the above considerations, I conclude that the arguments of the nosocomialists, though reasonable enough at the time they were made, do not hold up when a longer view is taken of the statistics. To a much more considerable degree than the nosocomialists were prepared to admit, the increase in the numbers of the insane did represent an increase in the real prevalence rate of insanity; and if the *prevalence* rate was increasing, then it was not unlikely that this was due, at least in part, to an increase in *incidence* rate.

Admission statistics

By the 1890s it had become generally accepted that 'the only true criterion of the increase or decrease of insanity is to be found in the number of first attacks' (Drapes, 1894), but it was later agreed that Hack Tuke's and the

Lunacy Commissioners' restriction of 'first attacks' to recent acute illness lead-ing directly to asylum admission was unfortunate. Data for 'first admissions' were available from 1869 though, as Tuke stressed, these were not first-ever admissions but only first admissions to a particular institution. First-ever admissions were not recorded until 1898, so that only a small series is available up to 1914. However, yearly figures for total admissions (excluding transfers and admissions to idiot establishments) are available from 1869 onwards, and there is reason to believe they can be of value. The 'first admissions' for each of the years 1869 to 1897 show a ratio to the total admissions which is constant within very narrow limits at about 88 per cent ($r = 0.992$). Similarly, there is an almost constant ratio between first-ever admissions and total admissions for the years 1898 to 1914 (about 82 per cent, $r = 0.995$), and this is true for each sex. In other words, there are very close correlations between first admissions, as variously measured, and total admissions. It is thus reasonable to suppose, I think, that the admission rate for total admissions during the period 1869 to 1914 gives a pretty accurate index for the 'first-ever admission' rate. With slightly less reliability, this argument can be extended back to the earliest date for which admission figures are available, 1859. Although we do not have the age-specific rates, I find it difficult to avoid the conclusion that between 1859 and 1900 there was a very considerable increase in the admission rate of new patients to institutions for the insane in England and Wales, and therefore a very considerable increase also of the incidence rate of insanity.

We might also notice here that the decade after the 1900 seems to have been a water-shed for lunacy statistics. Not only did the admission rate cease to rise (*Journal of Mental Science*, 1909; Commissioners, 1911), but two other distinct trends occurred: the asylum death rate, which had been essentially unchanged since 1860, began to fall; and the recovery rate (a less satisfactory statistic), which had been falling since about 1880, began to rise. We can only guess at the reasons for these phenomena, but they may explain why the question which so alarmed the nineteenth century—was insanity on the increase?—lost its urgency in the twentieth.

Explanations of the increase

The earlier evidence

The only other person, so far as I am aware, to have made a recent study of the nineteenth-century English lunacy statistics has come to the same conclu-sion as myself. In his book *Museums of Madness* (1979), Scull pointed out that the system of enumerating the insane remained substantially unchanged from 1846 onwards, and that this weighed against the view that registration became more accurate, i.e. that a pool of unrecognized cases was being mopped up. He argued that if accumulation of patients in asylums had been the main cause of increased prevalence, then patients in private hospitals should also have accumulated, for the mortality rate there was about the same as in the asylums and the recovery rates were even lower: but this did not happen. Scull also drew attention to the national statistical studies of the first half of the century, which had later been dismissed as inaccurate. He concluded

that they were carefully made and agreed with local studies, and that there
was no good reason to doubt their accuracy.

The rapid increase in prevalence rate shown by these early statistical studies
reflected a very general impression, dating from the late eighteenth century,
that insanity was becoming commoner. Jonathan Swift, like Maudsley after
him, provided a sum of money for the establishment of a hospital for the
mentally ill. But in his will, Swift expressed doubt that a sufficient number
of insane persons could be found to occupy the modest building he had in
mind, and so he directed that any spare places should be given over to physically
ill patients. That was in Dublin in 1747. Some 60 years later, William Halloran
(1810) undertook an inquiry 'into the cause of the extraordinary increase of
insanity in Ireland', having found that between 1789 and 1809 the numbers
of insane in the city of Cork (where he was asylum physician) had 'advanced
far beyond the extent upon which the humane founders had calculated'.

Similar impressions were being recorded in England. Thomas Arnold (1782)
referred to the 'vast increase of the disorder', which he could attribute only
to 'the present universal effusion of wealth and luxury'. William Perfect (1787)
referred to the belief that 'instances of insanity are at this day more numerous
in this kingdom than they were at any former period', and he suspected that
one factor might have been 'the epidemic catarrh, more generally known by
the name of the *Influenza*, which raged with such violence . . . in the year 1782'.
William Pargeter (1792) wrote that the lack of progress in understanding and
treatment of maniacal disorders was shown by this 'hideous malady which
so amazingly prevails at this day'.

Such observations continued into the nineteenth century. In his *Practical
Remarks* (1811), Bryan Crowther referred to insanity as 'an affection so rapidly
becoming prevalent among all orders of society', and Alexander Morrison
(1826) noted the recent increase of mental disorder both in Great Britain
and France (ascribing it to 'free governments and political commotions').
Prichard (1835) discussed the question at length, listing the differences of opinion;
he concluded that 'the apparent increase is everywhere so striking that it leaves
on the mind a strong suspicion . . . that cases of insanity are far more numerous
than formerly.' The remarkable output of treatises on insanity in the latter
part of the reign of George III (Pierce, 1919) was, one might think, as likely to
have been due to the general impression of its increasing prevalence as to the
more commonly accepted explanation of public interest in the King's illness.

This impressionistic and statistical evidence from the late eighteenth and
early nineteenth centuries, taken with the firmer evidence of the Reports of
the Lunacy Commissioners, makes it reasonable to suppose that the *prevalence*
rate of insanity in Britain was increasing throughout the nineteenth century.
There are no useful data on admission rates before 1859 and therefore none
on which the *incidence* of insanity before then can be estimated. Only by analogy
with later events could an argument for increasing incidence in the first half
of the nineteenth century be supported, but to my mind the analogy is a
fair one.

Why the admission rate increased

I now turn to consider possible reasons for such an increase, and in particular
why the 'first admission' rate to asylums should have increased during the

last four decades of the nineteenth century. There are two possibilities. The first, the one that understandably so frightened the public, is that the incidence of insanity increased without there being any diminution in the severity of the condition. The second, and more reassuring, possibility is that the increase was due to the admission of increasingly milder cases. We have no sure way of determining the relative contribution of these two factors. Scull, in his analysis, does not consider the first possibility at all: and he finds an adequate explanation solely in terms of milder cases. To the question why so many milder cases should be admitted when there was a continued pressure for new beds, Scull gives a sociological answer, which may be summarized in his statement that 'on the whole it was the existence and expansion of the asylum system which created the increased demand for its own services, rather than the other way around.'

Now while it is very probable that milder cases were being admitted—cases which would earlier have gone, in the first instance at any rate, to a work-house—I find it difficult to accept that the whole or even a large part of the increased number could for so long a period of time have simply been milder cases. In particular, Scull's view that the asylum system expanded first and then new patients were found to fill it up is hard to reconcile with the 'terrible discouragement and complaint' of the rate-payers faced with the demand for new asylums. One would suppose rather that the reasons for that demand must have been urgent, compelling and inescapable. Moreover, if milder cases had been the main cause of the increasing admission rate, then the asylum death rate should have decreased and the recovery rate increased, whereas in fact the death rate was static and the recovery rate declined markedly from the mid-1880s.

There is also other evidence that the prognosis of asylum cases was worsening. Granville (1877) believed that the proportion of patients who passed into a state of chronic dementia had increased (he blamed it on non-restraint). Savage (1890) was of the opinion that 'the form of insanity was worse' than formerly, though he could not back it up with statistics. The Commissioners in Lunacy (1899), noting that the recovery rate was falling although the appliances for skilled treatment were steadily mounting, concluded that this 'can only be due to the admission of less favourable cases'. The same idea was voiced in America, where Pliny Earle (1887) referred to 'the not improbable fact that insanity, as a whole, is really becoming more and more an incurable disease'.

From these considerations there appears to me to be a strong case for thinking that a considerable, perhaps a major, part of the increase in the asylum admission rate was due to a real increase in the incidence of insanity, of a kind not less severe than formerly.

Which disorders increased?

'If lunacy be on the increase', wrote Lockhart Robertson in 1871, 'it should be shown in which of its varieties the increase occurs.' He himself suggested that the increase might be in general paralysis, 'as it is in France'. But that was before separate statistics on general paralysis were published in the Blue Books, and it is evident from these that the admissions for general paralysis were only about 7 per cent or 8 per cent of the total (and only about 2 per cent for females), and that their proportion to the total did not change much over the years.

We can get an idea of the relative proportions of the different forms of insanity from the official statistics for the years 1909–1913 (Board of Control, 1914). These show that the group of conditions which we would now include in the term 'functional psychoses'—mania, melancholia, delusional insanity and secondary dementia—formed at least 75 per cent of the total. There is no reason to think that the organic cases could have been responsible for a major proportion of the overall increase in admission rate, and the conclusion must be that most of the increase was associated with the functional psychoses. But whereas we can say that delusional insanity, together with primary and secondary dementia, would have been closely related to what we now call the paranoid and schizophrenic psychoses, we have no way of distinguishing the relative proportions of schizophrenic and affective psychoses among the manias and melancholias, for the Kraepelinian delineation of *dementia praecox* had not then been adopted (Hare, 1981).

There is, however, some information to be gained from these figures. If the increase had been principally among the affective disorders, we should have expected an increase in the rates of recovery and readmission and a decrease in the death rate; but these did not occur. In fact, the evidence for the accumulation of chronic cases, together with the lack of any marked change in the death rate (until after 1905) suggests that it was the condition we now call schizophrenia which was most likely to have been the main cause of the increased admissions. Another piece of statistical evidence which seems to support this is the change which occurred in the relative proportions of admissions for mania and for melancholia. This change was, of course, recognized at the time. Clouston in 1891 noted 'the unprecedented increase' in the admissions for melancholia to the Royal Edinburgh Asylum. He attributed it to the influenza epidemic of 1889–90: 'the influenza poison burns up nervous energy and leaves the brain in some cases unable to recuperate'. Robert Jones (later Sir Robert Armstrong-Jones), in his presidential address of 1906, wondered whether the early physicians knew of the condition increasingly referred to as *dementia praecox*—a condition 'then apparently so rare, now so common'—and said that such cases almost invariably begin in depression. 'It was justifiable to conclude that they were classed as melancholia', he thought, and that would account for the rise in the relative proportion of admissions in that class.

I suggest therefore that there are reasons for thinking that, in so far as there was an increase in the incidence of insanity in Britain during the latter part of the nineteenth century, this increase was principally in that type of insanity which, in the 1890s, Kraepelin called *dementia praecox* and which we now call schizophrenia.

An epidemiological hypothesis

Now it is evident that if the incidence of schizophrenia was increasing during the second half—and perhaps also during the first half—of the nineteenth century, there would have been an earlier time when it was a comparatively rare condition. I think the commonly held view is that the incidence of schizo-phrenia has always been much the same: but that common opinion is certainly not based on historical evidence. In its acute stage, schizophrenia typically presents a striking clinical picture—of delusions, thought disorder and halluci-nations in a young adult, with no sign of mental confusion or physical disease—but one may search in vain for any such description before the nineteenth century. There were many British writers in the latter part of the *eighteenth* century who set themselves to describe in detail the various types of madness and their associated signs and symptoms, but I have been unable to find there, even in the first edition of Haslam's *Observations on Insanity* (1798), any account indicative of what we would recognize as acute schizophrenia. Andrew Harper, in 1789, said it was well known 'that young people are hardly ever liable to insanity and that the attack of this malady seldom happens before an advanced period of life', and in 1861 the Frenchman Renaudin remarked on the increasing number of cases where insanity had begun before the age of 20, adding that 'formerly, insanity of early age was a very rare exception'. It was also Tuke's impression in 1886, with which Savage concurred, that 'considerably more young people of both sexes break down mentally than there did formerly'. This question—whether descriptions of a disorder corres-ponding to schizophrenia can be found in the older literature, and if not why not—is debatable and I will not discuss it further here, although it does seem to me that those who believe schizophrenic-like disorders have always been with us, and always with about the same incidence rate, have yet to make a convincing case on purely historical grounds.

The view of schizophrenia as a perennial disease has been maintained on other grounds, and in particular it is implicit in the aetiological hypothesis put forward by Professor Manfred Bleuler (1978). On this hypothesis, schizo-phrenia is caused by the inheritance of an imbalance of normal genes, leading to the development of a type of schizoid personality which may later be tipped over into schizophrenia by the cumulative effect of traumatic psychological experiences. These experiences are non-specific and of a kind which will be unavoidable in the ordinary course of adult life. There are no important envir-onmental causes of a purely physical kind. This is a hypothesis which can neatly explain many facts about schizophrenia which have proved hard to explain otherwise.

But my inclination to search for an alternative hypothesis lies primarily in the hope of finding one less pessimistic than Bleuler's. For although in Bleuler's view the symptoms of schizophrenia may be alleviated by treatment, his hypothesis holds out no prospect of our ever being able to prevent schizo-phrenia by the elimination of some specific environmental cause or even—in the long term—of the genetic load being reduced by natural selection.

On Bleuler's hypothesis, schizophrenia is not an illness and the patient has no physical disorder. An alternative hypothesis, which brings schizophrenia properly into the realm of medicine, is that there *are* specific environmental factors of a physical kind, which have yet to be found. I am the more em-boldened to adopt this alternative in a Maudsley lecture because Maudsley him-self (1873) was a firm believer in the physical origin of mental disorder. Now once we think of schizophrenia as a disease with specific environmental causes, it becomes reasonable to accept that its manifestations and severity may have changed in the course of time and in response to changes in the prevalence or virulence of these causes and in the varying resistance to them which the prevailing conditions of human society permitted. The conclusion which I have drawn from my present study—that the incidence of schizophrenia increased in Britain during the nineteenth century—would come within the scope of such a causal hypothesis.

Dr Fuller Torrey (1980) was, I think, the first to put forward the idea that schizophrenia had been an uncommon disorder in Europe and America until towards the end of the eighteenth century, and that thereafter schizophrenia—or a particular type of it—became increasingly common. What I suggest now is that the lunacy statistics of Britain provide evidence in support of Torrey's idea. We then have the hypothesis of a slow epidemic of schizophrenia which in Europe, and perhaps also in the United States, began some 200 years ago and which can be attributed to the changing effect of some specific causal factor of a physical nature.

Comments

A hypothesis is useful in so far as it can explain a wide variety of observations and can point the way to further research. I should like to conclude by indicating some of the ways in which the 'slow epidemic' hypothesis provides a medical explanation of certain phenomena associated with schizophrenia which hitherto have received mainly psychological or sociological explanations.

A rapid increase in the incidence of schizophrenia, and therefore of 'insanity', at the end of the eighteenth century would very simply explain the abrupt development of interest in mental disease and the publication of numerous books on the subject at that time. It would also account in a most straightforward way for the asylum era: the real increase in insanity made urgently necessary the establishment and increasing provision of a specialized system of care. An increasing need for asylums occurred at about the same time in Britain, France and America, and perhaps also (though I have not specially studied it) in Germany and Russia, and it is not easy to see how the sociological explanations of the need for asylums can cover countries which had such widely different social and political systems.

The hypothesis would also explain why there are no satisfactory descriptions—or none that I have so far been able to find—in the medical or general literature before the nineteenth century of a disorder resembling acute schizophrenia. It would also account for the remarks by medical writers, whom I have quoted, on the former rarity of insanity in young persons.

A phenomenon which has proved difficult to account for on purely genetic grounds—and which would also be difficult to explain sociologically—is the apparent persistence of schizophrenia in spite of the low fertility of schizophrenics. This difficulty disappears on the hypothesis that schizophrenia (at least in the form best known to the industrialized world) was an uncommon disorder until about 200 years ago.

The hypothesis that the incidence of schizophrenia increased because of some change in the effect of a specific environmental factor carries the implication that further changes in incidence will probably occur; and by analogy with the history of epidemic disorders we might expect a period of rapid increase in incidence to be followed by a more gradual decrease and by changes in the severity and manifestations of the disorder. The change in the mania: melancholia ratio might be so explained—it would certainly be hard to explain in sociological terms. There has been no clear evidence of any change in the *incidence* of schizophrenia during the present century, though any comparatively slight change would be hard to demonstrate because of the problem of diagnosis. However, there is good evidence for a decrease in *severity*, as shown by improvement in prognosis; and Professor Ødegård, in his Maudsley Lecture of 1966 (published 1967), concluded that this amelioration had become apparent in the 1930s, a time when it could not easily be attributed to advances in treatment. There is, of course, well-documented evidence of changes in the *clinical manifestations* of schizophrenia.

During the past decade or two a great deal of research has suggested an association of schizophrenia—or one type of it—with pathological changes in the brain; and two aetiological hypotheses of a strictly environmental kind have been put forward, one implicating a dietary factor and the other an infective (viral) factor. The historical evidence, which I have suggested indicates a change in the incidence of a schizophrenia-like disorder in Britain during the nineteenth century, is certainly compatible with a somatic cause and may, I think, be considered as lending support to these aetiological hypotheses, particularly the infective one.

I am aware that the ideas I have put forward may seem speculative. What is clear, I think, is that in Britain during the second half of the nineteenth century the incidence of insanity, as measured by the asylum admission rate, showed a remarkable increase. The question then arises, how far this increase is to be explained in sociological terms, as the increasing admission of milder cases, and how far in medical terms as an epidemic of a mental disorder. In this essay I have wished only to suggest that a medical explanation of the asylum era is worth considering, as perhaps containing an element of truth. 'Truth', said Maudsley (1917) in his old age, 'is a pleasant abstraction, a visionary and ever-receding ideal to be pursued ... We shall not capture it; the joy lies in the pursuit.'

References

ARLIDGE, J. T. (1859) Review of the Twelfth Report of the Commissioners in Lunacy. *Journal of Mental Science*, **5**, 245–257.
—— (1862) Review of the Sixteenth Report of the Commissioners in Lunacy. *Journal of Mental Science*, **8**, 417–429.
ARNOLD, T. (1782) *Observations on the Nature of Insanity*, Vol. I, p. 27. Leicester: Ireland.
BLEULER, M. (1978) *The Schizophrenic Disorders: Long-term Patient and Family Studies*. New Haven: Yale U.P. (translated from the German by S. M. Clemens: first German edition 1972).
BOARD OF CONTROL (1914) *First Annual Report, for the year 1914*, Table VII. London: H.M.S.O. Page 33.
BOYD, R. (1871) Statistics of pauper insanity. *Journal of Mental Science*, **17**, 221–225.
BROWNE, C. (1871) quoted by Robertson, C. L. (1871) in: A further note on the alleged increase in lunacy. *Journal of Mental Science*, **16**, 473–497.
BRUSHFIELD, T. N. (1872) The alleged increase of insanity. *Journal of Mental Science*, **16**, 229.
BUCKNILL, J. C. (1855) Review of the Ninth Report of the Commissioners in Lunacy. *Journal of Mental Science*, **2**, 1–16.
CLOUSTON, T. S. (1891) Asylum reports. *Journal of Mental Science*, **37**, 598–599.

COMMISSIONERS IN LUNACY (1897) *Special Report on the Alleged Increase of Insanity*. London: H.M.S.O.

—— (1899) *Fifty-third Annual Report*, p. 10. London. H.M.S.O.

—— (1911) *Sixty-fifth Annual Report*, Chart No. 4. London: H.M.S.O.

CROWTHER, B. (1811) *Practical Remarks on Insanity*, p. v. London: Underwood.

DRAPES, T. (1894) On the alleged increase of insanity in Ireland. *Journal of Mental Science*, **40,** 519–561.

DUNHAM, H. W. (1971) Sociocultural studies in schizophrenia. *Archives of General Psychiatry*, **24,** 206–214.

EARLE, P. (1887) The curability of insanity. *American Journal of Insanity*, **33,** 483–533.

EATON, W. W. (1980) *The Sociology of Mental Disorders*, p. 174 *et seq*. New York: Praeger.

GOLDHAMER, H. & MARSHALL, A. W. (1953) *Psychosis and Civilization*. New York: Free Press.

GRANVILLE, J. M. (1877) *The Care and Cure of the Insane*, Vol. 2, p. 216. London: Hardwicke.

HALLORAN, W. (1810) *An Enquiry into the Causes Producing the Extraordinary Addition to the Numbers of the Insane*, pp. 9, 11. Cork: Edwards and Savage.

HARE, E. H. (1981) The two manias: a study of the evolution of the modern concept of mania. *British Journal of Psychiatry*, **138,** 89–99.

HARPER, A. (1789) *A Treatise on the Real Cause and Cure of Insanity*, p. 23. London: Stalker.

HASLAM, J. (1798) *Observations on Insanity*. London: Rivington.

HUMPHREYS, N. A. (1890) Statistics of insanity in England, with special reference to its alleged increasing prevalence. *Journal of the Royal Statistical Society*, **53,** 201–252.

JAMIESON, R. (1876) The increase of mental disease. *Journal of Mental Science*, **21,** 138–141.

JARVIS, E. (1852) On the supposed increase in insanity. *American Journal of Insanity*, **8,** 333–364.

JONES, K. (1955) *Lunacy, Law and Conscience 1744–1845*, pp. 116, 149. London: Routledge & Kegan Paul.

JONES, R. (1906) The evolution of insanity. *Journal of Mental Science*, **52,** 629–661.

JOURNAL OF MENTAL SCIENCE (1862) **7,** 534.

—— (1869) **15,** 557.

—— (1895) **41,** 498–512.

—— (1904) **50,** 797.

—— (1905) **51,** 733.

—— (1909) **55,** 96–112.

LANCET (1866) Increase of insanity, *Lancet*, **ii,** 675.

LUNIER, L. (1870) De l'augmentation progressive du chiffre des aliénés et de ses causes. *Annales Medico-Psychologiques*, **3** (5th series), 20–31.

MACCABE, F. (1869) On the alleged increase of insanity. *Journal of Mental Science*, **16,** 363–366.

MAUDSLEY, H. (1872) Is insanity on the increase? *British Medical Journal*, **i,** 36–39.

—— (1873) *Body and Mind*, p. 41. London: MacMillan.

—— (1877) The alleged increase of insanity. *Journal of Mental Science*, **23,** 45–54.

—— (1917) Optimism and pessimism. *Journal of Mental Science*, **63,** 1–16.

METROPOLITAN COMMISSIONERS IN LUNACY (1844) *Statistical Appendix to the Report of 1844*. London: H.M.S.O.

MORRISON, A. (1826) *Outlines of Lectures on Mental Diseases*, 2nd ed. pp. 65, 68. London: Longman.

ØDEGÅRD, Ø. (1967) Changes in the prognosis of functional psychoses since the days of Kraepelin. *British Journal of Psychiatry*, **113,** 813–822.

PARGETER, W. (1792) *Observations on Maniacal Disorders*, p. 1. London: Murray.

PERFECT, W. (1787) *Select Cases in the Different Species of Insanity, etc.* p. 118. London: Rochester.

PIERCE, B. (1919) Psychiatry 100 years ago: with comments on the problems today. *Journal of Mental Science*, **65,** 219–235.

PRICHARD, J. C. (1835) *A Treatise on Insanity and other Disorders Affecting the Mind*, p. 350. London: Sherwood.

RENAUDIN, E. (1861) Observations deduced from the statistics of the insane. *Journal of Mental Science*, **7,** 534–546.

ROBERTSON, C. L. (1869) The alleged increase of lunacy. *Journal of Mental Science*, **15,** 1–23.

—— (1871) A further note on the alleged increase in lunacy. *Journal of Mental Science*, **16,** 473–497.

ROBERTSON, GEORGE M. (1926) The prevalence of insanity—a preliminary survey of the problem. *Journal of Mental Science*, **72,** 455–491.

SANBORN, F. B. (1894) Is American insanity increasing? A study. *Journal of Mental Science*, **40,** 214–219.

SAVAGE, G. H. (1890) Discussion of Humphrey's paper. *Journal of the Royal Statistical Society*, **53,** 201–252.

SCULL, A. T. (1979) *Museums of Madness*, Chap. 6. London: Lane.

SWIFT, J. (1747) *A True Copy of the last Will and Testament of the Revd. Dr. Jonathan Swift.* Dublin: Bate.

TORREY, E. F. (1980) *Schizophrenia and Civilization,* Chap. 2. New York: Aronson.

TUKE, HARRINGTON (1873) Presidential address. *Journal of Mental Science,* **19,** 327–340 & 479–485.

TUKE, DANIEL HACK (1886) The alleged increase of insanity. *Journal of Mental Science,* **32,** 360–376.

—— (1894) Alleged increase of insanity. *Journal of Mental Science,* **40,** 219–231.

6 Was insanity increasing? A response to Edward Hare

ANDREW SCULL

One of the central paradoxes of the Victorian reforms in the treatment of the mentally ill was the curious fact that the 'scientific' discovery of mental illness and the adoption of a more rational approach based on this discovery—an approach which aimed at treating and curing the lunatic, rather than neglecting him or incarcerating him in a gaol or workhouse—were associated with an explosive growth in the number of insane people. **Hare** (**1983**) raises again the interesting question of whether or not this reflects a true increase in the incidence of mental illness in nineteenth century England. As he correctly notes, the aggregate data collected at the time do not allow a 'decisive answer', but I am pleased that his reassessment of the probabilities led him to endorse my prior conclusion that its incidence was indeed increasing (Scull, 1979).

Hare does dispute, however, the explanation I offered of this increase, which attributed much of it to the development of a more expansive view of madness. Instead of an expansion of the boundaries of what constituted mental illness, he argues that the growth in numbers reflects a real rise in the most serious forms of mental disorder, more specifically, 'a slow epidemic of schizophrenia' (**Hare, 1983**). The dispute between us is not purely an academic debate (in the bad sense of that term) since Hare argues that the adoption of his explanation provides some 'speculative' support for 'a medical explanation of the asylum era', and for a viral aetiology of schizophrenia (**Hare, 1983**). I should therefore like to point to some of the evidence which seems instead to favour my own hypothesis, recognizing (as does Hare) that in this matter we can at best obtain an approximation of the truth, given the data with which we have to work.

At least prior to the adoption of *DSM-III* in 1980, the research evidence demonstrates that even twentieth century psychiatric diagnoses lacked reliability and validity. Diagnosis remained dependent upon clinical supposition and consensus, with the consequence that 'the reliability of diagnoses of mental disorders, including those considered the most severe, measured by independent rater agreement, often failed to rise over 50 per cent' (Morse, 1982; see also Spitzer and Fleiss, 1974; Beck, 1962; Chapman and Chapman, 1969). Everything we know of the practice of nineteenth century psychiatrists suggests an even stronger reliance upon clinical experience to legitimize and certify the authenticity of the individual practitioners' decisions. Certainly, many of the leading men in the field devoted a good deal of their energies to the elaboration of complex nosologies, encompassing a plethora of sub-types and varieties of insanity, but as Henry Monro (1850) noted, those who tried to rely on these categories in their practice were soon obliged to abandon the attempt in despair:

All who have charge of asylums must well know how very different the clear and distinct classification of books is from that medley of symptoms which is presented by real cases ... It is useless to attempt to paint pictures with more vivid colours than nature presents, and worse than useless if practical men (or rather, I would say, men obliged to practice) receive these pictures as true representatives.

Notwithstanding all efforts to alleviate the situation, and with the exception of extreme cases of violent mania or complete dementia, alienists were forced to confess that 'the task of declaring this to be reason and that insanity is exceedingly embarassing and, to a great degree, arbitrary .. . no palpable distinction exists, no line of demarcation can be traced between the sane and the insane' (Browne, 1837). Thus, 'the practitioner's own mind must be the criterion by which he infers the insanity of any other person' (Haslam, 1809; see also Mayo, 1854).

'Such emphasis,' as Freidson (1970) has noted, 'is directly contrary to the emphasis of science on shared knowledge, collected and tested on the basis of methods meant to overcome the deficiencies of individual experience. And its efficacy and reliability are suspect.' In this instance, beyond the initial hard core of easily recognizable behavioural and/or mental disturbance, the boundary between the pathological and the normal was left extraordinarily vague and indeterminate. Hence the frequent and embarrassing disputes between alienists over individual cases in the courts (Smith, 1981). In the circumstances, the assumption that identifying who is and who is not mentally ill was an activity governed by some uniform, objective, and unchanging standard will not survive critical scrutiny.

As **Hare** (**1983**) notes, I have suggested that asylum doctors' professional self-interest provided one set of motives for the adoption of an expansionary view of madness. But other forces also prompted them to behave in this fashion. On humanitarian grounds, for example, since doctors were convinced that asylums were benevolent and therapeutic institutions, and believed that laymen were incompetent to cope with, and liable to maltreat the mentally ill, they were impelled to seek out still more cases rather than reject any who were proffered. Moreover, professional 'imperialism' provides only one—and to my mind by no means that most important—reason to suspect an ever-wider practical application of the term mental illness. The asylum provided a convenient and culturally legitimate alternative to coping with 'intolerable' individuals within the family, offering, if its proponents were to be believed, a level of care and possibilities of cure far beyond what even the most dedicated family could hope to provide in its midst. So far from being blamed, families were encouraged to place their mentally unbalanced relatives where they could receive professional care and treatment at the earliest possible moment. The attraction was obviously greatest for those with fewer resources for coping with the dependent and economically unproductive. Significantly, the statistics demonstrate that by far the largest portion of the increase in insanity occurred among those drawn from the lowest socio-economic classes.

Contemporary observers frequently commented on the dynamics of this process: the superintendent of the Northampton General Lunatic Asylum noted in his 1858 report that 'persons in humble life soon become wearied of the presence of their insane relatives and regardless of their age desire relief. Persons above this class more readily tolerate infirmity and command time and attention. The occasion may never occur in the one case, which is urgent in the other. Hence an Asylum to the poor and needy is the only refuge. To the man of many friends it is the last resort.' In the words of another asylum superintendent, 'Poverty, truly, is the great evil: it has no friends able to help. Persons in middle society do not put away their aged relatives because of their infirmities, and I think it was not always the custom for worn out paupers to be sent to the asylum ... It is one more of the ways in which, at this day, the apparent increase of insanity is sustained. It is not a real increase, since the aged have ever been subject to this sort of unsoundness' (Huxley, quoted in Arlidge, 1859).

One should note, moreover, that the level of disordered behaviour or dependency that a family could not or would not put up with was not fixed and immutable, but likely to vary over time, with individual circumstances and with the gradual growth of the perception that there existed alternatives to the retention of the disturbed and troublesome within a domestic setting. (Such a pattern is, however, much more difficult to reconcile with the hypothesis of a viral-induced epidemic of schizophrenia.) Finally, as Maudsley (1877) himself suggested, the central government contributed significantly to the process by enacting legislation 'whereby the government said in effect, to parish officials, "We will pay you a premium of four shillings a head on every pauper whom you can by hook or crook make out to be a lunatic and send into an asylum" [thus putting] a direct premium on the manufacture of lunacy.'

Hare makes much of the fact that recovery rates declined over time in Victorian asylums, arguing that 'milder' cases should have been more likely to recover. It is, however, not at all clear why we should accept this argument. First, there is no obvious warrant for the claim that Victorian psychiatry was more successful in treating milder cases (unless one tautologically assumes an identity between 'milder' and 'more treatable'). Indeed, 'mild' mental symptoms often co-existed with chronic and incurable underlying disease states. Bucknill, for example, while superintendent at the Devon County Asylum, found that:

Patients have been admitted suffering from heart disease, aneurism, and cancer, with scarcely a greater amount of melancholy than might be expected to take place in many sane persons at the near and certain prospect of death. Some have been received in the last stages of consumption, with that amount of cerebral excitement so common in this disorder; others have been received in the delirium or stupor of typhus; while in several cases the mental condition was totally unknown after admission, and must have been unknown before, since an advanced condition of bodily disease prevented speech, and the expression of intelligence or emotion, either normal or morbid. [quoted in Arlidge, 1859]

Second, there are other, at least equally plausible ways of accounting for the decline. Many Victorian critics of the asylum system, including Maudsley himself, thought that there was a clear connection between increasing size and decreasing therapeutic efficacy. As John Arlidge put it:

In a colossal refuge for the insane, a person may be said to lose his individuality and to become a member of a machine so put together, as to move with precise regularity and invariable routine; a triumph of skill adapted to show how such unpromising materials as crazy men and women may be drilled into order and guided by rule, but not an apparatus calculated to restore their pristine condition and their independent self-governing existence. In all cases admitting of recovery, or of material amelioration, a gigantic asylum is a gigantic evil, and figuratively speaking, a manufactory of chronic insanity. (Arlidge, 1859; see also Bucknill, 1880).

Modern research on 'institutionalism' (Wing, 1962; Wing and Brown, 1970; Barton, 1965; Belknap, 1956; Stanton and Schwartz, 1954) surely lends considerable credence to this hypothesis. And we know that the average size of English county asylums rose remorselessly through the course of the nineteenth century, from just over a hundred patients in 1827 to almost a thousand by the end of the century, paralleling the development of a steadily more hopeless and 'institutional' environment. Increasingly, within such mammoth institutions, 'the classification generally made is for the purpose of shelving cases; that is to say, practically it has that effect ... in consequence of the treatment not being personal, but simply a treatment in classes, there is a tendency to make whole classes sink down into a sort of chronic state ... I think they come under a sort of routine discipline which ends in their passing into a state of dementia' (Granville, in House of Commons, 1877).

Almost certainly, then, increasing size and the associated changes in the treatment of the inmate population had negative effects on cure rates. In turn, this provoked a steadily more pessimistic assessment of the prognosis for insanity among alienists themselves, forced to account for the falling rate of cures despite the advances of medical science. As explanations of mental illness were ever more frequently couched in terms of structural brain disease, defective heredity, and Morelian degeneration, so there emerged an entrenched expectation that most cases of mental illness would prove to be incurable. Expectations of this sort, through their effects on staff morale and the quality of care provided (to say nothing of the negative placebo effect), became a relentlessly self-fulfilling prophecy, further diminishing the underlying recovery rate while providing tautological 'proof' of their essential accuracy. I suggest it is this combination of factors rather than 'the admission of less favourable cases' (Commissioners in Lunacy, 1899, quoted in **Hare, 1983**) which accounts for the dismal therapeutic results of late nineteenth century asylum care— though for obvious reasons this was a conclusion that both the psychiatric profession and the Commissioners in Lunacy were reluctant even to consider.

Beyond this, a good deal of contemporary testimony supports my suggestion that the boundaries of what constituted committable madness expanded over the course of the nineteenth century. A wide range of nineteenth century observers commented on how much laxer the standards were for judging a poor person to be insane, and how much readier both local poor law authorities and lower class families were to commit decrepit and troublesome people to the asylum, individuals who, had they come from the middle and upper classes, would never have been diagnosed as insane. In the words of William Ley, superintendent of the Littlemore Asylum, 'Orders for the admission of Paupers into the County Asylum are given more freely than would be thought right as regards the imputation of Lunacy, towards persons equally debilitated in body and mind who have the means of providing for their own care' (Littlemore Asylum Annual Report, 1855). Over time, this tendency grew more marked. Just over twenty years later, John Joseph Henley, the General Inspector of the Local Government Board, informed a Select Committee of the House of Commons that in his inspectors' experience 'there is a disposition among all classes now not to bear with the troubles they may arise in their own houses. If a person is troublesome from senile dementia, dirty in his habits, they will not bear it now. Persons are more easily removed to an asylum than they were a few years ago' (House of Commons, 1877). Workhouse authorities, too, according to the medical inspector of the London workhouses, routinely used asylums to 'relieve their wards of many old people who are suffering from nothing else than the natural failing of old age' as well as to rid themselves of troublesome people in general (House of Commons, 1877; see also Commissioners in Lunacy Annual Report, 1861).

As a result, as Mortimer Granville (1877) noted, 'it is impossible not to recognize the presence of a considerable number of 'patients' in these asylums who are not lunatic. They may be weak, dirty, troublesome, but they are certainly no[t] ... affected with mental disease.' Those who had been acquainted with the county asylum system from its very earliest years could not help but notice the change in the implicit definition of mental illness, the enormous and striking difference 'between the inmates of the old madhouses and the modern asylum—the former containing only obvious and dangerous cases of lunacy, the latter containing great numbers of quiet and harmless patients whose insanity is often difficult to determine' (Bucknill, 1880). At least for these well placed observers, there could be no question but that:

... the law providing that madmen, dangerous to themselves and others, shall be secluded in madhouses for absolutely needful care and protection, has been extended in its application to large classes of persons who would never have been considered lunatics when this legislation was entered upon. Since 1845, medical science has discovered whole new realms of lunacy, and the nicer touch of a finikin civilization has shrunk from the contact of imperfect fellow-creatures, and thus the manifold receptacles of lunacy are filled to overflow with a population more nearly resembling that which is still at large. [Bucknill, 1880]

Hare argues that mild cases could not have provided the reservoir from which the increased asylum population was drawn, because such cases would not have seemed sufficiently urgent to warrant the construction of so many beds. But the definition of 'urgent' in this case is obviously a matter of complex social definition, not something engraved in stone. I see no reason to doubt that those committing patients in 1880 were convinced that their reasons for doing so were urgent and compelling—though one may reasonably question whether the same justifications would have seemed equally compelling some thirty or forty years earlier. Nor should it surprise us that what constituted adequate grounds for commitment should shift over time in this fashion. After all, the past quarter of a century has witnessed a move in just the reverse direction, towards a much more restricted view of the appropriate criteria for involuntary commitment (Scull, 1984).

Comment

Ultimately, of course, the most satisfactory way of deciding between the rival hypothesis offered by Hare and myself would be to look at a random sampling of admissions over time, to see whether the increase occurs among mild or severe cases. Unfortunately, there must be serious doubt about whether the quality of the records that have survived is adequate for this purpose. Case records for upper class asylums were extensive, as in the Ticehurst Asylum casebooks now at the Wellcome Institute. But, as Hare notes, almost none of the increase in the incidence of mental illness occurred among private patients, so that for our present purposes, these materials are unlikely to be very helpful. On the other hand, precisely because the county asylums were so overcrowded, and were filled with paupers, their individual case records are generally too skimpy to be useful for answering this question.

I would suggest, however, that the class-specific pattern of the increase in insanity does pose certain difficulties (though I grant these are not necessarily of an insuperable sort) for Hare's argument. Somehow, the slow epidemic of schizophrenia was a *class-specific* epidemic, so that on top of the highly speculative claim that it had a viral origin, one must add the further hypothesis that the upper classes—whether for constitutional or environmental reasons—were mysteriously immune to its ravages.

It may well be that we shall have to be satisfied with an assessment of the general plausibility of each argument, and the extent to which it makes sense of the wide variety of data and observations that *have* survived. However, since Hare felt free to draw on comparative data to buttress his case, perhaps I may be allowed to do the same. The one careful study we possess of the composition of asylum populations in this period is Fox's examination of legal commitments in California between 1906 and 1929 (1978). Using a random sample of commitments from San Francisco in this period, Fox demonstrates that:

Two thirds of those committed were odd, peculiar, or simply immoral individuals who displayed no symptoms indicating serious disability, or violent or destructive tendencies. The reported behavior of this 66 per cent included primarily nervous and depressive symptoms and a wide variety of fears, beliefs, perceptions, and delusions. In these cases the examiners noted that behaviors which they and various witnesses deemed inappropriate, but failed to indicate any reason why the individual, for his own protection or that of the community, had to be detained.

It goes almost without saying that this finding accords very well with my hypothesis and provides little or no support for Hare's.

References

ARLIDGE, J. T. (1859) *On the State of Lunacy and the Legal Provision for the Insane*. London: Churchill.
BARTON, R. (1965) *Institutional Neurosis*, 2nd edition. Bristol: Wright.
BECK, A. T. (1962) The reliability of psychiatric diagnosis: 1. A critique of systematic studies. *American Journal of Psychiatry*, **119**, 210–216.
BELKNAP, I. (1956) *Human Problems of a State Mental Hospital*. New York: McGraw Hill.
BROWNE, W. A. F. (1837) *What Asylums Were, Are, and Ought to Be*. Edinburgh: Black.
BUCKNILL, J. C. (1880) *The Care of the Insane and their Legal Control*. London: Macmillan.

CHAPMAN, L. J. & CHAPMAN, J. P. (1969) Illusory correlations as an obstacle to the use of valid psycho-diagnosis signs. *Journal of Abnormal Psychology*, **74**, 271–280.

COMMISSIONERS IN LUNACY (1861) *Annual Reports to the Lord Chancellor.*

Fox, R. W. (1978) *So Far Disordered in Mind.* Berkeley: University of California Press.

FREIDSON, E. (1970) *Profession of Medicine: A Study in the Sociology of Applied Knowledge.* New York: Dodd, Mead.

GRANVILLE, J. M. (1877) *The Care and Cure of the Insane*, 2 Vols. London: Hardewicke and Bogue.

HARE, E. (1983) Was insanity on the increase? *British Journal of Psychiatry*, **142**, 439–455.

HASLAM, J. (1809) *Observations on Madness and Melancholy*, 2nd edition. London: Callow.

HOUSE OF COMMONS (1877) *Report of the Select Committee on the Operation of the Lunacy Law.* London.

LITTLEMORE (OXFORDSHIRE) COUNTY LUNATIC ASYLUM (1855) *Annual Reports.*

MAUDSLEY, H. (1867) *The Physiology and Pathology of Mind.* London: Macmillan.

—— (1877) The alleged increase of insanity. *Journal of Mental Science*, **23**, 45–54.

MAYO, T. (1854) *Medical Testimony and Evidence in Cases of Lunacy.* London: Parker.

MONRO, H. (1850) *Remarks on Insanity, Its Nature and Treatment.* London: Churchill.

MORSE, S. J. (1982) A preference for liberty: The case against involuntary commitment of the mentally disordered. In *The Court of Last Resort: Mental Illness and the Law* (ed. C. A. B. Warren). Chicago: University of Chicago Press.

SCULL, A. (1984) The Theory and Practice of Civil Commitment. *University of Michigan Law Review* (Winter).

—— (1979) *Museums of Madness.* London: Allen Lane.

SMITH, R. (1981) *Trial by Medicine: Insanity and Responsibility in Victorian Trials.* Edinburgh University Press.

SPITZER, R. L. & FLEISS, J. (1974) A re-analysis of the reliability of psychiatric diagnosis. *British Journal of Psychiatry*, **125**, 341–347.

STANTON, A. H. & SCHWARTZ, M. S. (1954) *The Mental Hospital: A Study of Institutional Participation in Psychiatric Illness and Treatment.* New York: Basic Books.

WING, J. K. (1962) Institutionalism in mental hospitals. *British Journal of Social and Clinical Psychiatry*, **1**, 38.

—— & BROWN, G. W. (1970) *Institutionalism and Schizophrenia.* Cambridge University Press.

7 Schizophrenia: The sacred symbol of psychiatry

THOMAS S. SZASZ

Let us try to project ourselves back into the places and minds of physicians and psychiatrists in, say, 1900. When they spoke of disease, what did they mean? They meant, typically, something like syphilis. 'Know syphilis in all its manifestations and relations,' declared Sir William Osler (1849–1919), 'and all things clinical will be added unto you.' (Osler, quoted in Strauss, 1968). Obviously this is no longer true. Indeed, how many cases of syphilis do modern medical students see between the time they enroll in school and the time they graduate? In the United States, Osler's maxim has been replaced by another which asserts that 'mental illness is our number one health problem'. This would make schizophrenia—the most common and most disabling of the so-called mental diseases—the successor of Osler's syphilis, showing us immediately what a gulf separates us from him. For clearly, a physician may know all there is to know about schizophrenia, and yet be totally ignorant of medicine.

Still, the fascination which this medical image has exercised on the minds of psychiatrists, and hence its power over them, can hardly be exaggerated. At a 1974 international symposium on schizophrenia, Marvin Herz, Associate Professor of Clinical Psychiatry at Columbia University, is quoted as having alluded to 'the observation of Chicago psychiatrist Roy Grinker, who recalled at a recent meeting on schizophrenia that, as a young man, he had been told that if he knew schizophrenia, he would know psychiatry: "Well, the fact is that today I still don't know psychiatry," he confessed somewhat ruefully' (Herz, 1975).

The Oslerian image thus points to a lesson we forget at our own peril. That lesson is the agreement among modern physicians *qua* medical scientists that they must distinguish between complaints and lesions, between being a patient and having a disease; and the resolution to regard as diseases only those processes occurring in the body (human or animal) which they can identify, measure, and demonstrate in an objective, physico-chemical manner. This was one of the reasons why syphilis was the turn-of-the-century medical paradigm of disease. Another was that it was common. And a third was that the syphilitic infection could affect countless organs and body parts, causing discrete lesions which could be appropriately named, all of which were, nevertheless, due to, and were manifestations of, the general systemic disease called 'syphilis'. Thanks to the work of numerous medical investigators around the turn of the century, physicians finally grasped that such totally dissimilar biological phenomena as the genital chancre of primary syphilis, the dermatitis of secondary syphilis, and the general paralysis of the insane of tertiary syphilis were actually all different manifestations of the same disease process, called 'syphilis'.

What made these monumental medical discoveries important, besides the prophylactic and therapeutic benefits for which they were essential, was that they paved the way toward establishing the empirical and epistemological criteria for judging whether or not a person had syphilis (or any other disease). In other words, with the development of clear-cut anatomical, histological, biochemical, immunological, and clinical criteria for syphilis, it was possible to say not only that certain persons hitherto unsuspected of this disease were in fact syphilitics, but that others, suspected of it, were not.

These developments were of the most far-reaching importance for physicians, including psychiatrists, working at that time. By about 1900, European psychiatry was a well-established medical specialty. Its respectability, both scientifically and politically, thus depended on the medical perspective—perhaps we ought to say medical premise—that the psychiatrist's patients, like those of the surgeon or internist, suffered from diseases. The difference, in this view, between the non-psychiatric and the psychiatric patients was that whereas the diseases of the former caused them to have fevers and pains, those of the latter caused them to have hallucinations and delusions (Szasz, 1961). 'Mental diseases are brain diseases,' is the way Theodor Meynert (1833–1892), Freud's professor at the Medical School in Vienna, had put it. To Meynert it was clear that disease meant anatomical abnormality, and accordingly he searched for and postulated such abnormalities to account for all so-called mental diseases (Meynert, 1890). His 'vasomotor theory,' writes Zilboorg, '... permitted Meynert to offer a classification of mental diseases on a purely anatomical basis' (1941). Meynert thus sought to reduce psychiatry to neurology; revealingly, he objected not only to psychological explanations of so-called psychiatric illnesses, but even to the term 'psychiatry' itself.

The discovery of the syphilitic origin of paresis was a brilliant scientific confirmation of this organic-psychiatric hypothesis—namely, that persons whose brains are abnormal are likely to exhibit behaviour commonly judged to be abnormal. With paresis as its paradigm, psychiatry became the diagnosis, study, and treatment of 'mental diseases'—that is, of abnormal biological processes within the patient's head manifested by the psychological and social 'symptoms' of his illness. Psychiatry—whether organic or not, as Freud and his followers have subscribed to this model as slavishly as their organic opponents—thus became fatefully tied to medicine and its core concepts of illness and treatment. It is necessary that we should understand exactly how this happened.

There are experiences we may read about and know about intellectually, but cannot, without going through them personally, appreciate in their full human impact. People who are well cannot, in this sense, grasp what it is to be desperately ill; or those who are rich, what it is to be desperately poor.

In the same way, people—physicians and non-physicians alike—cannot now grasp the impact which neurosyphilis had exerted on modern institutional psychiatry during the crucial first four decades of its existence, that is, between 1900 and 1940. Most psychiatrists now practising in the major industrial socie- ties never see a patient with neurosyphilis. Many physicians have never seen one in their whole lives. For medical students, the disease has already become as legendary—in the sense of esoteric and extinct—as leprosy had been gener- ations ago.

It is against this contemporary background that we must re-inspect the frequency and reconsider the role of neurosyphilis during the formative decades of modern psychiatry. Until the advent of penicillin in the 1940s, a large propor- tion of patients admitted to mental institutions, throughout the world, suffered from general paresis. Here are some illustrative figures. In the mental hospital Dalldorf, in Berlin, between 1892 and 1902, from 22 to 32 per cent of the patients, both men and women, had paresis. At the Central State Hospital, in Indianapolis, Indiana, between 1927 and 1931, from 20 to 25 per cent of the newly-admitted patients were paretics. At the Tokyo Insane Hospital in 1930, 30 per cent of the patients admitted were paretics (Breutsch, 1959). And so it went throughout the world.

Is it any wonder, then, that in 1917 the great Kraepelin asserted, and no psychiatrist or psychoanalyst doubted, that:

The nature of most mental disorders is now obscured. But no one will deny that further research will uncover new facts in so young a science as ours; in this respect the diseases produced by syphilis are an object lesson. It is logical to assume that we shall succeed in uncovering the causes of many other types of insanity that can be prevented—perhaps even cured—though at present we have not the slightest clue ... [Kraepelin, 1917]

And is it any wonder, also, that the paradigm of paresis was deeply imprinted into the mind and memory of psychiatry? And that psychiatry still speaks with the accents of neurosyphilis on its lips? Or, to vary the metaphor, it is as if paresis had been a traumatic event, or indeed a series of such events, in the childhood of psychiatry. Now, while asleep, psychiatry still dreams about it; and while awake, it sees the world as if the spectre of paresis lurked behind every foolish face or troubled thought. Thus has the image of the crooked spirochaete making people mad been replaced, in the minds of many psychia- trists, by the image of the crooked molecule making them mad.

Viewed against this historical background, the story of the origin of the modern concepts of dementia praecox and schizophrenia appears, to me at least, in a quite different light from that in which it is usually presented.

The officially accepted form of this story is, briefly, that in the second half of the nineteenth century medical scientists began to be able to identify the precise morphological character and the material causes of many diseases; and that this led quickly to effective methods of prevention, treatment, and cure for some of these diseases. For example, physicians learned to identify many of the infectious diseases and their causes: puerperal fever, tuberculosis, syphilis, gonorrhoea, diphtheria, and so forth; they also learned to prevent and treat some of them. According to this version of the history of psychiatry, as some medical investigators discovered and identified diphtheria, so others— in particular, Bleuler—discovered and identified schizophrenia.

As I see it, this is not what happened at all. It is true, of course, that around the turn of the last century medical investigators discovered and identified a host of diseases—in particular, the major infectious diseases of that age. But it is not true that psychiatric investigators discovered and identified certain other diseases—in particular, dementia praecox, schizophrenia, or other so-called functional psychoses (or neuroses). Psychiatrists made no discoveries according to which the people allegedly suffering from these diseases would have qualified by Virchow's criteria—which were then the only ones that counted—as having a disease.

It cannot be emphasized enough, in this connection, that until Rudolf Virchow's (1821–1902) great work, *Die Cellularpathologie* (1858), the concept of disease was abstract and theoretical, rather than concrete and empirical; and that it became abstract and theoretical again with the introduction of psychopathological, psychoanalytic, psychosomatic, and psychodynamic concepts and terms into nosology (Virchow, 1974; Ackerknecht, 1953).

Before Virchow, the model of disease was 'humoral pathology'; since him, it has been 'cellular pathology'. More precisely, until about 1800, diseases were supposed to be due to an imbalance of the four fluid humours of the body—that is, blood, phlegm, yellow bile and black bile. This concept dated back to the ancient Greeks. In 1761, Giovanni Morgagni, an Italian anatomist, showed that diseases were due not to an imbalance of humours but to lesions in organs. Around 1800, Xavier Bichat, a French anatomist, demonstrated that the human body was composed of 21 different kinds of tissues, and suggested that in a diseased organ only some of its tissues might be affected. It was, however, not until 1858, when Virchow delivered his famous twenty lectures, published as *Die Cellularpathologie in ihrer Bergründung auf physiologische und pathologische Gewerbelehre* (*Cellular Pathology Based on Physiological and Pathological Histology*), that the model of disease as cellular pathology was firmly established. According to this view, 'disease of the body is a disease of cells. The cure of the body may be effected by curing the cells. The real question which the modern scientific physician puts to himself when called to treat a case is: what cells are out of order and what can be done for them?' (Virchow, 1935). This has been, and remains still, the basic concept and model of disease in Western countries and in scientific discourse throughout the world.

In short, Kraepelin and Bleuler discovered no histopathological lesions or pathophysiological processes in their patients. Instead, they acted *as if* they had discovered such lesions or processes; named their 'patients' accordingly; and committed themselves and their followers to the goal of establishing a precise identification of the 'organic' nature and cause of these diseases. In other words, Kraepelin and Bleuler did not discover the diseases for which they are famous; they invented them.

Because of the dominating role and importance of schizophrenia in modern psychiatry, it is easy to fall into the trap of believing that schizophrenia has always been an important problem in this field, and in the world. This is simply not so.

Actually, the concept of dementia praecox, as we now know it, was invented by Emil Kraepelin (1855–1926) in 1898. He has since been hailed as a great medical scientist, as if he had discovered a new disease or developed a new treatment; in fact, he did neither. What he did, according to Arieti—who is very respectful of his achievement—was this: 'Kraepelin's insight consisted in including three conditions under one syndrome' (Arieti, 1959). The three 'conditions' were catatonia, originally described by Karl Ludwig Kahlbaum (1828–1899); hebephrenia, partially described by Ewald Hecker (1843–1909); and 'vesania typica', or hallucinations and delusions, also previously described by Kahlbaum. The point I want to emphasize here is that each of these terms refers to behaviour, not disease; to disapproved conduct, not to histopathological change; hence, they may loosely be called 'conditions', but they are not, strictly speaking, medical conditions. If none of these three items is a disease, putting them together still does not add up to a disease. Nevertheless, the unpleasantness of the persons who displayed such 'psychotic' behaviour, the actual or seeming social incapacity of the 'patients', and the academic-scientific prestige of physicians such as Kraepelin sufficed to establish dementia praecox as a disease whose histopathology, aetiology, and treatment now awaited only the further flowering of medical science.

Before such developments could occur, the disease was put on even firmer footing. Its name was changed from Latin to Greek, that is, from 'dementia praecox' to 'schizophrenia'. And its incidence—that is, its epidemiological significance—was increased with the stroke of a pen. All this was done by Eugen Bleuler (1857–1939) who, again according to Arieti (1959):

> ... accepted the fundamental nosologic concept of Kraepelin but enlarged it to a great extent, because he considered as related to dementia praecox many other conditions such as psychosis with psychopathic personalities, alcoholic hallucinoses, etc. Furthermore, he thought that the largest number of patients are never hospitalized because their symptoms are not severe enough; that is, they are latent cases.

The imagery and vocabulary of syphilology are unmistakable here: 'severe cases' requiring confinement, and 'latent cases' lurking about without the patient realizing that he is ill. Since Bleuler, too, neither discovered a new disease nor developed a new treatment, his fame rests, in my opinion, on having invented a new disease—and, through it, a new justification for regarding the psychiatrist as a physician, the schizophrenic as a patient, and the place where the former confines the latter as a hospital.

Still, the question remained: just what was schizophrenia? Eugen Bleuler answered this question—at least to the satisfaction of most psychiatrists, past and present.

Before 1900, psychiatrists believed that paresis was due to bad heredity, alcoholism, smoking and masturbation. These beliefs are now only of historical interest, like the belief in demonic possession or exorcism. We celebrate and credit with discoveries the physicians—Alzheimer, Schaudinn, Wassermann, Noguchi and Moore—whose work demonstrated irrefutably that paresis was due to syphilis.

Today, psychiatrists believe that schizophrenia is similarly due to an organic disease of the brain. Batchelor's phrasing is illustrative: 'Both Kraepelin and

Bleuler believed that schizophrenia was the outcome of a pathological, anatomical, or chemical disturbance of the brain' (1969). But why, we might ask, should we care about what Kraepelin and Bleuler *believed*? Bleuler also believed in abstaining from alcohol and in the symbolic rather than literal interpretation of the Eucharist. These beliefs of Bleuler's are of no more consequence for the histology of schizophrenia than are Fleming's religious beliefs or disbeliefs for the therapeutic powers of penicillin. Why, then, do psychiatrists continue to record Kraepelin's and Bleuler's *beliefs* regarding the nature of schizophrenia? Why do they not emphasize instead Kraepelin's and Bleuler's utter inability to support their beliefs with a shred of relevant—that is, medical, histopathological—*evidence*?

Actually, Kraepelin and Bleuler were psychiatric clinicians, not medical investigators. Hence, they were not in a favourable position to generate any truly relevant evidence in support of their beliefs regarding the aetiology or pathology of schizophrenia. Instead, what they, and especially Bleuler, did was subtly to redefine the criterion of disease, from histopathology to psychopathology—that is, from abnormal bodily structure to abnormal personal behaviour. Since it was unquestionably true that most people confined in mental hospitals 'misbehaved', this opened the road toward charting the maps of psychopathology, thus identifying 'existing' mental diseases and 'discovering' new ones. It will repay us to review exactly how Bleuler achieved this scientific sleight of hand. My following quotations are from *Dementia Praecox or the Group of Schizophrenias*, published in 1911. Here is the definition of schizophrenia in Bleuler's original words:

> By the term 'dementia praecox' or 'schizophrenia' we designate a group of psychoses whose course is at times chronic, at times marked by intermittent attacks, and which can stop or retrograde at any stage, but does not permit a full *restitutio ad integrum*. The disease is characterized by a specific type of alteration of thinking ...

But 'alteration of thinking' is, from a strictly medical or physico-chemical, point of view, an irrelevant event. The fact that paresis is a brain disease could never have been established by studying the paretic's thinking. Then why study the schizophrenic's? Not, it seems to me, in order to prove that he is sick; that has already been established by the *presumption* of psychiatric authority whose power neither patient nor layman can match, and which no colleague dares to challenge. The schizophrenic's thinking is thus anatomized and pathologized in order to create a science of psychopathology, and then of psychoanalysis and psychodynamics, all of which serve to legitimize the madman as a medical (psychiatric) patient, and the alienist as a medical (psychiatric) doctor.

Throughout his book, Bleuler emphasizes that the schizophrenic patient suffers from a 'thinking disorder' manifested by a 'language disorder'. His book is full of illustrations of the remarks, pleas, letters, and other linguistic productions of so-called schizophrenic patients. He offers many comments about language, of which the following is typical:

> Blocking, poverty of ideas, incoherence, clouding, delusions, and emotional anomalies are expressed in the language of the patients. However, the abnormality does not lie in the language itself, but rather in its content. [Bleuler, 1911]

Here, and elsewhere, Bleuler goes to great lengths to protect himself against creating the impression that in describing a schizophrenic patient he is merely describing someone who speaks oddly or differently from the way he does, and with whom he disagrees. He never ceases to emphasize that this is not the case, that, on the contrary, the 'patient' is sick and his linguistic behaviour is only a 'symptom' of his 'illness'.

Thus, slowly and subtly, but surely indeed, Bleuler, Freud and Jung—and the other pioneer psychopathologists and psychoanalysts—brought about the great epistemological transformation of our medical age: from histopathology to psychopathology. It is now all too unappreciated how closely these three men worked together in the crucial few years before the outbreak of the First World War, and how intimately intertwined were the earliest developments of psychoanalysis and psychopathology. The first psychoanalytic journal, published in 1909, bore the title: *Jahrbuch für Psychoanalytische und Psychopathologische Forschungen* (*Yearbook for Psychoanalytic and Psychopathologic Investigations*). Its publishers were Eugen Bleuler and Sigmund Freud, and its editor was Carl Jung. Bleuler was then the professor of psychiatry, and Jung a *Privatdozent*, at the University of Zürich Medical School. The lead article in that issue was Freud's 'Analysis of a phobia in a five-year-old boy', which became known as the case of 'Little Hans' (McGuire, 1974).

Freud's fondness for pathologizing psychology—that is, life itself—had, of course, been clearly revealed eight years earlier in his popular work *The Psychopathology of Everyday Life* (1901). It was there that Freud developed, first and most fully, in James Strachey's words, 'his [Freud's] belief in the universal application of determinism to mental events. This is the truth which he insists upon in the final chapter of the book ...' (Strachey, 1960). Concepts such as 'idea', 'choice', and 'decision' all become, in Freud's hands, 'events', and all are 'determined'. 'I believe', he writes, 'in external (real) chance, it is true, but not in internal (psychical) accidental events.' (Freud, 1901). Thus have Bleuler and Freud transformed our image and idea of illness, and our vocabulary for describing and defining it: they had displaced lesion by language, disease by disagreement, pathophysiology by psychohistory—and, generally, histopathology by psychopathology.

Modern psychiatry began with the study of paresis and the efforts to cure it. It soon turned into the study of psychopathology and the efforts to control it. It has now become, the world over, the study of misbehaviour and the efforts to manage it. And schizophrenia is its sacred symbol—the largest grab-bag of all the misbehaviours which psychiatrists, coerced by society or convinced by their own zeal, are now ready to diagnose, prognose, and therapize. This ceremonial role of schizophrenia in psychiatry, indeed in the world at large, is illustrated by the publication, and the contents, of the prestigious *International Pilot Study of Schizophrenia* conducted under the auspices of the World Health Organization (1973).

The authors of this study list the following four characteristics—they call them 'inclusion criteria'—which, when observed about, or attributed to, a person by a psychiatrist, qualify that person as a schizophrenic: '(1) Delusions.

(2) Definitely inappropriate or unusual behaviour. (3) Hallucinations. (4) Gross psychomotor disorder; over- and under-activity. ... Inclusion criteria 1–4 automatically qualified the patient for inclusion, regardless of the severity of the symptomatology' (WHO, 1973).

We had better laugh at this, lest we weep. The briefest critical scrutiny of this list makes its scientific and medical pretensions vanish—like the frightened child's ghost dispelled by flicking on the light in the bedroom.

Delusions: We know what they are: believing that you are one of the Chosen People; or that Jesus is the son of God, who died, but is still alive; or that gold will always be worth $35 (US) an ounce.

Inappropriate or unusual behaviour: Well, we know that, too, when we see it: attacking Pearl Harbour, or invading Vietnam; having long hair or short hair or no hair; setting yourself on fire, committing hara-kiri, or jumping off the Golden Gate Bridge.

Hallucinations: No problem here, either: communicating with deities or dead people (and being unsuccessful at claiming a 'divine calling' or being a spiritualist); or seeing one's childhood or other long-past events (in one's mind's eye and relating it to someone who insists that the speaker 'actually' sees them).

Over- and under-activity: This is the easiest—travelling half-way across the world to attend a psychiatric meeting; falling asleep while listening to the papers.

I hope I will be excused for my levity. I am using it, at this point, deliberately in an effort to dramatize the degree and the depth to which psychiatry has been debauched by physicians who prefer to be detectives rather than doctors.

Medicine had been pregnant with psychiatry for a long time—for almost two hundred and fifty years, from the middle of the seventeenth century, when it was impregnated by the founding of madhouses, until the end of the nineteenth century, when Kraepelin and Bleuler gave birth to the living medical specialty of psychiatry. This birth was duly celebrated by a christening: the baby's last name was, of course, a double one, as befits a noble offspring: medicine, from the father, and psychiatry, from the mother. Hence the specialty of 'psychiatric medicine'. In addition, the child had to be identified by given names as well: these were bestowed upon it by its two great accoucheurs, Kraepelin and Bleuler, to whom we owe the names 'dementia praecox' and 'schizophrenia'. Their authoritative legitimization of all sorts of medically healthy (or non-sick) persons as sick—that is, as mentally sick—was the crucial event signifying the birth of modern psychiatry. This, briefly, is how it all happened.

When Kraepelin, Bleuler, and their contemporaries became psychiatrists, psychiatry was already an established form of medical and medico-legal practice. Moreover, the real locus of psychiatric practice was the insane asylum or mental hospital, just as the real locus of surgical practice was the operating room. What distinguished the important psychiatrist from his less important psychiatric colleagues and from his colleagues in other medical specialties was that he was the director or superintendent of an insane asylum or mental hospital. This meant that he had the authority, at once medical and legal, to keep innocent men and women—often thousands of them—under lock and key.

In addition, the medical and social definitions of madness being what they were (and still are), the majority of the patients brought to the attention of physicians like Kraepelin and Bleuler were considered to be mentally ill before, often long before, they reached these psychiatrists. The upshot was that these men reigned over hospitals full of people who were regarded—by their relatives, by other physicians, by the law—as *bona fide* patients. The pressure—both scientific and social—on them was therefore all one way: define the madman as sick and discover how he is sick!

Still, could these institutional psychiatrists have not taken a more independent, more scientifically honest position? Could they have not told themselves that, as medical scientists, one of their foremost duties was to asertain what was, and what was not, a disease? Which persons complaining or suspected of disease were, and were not, sick? And could they have not acted accordingly?

Had those physicians taken such a position, they could have also asked themselves whether it was not their first duty toward the inmates of their hospitals to examine them medically; and to declare, on the basis of their examination, whether they found them to be suffering from an illness or not? Actually, given the Virchowian criteria of disease which then prevailed, and given the social facts of psychiatry which also prevailed, I do not believe that Kraepelin, Bleuler, or the psychiatrists of that period could have assumed such a role, and got away with it. The reason is simple. Had they done that, they would have had to conclude that most of the 'patients' in their hospitals were not sick: at least they could not have found anything demonstrably wrong with the anatomical structure or physiological functioning of their bodies. But this would have dangerously undermined the justification for the patients' confinement.

It is, in fact, overwhelmingly clear that the institutional psychiatrists in the days of Kraepelin and Bleuler could not have declared their 'patients' as 'medically well', and have survived as professionals, as physicians and psychiatrists. Indeed, they still cannot do so. The 'patients'' relatives, physicians, and society generally, wanted to segregate certain disturbing persons and had done so in madhouses. This was a *fait accompli*—on a massive scale, at that—by the time Kraepelin and Bleuler arrived on the psychiatric scene. Had they said that their so-called patients (or many of them) were not sick, they would have cut the ground from under what was then the accepted justification for confining them. The medical profession, the legal profession, and society as a whole would not have stood for it. They would have got rid of such psychiatrists and would have replaced them with men who did what was expected of them. And they would have richly rewarded those who so fulfilled society's needs for social control and scapegoating—just as they had rewarded Kraepelin and Bleuler.

Accordingly, I regard Kraepelin, Bleuler and Freud as the conquistadors and colonizers of the mind of man. Society, their society, wanted them to extend the boundaries of medicine over morals and law—and they did so; it wanted them to extend the boundaries of illness from the body to behaviour—and they did so; it wanted them to conceal conflict as psychopathology, and confinement as psychiatric therapy—and they did so.

Schizophrenia, I have suggested, is the core concept of modern institutional psychiatry. This concept, and the problems it now poses for us, cannot be understood and unravelled except by a careful historical and epistemological re-examination of the origin and development of psychiatry.

The first step in the history of psychiatry was the building of madhouses or insane asylums. This created a population of institutional and institutionalized inmates whose conduct and condition created a demand for their description, and whose confinement cried out for justification.

The second step, generated by the first, was the identification and classification of the conduct and condition of the inmates of insane asylums. These acts of naming and ordering provided both a scientific rationalization for the fictions of the madhouse-keepers and for the fetters in which they confined their victims.

The third step—generated by the two previous steps, taken by Kraepelin, Bleuler and Freud, and heralding the birth of modern psychiatry—consisted of two interrelated moves. One was an ironclad, authoritative literalization of the psychiatric nomenclature built up in the course of the preceding decades. The names of psychiatric diseases were henceforth the unquestioned and unquestionable proofs of the existence of such diseases: because 'schizophrenia' was a disease, it was caused by lesions in the brain whose precise identification required only further refinements in medical science and technology. The second was an ironclad, authoritative justification of psychiatric confinement: because 'schizophrenics' (and other 'psychotics') were confined in nominally medical institutions, they were 'hospitalized', and the nature and function of closed psychiatric institutions became the sacred taboo of 'scientific' psychiatry. Henceforth, physicians and psychiatrists, as well as lawyers and laymen, averted their eyes from the world and fixed their gaze upon heaven: the more obvious it was that schizophrenics were imprisoned, the less attention psychiatrists, and others, paid to their imprisonment; and the more impossible it became to discover the brain lesions that caused schizophrenia, the more earnestly psychiatrists, and others, searched for them.

The fourth step—taken by so-called organic psychiatrists in our own day—was the systematic use of somatic treatments in schizophrenia. Since after a century of search, psychiatrists could still not demonstrate the characteristic histopathology, much less the organic aetiology, of schizophrenia, they now set out to 'prove' that it was a disease by subjecting schizophrenics to certain medical and surgical procedures called 'treatments'.

In all these ways, the development of modern psychiatry has not only differed from, but has been antithetical to, that of modern medicine. With the sole exception of the segregation of lepers (which occurred long before the birth of modern medicine), there has never been—in medicine and surgery—any kind of systematic involuntary institutionalizing of patients; nor has there been a systematic proliferation of disease names created independently of their anatomical, biochemical, microbiological, or physiological correlates. For example, until relatively recent times, physicians spoke of 'venereal diseases' collectively; genuine classification of these diseases occurred, only after discoveries in microbiology provided the necessary tools for it. The operation of the same principle is apparent in the identification and classification of all bodily diseases; that is, macroscopic pathological changes in organs, microscopic changes in tissues or cells, microbial invasions, and so forth are observed first; the precise naming of diseases comes next. It is just this sequence which has been systematically reversed and corrupted in psychiatry: the precise, or rather pseudo-precise, naming of alleged diseases came first; the existence of morphological pathology was postulated but never produced.

Hence the ceaseless manufacture of disease names in psychiatry, together with a total lack of evidence that any of them—from agoraphobia to schizophrenia—are caused by demonstrable brain lesions on the model of paresis. It is the greatest scientific scandal of our scientific age.

There is, in short, no such thing as schizophrenia. Schizophrenia is not a disease, but only the name of an alleged disease. Although there is no schizophrenia, there are, of course, individuals who are called 'schizophrenic'. Many (though by no means all) of these persons often behave and speak in ways that differ from the behaviour and speech of many (though by no means all) other people in their environment. These differences in behaviour and speech may, moreover, be gravely disturbing either to the so-called schizophrenic person or to those around him or to all concerned.

In the end, let us remember that physicians could not understand paresis until they accepted it as a disease—like any other, except that it affected the brain instead of the liver or kidney; and that they could not accept it as a disease until medical investigators demonstrated that the brain tissue of paretics, and of paretics only, harboured hordes of Treponema pallida. *Mutatis mutandis*, physicians will not understand schizophrenia until the so-called patients reassert themselves as agents, not objects; or until others—for example, politicians, legislators, or jurists—reaffirm that the role of the physician is to cure disease, not to control deviance; or, most generally and perhaps most importantly, until the dominant intellectual, economic, moral, and political institutions of society recognize and publicly acknowledge the differences between disease and disagreement.

References

ACKERKNECHT, E. H. (1953) *Rudolf Virchow: Doctor, Statesman, Anthropologist.* Madison: University of Wisconsin Press.
ARIETI, S. (1959) Schizophrenia: The manifest symptomatology, the psychodynamic and formal mechanisms. In *American Handbook of Psychiatry*, Vol 1 (ed. S. Arieti). New York: Basic Books.
BATCHELOR, I. R. C. (1969) *Henderson and Gillespie's Textbook of Psychiatry*, Tenth Ed. Oxford University Press.
BLEULER, E. (1911) *Dementia Praecox or the Group of Schizophrenias.* (Trans. by Joseph Zinkin, 1950.) New York: International Universities Press.
BREUTSCH, W. L. (1959) Neurosyphilitic conditions: general paralysis, general paresis, dementia paralytica, chronic brain syndrome associated with syphilitic meningoencephalitis. In *American Handbook of Psychiatry*, Vol II (ed. S. Arieti). New York: Basic Books.
FREUD, S. (1901) *The Psychopathology of Everyday Life.* In *The Standard Edition of the Complete Psychological Works of Sigmund Freud*, Vol. VI (1960). London: Hogarth Press.
HERZ, M. (1975) Quoted in 'Schizophrenia; specificity remains a very thorny issue, Roche Report (1975)'. *Frontiers of Psychiatry* (15 April), **5,** 5–6.
KRAEPELIN, E. (1917) *One Hundred Years of Psychiatry.* (Trans. by Wade Baskin, 1962.) New York: Philosophical Library.
McGUIRE, W. (ed.) (1974) *The Freud/Jung Letters: The Correspondence between Sigmund Freud and C. G. Jung.* (Trans. by R. Mannheim and R. F. C. Hull.) Princeton: Princeton University Press.

MEYNERT, T. (1890) *Klinische Vorlesungen über Psychiatrie auf wissenschaftlichen Grundlagen.* Wien: Wilhelm Braumüller.

OSLER, W. (1849–1919) Quoted in STRAUSS, M. B. (ed.) (1968) *Familiar Medical Quotations.* Boston: Little Brown.

STRACHEY, J. (1960) Introduction to *The Standard Edition of the Complete Psychological Works of Sigmund Freud,* Vol VI. London: Hogarth Press.

SZASZ, T. S. (1961) *The Myth of Mental Illness: Foundations of a Theory of Personal Conduct.* New York: Hoeber–Harper. (Revised edition—New York: Harper & Row.)

VIRCHOW, R. (1935) In *Funk and Wagnall's New Standard Encyclopaedia,* 6th ed, Vol. 10. Chicago: Standard Encyclopaedia Corp.

—— (1974) In *The Encyclopaedia Britannica: Macropaedia,* Vol. 19. Madison: University of Wisconsin Press.

WORLD HEALTH ORGANIZATION (1973) *Report of the International Pilot Study of Schizophrenia, Vol. 1: Results of the Initial Evaluation Phase.* Geneva: WHO.

ZILBOORG, G. (1941) *A History of Medical Psychology.* New York: Norton.

8 Schizophrenia and the theories of Thomas Szasz

MARTIN ROTH

The dichotomies of Dr Szasz

Anyone acquainted with Dr Thomas Szasz's previous writings about mental disorder, the nature of its relationship to the Law and to the problems of drug dependence (Szasz, 1961; 1963; 1970a; b; 1972; 1975) has learned to look in the first instance for the dualism, the poles of which are to be demonstrated as irreconcilable. For, as Glazer (1965) has pointed out, one of Dr Szasz's main conceptual devices is 'the dichotomy game'. A phenomenon may belong to category (x) or another category (y) but not to both. As a first step it is as well to examine the definitions of the categories in question. They are liable to prove inconsistent or idiosyncratic or just to be omitted. In other cases, as Professor Stone (1973) has shown in his detailed and telling dissection of the tortuous and confused logic pursued by Dr Szasz in *The Myth of Mental Illness*, the definitions are incomplete or erroneous and the implied antithesis dubious or false. Beginning with the equation that a lie is to a mistake as malingering is to hysteria, Szasz manages, following a maze of tortuous and self-contradictory arguments, to emerge at the conclusion that it would be '... more accurate to regard hysteria as a lie than as a mistake'.

In the paper he has devoted to schizophrenia, the categories depicted as being mutually exclusive are on the one hand 'Disease' or 'Illness' (x) in which there must be demonstrable histopathology or pathophysiology and on the other 'particular forms of personal behaviour' (y) such as schizophrenia for which an aetiological basis does not and cannot exist. In the case of (y) it is not only that organic factors are precluded by definition from any possible role or causation. The quest for possible psychological causes is also misconceived and a threat to human liberty. Freud is in the dock alongside Kraepelin and Bleuler as one of the '... conquistadors and colonizers of the mind of man. Society, their society, wanted them to extend the boundaries of medicine over morals and law ... and they did so; it wanted them to extend the boundaries of illness from the body to behaviour, ... and they did so; it wanted them to conceal conflict as psychopathology ... and they did so.'

Szasz seems to have no conception of the mental attitude an ordinary medical man takes up when he is first called to see a patient, and the mental processes that then ensue. Probably the very first thing the doctor becomes aware of is a global impression, that the patient is (or perhaps is not) obviously ill. By his history-taking and clinical examination he then confines the field of inquiry to perhaps one system. Step by step the diagnostic process works its way down to a syndrome, and eventually, perhaps, to a disease. Dr Szasz imagines it quite differently. As he supposes, the doctor first finds physical signs of macroscopic or microscopic cellular changes, proceeds from there to the naming of a disease and finally from the presence of the disease concludes that the patient must be ill. If the signs are not there, or are not found, he then says that there is no illness.

So it is that Kraepelin and Bleuler become the targets for Szasz's wrath and scorn. If they had only examined the patients in their asylums physically, finding nothing they would have been compelled, he says, to declare them free from illness by the medical criteria generally accepted at the time. They failed to do so, he says, through unwarranted and absurd pretensions to new discovery, intellectual cowardice and collusion with the agents of society in the coercion and control of deviant persons. It follows that when first described in the eighteenth century, Parkinsonism, according to Dr Szasz, could not have been a disease, nor did it qualify as such when James Parkinson wrote his famous *Essay on the Shaking Palsy* in 1817. In fact, discussing its causation, Charcot (1877) gave a prominent place to the 'violent moral emotions' commonly generated by the political disturbances which agitated France at the time. However, shortly before the First World War, European pathologists discovered lesions in the corpus striatum and neighbouring structures. Applying Dr Szasz's criteria, Parkinsonism was suddenly transmuted from category (y) into category (x) and those who suffered from it qualified overnight for treatment as patients.

Hippocrates had no right to claim in the fifth century BC that epilepsy has 'the same nature as other diseases and the cause that gives rise to individual diseases. It is also curable, no less than other illness' . . . and was not a state of sacred possession of the mind as was generally believed (Adams, 1849). For some two thousand four hundred years it was a non-disease until lesions were discovered in a minority of cases in the last century. Those who had been thus afflicted could then be correctly judged as having been ill. However, 'idiopathic' epilepsy remained a non-disease until the discovery of the EEG which showed that specific abnormalities were to be found in the electrical discharges recorded from the brain even in those cases in which cerebral lesions could not be found.

Szasz focuses his attention on syphilis as the paradigm of disease at the turn of the last century. It happens to suit his argument well. Other forms of affliction would have proved more awkward. Micro-organisms such as the streptococcus or tubercle bacillus cause fatal infections in some individuals and live harmlessly in others. As the latter do not suffer pain or incapacity we do not diagnose disease or regard them as ill. Moreover, there are good examples of diseases for which a definite physical lesion was long believed to be responsible until the advance of knowledge proved this theory false. Forty years ago, textbooks of medicine and physiology carried pictures of extremely emaciated young girls who suffered from a condition called Simmonds' Disease which was attributed to deficiency of the anterior pituitary gland. The diagnosis and treatment of such cases of indubitable illness was then presumably justified. But the inquiries of psychiatrists and endocrinologists showed the previously held explanation for the disease to have been mistaken. There is no primary lesion in the pituitary gland or anywhere else. Some subtle derangement in endocrine function is suspected, but proof is lacking. On the other hand, there are usually problems in maturation, the family environment is disturbed and the relationship of the parents ill-balanced. By Szasz's criteria these girls no longer suffer from a disease but merely show some 'particular forms of personal behaviour'. The fact that untreated, a high proportion die within a few years is irrelevant for his order of things.

The status of a whole host of conditions has to be reconsidered. Tic douloureux, narcolepsy, migraine and all forms of severe mental subnormality for which no cerebral or biochemical basis has as yet been demonstrated are non-disease. In fact, as virtually no physical causes or lesions had been established until about a century ago, 'disease' was rare in the extreme. But suffering in body and mind culminating in death during childhood and early life was very common.

This is to labour the obvious. But it is necessary to spell out issues because Szasz is a brilliant writer who, working behind a smoke-screen of erudition, savages facts in the manner of Procrustes and disguises absurdities so that they appear to many lay and some medical people as self-evident and axiomatic truths. Psychiatrists are once again accused of 'inventing' or 'manufacturing' mental disorder for ignoble reasons. The poets and novelists who anticipated many discoveries of modern psychiatry must have sinned in similar fashion. Szasz would say it is not insight and compassion we find in the words of Macbeth—

> Canst thou not minister to a mind diseased,
> Pluck from the memory a rooted sorrow,
> Raze out the written troubles of the brain,
> And with some sweet oblivious antidote
> Cleanse the stuff'd bosom of that perilous stuff
>   Which weighs upon the heart?

—but an early version of the medical model with its depraved pharmacological practices.

Of course, if illness is a matter of lumps, lesions and germs most schizophrenics are perfectly healthy. But such definition of disease would be repudiated even by physicians as too arid and restrictive for general medicine. For psychiatry which is primarily concerned with mental suffering, its mitigation and prevention irrespective of cause, they are even more relevant. It is with the tribulations of people that the analysis of the scope and limitations of psychiatry has to begin. 'Disease' is a highly complicated concept, and to impose upon the word the concreteness of hard fixed objects of one's personal choice is something different from understanding. The Greeks recognized it as a form of sophistry.

It is time to turn to the definition of the other category in Dr Szasz's dichotomy. It is apparent from the outset that schizophrenia is to be proved one way or another to be a myth. One looks, therefore, for a definition of those states of mind which Szasz believes that psychiatrists designate as 'schizophrenia' and which is to be demonstrated in due course to be non-existent in the sense of 'disease'. He describes schizophrenia as '... a particular form of personal behaviour'. As he does not particularize, this is of little help. Nor does the statement 'many of the persons given this diagnosis by psychiatrists often behave and speak in ways that differ from others in their environment' provide a clear picture of phenomena about which he is writing.

However, a study of the International Pilot Study of Schizophrenia (WHO, 1973), provides him with an opportunity to specify more clearly the type of disorder to which his paper is devoted. It enables him also to 'dramatize the degree and the depth to which psychiatry has been debauched by physicians who prefer to be detectives rather than doctors'.

To the accompaniment of much merriment, for which he begs to be excused, he describes the first four 'inclusion criteria' which were allegedly used in this inquiry for the diagnosis of schizophrenia. But the clinical features to which he refers were not intended to select schizophrenic patients. That 'hallucinations' and 'delusions' do not define any one form of psychiatric disorder would have been obvious to anyone familiar with an elementary textbook of psychiatry. The criteria in question were, in fact, utilized as a screen for the selection of 125 patients with any form of functional psychosis at each centre that participated in the inquiry. Manic and depressive psychoses and paranoid states were intended for inclusion as well as all the different forms of schizophrenia.

There was a cluster of features which commanded a consensus from psychiatrists of different countries as being schizophrenic. But this bore little relationship to the symptoms and behaviours with which Szasz makes such free and jocular play. The report of the International Pilot Study is quoted among the references. But Szasz cannot have read it. This will not surprise anyone who has submitted his previous polemical excursions to careful scrutiny (Stone, 1973). Of greater importance in the present context is the fact that Szasz's knowledge could hardly be more vague concerning the condition to which the majority of psychiatrists in the world would give a diagnosis of schizophrenia. This does not deter him from writing a paper with numerous references to the historical, pathological, clinical and psychoanalytic literature and relegating the disorder to non-existence.

Szasz and the history of medicine

Szasz's account of the history of medicine in the nineteenth century contains heroes and villains, true creative spirits and mythologists. Medical science is depicted as having made rapid strides discovering the causes of a multitude of infectious and other diseases. The sequence of events that culminated in these discoveries is exhibited by a consistency that enables Szasz to enunciate a general principle which is exemplified in all advances in knowledge of causation of true disease. In the first instance pathological changes are discovered '... macroscopic pathological changes in organs, microscopic changes in tissues or cells, microbial invasions, and so forth are observed first; the precise naming of diseases comes next.' He complains that the sequence has been 'reversed and corrupted in psychiatry' by the observation, description or classification of disorders. As the main burden of Szasz's thesis is that disorders like schizophrenia have nothing in common with bodily illness, it is unclear why the course of events followed by medical discovery should be held up as a paradigm for psychiatry to emulate. Whatever the reasons that led him to draw this particular comparison, he stands the history of medicine on its head to argue his case.

General paralysis, to which he devotes such a large part of his paper, provides a case in point. The pathological changes and the evidence of infection by micro-organisms are said to have come first, the precise naming of the disease thereafter. The true story is quite different. The principal features of the disorder were described 150 years ago. The relationship with syphilis was suspected but remained for decades the subject of embittered controversy until the discovery of the Wassermann test. Henry Maudsley (1879) attributed general paralysis to sexual excess which '... by degrees sapped the vitality of the nervous system'. Some physicians held such views with an unshakeable conviction that has a familiar ring. But there were some prescient workers who suspected the syphilitic origin of the disorder decades before Noguchi's discovery and whose views were rejected by eminent contemporaries. Had the opinions of those who insisted that there was nothing to investigate—a moral problem and not a biological one—gained general acceptance, knowledge of the causes and treatment of general paralysis might have been delayed for decades. The moral of the story is clear. Those who observed and recorded what happened to patients made a valuable contribution and, so did those who advanced hypotheses that had testable consequences. Those who made dogmatic assertions contributed nothing.

The scientific achievement of Virchow wins Szasz's unstinted praise. His summary goes like this: Before the publication of *Die Cellularpathologie*, abstract and theoretical concepts prevailed. The work of Virchow initiated a period of sturdy empiricism with concrete concepts, until the nebulous theories of psychopathology, psychoanalysis and psychosomatic medicine once again obscured the light of day. The basic scientific 'concept and model of disease' is summarized in Virchow's famous statement '... the real question which the modern scientific physician puts to himself when called to treat the case is: what cells are out of order and what can be done for them?' In contrast to the scientific physicians who observed histopathology and thereby earned the right to name diseases and the credit for making discoveries, Kraepelin and Bleuler did not discover the diseases for which they became famous. They merely invented new words such as 'dementia praecox' and 'schizophrenia'.

What Szasz does not tell the reader is that the question posed by Virchow had to go unanswered in relation to the overwhelming majority of patients seen by scientific physicians who practised in his day. And more than a century later the question has to go unanswered in most patients treated. Even when certain cells can be shown to be the seat of pathological change further questions are posed rather than the aetiological problem resolved. The coronary vessels may show marked atheroma in a man of 45 who has had a myocardial infarct. But one learns more about the reasons why he had it from the number of cigarettes he smokes a day and the sort of life he leads than from the degree of occlusion of vessels.

And if the clinical descriptions of Kraepelin, Bleuler and Freud are to be reckoned as no achievement the same verdict has to be passed on Hippocrates, Sydenham, Laennec, Heberden, Graves, Charcot, Addison, Gowers and Parkinson. For the large part they were able to provide no more than clinical descriptions. But the fact that they could see what others could not laid the foundation for the knowledge of causes that followed.

The advances in understanding and treatment of infectious disease are greeted with enthusiasm as real achievements of medical science. But they did not come out of the blue. Szasz does not appear to have heard of Sydenham who first studied the natural history of infectious diseases. In claiming that histopathology and microbiology came first and the naming of diseases afterwards, Szasz has surely turned the story upside down.

The account we are given of the history of medical science in the 18th and 19th centuries makes no reference to the emergence of medical statistics or public health, to Farr or Florence Nightingale or to the contributions of improved nutrition and housing to health and to the decline in rates of mortality.

The dualism of Szasz's concept of schizophrenia

If the concept of 'disease' is confined by arbitrary definition to conditions in which physical lesions have been found, all forms of mental suffering are neatly consigned to the category of 'non-disease'. That it is impossible to reconcile such a sharp line of demarcation with the existing facts, does not impede the argument; for the observations that bear upon the validity of the concept of disease are nowhere considered.

For example, patients suffering from the commonest forms of 'non-disease' seen by psychiatrists, the neuroses and affective disorders, have been shown in a number of clinical and epidemiological inquiries (Roth and Kay, 1956; Kay et al, 1964a; 1964b; Hare and Shaw, 1965; Shepherd et al, 1966) to exhibit a significant excess of somatic illness. Among the aged the excessive prevalence of physical disease is partly responsible for the markedly diminished life expectation of elderly depressives (Kay and Bergmann, 1966). But this is not the whole explanation. For the emotional disturbance with the typical features of a 'non-organic' psychiatric disorder may be the early harbinger of malignant disease (Kerr et al, 1969). In some measure the association stems from the emotional response to physical disablement. But it is a far more complicated matter than this; there is no single formulation that satisfactorily covers all cases. That the association is highly significant both clinically and statistically is beyond reasonable doubt. And it is plain that the personality setting, heredity psychodynamic factors, physical disablement and its significance for the patient are intertwined in varying combinations in the genesis of emotional disorder.

This complexity both of physical and mental disorder in their commonest forms is incompatible with Szasz's 'all or none' concepts. But he gives no indication as to how he deals with it. Is the physical lesion 'disease' and the depression 'non-disease'? The majority of modern physicians, the real doctors, towards whom Szasz adopts an attitude of such profound respect, would regard such dismemberment of the sick person into mind and body as archaic and irrational.

The situation is not essentially different in relation to schizophrenia. Painstaking investigations have shown that a closely similar syndrome, often with 'nuclear' features, occurs in significant excess among those with temporal lobe lesions of long-standing (Slater *et al*, 1963). Among elderly schizophrenics cerebral lesions have been demonstrated in a substantial minority; they appear to potentiate the effects of hereditary factors (Kay and Roth, 1961; Post, 1966). Decades of investigation have served to establish in an indubitable manner that lesions in certain areas of the cerebrum are associated with excessive prevalence of a syndrome that has by phenomenological criteria to be diagnosed as schizophrenic (Davison and Bagley, 1969). And a specific chronic intoxication, i.e. with amphetamine, will often closely simulate the clinical picture of paranoid schizophrenia.

Such identifiable organic factors are not to be found in the majority of cases of schizophrenia. But the testimony provided by the 'symptomatic' cases cannot be brushed aside in any objective evaluation of the status of the disorder that most psychiatrists describe as 'schizophrenic'.

Moreover, as the contribution of genetic factors to the causation of schizophrenia has been clearly established in recent years, the feat of denying that it has some specific biological basis can be achieved only by turning a blind eye on any evidence that fails to accord with preconceived notions. The hereditary factors do not make schizophrenia into a wholly organic disease. It is clear that a wide range of factors, biological, familial and psychological are involved. But genes are concrete biological entities. That they are necessary for the development of a substantial proportion of those identified as schizophrenic has to be conceded by those who treat evidence as scholars and scientists can be expected to treat it. Dr Szasz refers neither to the older evidence relating to heredity, nor to the recent investigations into the fate of children adopted shortly after birth to schizophrenic and normal mothers (Heston, 1966; Kety *et al*, 1968; Rosenthal *et al*, 1968; Wender *et al*, 1968) which have conclusively established the role of heredity in schizophrenia. Nor does he explain how the theory concerning the nature of schizophrenia, implicit in his writings is to be reconciled with the fact that it has been described in every country, culture, race and social class investigated. Szasz would say, no doubt, that all over the world, where schizophrenia is found at approximately the same incidence, in India, Africa, Asia, Europe and the Americas, 'professional degraders' are at work, with equal intensity, doing the diagnosing. We had best laugh at this, lest we weep.

Szasz's theory of schizophrenia

Although Szasz rejects all the theories that have been advanced for the causation of schizophrenia, whether genetical, familial, psychodynamic or biochemical, and by implication all theorizing about it, he insinuates a theory of his own. This purports to explain how it comes about that certain individuals are examined by psychiatrists and given a diagnosis of 'schizophrenia'. These individuals differ from other people in society only in so far as they deviate from them in mode of speech or conventional standards of conduct. Psychiatrists are agents specially trained to silence all those who transgress against the prevailing power interests in contemporary society. They now fulfil the role assigned to them by pronouncing 'defamation disguised by diagnosis' or 'the manufacture, with state approval, of stigmatized individuals and classes by professional degraders' (Szasz, 1970). Those who enter into conflict with it can be labelled, dehumanized and then imprisoned. The 'most denigrating diagnostic label' applied is the diagnosis of schizophrenia. In such a context 'treatment' is a euphemism for 'torture' and 'rape' (Szasz, 1975). As he has repeatedly explained in a long series of publications, but particularly in *The Manufacture of Madness* (1970), there is treatment administered by physicians and there are the disguised forms of coercion and brain-washing inflicted by psychiatrists upon the oppressed on behalf of the oppressors. There is real psychotherapy administered for fees privately by Dr Szasz, and there are the therapies of institutional psychiatry which consist of the 'Dehumanization of Man'.

We are not informed about the precise identity of the power interests psychiatrists serve. In some cases institutional psychiatry appears to act on behalf of the 'dominant ethic'. Elsewhere it favours prevailing 'religious beliefs', or acts to keep the poor and ill-educated in their proper station of subordination to the rich.

Szasz's theory about schizophrenia is, therefore, conspiratorial. Here arguments and explanations begin and end with the sinister and ignoble motives imputed to those whose opinions differ from one's own. They hold such views because they and those they serve stand to gain from them. No evidence is presented. Indeed it is implicit in the argument that the psychiatrists' quest for evidence is itself part of the politically motivated endeavour in which they have been engaged since Kraepelin first advanced the concept of dementia praecox. Such an attitude of mind precludes discussion and makes it impossible to arrive at the truth. For there is no public criterion by which the veracity of such statements can be tested.

In short, Szasz advances an essentially Marxist theory which explains the existence of schizophrenia in the following terms. The true nature of the behaviour of certain individuals who come into conflict with society has to be disguised as something different. The reasons that necessitate camouflage for such dissident acts are socio-economic in character. The ruling classes in a given society are thereby protected from the danger of direct confrontation with their critics. A class of professional defamers is, therefore, created. Their task is to affix labels on all individuals whose deviance threatens the power of the ruling classes. These labels have the effect of invalidating the actions of deviants and concealing or nullifying their political significance. Whether psychiatrists fulfil the social role assigned to them consciously or unwittingly is immaterial.

The question is under what circumstances could such a theory clash with evidence? What are its consequences? What testimony would serve to falsify it or call it in question? The answer is that the theory is immune from any such challenge from independent observation. It remains for ever impregnable. It explains all disease in all cultures and races at all times. It follows that it can explain nothing. But the fact that he can 'explain' everything and anything is one of the reasons for Szasz's remarkable achievement. Over a period of thirty years, in which he has placed no observations of his own on record but has published a large number of books and papers in many languages, flashing rays of darkness upon the entire field of psychiatry, he has made a remarkable number of converts.

Szasz and the treatment of schizophrenia

The fourth step of Szasz's version of the history of modern psychiatry was the 'systematic use of somatic treatments in schizophrenia'. He complains that psychiatrists have 'set out to prove' that schizophrenia is a disease by 'subjecting schizophrenics to certain procedures... called treatment, despite the fact that... after a century of search psychiatrists could still not demonstrate the characteristic histopathology, much less the organic aetiology of schizophrenia'. There would probably be no purpose in trying to convince Szasz that controlled therapeutic trials are designed not to 'prove' but to disprove the beneficial effects attributed to them. It would have been possible for the best clinical trials of phenothiazine compounds to have disposed of the early claims made on their behalf. In the event they survived the tests, and their efficacy, both in the acute and chronic stages of schizophrenia, was substantiated; (Leff and Wing, 1971; Hirsch *et al*, 1972).

Szasz's tone changes to deep respect when he refers to medical diagnosis and treatment. Yet many forms of treatment in medicine are no less empirical than those used in psychiatry. The causation of trigeminal neuralgia, migraine and idiopathic epilepsy, torticollis and many other forms of involuntary movement is unknown and the treatments employed are empirical, symptomatic or of dubious efficacy. The aetiological basis of virtually all serious illnesses in medicine, including myocardial infarction, hypertension, cerebrovascular disease and peptic ulcer is poorly understood or completely obscure, and the main therapies employed are palliative.

Physicians nowadays try to devote effort to reducing the prevalance of smoking and obesity, since these have proved to be correlated with an overall decrease in life expectation and with a number of diseases which carry a high mortality. If the underlying basis of the associated states of dependence were better understood, the results of intervention would be more impressive than they are. In the meantime physicians can only travel hopefully. If they should hit upon a new finding, whether positive or negative, they will be expected to back it with evidence when they try to place it on record.

Szasz has been more or perhaps less fortunate. Over a period of 30 years, he has made numerous pronouncements about the care and treatment of patients. But in no case has he submitted his views to formal tests that could have disposed of them or substantiated them. Yet his statements about the treatment of schizophrenic patients imply that individuals so 'labelled' fare better without treatment than under the care of those who employ modern psychiatric therapy. Here is a clear hypothesis that could be submitted to critical evaluation. Even more interesting would be an experiment in which the fate of patients treated by the majority of clinical psychiatrists could be compared with the fate of those managed under the aegis of Dr Szasz.

Indeed, as Szasz dispenses with diagnosis and accepted forms of treatment and yet continues to practise as a psychiatrist and to profess his subject, the methods he employs are of the greatest possible interest. How does he manage the problems of those who complain that their innermost secrets are broadcast to the world at large or that voices, which they feel a compelling urge to obey, tell them to mutilate themselves? What form of help does he provide for men who show him imaginary seminal stains on their wives' underclothes, and what steps does he take to protect lives so endangered? Does he tell such clients that they suffer from having been declared outsiders and deviants by a society with debased moral standards? What are the exact means used to encourage those who seek Dr Szasz's aid 'to adopt a critical attitude towards all rules of conduct significant to him and to maximize his free choice in adopting either socially accepted or unaccepted rules of conduct' (Szasz, 1965). And what are the results obtained? We seek in vain among Szasz's multitudinous pages for an answer. His discourse with himself takes place in a realm where the effects of making diagnoses and administering treatment or withholding them have to undergo no tests and where conjectures concerning the nature of disease, or anything else for that matter, run no risk of exposure to challenge or refutation.

Negations and affirmations

Such words as Szasz has set down for the guidance of those whose main concern is to mitigate mental suffering, have been few and uninformative. He has nothing positive to offer. Psychiatric disorders are 'problems of living'. So are wars, earthquakes, floods, famines, bad digestion and a cold climate. The plight of psychiatric patients, whom he classes among the oppressed, derives from the misdeeds of the oppressors and their agents, but he does not divulge who these oppressors are. Elsewhere (*The Manufacture of Madness*, 1970) it is stated that the function of psychiatrists is to protect 'the rich and well educated'. The remedies are, therefore, to be sought in some different form of social organization. But we are not provided even with the faintest glimpse of that just, equitable and better-ordered society in which mental distress could be expected to be less than it is. For an indefinite time ahead we have to resign ourselves to the irreconcilable opposition of oppressors and oppressed and the anguished states of mind this engenders.

Szasz is far more explicit and eloquent in negation. He says 'no' to the 'medical model' and 'no' to psychiatrists who are, he says, professional hirelings of the dominant classes. He gives an equally emphatic 'no' to psychoanalysis; the concept of mental pathology inherent in it is spurious. Psychiatric diagnosis is falsehood and the description of such a condition as schizophrenia is 'the greatest scientific scandal of our time'. Psychiatric hospitals, he maintains, are prisons, and the psychiatrists who work in them are jailers and torturers. One would suppose that it could only be by an effort of will that he shuts his eyes to the manifest facts: that these are places of asylum, of refuge; that a great number (in Britain nearly all) of those who go there go voluntarily for help; that their troubles are desperate, their sufferings extreme; that, indeed, they feel, and are, very ill; that the psychiatrists who care for them are not guilty conspirators but earnest and compassionate men and women, trying to do what they can to help the sufferer in each individual case.

There are numerous examples of simplistic philosophies with close affinities to that of Szasz, which provide simple explanations for complex and painful human predicaments in terms of the deeds of exploiters, oppressors, conquistadors, their hirelings and dupes. It requires no leap of the imagination to perceive how, by revealing 'the truth' to multitudes of people in a blinding flash, their influence spreads far and wide.

A philosophy with similar ingredients was the main weapon of the 'Spirit of Negation' who dominated the nightmare of Bertrand Russell's metaphysician (1954): 'He himself is the most complete improbability imaginable, he is pure nothing, total non-existence, and yet continually changing ... Before going forth he clothes himself in shining white armour, which completely conceals the nothingness within. Only his eyes remain unclothed and from his eyes piercing rays of nothingness shoot forth seeking what they may conquer. Wherever they find negation, wherever they find prohibition, wherever they find the cult of not-doing, there they enter into the inmost substance of those who are prepared to receive him. Every negation emanates from him and returns with a harvest of captured frustrations.'

Russell's metaphysician uses a simple device for disposing of the argument of the Prince of Darkness that non-existence is the only reality. Their fallacies serve to reveal to the philosopher a profound truth. He concludes that the word 'not' is superfluous. Thereupon, he proceeds to expunge all words expressing negation from his dictionary, saying: 'My speech shall be composed entirely of the words that remain. By the help of these words ... I shall be able to describe everything in the universe.' When the Spirit of Negation was thus denounced as a bad linguistic habit, '... there was a vast explosion, the air gushed in from all sides and the horrid shape vanished. The murky air which had been due to inspissated rays of nothingness cleared as if by magic'.

Szasz has exhibited no tendency, over the decades, to follow the examples of Russell's metaphysician. He appears unlikely to expunge any words from his now familiar vocabulary. For, as a philosopher, he is untroubled by the uncertainties of those compelled by evidence to abandon arrogant dogmatism and 'to travel into the region of liberating doubt' (Russell, 1959). He never concludes that perhaps there may be some substance in the views of those who dissent from his view. This endows him with powerful advantages in his polemical excursions as compared with scholars, scientists or philosophers in the broad sense of the term.

Szasz's meteoric rise, his growing influence and world renown are not, therefore, unexpected. The reasons are perhaps to be found in the verdict, 'I think that bad philosophers may have a certain influence, good philosophers never.'

Comment

Why then, do psychiatrists continue to record Thomas Szasz's *beliefs* regarding the nature of schizophrenia? Why do they not emphasize instead his utter inability to support his belief in its non-existence as an illness with a shred of relevant—i.e. biological, epidemiological, clinical—*evidence*? Why? Perhaps one can put one's finger on the answer.

Although he has called psychiatrists 'professional degraders', we must not think of him as a professional mountebank. Under his specious argumentation he is deeply sincere. He has not only the gift of words but fire in the belly. Although he takes care not to show it, he is in fact a very angry man; and one can deduce what he is angry about from the effects he has produced. His philosophy has been widely influential. He has led psychiatrists, always unsure of themselves and aware of the extreme limitation of their knowledge, to undertake a critical reappraisal of their practices and the principles underlying them. He has made explicit the danger that in certain roles they may have double allegiance, to their patient and to the community. Among his achievements may be reckoned the right for better or worse, now enjoyed by certain citizens of the United States to commit suicide. He has been a powerful fighter for the freedoms, rights and responsibilities of psychiatric patients. The attitude of the law and the legal profession to psychiatry and mental disorder has been transformed by the writings of Thomas Szasz, in the USA. He is obsessed by the need he feels for psychiatric patients, psychotic or neurotic, to be accepted by us all as human beings of no less value than ourselves, and therefore not ill; for if they are thought of as mentally ill, they cannot but be devalued, dehumanized, degraded. This is the conclusion at which he *has* to arrive; and hence comes the necessity to stand logic on its head in order to get there.

References

ADAMS, F. (1849) *The Genuine Works of Hippocrates*. London: The Sydenham Society.

CHARCOT, J. M. (1877) *Lectures on the Diseases of the Nervous System*. London: The New Sydenham Society.

DAVISON, K. & BAGLEY, C. R. (1969) Schizophrenia-like psychoses associated with organic disorders of the central nervous system: a review of the literature, In *Current Problems in Neuropsychiatry. British Journal of Psychiatry Special Publication No. 4*. Ashford, Kent: Headley Bros.

GLAZER, F. (1965) 'The dichotomy game'. *American Journal of Psychiatry*, **122**, No. 8, 1069.

HARE, E. H. & SHAW, G. (1965) *Mental Health in a New Housing Estate*. Maudsley Monograph No 12. London: Oxford University Press.

HESTON, L. L. (1966) Psychiatric disorders in foster-home reared children of schizophrenic mothers. *British Journal of Psychiatry*, **112**, 819–852.

HIRSCH, S. R., GAIND, R. & ROHDE, P. (1972) The clinical value of fluphenazine decanoate in maintaining chronic schizophrenics in the community. Presented at the International Symposium on Rehabilitation in Psychiatry, Belgrade, Yugoslavia.

KAY, D. W. K., BEAMISH, P. & ROTH, M. (1964a) Old age mental disorders in Newcastle upon Tyne. I. A study of prevalence. *British Journal of Psychiatry*, **110**, 146–158.

—— —— —— (1964b) Old age mental disorders in Newcastle upon Tyne. II A study of the possible social and medical causes. *British Journal of Psychiatry*, **110**, 668–682.

—— & BERGMANN, D. (1966) Physical disability and mental health in old age. *Journal of Psychosomatic Research*, **10**, 3–12.

—— & ROTH, M. (1961) Environmental and hereditary factors in the schizophrenias of old age ('late paraphrenia') and their bearing on the general problem of causation in schizophrenia. *Journal of Mental Science*, **107**, 649–686.

KERR, T. A., SCHAPIRA, K. & ROTH, M. (1969) The relationship between premature death and affective disorders. *British Journal of Psychiatry*, **115**, 1277–1282.

KETY, S. S., ROSENTHAL, D., WENDER, P. H. & SHULSINGER, F. (1968) The types and prevalence of mental illness in the biological and adoptive families of adopted schizophrenics. In *The Transmission of Schizophrenia* (eds. D. Rosenthal and S. S. Kety). Oxford: Pergamon Press.

LEFF, J. P. & WING, J. K. (1971) Trial of maintenance therapy in schizophrenia. *British Medical Journal*, *iii*, 599.

MAUDSLEY, H. (1879) *The Pathology of Mind*. London: Macmillan & Co.

PARKINSON, J. (1817) *Essay on the Shaking Palsy*.

POST, F. (1966) *Persistent Persecutory States of the Elderly*. London: Pergamon.

ROSENTHAL, D., WENDER, P. H., KETY, S. S., SCHULSINGER, F., WELNER, J. & OSTERGAARD, L. (1968) Schizophrenics' offspring reared in adoptive homes. In *The Transmission of Schizophrenia* (eds. D. Rosenthal and S. S. Kety). Oxford: Pergamon Press.

ROTH, M. & KAY, D. W. K. (1956) Affective disorders arising in the senium. II Physical disability as an aetiological factor. *Journal of Mental Science*, **102**, 141–150.

RUSSELL, B. (1954) *Nightmares of Eminent Persons*. The Bodley Head.

—— (1959) *The Problems of Philosophy*. Oxford University Press.

SHEPHERD, M., COOPER, B., BROWN, A. A. & KALTON, G. W. (1966) *Psychiatric Illness in General Practice*. London: Oxford University Press.

SLATER, E., BEARD, A. W. & GLITHERO, E. (1963) The schizophrenia-like psychoses of epilepsy. I–V. *British Journal of Psychiatry*, **109,** 95–150.

STONE, A. A. (1973). Psychiatry kills: a critical evaluation of Dr Thomas Szasz. *Journal of Psychiatry & Law*, **1,** 23–37.

SZASZ, T. S. (1961) *The Myth of Mental Illness: Foundations of a Theory of Personal Conduct*. New York: Hoeber-Harper.

—— (1963) *Law, Liberty and Psychiatry*, New York: The Macmillan Co. Ch 8, esp. p 104.

—— (1965) *Psychiatric Justice*. New York: The Macmillan Co. Ch. 9, esp. pp 266–269.

—— (1970a) *Ideology and Insanity: Essays on the Psychiatric Dehumanization of Man*. New York: Anchor.

—— (1970b) *The Manufacture of Madness*. New York: Harper & Row.

—— (1972) The ethics of addiction. *International Journal of Psychiatry*, **10,** 51–61.

—— (1975) Georgetown University Law School Symposium on 'Basic Issues of the Therapeutic State'. Report in *Psychiatric News*, November 5, 1975.

WENDER, P., ROSENTHAL, D. & KETY, S. S. (1968) A psychiatric assessment of the adoptive parents of schizophrenics. In *The Transmission of Schizophrenia* (eds. D. Rosenthal and S. S. Kety). Oxford: Pergamon Press.

WORLD HEALTH ORGANIZATION (1973) *Report of the International Pilot Study of Schizophrenia, Vol I: Results of the Initial Evaluation Phase*. Geneva: WHO.

II. Classification and phenomenology

9 The classification and phenomenology of schizophrenia: Overview

R. E. KENDELL

A dramatic resurgence of interest in classification and the observable phenomena of mental illness took place in the 1970s, particularly in the United
States. This new outlook was heralded by the publication, by the Washington
University Department of Psychiatry at St Louis, of strict operational criteria
for the diagnosis of 15 major syndromes (Feighner *et al*, 1972) and then proclaimed eight years later by DSM-III, the radically revised and greatly
enlarged third edition of the American Psychiatric Association's *Diagnostic
and Statistical Manual of Mental Disorders* (American Psychiatric Association,
1980). The emphasis on reliability and on observable phenomena rather than
psychodynamic inference, which these methodological innovations repre
sented, was primarily a response to the evidence that had accumulated in
the 1960s that the reliability of psychiatric diagnoses was alarmingly low,
and that serious international differences in usage had developed, particularly
between North America and Europe (**Leff,1977**). It was also a manifestation
of a fairly explicit attempt to reassert psychiatry's identity as a branch of
medicine and its acceptance of traditional medical concerns for the delineation
of syndromes and disease entities and the biological abnormalities underlying
them.

   This laudable concern for reliability and general acceptance of the importance of unambiguous 'rules of application', or operational definitions as a
means of achieving adequate reliability, had by 1980 resulted in the publication
of over a dozen operational definitions of schizophrenia and other major syndromes. It rapidly became clear that these competing definitions often
embraced quite different populations of patients. It therefore became necessary
to choose between them, a situation which immediately drew attention to
the lack of any adequate criterion of validity with which to assess them. It
was suggested that long-term prognosis might, *faute de mieux*, be an acceptable
criterion and that definitions which successfully identified patients with a poor
long-term prognosis were to be preferred to those which also embraced many
patients who made a full recovery. The Feighner and DSM-III definitions
proved to be much more successful in this respect than most of their rivals
(Helzer *et al*, 1981). Schneiderian first rank symptoms, on the other hand,
and the CATEGO criteria derived from them, turned out to be surprisingly
poor predictors of long-term outcome (see, for example, Kendell *et al*, 1979).
At the same time it was pointed out by Shields and Gottesman (1973) that,
as schizophrenia is genetically transmitted, definitions with high heritability

would be more likely to identify patients possessing the biological abnormality assumed to underlie the clinical syndrome than those with lower heritability. Unfortunately, accurate calculation of comparative heritabilities requires data from a large, well documented and representative population of psychotic twins, and so far only preliminary comparisons have been carried out (McGuffin *et al*, 1984).

Partly because they are favoured by the clinical research workers and epidemiologists in the United States who have been the main force behind this new interest in classification, and partly because their reliability and ability to predict poor long-term prognosis compare favourably with their rivals, the most widely used definitions of schizophrenia at present, for research purposes at least, are all American in origin. They are the original St Louis definition (Feighner *et al*, 1972), the RDC definition (Spitzer *et al*, 1975), and the DSM-III definition derived from these. As **Fox (1981)** points out, the DSM-III concept and definition of schizophrenia is much narrower than its predecessors. It excludes most patients with extensive depressive or manic symptoms, all patients with a symptom duration of less than six months, and anyone whose illness begins after the age of 45. It also requires solid evidence of psychotic phenomena at some stage in the illness. It therefore excludes four of the international classification's eight varieties of schizophrenia, the simple (ICD 295.0), latent (295.5) and schizoaffective (295.7) types, and acute schizophrenic episodes (295.4). As a result the current American concept of schizophrenia is far narrower than it was a generation ago, and if the Anglo-American comparisons reviewed by **Leff (1977)** were to be repeated now, American usage might well prove to be more restricted than that of British psychiatrists. Much would depend on whether or not the majority of American psychiatrists have really abandoned the broad criteria and psychodynamic assumptions they learnt as residents and used for much of their careers and are now using instead the restricted criteria officially adopted by the American Psychiatric Association. Most research workers and psychiatric residents are probably doing so but, as **Mukherjee (1983)** says, there must be some doubt whether the silent majority has yet been either able or willing to make the major conceptual changes required.

Moving the boundaries of schizophrenia as the Feighner and DSM-III definitions have done has important implications for the definition, and even for the independent existence of several other syndromes. The many patients who develop schizophrenic and affective symptoms simultaneously have either to be regarded as suffering from affective illnesses or assigned to a separate schizoaffective category whose status remains unresolved. The exclusion of those whom Eugen Bleuler regarded as suffering from simple or latent schizophrenia effectively creates two new types of personality disorder, known in DSM-III as schizotypal and borderline personality disorders. And the exclusion of those becoming psychotic for the first time after the age of 45 focuses renewed interest on the so-called paranoid psychoses. These have long been a neglected group of disorders partly because, as **Munro (1982)** points out, English speaking psychiatrists have come to equate the term paranoid with persecutory, whereas its original German meaning was far wider, embracing grandiose, jealous, somatic and hypochondriacal delusions as well. Although DSM-III perpetuates this mistaken assumption, Winokur has recently resuscitated

Kraepelin's paranoia under the title of 'delusional disorder'. He has shown that there exists a small group of patients who develop delusional systems in middle age without hallucinations or other psychopathology (Winokur, 1977), and Kendler *et al* (1981) have produced some evidence to suggest that these illnesses are unrelated to schizophrenia.

The most fundamental reason why we have such difficulty deciding where to draw the boundaries of schizophrenia, and most of the other syndromes we recognize, is that the clinical phenomena we use to recognize and define these syndromes are not obviously distributed in discrete clusters. One syndrome merges into another, forcing us, or at least inviting us, to use terms such as schizoaffective, borderline state and anxiety depression. Because terms like schizophrenia and melancholia are the names of elements in a categorical classification or typology, and because a typology treats its constituent elements *as if* they were independent entities, it is dangerously easy to assume that this has been established. In reality, although references to 'disease entities' and claims that this or that syndrome is a 'genuine entity' are commonplace in psychiatric writing, the meaning of such terms is rarely defined and the kind of evidence needed to establish that a given condition is an entity is rarely discussed. Moran (1966) and Kendell (1975) have suggested that a 'point of rarity'—a bimodal distribution of scores on a discriminant function— has to be demonstrated before it can be assumed that any syndrome is a discrete entity. An alternative approach based on the demonstration of a non-linear relationship between symptomatology and an independent variable such as outcome was suggested by Kendell and Brockington (1980), but they failed to demonstrate any such relationship for schizophrenia. Whether syndromes like schizophrenia and melancholia are indeed discrete entities, or whether we are dealing for the most part with phenomena which lack natural boundaries is one of psychiatry's most important theoretical issues, with major implications for theories of aetiology as well as classification. The claim recently made by Cloninger *et al* (1985) to have demonstrated a point of rarity between schizophrenia and other mental disorders is therefore of considerable importance.

Interest in the phenomenology of schizophrenia in the last decade has largely been secondary to interest in the classification or aetiology of the disorder. Most Anglo-Saxon psychiatrists would defend this as a sensible ordering of priorities. But Berner, speaking for an old and distinguished continental tradition, laments British psychiatrists' lack of interest in phenomenology (Berner and Küfferle, 1982). He also deplores our use of the term to refer loosely to all the phenomena of mental illness, behavioural and subjective, rather than in the restricted subjective sense of Husserl and Jaspers. Others, like Huber, would do the same. It is at least open to doubt, though, whether a detailed study of phenomenology in the Jasperian sense would lead to important insights or practical benefits. Certainly where schizophrenia is concerned the available evidence suggests that the course and prognosis of the illness are determined by the mode of onset, the premorbid personality and the presence or absence of affective symptoms rather than by the precise psychopathological phenomena experienced.

In the 1960s Kurt Schneider's 'symptoms of the first rank' were seized upon rather uncritically by a generation of German and British psychiatrists searching for unambiguous and reliable criteria to which the diagnosis of schizophrenia could be anchored. Schneiderian symptoms are indeed easier to define than such Bleulerian symptoms as thought disorder, autism and blunting of affect, and can therefore be rated more reliably. But they do not constitute the talisman they are sometimes taken for. As Schneider himself emphasized, they have no theoretical status; and as **Koehler** (**1979**) has pointed out, the precise range of psychopathological phenomena embraced by several of the symptoms is ambiguous and interpreted in different ways by different authorities. Worse still, several follow-up studies of schizophrenic populations have found them to have little or no prognostic significance, thereby undermining their claim to be of special diagnostic significance. **Mellor** (**1982**) may possibly be right in suggesting that structured interviews like the Present State Examination, or their users, may be incapable of eliciting Schneiderian symptoms accurately enough for final decisions to be made about their prognostic significance. But the burden of proof must lie with him, particularly as the definitional problems described by Koehler remain unresolved.

As interest in first rank symptoms increased, interest in thought disorder waned. It had always been an ill-defined concept, difficult to recognize or rate reliably, and half a century of research had failed to clarify its origins or the psychological mechanisms involved. Worse still, the Bleulerian assumption that thought disorder could be elicited in all true schizophrenics and in no other condition had become impossible to reconcile with empirical findings. More recently, though, interest has started to return. Andreasen (1979) has defined 18 of the main components of what she prefers to call 'disorders of thought, language and communication'. She has also shown that most of these can be rated reliably, and explored their distribution in mania and schizophrenia. Perhaps of greater significance, attempts are now being made to subject schizophrenic speech to detailed linguistic analysis and to replace clinical metaphors like derailment and 'knight's move' thinking with modern linguistic concepts like cohesion, depth of embedding and redundancy (Morice and Ingram, 1982).

Probably the most important exploration of schizophrenic phenomenology in this last decade has been Crow and Stevens demonstration of age disorientation and other widespread cognitive deficits in many chronic patients (Stevens *et al*, 1978; Crow and Stevens, 1978). This was not a novel observation; but previous reports had passed unnoticed, partly because their authors had not been prepared to challenge Bleuler's authority and his dictum that cognitive functions remain intact in schizophrenia. Johnstone's demonstration of enlarged lateral ventricles (Johnstone *et al*, 1978) suddenly made it much easier to regard schizophrenia as a progressive brain disease, and therefore as a disease in which cognitive deficits were to be expected. And when cognitive deficits were sought, they were found. The history of science contains many examples of mistaken assumptions preventing men from seeing what was staring them in the face, from the parabolic trajectory of an arrow to the eccentric position of the lens in the human eye, but it is none the less disconcerting to find the same blindness suddenly exposed in ourselves.

References

AMERICAN PSYCHIATRIC ASSOCIATION (1980) *Diagnostic and Statistical Manual of Mental Disorders*, 3rd Ed. (DSM-III). Washington D.C.: American Psychiatric Association.

ANDREASEN, N. C. (1979) Thought, language, and communication disorders. *Archives of General Psychiatry*, **36**, 1315–1321; 1325–1330.

BERNER, P. & KÜFFERLE, B. (1982) British phenomenological and psychopathological concepts: a comparative review. *British Journal of Psychiatry*, **140**, 558–565.

CLONINGER, C. R., MARTIN, R. L., GUZE, S. B. & CLAYTON, P. J. (1985) Diagnosis and prognosis in schizophrenia. *Archives of General Psychiatry*, **42**, 15–25.

CROW, T. J. & STEVENS, M. (1978) Age disorientation in chronic schizophrenia: the nature of the cognitive deficit. *British Journal of Psychiatry*, **133**, 137–142.

FEIGHNER, J. P., ROBINS, E., GUZE, S. B., WOODRUFF, R. A., WINOKUR, G. & MUNOZ, R. (1972) Diagnostic criteria for use in psychiatric research. *Archives of General Psychiatry*, **26**, 57–63.

FOX, H. A. (1981) The DSM-III concept of schizophrenia. *British Journal of Psychiatry*, **138**, 60–63.

HELZER, J. E., BROCKINGTON, I. F. & KENDELL, R. E. (1981) The predictive validity of DSM-III and Feighner definitions of schizophrenia: a comparison with RDC and CATEGO. *Archives of General Psychiatry*, **38**, 791–797.

JOHNSTONE, E. C., CROW, T. J., FRITH, C. D., STEVENS, M., KREEL, L. & HUSBAND, J. (1978) The dementia of dementia praecox. *Acta Psychiatrica Scandinavica*, **57**, 305–324.

KENDELL, R. E. (1975) *The Role of Diagnosis in Psychiatry*. Oxford: Blackwell Scientific Publications.

—— & Brockington, I. F. (1980) The identification of disease entities and the relationship between schizophrenic and affective psychoses. *British Journal of Psychiatry*, **137**, 324–331.

—— —— & LEFF, J. P. (1979) Prognostic implications of six alternative definitions of schizophrenia. *Archives of General Psychiatry*, **36**, 25–31.

KENDLER, K. S., GRUENBERG, A. M. & STRAUSS, J. S. (1981) The relationship between paranoid psychosis (delusional disorder) and the schizophrenia spectrum disorders. *Archives of General Psychiatry*, **38**, 985–987.

KOEHLER, K. (1979) First rank symptoms of schizophrenia: questions concerning clinical boundaries. *British Journal of Psychiatry*, **134**, 236–248.

LEFF, J. (1977) International variations in the diagnosis of psychiatric illness. *British Journal of Psychiatry*, **131**, 329–338.

MCGUFFIN, P., FARMER, A. E., GOTTESMAN, I. I., MURRAY, R. M. & REVELEY, A. M. (1984) Twin concordance for operationally defined schizophrenia. *Archives of General Psychiatry*, **41**, 541–545.

MELLOR, C. S. (1982) The present status of first-rank symptoms. *British Journal of Psychiatry*, **140**, 423–424.

MORAN, P. A. P. (1966) The establishment of a psychiatric syndrome. *British Journal of Psychiatry*, **112**, 1165–1171.

MORICE, R. D. & INGRAM, J. C. L. (1982) Language analysis in schizophrenia: diagnostic implications. *Australian and New Zealand Journal of Psychiatry*, **16**, 11–21.

MUKHERJEE, S. (1983) Reducing American diagnosis of schizophrenia: will the DSM-III suffice? *British Journal of Psychiatry*, **142**, 414–418.

MUNRO, A. (1982) Paranoia revisited. *British Journal of Psychiatry*, **141**, 344–349.

SHIELDS, J. & GOTTESMAN, I. I. (1973) Cross-national diagnosis of schizophrenia in twins: the heritability and specificity of schizophrenia. *Archives of General Psychiatry*, **27**, 725–730.

SPITZER, R. L., ENDICOTT, J. & ROBINS, E. (1975) *Research Diagnostic Criteria, Instrument No. 58.* New York: New York State Psychiatric Institute.

STEVENS, M., CROW, T. J., BOWMAN, M. J. & COLES, E. C. (1978) Age disorientation in schizophrenia: a constant prevalence of 25 per cent in a chronic mental hospital population? *British Journal of Psychiatry*, **133**, 130–136.

WINOKUR, G. (1977) Delusional disorder (paranoia). *Comprehensive Psychiatry*, **18**, 511–521.

10 International variations in the diagnosis of psychiatric illness

JULIAN LEFF

The virtual absence of pathognomonic laboratory investigations for psychiatric conditions forces the psychiatrist to base his diagnosis firmly on the clinical interview. Shepherd *et al* (1968) identified four major components of the psychiatric interview: (i) the interviewing technique of the psychiatrist; (2) perception of the patient's speech and behaviour; (3) inferences and decisions made by the psychiatrist on the basis of what he has perceived; (4) attachment of a particular diagnostic label to the patient. These are useful distinctions and will be employed to structure this review. However, they are not strictly compartmentalized and in practice are subject to mutual influences. In particular, the psychiatrist's diagnostic scheme strongly determines his interviewing technique and, as we shall see, affects his perception of what the patient says and does, in addition to his decisions about the presence of symptoms. The importance of this pervasive influence cannot be over-estimated, since it has been shown that psychiatrists confidently reach a conclusion about the diagnosis within the first few minutes of the interview (Sandifer *et al*, 1970; Kendell, 1973). For these reasons, although this review is primarily concerned with international variations in diagnosis, the subject cannot be adequately dealt with unless some consideration is given to the individual components of the clinical interview.

Interviewing technique

Patients express some of their symptoms spontaneously, but by no means all of them, and then not usually in great detail. This allows the interviewer considerable latitude as to how far he will probe to elicit and clarify the patient's abnormal experiences. The importance a psychiatrist attaches to careful questioning about the phenomena of illness is largely determined by his theoretical frame of reference. For example, an interviewer working within a psychoanalytic framework is likely to accept a patient's statement that people stare at him as sufficient evidence for the utilization of projective mechanisms. A phenomenologist, by contrast, will want to question the patient closely until he has determined whether the statement indicates a social phobia, a simple idea of reference, or a delusion of reference. On the other hand, the analytic interviewer will attempt to delineate the patient's relationships with his parents in great detail, an area which the phenomenologist will probably skim over.

Hence the psychiatrist's theoretical orientation determines the structure of the interview and the kind of information elicited.

Even the psychiatrist who is primarily concerned with phenomenology will not attempt to cover the whole range of possible symptoms in the usual clinical interview. The exigencies of a busy clinic lead the psychiatrist to cut corners. Thus, once he has confidently made a diagnosis of schizophrenia, the clinical psychiatrist is unlikely to press on further and explore neurotic symptomatology in any depth. The research psychiatrist, however, is usually committed by the nature of a structured interview to cover the whole range of possible pathology regardless of diagnosis. He soon learns that schizophrenic patients often prove to have a multiplicity of neurotic symptoms when these are enquired about specifically. The importance of this in relation to the topic of this review is that the psychiatrist who brings the interview to a premature end may fail to elicit symptoms that could cause him to modify his diagnosis.

Perception of the patient's speech and behaviour

There is an extensive body of work by social psychologists demonstrating that subjects' preconceptions or prejudices can influence their perception of stimuli. This applies as much to the psychiatrist as to the naïve subject of a psychological experiment. The psychiatrist's perception of pathology is affected by his diagnostic preconceptions and by his expectations built up by previous experience. The interviewer's judgement of the *level* of pathology exhibited by the patient depends to some degree on his theoretical background and training.

Influence of diagnostic preconceptions

Most people applying a scheme for classification, such as diagnosis, prefer to encounter phenomena that fit neatly into one or other of their categories rather than overlapping several categories. This is probably because phenomena that overlap categorical boundaries challenge the validity of the classificatory scheme. So that psychiatrists encountering symptoms in a patient that do not fit with the diagnosis that has already taken shape in their mind are likely to ignore such symptoms or even misperceive them. Shepherd *et al* (1968) give as an example the patient with a relatively immobile face. This could be interpreted as the affective blunting of schizophrenia or the mask-like facies of depression, depending on the diagnosis the interviewer has decided on. They point out that this is an example of the 'halo' effect.

Their example proved to be well-chosen, as it received confirmation in a study by Katz *et al* (1969). These workers showed short cine films of psychiatric interviews to audiences of psychiatrists. For two of the patients, audiences showed significant variations in their rating of 'apathy' on a standardized rating scale. High ratings of apathy were found to be associated with a diagnosis made by the rater of schizophrenia.

Influence of prior expectations

This has been most clearly shown in relation to the patient's expression of affect. Leff (1973) analysed data from the International Pilot Study of Schizophrenia (WHO, 1974) and found that patients from developed countries showed a greater ability to differentiate between unpleasant emotional states than those from developing countries. The data on which the finding was based were scores derived from the sections on Depression, Anxiety and Irritability in the Present State Examination (PSE), a semi-structured psychiatric interview (Wing *et al*, 1974). In a subsequent paper (Leff, 1974), reliability exercises from the same study were used to compare the ratings of psychiatrists from developed and developing countries. The psychiatrists rated videotaped, filmed and live interviews of patients from the various centres involved in the study. This made it possible to derive measures of emotional differentiation from their ratings of patients from developed and developing countries. It was found that both groups of psychiatrists agreed in rating patients from developed countries as showing a high degree of emotional differentiation; but they differed significantly in their ratings of patients from developing countries: psychiatrists from developing countries rated these patients as showing a low degree of differentiation between Depression, Anxiety and Irritability, whereas psychiatrists from developed countries rated *the same patients* as showing a pattern of emotional differentiation which was much closer to that exhibited by patients from developed countries. The most plausible explanation is that developed centre psychiatrists were imposing a greater differentiation on developing centre patients because this is what they were led to expect from their experience with patients from their own developed centres. It must be emphasized that the differences in ratings of the psychiatrists involved in the reliability exercises imply different perceptions of the patients' responses, since they were all exposed to the same interviews.

Influence of theoretical background

The influence this has on the interviewers' perception of the level of pathology exhibited by the patient has been studied in relation to American and British psychiatrists. The development of videotape equipment has been a great spur to the advancement of this area, as it greatly facilitates international comparisons of ratings of the same interview. It is hardly surprising that American and British comparisons predominate in this work, since there is no apparent language barrier to surmount. Katz *et al* (1969) asked audiences of American and British psychiatrists to rate films of psychiatric patients on the IMPS scales (Lorr and Klett, 1967). The scores of British psychiatrists were found to be lower on eight of the nine IMPS scales than those of American psychiatrists. Sandifer *et al* (1969) conducted a very similar exercise. They filmed interviews with 23 patients in a public mental hospital in America and showed them to 33 American and 8 British psychiatrists. Each observer was provided with a checklist of 39 common psychiatric symptoms, such as 'suspicious', 'grandiose', and 'bizarre behaviour', and 16 diagnostic clues, such as 'sex of patient' and 'response to previous treatment'. Items were generally rated on a present-absent basis. The American raters reported almost twice as many symptoms as the British raters, the mean number of symptoms per case being 11.2 and 6.2 respectively. Only three symptoms were rated more often as present by the British observers. One of these was 'elated mood', which is in keeping with the fact that the British psychiatrists diagnosed manic-depressive disorder in 26 per cent of cases compared with 12 per cent diagnosed by the American psychiatrists. This is another example of the way in which diagnostic preconceptions can influence the perception of symptoms.

Sandifer *et al* point out that the main finding of the lower reporting of symptoms by British observers could be the consequence of a higher threshold for the recognition of pathology. Alternatively it might result from caution in diagnosing pathology in patients from another culture (i.e. American as opposed to British). One way to distinguish between these explanations is to show both American and British patients to psychiatric raters of both nationalities. This is what Kendell *et al* (1971) did, using videotapes of five interviews with British patients and three with American patients. The patients portrayed a wide range of symptoms and a variety of clinical problems. The tapes were rated by a maximum of 200 British and 120 American psychiatrists, with an average length of experience of between 12 and 15 years. More of the American than of the British psychiatrists had received a formal training in psychotherapy. The raters completed 89 items from the IMPS and a checklist of 116 technical terms, as well as making a diagnosis. The tendency of the British psychiatrists to rate less pathology than the Americans was apparent in their assessments of the British patients as well as in those of the American patients (Kendell, personal communication). Hence the findings of this series of studies are explained by a higher threshold among British psychiatrists for rating pathology. This is likely to stem from the difference in training alluded to by Kendell *et al*. A formal training in psychotherapy sensitizes the trainee to what may lie behind the symptoms. He focuses as much on hypothetical psychological mechanisms and personality structures as on the observable phenomena. Since the same mechanisms and structures are postulated to underlie both mild symptoms and severe symptoms, the trainee's sensitivity to possible pathology is increased and his threshold for rating its presence is lowered.

Inferences and decisions

This stage of inferring pathology on the basis of what has been perceived is subject to the psychiatrist's ethnocentric bias. This increases in proportion to his ignorance of the culture to which his patient belongs. The definition of a delusion includes a vital clause, namely that the false belief shall be inconsistent with the patient's cultural background. Consequently, the psychiatrist cannot make a firm assertion that a delusion is present without a thorough knowledge and understanding of the beliefs and values of the patient's culture. This is an unusual circumstance when the psychiatrist belongs to a different culture from the patient. The mistakes in diagnosis that can be made out of ignorance of the patient's culture are exemplified by *koro* and possession states. *Koro* is one of the so-called 'culture-bound psychoses' and is usually discussed in company with *amok*, *latah* and *whitigo*. It is confined to South-East Asia and is characterized by a state of panic occurring in males who believe that their penis is in danger of disappearing into their abdomen, leading to their death. So overwhelming is this fear that the sufferer may secure his penis to a large boulder with wire, or may recruit his relatives to hold on to it in relays. This belief seems bizarre and incomprehensible to the Western psychiatrist and viewed in isolation appears to have the hallmarks of a delusion. However, it has to be judged against the background of the belief, widely held in the same area, that ghosts have no sexual organs. Furthermore, the fact that relatives can be persuaded by the patient to do their best to prevent the dreaded happening informs us that they accept the fear as realistic. Hence, knowledge about local beliefs concerning spirits corrects the impression that *koro* is characterized by delusions and should be classed with the psychoses. Instead, as Yap (1965) points out, it is much closer to hypochondriacal neurosis in the West.

A similar lesson is provided by possession states. Subjects undergoing 'possession' are found in virtually every culture in the world. Bourguignon (1976) surveyed 488 societies weighted towards traditional cultures, and found that 90 per cent of them had institutionalized some state of altered consciousness; trance, possession-trance, or both. 'Possessed' subjects behave in unusual ways and may speak in a different voice from usual. They may claim at the time or afterwards that an alien spirit has entered into them and is controlling their will, their actions and their speech. These assertions fulfil Schneider's (1957) criteria for a delusion of control, one of his first-rank symptoms of schizophrenia; but it would be a mistake to diagnose the possessed person as suffering from schizophrenia or any other psychosis. As Bourguignon points out, the possession state occurs in the presence of and for the benefit of an audience. These members of the subject's own culture accept the reality of spirit possession and indeed have often taken part in a ritual which is specifically designed to lead to this end. The subject's apparent delusions are completely in harmony with the beliefs of his fellow men, who would not view his altered behaviour as being indicative of pathology. It is understandable that Western psychiatrists occasionally mistake possession states for schizophrenia, but, surprisingly, psychiatrists from the subject's own culture sometimes fall into the same error; this must result from the distance that a Western education interposes between them and the local beliefs and values.

Attachment of a diagnostic label

We have seen from the foregoing that the psychiatrist's diagnostic framework can influence what he tries to elicit from the patient, how he perceives what has been elicited, and how he interprets what he has perceived. These various processes form reverberating circuits which in turn influence the diagnosis. It is all too easy, therefore, for a diagnostic framework to became a tautology from which it is impossible for the psychiatrist to escape, even when it bears little relation to the observable phenomena. In this section we will consider studies which have compared the diagnostic frameworks of different national groups. This field is dominated by two large-scale international programmes, the US:UK Project (Cooper *et al*, 1972) and the International Pilot Study of Schizophrenia (WHO, 1974). Before discussing these, one of the earliest and simplest international studies of the diagnostic process should be mentioned.

Rawnsley (1968) selected a set of 59 case records of psychiatric in-patients from hospitals in England and Wales. Summaries of not more than 400 words were prepared from them and were sent to 205 psychiatrists in England and Wales to provide diagnoses for them. The 30 summaries on which these psychiatrists were in broad agreement were then sent to 260 psychiatrists in America, 30 in Denmark, 28 in Norway and 18 in Sweden. In 22 of the 30 cases there was fairly high agreement between the international panel if broad diagnostic categories were employed to classify the individual labels. However, there was a marked propensity for American psychiatrists to diagnose schizophrenia, where the European psychiatrists assigned diagnoses of depression, obsessional disorder, or paranoid psychosis not specified as schizophrenia. The Scandinavian psychiatrists, in particular the Norwegians, exhibited an idiosyncratic use of the term 'psychogenic psychosis', which was hardly used at all by American and British psychiatrists, who tended to call the same cases neurotic. The results for the American psychiatrists foreshadow the findings of the large-scale international programmes, but it must be borne in mind that the presentation of clinical material in the form of case summaries cuts out a major source of variation in diagnosis, namely the preliminary stage of observation of symptoms.

The US:UK Project

The US:UK Project was stimulated by the earlier studies presented above and by striking differences in the mental hospital statistics from England and America. For example, Kramer (1961; 1969a; 1969b) showed that the first-admission rate for manic-depressive disease in the age-group 55–64 years was 20 times as high for England and Wales as for America. Differences of this degree could provide an excellent opportunity to search for the causes of these conditions if one could be certain that the diagnoses were being made in the same way on both sides of the Atlantic. This issue comprised one of the major aims of the US:UK Project. It was tackled by assembling a team of research psychiatrists and training them to assess symptoms in a standardized way and to apply, as far as possible, the same diagnostic framework to the symptoms. Ideally the Project team should then have been capable of acting as a standardized measuring instrument, whose component parts (the individual psychiatrists) were interchangeable and could be employed in an identical way to assess patients in America or England. The basic instrument for assessing patients' clinical state was the Present State Examination (Wing *et al*, 1974), an interview with a demonstrably high reliability. The diagnostic procedure was not standardized in the sense that a set of rules was laid down for processing the symptoms; but great care was taken to ensure that Project diagnoses were made with identical criteria on both sides of the Atlantic by an exchange of interviewers between London and New York and by numerous statistical checks on consistency. Thus we can conclude that although the diagnostic procedure was not standardized in the strict sense it was homogenized. Since four of the six members of the Project team had received their psychiatric training at the Maudsley Hospital, it could be anticipated that Project diagnoses would approximate to British rather than American practice. This might appear to introduce a source of bias into the study, but a consideration of the following analogy should dispel that impression. Suppose that there is a line drawn on the pavement in Trafalgar Square, London, and another one in Times Square, New York. The Londoners assert that their line is 6 cubits long, whereas the New Yorkers maintain that their line measures 3 cubits. Unfortunately we know that the cubit is a variable unit, being defined by the length of the Queen's forearm in England and the President's forearm in America. It is therefore necessary, in order to compare the length of the lines, to construct a ruler marked out in cubits which can be used on both sides of the Atlantic. It is immaterial whether the ruler is calibrated in American or English cubits, since the issue is not the absolute length of the lines but a comparison of their lengths relative to each other. The diagnostic framework of the Project team acts as just such a transportable ruler, which happens to be calibrated in British units.

The first cross-national comparison in the Project was made by interviewing 250 recently admitted patients in Netherne Hospital, near London, and the same number in Brooklyn State Hospital, New York. In order to avoid contamination of the diagnosis either way, there was no communication on the cases between Project psychiatrists and hospital staff. The Project psychiatrists were constrained by the design of the study to use for their diagnoses the 8th edition of the International Classification of Diseases. The hospital diagnoses of the Brooklyn and Netherne patients were taken from the official returns and were combined into ten broad groupings. Table I shows a comparison of the most important diagnostic categories.

TABLE I

A comparison of the hospital and Project diagnoses of the Brooklyn and Netherne patients. The figures represent percentages of the total sample

	Brooklyn patients		Netherne patients	
	Hospital diagnosis	Project diagnosis	Project diagnosis	Hospital diagnosis
Schizophrenia	65.2†	32.4	26.0	34.0†
Depressive psychosis	7.2†	20.0*	28.0*	32.8†
Mania	0.8	6.8	3.6	1.6
Personality disorder	0.8†	2.4	4.4	8.4†

† P < 0.01; * P < 0.05
Significance levels relate to comparison of the two sets of hospital diagnoses with each other, and the two sets of Project diagnoses with each other.
Adapted from Cooper *et al* (1972).

It can be seen that the hospital diagnoses differ in distribution highly significantly for three out of the four categories shown. Schizophrenia, in particular, appears to be almost twice as common among Brooklyn patients as among Netherne patients, whereas depressive psychosis is diagnosed more than four times as frequently by the Netherne psychiatrists. By contrast, the Project diagnoses for the two hospitals are much more similar, only the difference in proportion of depressive psychosis reaching significance. As anticipated, the Project diagnoses are much closer to the diagnoses of the Netherne psychiatrists than to those of the Brooklyn psychiatrists.

These striking results were obtained from a comparison of only two hospitals. It was considered necessary to broaden the study to include a representative sample of newly admitted patients from the whole of New York and the whole of London. This was achieved by randomly selecting between 150 and 200 admissions to all nine psychiatric hospitals serving New York, and nine representative hospitals serving the London area. The procedures were exactly the same as in the Brooklyn-Netherne comparison. The main findings are presented in Table II.

TABLE II

A comparison of the hospital and Project diagnoses of the New York and London patients. The figures represent percentages of the total sample

	New York patients		London patients	
	Hospital diagnosis	Project diagnosis	Project diagnosis	Hospital diagnosis
Schizophrenia	61.5†	29.2	35.1	33.9†
Depressive psychosis	4.7†	19.8	22.3	24.1†
Mania	0.5†	5.7	6.3	6.9†
Personality disorder	1.0*	4.2	2.9	4.6*

† P < 0.01; * P < 0.05
Significance levels relate to comparison of the two sets of hospital diagnoses with each other, and the two sets of Project diagnoses with each other.
Adapted from Cooper *et al* (1972).

The results are very similar to the Brooklyn-Netherne comparison, though perhaps even more remarkable. The distributions of all four major diagnostic groups given differ significantly when the hospital diagnoses are compared. All these significant differences disappear when the Project diagnoses are compared, and in fact the Project diagnoses on both sides of the Atlantic are remarkably similar in their distribution.

This work confirms and underlines previous findings that the American diagnosis of schizophrenia is much broader than the British diagnosis. It includes most of what the British psychiatrist would call mania, which is hardly recognized at all by the New York psychiatrists. It also encompasses substantial parts of what the British psychiatrists would regard as depressive illness, neurotic illness and personality disorder. This is an alarming state of affairs for transatlantic communication about psychiatric conditions, but Cooper *et al* sound a slightly hopeful note. They suggest that New York psychiatrists may not be typical of the United States as a whole, and that overall Anglo-American differences may be somewhat less substantial than the Project results indicate.

This qualified optimism gains some support from a study of American, British and Canadian psychiatrists, which was stimulated by the results of the US:UK Project. Sharpe *et al* (1974) showed videotapes of interviews with three patients to psychiatrists from many parts of the US, the UK and Canada. These videotapes had been found in previous international studies to provoke considerable diagnostic disagreement among psychiatrists. Each rater was required to record the psychopathology on a list of 116 items, to fill in the IMPS, and to select a diagnosis from the 8th edition of the ICD. Two of the patients exhibited a mixture of schizophrenic and affective symptoms, while the third showed symptoms which British psychiatrists tended to call 'hysterical' and American psychiatrists schizophrenic. For one of the 'schizoaffective patients' the diagnosis of schizophrenia was made by 86 per cent of American psychiatrists, 70 per cent of British, and 56 per cent of Canadians. For the other, schizophrenia was favoured by 82 per cent of Americans, 66 per cent of British, and 81 per cent of Canadians. For the third patient, schizophrenia was diagnosed by 53 per cent of Americans, 2 per cent of British, and 27 per cent of Canadians.

Thus, in terms of the use of the diagnosis of schizophrenia, the Canadian psychiatrists tended to occupy a position between American and British psychiatrists. This is probably a reflection of the fact that some of them received their psychiatric training in Britain and others in the US. In terms of their perception of a high level of psychopathology and their ratings of items such as 'ambivalence' and 'projection', the Canadians were much closer to the American psychiatrists than to the British. This interesting observation suggests that the influence of a formal training in psychotherapy can lower the threshold for perceiving psychopathology without necessarily broadening the diagnostic concept of schizophrenia. These results, however, only derive from a small series of patients, and a much more extensive study would be required to investigate this proposition.

The International Pilot Study of Schizophrenia (IPSS) (WHO, 1974)

This study was broader in scope than the US:UK Project in that it included centres in nine different countries, but narrower in that it concentrated almost exclusively on the diagnosis of schizophrenia. There are similarities in the design of the two studies, both involving the training of research psychiatrists in the use of the Present State Examination in order to assess symptoms in a standardized way. But here the similarity ends, for in the US:UK Project a deliberate attempt was made to standardize the diagnostic habits of the Project psychiatrists. By contrast, in the IPSS the variation in the diagnostic habits of the research psychiatrists in the nine centres was one of the main objects of study. A central issue in this project was to determine whether psychiatrists in various countries thoughout the world use the term schizophrenia to group together patients with similar patterns of symptoms. To investigate this question, it was first necessary to ensure that the research psychiatrists were assessing symptoms in the same way. This was achieved by translating the PSE from English into the seven other languages used in the IPSS centres. These were sited in Aarhus, Agra, Cali, Ibadan, London, Moscow, Prague, Taipei and Washington. Only two of the languages, Yoruba in Ibadan and Chinese in Taipei, do not belong to the Indo-European family of languages. Some difficulty was experienced in translating words for various emotions into these two languages (Leff, 1973), but otherwise the translations went smoothly.

The trained psychiatrists then used the translated versions of the PSE to interview a consecutive series of about 100 psychotic patients admitted to their local psychiatric facility. The screening net for 'psychosis' was deliberately very broad in order to include a wide variety of patients who might receive a diagnosis of schizophrenia. In all, 1,202 patients were included in the study from the nine centres, and 77.5 per cent of them were given a diagnosis of schizophrenia by the research psychiatrists. One way of looking for possible differences in the use of this diagnosis in the various centres is to compare the symptom profiles of patients diagnosed as schizophrenic. This comparison revealed close similarities between the groups of patients from each centre given a diagnosis of schizophrenia.

However, for a more detailed examination of possible differences it is most informative to use a reference classification. This is equivalent to the Project diagnoses in the US:UK study, but in the IPSS a strictly standardized diagnostic procedure was used. This was the CATEGO program (Wing *et al*, 1974), which embodies a set of rules for condensing the PSE items and weighting them differentially to yield a diagnosis. This set of rules stems from the clinical judgements of the psychiatrists constructing the program, and represents a conservative English diagnostic approach, which itself owes a great deal to German psychiatry.

The PSE findings on all the patients from the nine centres were fed into a computer and processed by the CATEGO program. The CATEGO diagnoses, resulting from the application of an explicit set of rules, can be compared with the centre diagnoses to throw light on the diagnostic process in each centre. This comparison is shown in Table III. CATEGO classes S, P and O are equivalent to schizophrenia and paranoid psychoses, Class M to mania, and classes D, R and N to depressive psychoses and neuroses.

The overall discrepancy between CATEGO classes and centre diagnoses is smallest for the London centre. This is hardly surprising, as the present author made virtually all the diagnoses on the London patients and works closely with Wing. What is remarkable, though, is that the discrepancy between CATEGO and the Taipei psychiatrists is almost as small. In fact, in only two centres, Moscow and Washington, is the discrepancy large enough to suggest a substantial difference in diagnostic rules. If these two centres are excluded, the overall agreement between the seven remaining centres and CATEGO is 95.5 per cent on schizophrenia and 86.2 per cent on affective psychoses and neuroses. For Moscow and Washington combined, the agreement with CATEGO is only 70.5 per cent. It is evident from Table III that in both Moscow and Washington substantial proportions of the patients given a centre diagnosis of schizophrenia are assigned by CATEGO to mania or depressive psychoses and neuroses. The results for the Washington centre confirm the findings from the US:UK Project. The Moscow psychiatrists also have an unusually broad concept of schizophrenia but this stems from a different approach to that of American psychiatrists.

The Moscow centre psychiatrists all came from the same Institute headed by Professor Snezhnevsky. A school of psychiatry has developed under his leadership which places great emphasis on the course of psychiatric conditions. In making a diagnosis of schizophrenia, the symptoms exhibited during episodes are less important than the recurrent or chronic nature of the illness and the impairment of the patient's social adjustment between episodes. The Moscow psychiatrists provided some detailed case histories to illustrate their diagnostic method. It is clear from these that their diagnosis of individual episodes is firmly based on the phenomenology and is quite close to British practice. Thus one patient was described as suffering episodes characterized

TABLE III

A comparison of centre diagnoses and CATEGO classes

CATEGO classes	Aarhus	Agra	Cali	Ibadan	London	Moscow	Taipei	Washington	Prague
Centre Schizophrenia and Paranoid Psychoses									
S, P, O	73	92	97	117	100	52	107	75	73
M	—	5	4	5	1	10	—	11	8
D, R, N	4	3	1	—	—	21	—	10	7
Centre Mania									
S, P, O	4	2	—	1	1	1	1	—	—
M	18	18	3	3	6	—	5	4	9
D, R, N	—	—	—	—	—	2	—	1	—
Centre Depressive Psychoses and Neuroses									
S, P, O	4	6	2	7	3	4	4	3	2
M	5	2	1	1	—	1	1	1	—
D, R, N	15	9	6	9	16	20	13	16	25
Total patients	123	137	114	143	127	111	131	121	124
% Discrepancy	13.8	13.1	7.0	9.8	3.9	35.1	4.6	21.5	13.7

Adapted from WHO (1974).

by affective symptoms, but because of the recurrent nature of the illness and a deterioration of the patient's work record between attacks plus an increasing apathy the overall diagnosis was recurrent schizophrenia.

It is worth noting that the Moscow school by no means sets its stamp on the whole of Russian psychiatric practice, and that in Leningrad psychiatric diagnosis is much closer to that in the West.

For the seven centres other than Moscow and Washington, it is evident that the rules used by the centre psychiatrists to diagnose schizophrenia must be similar to those embodied in the CATEGO program. This has a hierarchical structure, with the greatest weight given to the first-rank symptoms of Schneider (1957). It is not surprising, therefore, that when these symptoms are present in IPSS patients there is a very high probability of the centre psychiatrists making a diagnosis of schizophrenia. These probabilities can be calculated exactly and are 95 per cent for third-person auditory hallucinations, 95 per cent for voices commenting on the patient's thoughts or actions, 97 per cent for thought broadcast, insertion or withdrawal, and 97 per cent for delusions of control.

Other studies

The relationship between the diagnostic habits of British and German psychiatrists has been explored by Kendell *et al* (1974); they also included a group of French psychiatrists in the comparison. Videotapes were made of brief diagnostic interviews, lasing five minutes each, with a series of 27 patients at the time of their admission to the Maudsley Hospital. These were shown to audiences of experienced psychiatrists in London, Munich and Paris. Raters had to indicate the presence of symptoms on a checklist and make a diagnosis from the 8th edition of the ICD. There was substantial diagnostic agreement between all three national groups in 17 of the 27 cases. Agreement was closest between the English and German raters and least between the English and French. There was generally good agreement on the diagnosis of schizophrenia, but striking differences for manic-depressive disorder. The English psychiatrists used this label for 23 per cent of cases, the Germans for 14 per cent, and the French for only 5 per cent. The French raters had a lower threshold for the recognition of symptoms than either the English or the Germans. They showed particularly high ratings relative to the others on 'odd or inappropriate behaviour', 'perplexity', and 'bizarre or inappropriate remarks'.

Comments

The influence of the German school of psychiatry on diagnostic practice appears to have spread around the world, reaching places as widely scattered as Taipei, Agra and Cali. The main emphasis is on the observable phenomena of psychiatric illness, the threshold for the recognition of pathology being relatively high. The diagnosis of schizophrenia is based directly on observable symptoms and is relatively narrow. This allows room for a relatively wide concept of affective disorders.

In contrast to this is American diagnostic practice, which appears to have been influenced by the ascendancy of psychoanalysis in the US. Emphasis is placed on psychological mechanisms which are inferred from the observable symptoms. This leads to a relatively low threshold for the recognition of pathology and a relatively broad concept of schizophrenia, leaving little scope for the diagnosis of affective disorders. French diagnostic practice appears to be much closer to American than to German practice. Canadian psychiatrists are in the interesting position of being influenced by American, British and French psychiatry; their diagnostic practice appears to lie mid-way between the American and British, which itself is very close to the German.

Muscovite practice is idiosyncratic, involving a heavy emphasis on course of illness and social adjustment at the expense of phenomenology, which is not shared by any other school.

It must be emphasized that there can be no rights or wrongs about these different diagnostic schemata at this point in time. Until there is some way of validating diagnosis which is not part of a tautology, we must be content to allow a hundred flowers to bloom together.

References

Bourguignon, E. (1976) Possession and trance in cross-cultural studies of mental health. In *Culture-Bound Syndromes, Ethnopsychiatry, and Alternate Therapies* (ed. W. P. Lebra). Honolulu: University Press of Hawaii.

Cooper, J. E., Kendell, R. E., Gurland, B. J., Sharpe, L., Copeland, J. R. M. & Simon, R. (1972) *Psychiatric Diagnosis in New York and London.* Maudsley Monograph No. 20. Oxford University Press.

Katz, M., Cole, J. O. & Lowery, H. A. (1969) Studies of the diagnostic process: the influence of symptom perception, past experience and ethnic background on diagnostic decisions. *American Journal of Psychiatry*, **125,** 937–947.

Kendell, R. E. (1973) Psychiatric diagnoses: a study of how they are made. *British Journal of Psychiatry*, **122,** 437–445.

—— Sharpe, L., Cooper, J. E., Gurland, B. J., Gourlay, A. J. & Copeland, J. R. M. (1971) Diagnostic criteria of American and British psychiatrists. *Archives of General Psychiatry*, **25,** 123–130.

—— Pichot, P. & Von Cranach, M. (1974) Diagnostic criteria of English, French and German psychiatrists. *Psychological Medicine*, **4,** 187–195.

Kramer, M. (1961) Some problems for international research. In *Proceedings of the Third World Congress of Psychiatry, Vol 3.* Montreal: University of Toronto Press.

—— (1969a) Cross-national study of diagnosis of the mental disorders: origin of the problem. *American Journal of Psychiatry*, **125** (Suppl), 1–11.

—— (1969b) Statistics of mental disorders in the United States: current status and future goals. In *Comparative Epidemiology of the Mental Disorders* (eds P. Hoch and J. Zubin). New York: Grune and Stratton.

Leff, J. P. (1973) Culture and differentiation of emotional states. *British Journal of Psychiatry*, **123,** 299–306.

—— (1974) Transcultural influences on psychiatrists' rating of verbally expressed emotion. *British Journal of Psychiatry*, **125,** 336–340.

Lorr, M. & Klett, C. J. (1967) *In-patient Multidimensional Psychiatric Scale.* Palo Alto: Consulting Psychologists Press.

Rawnsley, K. (1968) An international diagnostic exercise. In *Proceedings of the Fourth World Congress of Psychiatry, Vol 4.* Amsterdam: Excerpta Medica Foundation.

Sandifer, M. G., Hordern, A., Timbury, G. C. & Green, L. M. (1969) Similarities and differences in patient evaluation by U.S. and U.K. psychiatrists. *American Journal of Psychiatry*, **126,** 206–212.

—— —— & Green, L. M. (1970) The psychiatric interview: the impact of the first three minutes. *American Journal of Psychiatry*, **126,** 968–973.

Schneider, K. (1957) Primäre und sekundäre Symptome bei der Schizophrenie. *Fortschritte der Neurologie und Psychiatrie*, **25,** 487–490.

Sharpe, S., Gurland, B. J., Fleiss, J. L., Kendell, R. E., Cooper, J. E. & Copeland, J. R. M. (1974) Comparisons of American, Canadian and British psychiatrists in their diagnostic concepts. *Canadian Psychiatric Association Journal*, **19**, 235–245.

Shepherd, M., Brooke, E. M., Cooper, J. E. & Lin, T. (1968) An experimental approach to psychiatric diagnosis. *Acta Psychiatrica Scandinavica*, Suppl 201.

Wing, J. K., Cooper, J. E. & Sartorius, N. (1974) *Measurement and Classification of Psychiatric Symptoms*. Cambridge University Press.

World Health Organization (1974) *The International Pilot Study of Schizophrenia*. Vol 1. Geneva: WHO.

Yap, P. M. (1965) Koro—a culture-bound depersonalization syndrome. *British Journal of Psychiatry*, **111**, 43–50.

11 The DSM-III concept of schizophrenia

HERBERT A. FOX

The DSM-III concept of schizophrenia differs in important ways from the DSM-II concept of the disorder. This paper will critically examine the elements of the DSM-III concept and describe the aims and perspectives of its authors.

The most important influence on the character of DSM-III was the work of Eli Robins and his research group at the Washington University in St Louis. Robins *et al* worked for many years to develop a valid and reliable system of diagnostic classification for psychiatry that would allow a meaningful comparison of research findings among different investigators. The achievement of such comparison required the common use of formal diagnostic criteria. Robins and his colleagues believed that these should be based upon research findings rather than simply upon clinical judgement and experience. Accordingly, they conducted a large number of studies over several years and, on the basis of their data, derived a series of specific diagnostic criteria for 14 psychiatric disorders. These criteria have come to be known as the Feighner criteria, named after the senior author of the paper describing their work (Feighner *et al*, 1972).

The Feighner criteria are rigorous ones, reflecting the authors' research interest in establishing homogeneous diagnostic groups. It is generally assumed that homogeneity is a requirement for sound research design (Buchsbaum and Haier, 1978). The purer the groups being compared, the more significant and valuable are the results of research.

The Feighner criteria were derived on the basis of Robins's five criteria for establishing diagnostic validity (Robins and Guze, 1970): (1) Clinical description—by considering aspects of the clinical picture other than signs and symptoms, e.g. age at onset, sex, race, etc., a disorder can be more precisely and narrowly defined; (2) Laboratory study—this is obviously of great importance in establishing validity. Unfortunately consistent studies are not yet available for psychiatric disorders; (3) Delimitation from other disorders—by providing specific exclusion criteria for each diagnosis, disorders with similar symptoms can be more clearly distinguished; (4) Follow-up studies—the persistence of a diagnosis over time suggests its validity. Markedly different outcomes for a given disorder question its validity; (5) Family study—increased incidence of a disorder among family members supports its validity. These five criteria, as will be seen, play a central role in the structure of DSM-III.

The next major step in the development of DSM-III was the creation of the Research Diagnostic Criteria (RDC). Working in collaboration with Robins and Endicott, Spitzer developed the RDC for use in a National Institute of Mental Health (NIMH) collaborative project on the psychobiology of depression. The RDC is an elaboration, expansion and modification of the Feighner Criteria. It added 16 categories, provided non-mutually exclusive sub-categories, and refined the inclusion and exclusion criteria. The purpose of the RDC was to enhance diagnostic agreement among research centres. Since diagnostic disagreement results primarily from the use of different criteria, the development of widely accepted, sound, operationally defined, and reliable criteria was considered crucial (Spitzer *et al*, 1975).

The criteria developed for the RDC have been utilized—with modifications—in DSM-III. In general, DSM-III criteria are less stringent, reflecting their general clinical rather than specific research purposes. Several studies have confirmed their relatively high reliability (Spitzer *et al*, 1978b).

Schizophrenia

DSM-III defines schizophrenia as a mental disorder with a tendency toward chronicity which impairs functioning and which is characterized by psychotic symptoms involving disturbances of thinking, feeling and behaviour.

The definition was shaped by a number of different goals: to improve reliability; to reflect recent research findings; to relate diagnosis more closely to prognosis and treatment; to minimize the stigma of labelling; to achieve clinical acceptability while reducing differences with European colleagues; and to allow the clinician to express diagnostic uncertainty (Spitzer *et al*, 1978a).

There are six specific criteria for the diagnosis of schizophrenia: (a) certain psychotic symptoms (see below); (b) deterioration from a previous level of functioning in such areas as work, social relations and self-care; (c) continuous signs of the illness for at least six months, including an active phase of psychotic symptoms—the six months may include prodromal and residual phases during which symptoms like withdrawal, peculiar behaviour, impaired functioning and blunted affect are present, but overt psychotic symptoms are absent: (d) onset before age 45; (e) not due to affective disorder; (f) not due to organic mental disorder or mental retardation.

The list of specific symptoms—any one of which is sufficient to satisfy the symptom criterion—is very broad and is drawn from a number of sources including the work of Bleuler (1911), Schneider (1959) and the IPPS (Carpenter *et al*, 1973). The symptoms can be grouped in the following four categories: (1) Any delusion, except jealousy or persecution—most of Schneider's first-rank symptoms (delusions of control, thought broadcast, thought insertion and thought withdrawal) and other bizarre delusions are emphasized; (2) Delusions of jealousy or persecution, if accompanied by auditory hallucinations; (3) Any repeated auditory hallucinations of more than one or two words whose content is not related to depression or elation. Again, two of Schneider's most important auditory hallucinations are emphasized (two or more voices, and voices keeping up a running commentary on the person's thoughts or behaviour); (4) A formal thought disorder (incoherence, loosening of associations, markedly illogical thinking, or marked poverty of content of speech), if accompanied by flat or inappropriate affect, hallucinations or delusions (of any kind), or catatonic or other grossly disorganized behaviour. A thought disorder alone—presumably because of its low reliability– is not sufficient. Similarly, bizarre behaviour and flat or inappropriate affect alone are excluded for purposes of diagnosis.

The DSM-III definition of schizophrenia eliminates several entities included in the DSM-II concept of the disorder. Syndromes which look like schizophrenia, but which last less than six months are called schizophreniform disorder, and are classified elsewhere. Schizophreniform disorder has been separated from schizophrenia because of research evidence that it may be associated with a greater likelihood of emotional turmoil and confusion; a better prognosis; a tendency toward acute onset and resolution; more likely recovery to premorbid level of functioning; and no increased incidence of schizophrenia among family members (Task Force, 1980). Psychotic syndromes of less than two weeks duration which follow a significant psychosocial stressor are also excluded and are called brief reactive psychosis.

Borderline or latent schizophrenia and simple schizophrenia, as they lack psychotic symptoms, are also excluded. These entities are diagnosed borderline or schizotypal personality disorder. Schizophrenia-like syndromes of late onset—particularly the involutional paraphrenias—are excluded as well. Such entities will be diagnosed paranoid disorder or atypical psychosis.

Organic mental disorder or mental retardation, and affective disorder are specifically excluded. The exclusion of the former is relatively obvious and straightforward. The exclusion of affective disorder is complicated and problematic. This exclusion raises the question of how syndromes with features suggestive of both schizophrenia and affective disorder are to be classified.

The term schizoaffective was coined by Kasanin (1933) to describe such cases. Ever since, controversy has raged over whether schizoaffective disorder (SAD) represents a variety of schizophrenia, a variety of affective disorder, some combination of both, or a completely distinct third psychosis. Part of the confusion has been the failure to define SAD precisely.

In an earlier draft (Task Force, 1978) DSM-III defined SAD as a disorder in which a full affective syndrome (depression or mania) preceded or developed concurrently with typical schizophrenic symptoms (e.g. delusions of control). Preoccupation with non-affective hallucinations or delusions, or the persistence of such symptoms after the resolution of affective symptoms, also established the diagnosis.

In the final draft of DSM-III the category schizoaffective disorder was significantly narrowed. Most patients with mixtures of schizophrenic and affective symptoms are now to be diagnosed schizophrenia or affective disorder. The category schizoaffective disorder has been left devoid of criteria (the only such diagnosis in the nomenclature) because of the authors' inability to achieve consensus on its definition. It is a wastebasket category for cases in which 'the clinician is unable to make a differential diagnosis with any degree of certainty between affective disorder and schizophreniform disorder or schizophrenia.' (Task Force, 1980, p. 202).

DSM-III asserts that affective symptoms are consistent with a diagnosis of schizophrenia and that schizophrenic symptoms are consistent with the diagnosis of affective disorder. The distinction for syndromes with both kinds of symptoms rests upon course. If schizophrenic symptoms precede, or follow a brief course of affective symptoms, the diagnosis is schizophrenia (or schizophreniform disorder) or schizophrenia with superimposed atypical affective disorder. In general, use of such multiple diagnoses is encouraged. If affective symptoms precede schizophrenic symptoms, the diagnosis is affective disorder (bipolar manic or major depression) with mood incongruent psychotic symptoms. Mood incongruent means not typically associated with a mood disturbance (e.g. persecutory delusions, bizarre delusions). Finally, if the mood incongruent psychotic symptoms dominate the clinical picture when the affective symptoms are no longer present, the diagnosis is schizoaffective disorder.

The DSM-III codes for subtypes of schizophrenia essentially retain the standard subtypes, despite an absence of data to substantiate their usefulness or validity (Carpenter and Stevens, 1979). Based upon cross-sectional symptom profiles, schizophrenia may be classified as disorganized (hebephrenic), catatonic, paranoid, undifferentiated, and residual. The latter category is reserved for patients with a history of at least one episode of schizophrenia with psychotic symptoms who present with some continuing evidence of the illness (e.g. blunted affect, withdrawal, etc.) but without prominent psychotic symptoms.

Finally, DSM-III allows for the classification of the course of the illness: subchronic (less than two years); chronic (more than two years); subchronic with acute exacerbation; chronic with acute exacerbation; and in remission. The latter category is for patients with a history of schizophrenia who are currently free of all signs of the illness.

Discussion

The DSM-III concept of schizophrenia entails resolutions to several controversies. These resolutions are heuristic and for the most part unvalidated. Generally they reflect the authors' assessment of current schizophrenia research. They also reflect the compromise of varying aims, interests and perspectives.

The classic controversy in the study of schizophrenia involves the narrow, Kraepelinian definition of the disorder (a deteriorating disease) versus the broader, Bleulerian definition (a disease with several possible outcomes). The DSM-III resolution falls somewhere in-between. By requiring six months' duration, the authors suggest that schizophrenia is a disorder with a tendency toward chronicity. On the other hand, deterioration is not considered inevitable.

A variation of this controversy involves the universal observation that some schizophrenic patients do poorly and others do well. Are both groups truly schizophrenic or do those with more favourable outcomes suffer a different illness? By classifying schizophreniform disorder among the 'psychoses not elsewhere classified' rather than among the schizophrenias, DSM-III tilts toward the latter position. Since patients with schizophrenia can have favourable outcomes, however, the distinction is blurred.

Another related question is whether the briefer and more chronic forms of the disorder (or the two separate disorders) are distinguishable on the basis of symptoms. Langfeldt, who coined the term schizophreniform disorder, thought so (Fox, 1978). DSM-III says no. Schizophrenia and schizophreniform disorders are distinguished by duration alone.

Kraepelin set the stage for the second major controversy by dichotomizing functional mental disorder as dementia praecox and manic-depressive disease. How are conditions with features suggestive of both to be classified? The DSM-III resolution again temporizes. By classifying most patients with mixtures of schizophrenic and affective symptoms as schizophrenia or affective disorder, the Kraepelinian dichotomy is reinforced. On the other hand, by defining a narrow entity called schizoaffective disorder and classifying it separately the principle of a separate, or third psychosis is suggested.

Comment

DSM-III's atheoretical approach to classification, extensive descriptions of disorders, and multi-axial system constitute significant nosologic advances. Its most important innovation is the provision of specific operational criteria for diagnosis. Use of the criteria—based as they are upon research findings and modified through extensive field trials and the involvement of large numbers of organizations and individuals—is likely to render American diagnostic practice more thoughtful, more precise, more valid and more reliable.

The value of the narrowed DSM-III concept of schizophrenia is moot. The increased homogeneity of this group will likely contribute to more meaningful schizophrenia research. On the other hand, the validity of the concept remains to be firmly established. Moreover, the categories of affective disorder and atypical psychosis to which many of those excluded will be re-assigned, will burgeon.

The least satisfactory aspect of the DSM-III treatment of the psychoses is the classification of those acute and episodic disorders with features suggestive both of schizophrenia and affective disorder. By assigning most such cases to schizophrenia or affective disorder, DSM-III may obscure the uncertainty surrounding such patients, and diminish the possibility of further clarifying their correlates (McGlashan and Carpenter, 1979).

No system of classification is perfect. Nosologic systems are approximations which reflect changing ideas and knowledge (Campbell, 1974). The authors of DSM-III acknowledge that disorders cannot be sharply distinguished one from another, and that boundaries are often vague and imprecise. Not surprisingly, DSM-III is least satisfactory where the state of the art is most confused. Nonetheless, DSM-III is a powerful and significant achievement.

References

BLEULER, E. (1911) *Dementia Praecox or the Group of Schizophrenias.* Eng. transl. 1950. New York: International Universities Press.

BUCHSBAUM, M. S. & HAIER, R. J. (1978) Biological homogeneity, symptom heterogeneity, and the diagnosis of schizophrenia. *Schizophrenia Bulletin,* **4,** 473–475.

CAMPBELL, R. J. (1974) The nosology of psychiatry. In *American Handbook of Psychiatry,* Second Edition (ed. S. Arieti). New York: Basic Books.

CARPENTER, W. T., STRAUSSS, J. S. & BARTKO, J. J. (1973) Flexible system for the diagnosis of schizophrenia: Report from the WHO International Pilot Study of Schizophrenia. *Science,* **182,** 1275–1277.

—— & STEPHENS, J. (1979) An attempted integration of information relevant to schizophrenic subtypes. *Schizophrenia Bulletin,* **5,** 490–504.

FEIGHNER, J. P., ROBINS, E., GUZE, S. B. *et al* (1972) Diagnostic criteria for use in psychiatric research. *Archives of General Psychiatry*, **26**, 57–62.

Fox, H. A. (1978) Bleuler, Schneider and schizophrenia. *Journal of Clinical Psychiatry*, **39**, 30–35.

KASANIN, J. (1933) Acute schizoaffective psychosis. *American Journal of Psychiatry*, **90**, 97–126.

McGLASHAN, T. H. & CARPENTER, W. T. (1979) Affective symptoms and the diagnosis of schizophrenia. *Schizophrenia Bulletin*, **5**, 457–553.

ROBINS, E. & GUZE, S. B. (1970) Establishment of diagnostic validity in psychiatric illness: Its application to schizophrenia. *American Journal of Psychiatry*, **126**, 983–987.

SCHNEIDER, K. (1959) *Clinical Psychopathology*. New York: Grune & Stratton.

SPITZER, R. L., ENDICOTT, J. & ROBINS, E. (1975) Clinical criteria for psychiatric diagnosis and DSM-III. *American Journal of Psychiatry*, **132**, 1187–1192.

—— ANDREASEN, N. C. & ENDICOTT, J. (1978a) Schizophrenia and other psychotic disorders in DSM-III. *Schizophrenia Bulletin*, **4**, 489–495.

—— ENDICOTT, J. & ROBINS, E. (1978b) Research diagnostic criteria. *Archives of General Psychiatry*, **35**, 773–782.

TASK FORCE ON NOMENCLATURE AND STATISTICS OF THE AMERICAN PSYCHIATRIC ASSOCIATION (1978) *Diagnostic and Statistical Manual of Mental Disorders*. Draft, 1/15/78. Washington, D.C.: American Psychiatric Association.

—— (1980) *Diagnostic and Statistical Manual of Mental Disorders*. Washington, D.C.: American Psychiatric Association.

12 Reducing American diagnosis of schizophrenia: Will the DSM-III suffice?

SUKDEB MUKHERJEE

At the turn of the century Kraepelin brought together the disparate syndromes of hebephrenia, dementia paranoides, and catatonia under the rubric of dementia praecox. At the same time he crystallized the concept of manic-depressive illness as an entity discrete and separate from the former syndrome. In the years since Kraepelin's classification first came to be adopted, the definitions and descriptions of these two major disorders have undergone many changes. In an attempt to comprehend the meaning and the mechanism of the psychoses, Bleuler was drawn by the emergent theories of psychoanalysis to extend Kraepelin's clinical observations into the realm of psychology. He renamed dementia praecox the schizophrenias, thus emphasizing his idea that the splitting of associative processes was a fundamental feature of the syndrome; and he added the subcategory of simple schizophrenia. American psychiatry, dominated until recently by psychoanalytic concepts, has been influenced more by Bleulerian than Kraepelinian contributions. However, it has not restricted itself to Bleulerian notions. As **Kety (1980)** remarked in his Maudsley Lecture, great liberties have been taken with the syndrome of schizophrenia; the essential features have been altered, primarily by an expansion of its boundaries.

As thinking about the schizophrenic syndrome broadened, there was a simultaneous narrowing of the concept of manic-depressive illness, particularly in its psychotic forms. **Leff (1977)** commented that with the ascendancy of psychoanalytic theories, American diagnostic practice stressed hypothetical psychological mechanisms inferred from observable behaviour. This resulted in both a relatively low threshold for the recognition of pathology and a broad concept of schizophrenia; and thereby left little scope for the diagnosis of affective disorders.

From a different perspective, Klerman (1981) wrote that attention to diagnosis and classification fell into disrepute among American psychiatrists in the 1940s and 1950s during the height of the era of psychodynamic influence, when all patients were candidates for psychotherapy—the preferred treatment. The recent advent of pharmacotherapy, with specific treatments for affective disorders, has revived the importance of differentiating between the affective disorders and schizophrenia. The greatest pull in this direction has probably been the demonstration of the efficacy of lithium in the treatment and prophylaxis of bipolar affective disorders. Consequently, proper diagnosis of the patient's condition became imperative.

The last two decades have witnessed a resurgence of interest in psychiatric nosology in the United States, and the difference between schizophrenia and other psychotic disorders, particularly the affective disorders, has regained importance. Various studies both national (Mendlewicz *et al*, 1972; Simon *et al*, 1973; Taylor and Abrams, 1973) and cross-national (Edwards, 1972; Cooper *et al*, 1972) drew attention to the significant over-use of the diagnosis of schizophrenia, and the corresponding under-use of the diagnosis of affective disorder (particularly mania) in American psychiatric practice. This trend was particularly evident when contrasted to diagnostic practice in the United Kingdom, and was documented in a series of carefully planned studies (Cooper *et al*, 1972). The problem of diagnosis was recently comprehensively reviewed by Pope and Lipinski (1978).

In addition to compromising patient treatment and causing unnecessary exposure to the long-term hazards of maintenance neuroleptic therapy, such diagnostic unreliability also raises questions about the validity of some research on schizophrenia. For example, it was estimated that contamination from the inclusion of non-schizophrenic cases in some early studies of schizophrenia was as high as 40 per cent (Pope and Lipinski, 1978). An extreme example of diagnostic unreliability was seen in a report (Taylor and Abrams, 1973), in which, of 52 patients found to meet research criteria for mania, none had been so diagnosed on admission and 48 had been given a diagnosis of schizophrenia.

Concerns such as these led some American investigators to develop more reliable diagnostic methods using operationally defined criteria (Feighner *et al*, 1972; Spitzer *et al*, 1975a). The American Psychiatric Association, addressing itself to the problem of diagnostic unreliability, revised the *Diagnostic and Statistical Manual of Mental Disorders*. The third edition of this manual, popularly known as DSM-III (American Psychiatric Association, 1980), was a consequence of the aforementioned efforts to improve diagnostic reliability. Unlike its predecessors, DSM-III advocates the use of operationally defined phenomenological criteria to arrive at a diagnosis.

The concept of schizophrenia has been markedly narrowed in DSM-III, relative to previous American diagnostic standards. The following are the DSM-III criteria for schizophrenia: onset of illness before the age of 45 years; the presence of specific psychotic symptoms during an acute phase; duration of illness of at least six months, including prodromal and residual manifestations which are clearly specified and which should occur in the absence of a mood disorder or substance use disorder; the absence of a full affective syndrome; or, if such is present, the development occurring after the onset of psychosis, or the duration brief in relation to that of the psychosis; finally, the exclusion of organic mental disorders or mental retardation.

In contrast, the concept of affective disorders has been considerably broadened and admits any psychotic symptoms, including Schneiderian first rank symptoms, if these occur during a full affective syndrome. Also, certain categories previously subsumed under the schizophrenias have been removed to non-schizophrenic categories. Schizoaffective schizophrenia has been changed to schizoaffective disorder and classified under the non-specific category of *psychotic disorders not elsewhere classified*. Acute schizophrenic episode, similarly, comes under the DSM-III categories of schizophreniform disorder or brief reactive psychosis, both *psychotic disorders not elsewhere classified*. The latent and simple schizophrenias have likewise been deleted, on the assumption that patients previously classified under these categories may be reassigned by DSM-III criteria to schizotypal personality disorder.

The lack of a clear understanding of the aetiological factors and pathophysiology of schizophrenia limits statements about the validity of any particular diagnostic schema, DSM-III included. However, the reliability of a diagnostic system is important, and DSM-III is addressed to this end. Although a reliable diagnostic system is not necessarily valid, validity is perforce limited by the lack of reliability (Spitzer and Fleiss, 1974). In an analysis of the cause of diagnostic unreliability, Spitzer *et al* (1975b) mention five variances: subject, occasion, observation, information and criterion variance. They point out that the first two represent real differences in clinical presentations, and should be recognized as such. Of the remainder, they consider the last one, criterion variance, to be the most important cause of diagnostic unreliability. Observation and information variances are important; but, they can be controlled for by training and the use of structured interviewing techniques, and so are less of a problem. Therefore, the emphasis falls on the need for clearer and more explicit diagnostic criteria. The DSM-III is a reflection of this position.

There is little doubt that the use of DSM-III will significantly reduce the diagnosis of schizophrenia. However, this requires the reasonable control of information and observation variances as a *sine qua non*. It has been shown (Weitzel *et al*, 1973) that the use of an operationally defined interview is more efficient than a free form one. A structured interview (Spitzer *et al*, 1975b) may well significantly reduce observation and information variances. But, such interviewing techniques are time consuming, and neither widely known, nor used in American psychiatric practice (outside academic research settings). In the absence of this control, other biases from the past which favour a broad definition of schizophrenia will continue to affect the diagnostic process.

In a historiographic investigation of the development of science, Thomas Kuhn (1970) introduced his concept of the paradigm. A paradigm is a construct or artefact which is used as a conceptual frame of reference, and within which the observer approaches the immediate problem. In essence, it is a concrete way of seeing. It is naive to assume that an observer might be free of bias from his conceptual frame of reference. As Turner (1965) stated, 'We perceive according to our inclinations, our beliefs, predispositions, sets ... One does not arrive on the scene as a naive observer recording facts on a blank tablet wherein such facts are to repose in their own pristine integrity.' **Leff (1977)**, writing about the psychiatric interview, pointed out that the importance a psychiatrist attaches to the phenomena of illness is largely determined by his theoretical frame of reference. This is an important point when considering the effects of introducing DSM-III to American psychiatrists.

The theoretical tradition of American psychiatry strongly inclines toward a psychodynamic, rather than phenomenological, paradigm. However, DSM-III operates within a phenomenological paradigm, and assumes an atheoretical descriptive position, with no reference to the aetiology of the schizophrenic and major affective disorders. Whereas, a psychodynamic approach assumes the presence of certain specific, albeit hypothetical, psychological mechanisms of aetiological and pathophysiological import. In the context of diagnosis based on a phenomenological approach, this is a disadvantage. In the words of Jaspers

(1963), 'We are not concerned at this stage with connections nor with the patients' experience as a whole and certainly not with any subsidiary speculations, fundamental theory or basic postulate . . . Conventional theories, psychological constructions, interpretations and evaluations must be left aside.'

Except for a small, though growing, number of psychiatrists trained in the phenomenological approach, most American psychiatrists have been groomed in the psychodynamic tradition with a broad concept of schizophrenia. This is epitomized by the statement that even a touch of schizophrenia is schizophrenia (Lewis and Piotrowski, 1954). Moreover, Sandifer *et al* (1970) demonstrated that most psychiatrists tend to arrive at a diagnostic decision within the first few minutes of an interview, and that in about two-thirds of the interviewers this initial opinion is not changed by subsequent information. In fact, once an initial impression is accepted, psychiatrists often neither seek nor give heed to evidence that may contradict it. Many American psychiatrists might thereby move towards diagnostic unreliability and in the direction of over-diagnosing schizophrenia. The DSM-III may not fully succeed in dealing with this problem as it has no mechanism for controlling such bias.

Five well known widely read American accounts of schizophrenia were recently reviewed in the light of DSM-III (North and Cadoret, 1981); none qualified for a schizophrenic diagnosis by DSM-III criteria. Other studies have documented a similar diagnostic shift. In one study (Silverstein *et al*, 1982), only 55 per cent of previously diagnosed schizophrenics were found to meet DSM-III criteria for schizophrenia, and 20 per cent of the same sample met DSM-III criteria for major affective disorders. No patient with previously diagnosed major affective disorder, unipolar or bipolar, was reclassified to a DSM-III schizophrenic category. Another study (Stephens *et al*, 1982) compared nine ways of diagnosing schizophrenia and found that only 37 per cent of 283 previously diagnosed schizophrenics met DSM-III criteria for that disorder. Although the DSM-III criteria were the narrowest of the systems compared, they were the most prognostically predictive.

Naturalistic investigations of routine clinical practice tell a different story. In a survey of 100 consecutive admissions to a New York hospital clinic in 1981—18 months after the formal acceptance at the clinic of DSM-III, and following a series of seminars on its use—we found that the proportion of schizophrenic diagnoses had not decreased when compared to a pre-DSM-III sample of 237 patients from the same clinic in 1976–77 (unpublished data). This finding was remarkable because a number of papers written by psychiatrists at that hospital have drawn attention to the high rate of misdiagnosis of affective disorder as schizophrenia (Taylor and Abrams, 1973). With a different approach, Lipkowitz and Idupuganti (paper read at the Annual Meeting of the American Psychiatric Association, 1982) conducted a questionnaire survey among psychiatrists to assess their criteria for diagnosing schizophrenia in 1981. Only 1 out of 298 respondents used all the DSM-III criteria; 80 per cent did not mention that they excluded affective disorder before diagnosing schizophrenia. These examples clearly illustrate the difficulty many American psychiatrists experience in the adoption of the phenomenological methods of DSM-III.

Furthermore, another aspect of the problem is seldom considered. Will the established psychiatrist who has always used a broad definition of schizophrenia concede that he has been in diagnostic error merely on account of DSM-III? Will the professor who has long taught that mania is a rare condition, seldom encountered in clinical practice, and, that virtually all psychotics are schizophrenic, be easily able to shift to DSM-III's narrower concept of schizophrenia? Is the psychiatrist who has based his understanding of schizophrenia on psychoanalytical theories ready to accept the narrower phenomenological DSM-III definition of the disorder, together with the implication that his former understanding evolved from the study of non-schizophrenic cases?

DSM-III has introduced a new paradigm into American psychiatric practice. Many may not be prepared conceptually to assimilate the new arrival, for the phenomenological approach is not simple. As Jaspers (1963) stated, 'We refuse to prejudge when studying our phenomena, and this open-mindedness, so characteristic of phenomenology, is not something which one just has, but it has to be acquired painfully through much critical effort and frequent failure... Phenomenological orientation is something we have to attain to again and again and involves a continual onslaught on our prejudices.' Habits of thought are not easily changed in most people, psychiatrists being no exception. As long as psychiatrists' conceptual frameworks fail to convert to the new paradigm of phenomenology, observation and information variances will continue to play a significant role in diagnostic unreliability and the consequent over-diagnosis of schizophrenia in American psychiatric practice. In his introduction to *The Born-Einstein Letters*, Werner Heisenberg (1971) wrote, 'All scientific work is, of course, based consciously or subconsciously on some philosophical attitude; on a particular thought structure which serves as a solid foundation for further development... Most scientists are willing to accept new empirical data and to recognize new results, provided they fit into their philosophical framework. But in the course of scientific progress it can happen that a new range of empirical data can be understood only when the enormous effort is made to enlarge this framework and to change the very structure of the thought processes.' If such a shift were difficult for physical scientists, it will be many times more difficult for psychiatrists, particularly those groomed in a metaphysically oriented psychodynamic paradigm.

If an adjustment from a psychodynamic to a phenomenological paradigm is to succeed, an enormous effort is required of those who advocate it. A smooth transfer of intellectual allegiance cannot be presumed purely on the basis of prescription. Max Planck (1949) wrote 'A new scientific truth does not triumph by convincing its opponents and making them see the light, but rather because its opponents eventually die, and a new generation grows up that is familiar with it.' So it may be with DSM-III, American diagnostic practice, and trans-Atlantic diagnostic differences.

References

AMERICAN PSYCHIATRIC ASSOCIATION (1980) *Diagnostic and Statistical Manual of Mental Disorders.* Third edition. Washington, D.C.: American Psychiatric Association.

COOPER, J. E., KENDELL, R. E., GURLAND, B. J., SHARPE, L., COPELAND, J. R. M. & SIMON, R. (1972) *Psychiatric Diagnosis in New York and London.* Maudsley Monograph no 20. Oxford University Press.

EDWARDS, G. (1972) Diagnosis of schizophrenia: An Anglo-American comparison. *British Journal of Psychiatry*, **120**, 385–390.

FEIGHNER, J. P., ROBINS, E., GUZE, S. B., WOODRUFF, R. A., WINOKUR, G. & MUNOZ, R. (1972) Diagnostic criteria for use in psychiatric research. *Archives of General Psychiatry*, **26**, 57–63.

HEISENBERG, W. (1971) Introduction. In *The Born-Einstein Letters*. (Translated by I. Born). New York: Walker & Co.

JASPERS, K. (1963) *General Psychopathology*. (Translated by J. Hoenig and M. W. Hamilton). Manchester: Manchester University Press.

KETY, S. S. (1980) The syndrome of schizophrenia: Unresolved questions and opportunities for research. *British Journal of Psychiatry*, **136**, 421–436.

KLERMAN, G. L. (1981) The spectrum of mania. *Comprehensive Psychiatry*, **22**, 11–20.

KUHN, T. (1970) *The Structure of Scientific Revolutions*. Second edition. Chicago: The University of Chicago Press.

LEFF, J. (1977) International variations in the diagnosis of psychiatric illness. *British Journal of Psychiatry*, **131**, 329–338.

LEWIS, N. D. C. & PIOTROWSKI, Z. A. (1954) Clinical diagnosis of manic-depressive psychosis. In *Depression* (eds. P. Hoch and J. Zubin). New York: Grune & Stratton.

MENDLEWICZ, J., FIEVE, R. R., RAINER, J. D. & FLEISS, J. L. (1972) Manic-depressive illness: A comparative study of patients with and without a family history. *British Journal of Psychiatry*, **120**, 523–530.

NORTH, C. & CADORET, R. (1981) Diagnostic discrepancy in personal accounts of patients with 'schizophrenia'. *Archives of General Psychiatry*, **38**, 133–137.

PLANCK, M. (1949) *Scientific Autobiography and Other Papers*. (Translated by F. Gaynor). Westport, Connecticut: Greenwood Press.

POPE, H. G. & LIPINSKI, J. F. (1978) Diagnosis in schizophrenia and manic-depressive illness. *Archives of General Psychiatry*, **35**, 811–828.

SANDIFER, M. G., HORDERN, A. & GREEN, L. M. (1970) The psychiatric interview: The impact of the first three minutes. *American Journal of Psychiatry*, **126**, 968–973.

SIMON, R. J., FLEISS, J. L., GURLAND, B. J., STILLER, P. R. & SHARPE, L. (1973) Depression and schizophrenia in hospitalized black and white mental patients. *Archives of General Psychiatry*, **28**, 509–512.

SILVERSTEIN, M. L., WARREN, R. A., HARROW, M., GRINKER, R. R. & PAWELSKI, T. (1982) Changes in diagnosis from DSM-II to the Research Diagnostic Criteria and DSM-III. *American Journal of Psychiatry*, **139**, 366–368.

SPITZER, R. L., ENDICOTT, J. & ROBINS, E. (1975a) *Research Diagnostic Criteria (RDC) for a Selected Group of Functional Disorders*. New York: New York State Department of Mental Hygiene, New York State Psychiatric Institute, Biometrics Research.

—— —— —— (1975b) Clinical criteria for psychiatric diagnosis and DSM-III. *American Journal of Psychiatry*, **132**, 1187–1192.

—— & FLEISS, J. L. (1974) A reanalysis of the reliability of psychiatric diagnosis. *British Journal of Psychiatry*, **125**, 341–347.

STEPHENS, J. H., ASTRUP, C., CARPENTER, W. T., SHAFFER, J. W. & GOLDBERG, J. (1982) A comparison of nine systems to diagnose schizophrenia. *Psychiatry Research*, **6**, 127–143.

TAYLOR, M. A. & ABRAMS, R. (1973) The phenomenology of mania. *Archives of General Psychiatry*, **29**, 520–522.

TURNER, M. B. (1965) *Philosophy and the Science of Behavior*. New York: Appleton-Century-Crofts.

WEITZEL, W. D., MORGAN, D. W., GUYDEN, T. E. & ROBINSON, J. A. (1973) Toward a more efficient mental status examination. *Archives of General Psychiatry*, **28**, 215–218.

13 First rank symptoms of schizophrenia: Questions concerning clinical boundaries

KARL KOEHLER

In the present paper the main purpose will be to examine comparatively four detailed sets of first rank symptoms (FRS) definitions as found in the writings of selected modern Anglo-American researchers (Fish, 1962; 1967; 1969; Mellor, 1970; Taylor and Heiser, 1971; Wing *et al*, 1974). These authors have been chosen for closer scrutiny because their criteria have generated the most important operationally oriented FRS research of recent years (Koehler, 1977). Their sets of definitions are all ultimately based on Schneider's *Clinical Psychopathology* (1959), and therefore must necessarily share many essential similarities. And yet, it is often enough phenomenologically irksome trying to reconcile their positions on whether a particular phenomenon is or is not to be regarded as of first rank quality. However, the same holds true when reading FRS views held by various German writers, including some of Schneider's pupils (Koehler and Witter, 1976).

The primary contention of this paper is that the phenomenological difficulties encountered when comparing the FRS views of the above mentioned English-speaking researchers can be traced to clearly demonstrable FRS descriptive discrepancies. It must be emphasized that the point at issue cannot be: Who has the right views on first rank symptoms? Such a question is meaningless. Rather, the point at issue must be: Can divergent views on individual FRSs be documented or not? Thus, Tables I and II highlight the important areas of Anglo-American phenomenological disagreement; however, Schneider's (1971) views or those of other prominent German authors have not been formally interpreted and incorporated into the Tables. Hopefully what follows will redirect some attention to a systematic reappraisal of certain familiar phenomenological criteria.

A provisional first rank continuum

For Kurt Schneider (1959; 1971) the primacy of first rank symptoms was not a theoretical matter but rather FRSs were regarded as primary only in the practical diagnostic decision-making sense. In fact, he stressed that he had no desire to speculate on a 'common structure' for all such phenomena. However, Schneider at one point did mention that those first rank symptoms usually subsumed under the term passivity or made experiences might be viewed as due to a kind of 'permeability of the ego-world boundary', whereas

TABLE I

Passivity experiences: their interpretations as first rank symptoms of schizophrenia by various Anglo-American authors

Passivity phenomena	Fish (1962, 1967, 1969)	Mellor (1970)	Taylor & Heiser (1971)	Wing et al (1974)
Influenced thought	+	−	+	−
Alienated thought (thought insertion)	+	+	+	+[1]
Influenced impulses	+	−[2]	+	○
Alienated impulses	+	+	+	○
Influenced volit. acts	+	+	+	−[2]
Alienated volit. acts	+	−	+	○
Influenced will	+	○	+	−
Alienated will	+	○	+	+[1]
Influenced feelings	+	−	+	−
Alienated feelings	+	+	.+	+
Non-shared thought broadcast	−	+	+	−
Shared thought broadcast	+	+	−	+[1]
Pure thought block	−[3]	−	○	+
Alienated thought (thought withdrawal)	+	+	○	+[1,4]
Influenced bodily sensations	+	+	+	−[2]
Alienated bodily sensations	+	+	+	−[2]

Plus indicates that the phenomenon actually seems to be or is assumed to be of the first rank. Minus indicates that it is not of the first rank. Circle indicates no easy interpretation possible (various reasons).

[1] Part of their schizophrenic nuclear syndrome.

[2] Where a passivity phenomenon actually seems to be or is assumed to be the result of secondary elaboration of another experience, it is not given first rank status in this paper (see 4).

[3] Thought block was for Fish, in contrast to Wing et al, an objective sign and not an experience.

[4] Apparently given first rank status although described as secondary, in the sense of an explanatory delusion, to 'pure thought block'.

first rank phonemes and delusional perception could not be understood in the same light.

In contrast to Schneider, some important German clinicians, apparently impatient with the Jasperian (1912a; 1968) static-descriptive approach to phenomenology, have attempted to understand some first rank phenomena in a more dynamic way (Matussek, 1952; 1953; Conrad, 1957; Janzarik, 1959; 1968; Kisker, 1960). Conrad (1957), in his monograph on acute schizophrenia, tried to demonstrate, on the basis of Gestalt psychological ideas, that dynamic phenomenological transitions between FRSs frequently occurred. Fish (1960) later reviewed Conrad's views in this area and also pointed out their possible heuristic value (Fish, 1961).

Indeed, as the writings of these last mentioned German authors imply, first rank and similar symptoms may interchange with one another in the dynamic manner they suggest. Obviously such so-called dynamic approaches represent

TABLE II

Sense deceptions and delusional phenomena: their interpretations as first rank symptoms of schizophrenia by various Anglo-American authors

Sense deceptions + Delusional phenomena	Fish (1962, 1967, 1969)	Mellor (1970)	Taylor & Heiser (1971)	Wing et al (1974)
Pseudo-hallucinatory audible thoughts	+	−	−	+[1]
Hallucinatory audible thoughts	+	+	+	−
Pseudo-hallucinatory voices (arguing, discussing, commenting)	+	−	−	+[1]
Hallucinatory voices (arguing, discussing, commenting)	+	+	+	+[1]
Delusional notion linked to a perception	−	○	○	○
Delusional perception	+	+	+	+[1]

Plus, minus, and circle as in Table I.
[1] A part of their schizophrenic nuclear syndrome.

theoretically biased continuum views whereby FRSs are seen as more or less easily recognizable *Prägnanztypen* on any such continuum. A study of their work, however, reveals a lack of operational sharpness in the definition of the individual FRS phenomena.

Although the various psychological theories proposed offer solutions to the problems of FRS phenomenology they are not very practical in a clinical sense. For such a purpose a simplified continuum with the main stress placed on the static-descriptive aspects of certain phenomena considered as arbitrary points seems more appropriate. Table III presents a possible scheme for use in clinical practice. It is important to note that the definitions provided in this Table are meant only to serve as provisional phenomenological hints and make no claim to represent exhaustive criteria of such symptoms.

The first rank continuum in Table III is non-theoretical in the sense that no overriding, non-clinical, psychological principle governs the arrangement of the phenomena from F1 to F12. Furthermore, the order of the arrangement does not imply any corresponding degree of severity nor does the arrangement mean that these phenomena actually interchange with one another on a sort of dynamic sliding scale. Rather, the continuum suggested is best seen as a clinical common-sense device for arranging first rank and FRS-like symptoms according to phenomenological principles.

In this sense Table III can offer a provisional operational understanding of how the phenomena might be linked to one another. Moreover the broken lines of Table III arbitrarily divide the first rank continuum into three major phenomenological areas, which can conveniently be labelled the delusional, the passivity and the sense deception continua respectively. Although such a phenomenological tripartite breakdown is meant to be theoretically and noso-logically neutral, representatives of the dynamic school, such as Conrad (1957) and Janzarik (1968), view the progression of an acute schizophrenic illness in terms of severity from the delusional perception through passivity experiences to phonemes.

As Strauss (1969) has aptly pointed out: 'It is one thing, of course, to stress the need for describing, rating, and conceptualizing symptoms on continua and yet another to describe in a simple and operational way the major factors

TABLE III

A provisional, phenomenologically oriented, non-theoretical, clinical continuum of first rank and associated symptoms

Delusional continuum

F1. *Delusional mood (Wahnstimmung)*: The subject perceives something in the outside world and feels that something is 'going on' in the sense that he is more or less aware that something is happening to or in his familiar surroundings, that these may have specially or significantly changed in an odd, strange or puzzling way, but he is as yet not certain if or what or how this may be occurring.

F2. *Delusional notion linked to or provoked by a perception (Wahrnehmungsgebundener Wahneinfall)*: The subject perceives something in the outside world and this triggers a special, significant relatively non-understandable meaning of which he is certain and which is more or less loosely linked to the triggering perception; that is, the meaning is not contained within this particular perception itself.

F3. *Delusional perception (Wahnwahrnehmung)*: The experience is like F2 except for the fact that the special, significant relatively non-understandable meaning is contained within, not merely linked to, the perception itself.

Passivity continuum

F4. *Passivity mood (Beeinflussungsstimmung)*: The subject experiences that something is 'going on' in his inner world in the sense that he is more or less aware that something may be impinging upon the integrity of his self or aspects of the self, but he is not as yet certain if or what or how this may be occurring.

F5. *General experience of influence (Allgemeines Beeinflussungserlebnis)*: The experience is like F4 but now the subject is quite certain that there is some general control or influence being exerted on him from without.

F6. *Specific experience of influence (Spezifisches Beeinflussungserlebnis)*: The experience is like F5 but now the subject is quite certain about which specific ego areas, for example *his own* thoughts, feelings and so on, are being controlled or influenced by an outside force.

F7. *Experience of influenced depersonalization (Beeinflussungs-Depersonalization)*: This represents a combination of the more usual experience of depersonalization of the self or aspects of the self, such as thoughts, feelings and so on, with the above-mentioned specific experience of influence (F6).

F8. *Positive experience of alienation (Beeinflussungerserlebnis mit Ersatz-Qualität)*: The experience is like F6 but now the subject is quite certain of 'positively' experiencing completely alien or foreign thoughts, feelings and so on; that is, those that are definitely *not his own* have been imposed upon him from outside (e.g. thought insertion).

F9. *Negative-active experience of alienation (Beeinflussungserlebnis mit aktiver Verlust-Qualität)*: The experience is like F6 but now the subject is quite certain of 'negatively' being aware that he has lost *his own* thoughts, feelings and so on because they have been actively taken away from without (e.g. thought withdrawal).

F10. *Negative-passive experience of alienation (Beeinflussungserlebnis mit passiver Verlust-Qualität)*: The experience is like F6 but now the subject is quite certain of 'negatively' being aware that he has lost *his own* thoughts, feelings and so on because in some way they passively diffuse into or are lost to the outside world against his will (e.g. thought broadcasting).

Table III *(contd.)*

Sense deception continuum

F11. *Pseudo-hallucinatory voices* (*Pseudohalluzinatorische Stimmen*):

    (a) The integrity of the ego areas is no longer experienced by the subject as being influenced or alienated from without, but rather he hears a voice or voices commenting on his actions, or voices arguing or discussing among themselves, and this experience takes place in his head, that is, in his inner world and not in external space.

    (b) Like F11a but now the voice or voices speak his own thoughts (*Pseudo-hallucinatory audible thoughts* or *Gedankenlautwerden*).

F12. *Hallucinatory voices* (*Halluzinatorische Stimmen*):

    (a) Like F11a but now the experience takes place not in his head but rather in external space, although there is no actual source for these voices in the outside world.

    (b) Like 12a but now the voice or voices speak his own thoughts. (*Hallucinatory audible thoughts* or *Gedankenlautwerden*).

---

that determine the position of an experience on these continua'. In other words, the components of any suggested operational definition for individual FRSs and similar symptoms representing arbitrary points on a FRS continuum, in turn actually consist of many complex continua of their own. Theoretically, such phenomena are probably best viewed on the basis of a multidimensional model of psychopathological disorder.

However, the criteria of any continuum meant to be actually used in routine clinical work must necessarily be more primitive by comparison. That this is so can be seen by the fact that in practice the arbitrary separation of the various FRSs is often made by means of rather simplified forced dichotomizations in the various areas of continua function considered phenomenologically relevant.

At first glance the arrangement of Table III might seem a sort of phenomenological procrustean bed. Of course it would be possible to tease out further distinct phenomena as arbitrary points located on such an operational clinical continuum (e.g. *alienated depersonalization, positive-passive experiences of alienation*). However, the arbitrary selection of the items in Table III represents the present author's own bias as to what he considers to be relevant. Other writers might favour the use of a greater or lesser number of such phenomena, a different arrangement of them or another terminology. Nevertheless the phenomenological distinctions proposed in Table III and their corresponding terms appear useful not only in clinical work, but also for the provisional framework that they offer in order to conceptualize and compare various sets of FRS criteria. In the FRS discussions of the following three sections, the major subheadings make use of Mellor's more familiar terminology for eleven Schneiderian FRSs; the corresponding analyses of the four sets of FRS criteria, however, are carried out in the light of the terminology and definitions suggested in Table III.

The delusional continuum

Jaspers' (1962; 1965) three basic criteria for delusional phenomena as well as his dichotomy of understandable, secondary delusion-like ideas or notions (*wahnhafte Ideen*) and the non-understandable, primary delusion itself (*echter Wahn*), are well known. His breakdown of this latter phenomenon into delusional perception (*Wahnwahrnehmung*), delusional ideas (*Wahnvorstellungen*) and delusional awareness (*Wahnbewusstheiten*) was later abbreviated by Kurt Schneider into the delusional notion (*Wahneinfall*) and the delusional perception (Berner and Naske, 1973). However, Schneider (1971) had also described another largely neglected intermediate phenomenon called the delusional notion linked to a perception (*wahrnehmungsgebundener Wahneinfall*); furthermore, another experience, obviously secondary, called the delusion-like notion linked to a perception (*wahrnehmungsgebundener wahnhafter Wahneinfall*) can also be conceptually separated from this latter phenomenon (Koehler, 1976).

The present writer, in agreement with Fish (1962, p. 121), regards the differentiation of the delusional notion provoked by a perception from a delusional perception itself as the crucial issue. Assuming that one does not subscribe to an extremely wide concept of schizophrenia, the clinical impression is that the former phenomenon often appears in both affective and schizophrenic disorder, whereas the latter symptom, when narrowly defined as in this paper, occurs much less frequently and then almost only in schizophrenia. In an attempt to clarify the distinction, Schneider (1971) offered the following suggestion: in the case of the delusional notion linked to a perception, the abnormal new meaning was only linked to (*angeknüpft*) the perception but in the true delusional perception the abnormal meaning was contained in (*beigelegt*) the perception itself. Schneider's German text and examples clearly demonstrate that the precise relationship of abnormal meaning to perception was a decisive criterion in such instances (Koehler, 1976).

In connection with a critique of some Present State Examination (PSE) criteria and the phrasing of some PSE questions relating to delusional phenomena (Wing *et al*, 1974), the example in the PSE glossary (pp. 153–4) of a delusion of reference was recently used as the point of departure to analyse further such phenomena in terms of the above-mentioned clinically crucial distinction (Koehler, 1976): (1) Did the fact that someone crossed his legs set off a train of associations that made you believe that other people thought you were homosexual? and (2) Did the crossing of the legs in itself contain the meaning that people thought this? Assuming that the symptom was not obviously secondary to some basic psychic phenomenon, especially to major mood change, then the so-called delusion-like notion linked to a perception can be dropped from consideration and one would opt for a delusional perception if the answer to the second question, or perhaps to both questions, were positive. On the other hand, if only the first question were answered affirmatively then a delusional notion linked to a perception would seem more likely.

Delusional perception (Table II): As mentioned, the essential distinction between the delusional notion linked to a perception (F2) and the delusional perception (F3) had been seen by Fish. In his book on schizophrenia (Fish, 1962; p. 121) he stressed the differential diagnosis from affective disorder and stated: 'Often it is difficult to be sure that a patient has a delusional perception ...' and in the next sentence we read: 'Thus ... in (some patients) an apparent delusional perception may turn out to be ... a sudden delusional idea provoked by a perception'. Unfortunately, no further help is then given for making this distinction in the concrete case. Moreover, there is no mention at all of the delusional idea provoked by a perception in the long discussion of delusional symptomatology in his monograph in schizophrenia (Fish, 1962, pp. 29–35), his *Clinical Psychopathology* (Fish, 1967, pp. 39–48) or in his article on the diagnosis of acute schizophrenia (Fish, 1969).

In all these cited references, Fish pointed out the difference between the delusional perception and what he called the delusional misinterpretation (Fish, 1962, pp. 30–1; 1967, pp. 40–1; 1969, p. 42), whereby the latter was obviously defined in terms of a Jasperian secondary phenomenon; indeed, his delusional misinterpretation is identical with the concept of the delusion-like notion linked to a perception mentioned earlier (Koehler, 1976). Mellor, Taylor and Heiser and Wing and his co-workers (pp. 172, 214, 218), all appear to follow Schneider in defining delusional perception (called primary delusion by Wing *et al*); all apparently stress the presence of a real perception and the special meaning connected with this perception. Although in all three definitions it is suggested that the delusional special meaning is somehow contained within the perception itself, no explicit statement is made regarding the exact nature of the special meaning to perception relationship in the light of the distinction between the delusional notion linked to a perception and the delusional perception itself.

The passivity continuum

The German terms for *gelenkte, gemachte oder beeinflusste Erlebnisse* have been variously translated into English as *made, fabricated* or *passivity experiences* as well as by *experiences of influence or alienation*. In most instances, German and non-German writers use such terms interchangeably, seemingly not recognizing any phenomenological differences, or, when aware of possible distinctions, failing to assign them any particular significance. It was therefore of interest that Taylor and Heiser's (1971) list of FRSs clearly differentiated between what they arbitrarily called *experiences of influence* and *experiences of alienation*. *Influenced experiences* were defined as those in which the patient knew that *his own* thoughts, feelings, impulses, volitional acts or actual somatic sensations were controlled or imposed upon him by some external agency. In contrast, *alienated experiences* were described as the patient's awareness that thoughts, feelings and so on were *not his own* in the sense that they were coming from an outside source.

A further important phenomenon can be considered as intermediate between the *influenced* and *alienated* experiences just mentioned. Thus, the subject may be aware of *his own* thoughts and feelings as if in some way they were *not his own*, while simultaneously experiencing that all this is due to some outside influence. This phenomenon seems to be a depersonalization experience, in which the patient experiences himself or aspects of the self as not belonging to himself, in combination with the experience that this is happening because of being controlled by an external source. Despite its clumsiness, the expression *influenced depersonalization* (F7) seems suitable for this experience. Fish's (1967) term *schizophrenic depersonalization* cannot properly be used in this context since, conceptually, it actually encompassed all the passivity experiences under discussion here.

In his *Klinische Psychopathologie*, Kurt Schneider (1971, p. 121) stated: '...
dass die eigenen Akte und Zustände nicht als solche eigene, sondern als von
andern gelenkte und beeinflusste erlebt werden', and Fish (1967, p. 84) con-
veyed Schneider's uncharacteristically vague German text regarding such passivity phenomena into English by stressing that the patient was aware that
his own thoughts, feelings and so on were being experienced as being foreign
or manufactured against his will by some outside influence. By closely analysing
the exact wording used by Schneider and Fish to describe the essence of these
so-called specific schizophrenic ego disturbances, one could conclude that their
criterion was vague enough to allow for phenomenological interpretations
covering *influenced experiences, alienated experiences* and *influenced depersonalization*
as already defined. The attempt to break down Schneider's and Fish's description of passivity into various phenomenological components may seem like
unnecessary hair-splitting; however, such distinctions assume no little importance when one realizes that there are authors, as Table I shows, who separate
some *influenced experiences*, as defined above, from the other ego disturbances
and then proceed to deny the former first rank status.

For the most part, German writers have followed Schneider's (1971) general
position on the schizophrenic ego disturbances. However, Jaspers (1965), in
his discussion of thought insertion, had actually foreshadowed the Taylor-
Heiser dichotomy of *influenced* versus *alienated* experiences (Koehler and Witter,
1976). Unfortunately, after breaking down the phenomenon of thought insertion into the influencing of the patient's own thoughts from without and the
more specific insertion of alien thoughts by an external agency, Jaspers failed
formally and systematically to transfer these phenomenological insights into
other psychopathological areas.

Recently, a provisional phenomenological breakdown, based on Taylor and
Heiser's *influenced* versus *alienated* differentiation, of ideally typical pathological
ego disturbances into four main phenomenological areas lying on a passivity
continuum has been suggested (Koehler and Witter, 1976). In the present
paper, this latter clinical continuum view has been modified and extended
into an arbitrary passivity continuum representing part (F4–F10) of the first
rank continuum shown in Table III.

Thoughts ascribed to others or thought insertion (Table I): For Fish (1967,
p. 39), the term *thought alienation* was a more general concept meant to cover
thought insertion, thought deprivation (withdrawal) and *thought broadcasting*. He
defined *thought alienation* as the subject's experience that 'his thoughts are under
the control of an outside agency, or that others are participating in his thinking',
a description obviously vague and wide enough to cover not only positive
alienation of thought (F8), negative-active (F9) and negative-passive (F10)
thought alienation (see later), but also the specific experience of influenced
thought (F6). However, his description of thought insertion (Fish, 1967,
p. 39) was clearly couched in terms of a positive experience of thought alienation
(F8): '... he knows that thoughts are being inserted into his mind, and he
recognizes them as being foreign and coming from without'. In defining thought
insertion, Mellor similarly selected criteria unmistakably pointing to positive
thought alienation (F8): the subject 'experiences thoughts which have not
the quality of being his own' and complains that some external agency is
imposing these thoughts.

Although Taylor and Heiser did not use the term thought insertion as such, they obviously distinguished between first rank experiences of specific influence of thought (F6) and first rank experiences of positive thought alienation (F8), the latter clearly equivalent to thought insertion as defined by Fish and Mellor. As for the more recent description of thought insertion given by Wing *et al* (pp. 160–1), it is no different since the criteria are also framed in terms of positive thought alienation (F8): the subject 'experiences thoughts which are not his own intruding into his mind. The symptom is not that he has been caused to have unusual thoughts, but that the thoughts themselves are not his'.

Thus, a sharp separation of thought insertion (F8) from influenced thought (F6) is obviously carried out. Interestingly, Wing and colleagues also rate positively for thought insertion in those cases where the patient, although quite certain the thoughts are not his own, does not as yet know that they originate from an external agency; this would therefore represent another of the possible intermediate experiences that could be placed on the passivity continuum.

Made impulses (drives) and made volitional acts (Table I): Fish's (1967, p. 78) description of alienation of personal action (e.g. 'his actions are under the control of some external power' and 'knows his actions are not his own and may attribute this control to ...') can easily be interpreted as covering not only specific experiences of influenced volitional acts (F6) but also positively alienated (F8) experiences in this area. It can be assumed that these broad views would also govern Fish's position on influenced and alienated experiences of impulses and of the will, phenomenological areas he apparently did not explicitly treat.

The definition given by Mellor of made impulses is quite complex, appearing to combine an experience of positive impulse alienation (F8) with the secondary experience of an influenced volitional act (F6-like): 'The impulse to carry out the action is not felt to be his own, but the actual performance of the act is', and 'the impulse is made by an external agency'. In contrast, Mellor's position on made volitional acts, as it stands, clearly described a primary experience of influenced volitional acts (F6): the subject 'experiences his own actions as being completely under the control of an external influence'.

Taylor and Heiser distinguished between specific influenced impulses and volitional acts (F6), on the one hand, and the positive alienation of impulses and volitional acts (F8) on the other. To cover the psychopathological area under discussion here, Wing *et al* (p. 167) introduced the expression *delusions of control*. Indeed, their definition remained quite narrow, being obviously formulated only in terms of positive alienation of the will (F8): the subject 'experiences that his will is actually replaced by that of some other force or agency'. However, they also highlighted the various elaborations that this phenomenon might take on; for example, the patient may feel 'even his bodily movements being willed by some other power'. Apparently, this latter elaboration represents a combination of an experience of primary positive alienation of the will (F8) with the secondary experience of influenced volitional acts (F6-like).

Made feelings (Table I): Fish's (1967) views on made feelings are similar to those he actually held or can be assumed to have held on made volitional acts, impulses and will. Mellor apparently defined made feelings in terms of positive alienation of feelings (F8): the subject 'experiences feelings which do not seem to be his own' and 'thus they are attributed to some external source'. Once again, Taylor and Heiser sharply differentiated between influenced feelings (F6) and positively alienated feelings (F8).

In the ninth edition of their Present State Examination, Wing and colleagues made no mention of made feelings. However, one can probably assume that their views on thought insertion and made will (delusions of control) would also be applicable to made feelings; that is, they would most likely define the latter phenomenon as a primary experience of positively alienated feelings (F8).

Diffusion or broadcasting of thoughts (Table I): Fish's definition of this phenomenon seemed rather narrow: the subject 'knows that as he is thinking everyone else is thinking in unison with him (Fish, 1967, p. 39),' that is, he has 'the certain knowledge that everyone else is participating in his thoughts (Fish, 1962, pp. 28–9)'. Apparently the actual sharing of thoughts remains an essential criterion in his description so that the mere diffusion of thoughts from the patient's head would not suffice to merit a positive rating. At any rate, Fish's concept of thought broadcasting represents an experience of negative-passive thought alienation (F10). Earlier, Fish (1962, p. 29) had also mentioned that thought broadcasting 'may form the basis of the delusion that his thoughts are being read'. However, in a later discussion (Fish, 1969), the primary-secondary roles of these two phenomena are apparently reversed, that is, thought broadcasting now appears to be the secondary explanation for thought reading.

In contrast to Fish, Mellor's definition of thought broadcasting was not as narrow in the sense that for him the criterion of actual sharing was not absolutely necessary: the subject experiences not only that 'thoughts escape from the confines of the self into the external world' but then 'they may be experienced by all around'. This phenomenon, obviously, is also a negative-passive experience of alienated thought (F10).

Taylor and Heiser separated thought broadcasting not only from all other general and specific experiences of influence (F5 + F6), but also from all other experiences of positive alienation (F8). In their example, a description of an initiating experience of influenced thought (F6) is also given, for they spoke of 'the machines' (from outside) being used to broadcast the patient's thoughts; indeed, in this instance, thought broadcast is actually described in terms of a secondary experience of negative-passive alienation of thought (F10-like). However, their formal definition of thought broadcast can be regarded in terms of primary negative-passive thought alienation (F10): the subject has 'the experience that as his thoughts occur they are escaping from his head into the external world'. It is also very important to note that for Taylor and Heiser the actual sharing of the diffused thoughts was not considered an essential requirement for a positive rating. Moreover, their description of thought broadcast did not seem clearly to separate it from hallucinatory audible thoughts (F12b).

On the basis of their definition of *thought broadcast* or *thought sharing*, Wing and colleagues (p. 161) evidently considered pseudo-hallucinatory *Gedanken-lautwerden* or audible thoughts (F11b) as some sort of prior stage to thought broadcasting. As for their description of thought broadcast itself, this was clearly framed in terms of negative-passive thought alienation (F10). Indeed, their definition was as narrow as Fish's concept since they also insisted that only when the subject actually experiences his thoughts being shared with others, irrespective of the mechanism, could a positive rating be made. As for delusions of thoughts being read, these, for Wing and his colleagues, could at times represent a possible secondary elaboration of thought broadcast.

Thought withdrawal (Table I): Fish (1967, p. 39) defined thought deprivation (withdrawal) as an experience of negative-active alienation of thought (F9): the subject finds that 'as he is thinking his thoughts suddenly disappear and are withdrawn from his mind by a foreign influence'. Of interest is the fact that for Fish (1967, p. 38) thought blocking was 'an objective sign', that is, an abnormality of expression or behaviour (*Ausdruckssymptom*) and not defined in terms of an experience (*Erlebnissymptom*). Thus, he suggested that thought deprivation was 'the subjective experience of thought blocking'. These views become important when compared with those of Wing and colleagues on 'pure thought block' (see below).

Mellor also defined thought withdrawal in the sense of an experience of negative-active thought alienation (F9): the subject simultaneously experiences a cessation of his own thoughts and their being withdrawn by some external force. Surprisingly, neither Taylor and Heiser's description of influenced thought (F6) nor of alienated thought (covering only F8 and F10) made any allowance for the phenomenological possibility of thought withdrawal viewed as an experience of negative-active alienation of thought (F9). Indeed, they made no separate mention of thought withdrawal as had been the case with the separate listing of thought broadcast.

Wing and colleagues (p. 162) used the expression thought block or thought withdrawal as if both components were merely different terms for the same phenomenon. In their descriptions, pure thought block, the experience of a sudden stopping of the subject's own thoughts quite unexpectedly, was clearly separated from what they called the 'explanatory delusion of thought withdrawal', that is, the experience that 'his thoughts have been removed from his head so that he has no thoughts'. This latter elaboration actually represents a secondary negative-active experience of alienated thought (F-9-like); however, despite the obvious secondary nature of their description, the impression is still given that thought withdrawal is considered to have primary first rank status (F9).

Influences playing on the body or somatic passivity (Table I): In his discussion of bodily or somatic hallucination, Fish (1969) stressed that 'one must make sure that the patient actually experiences bodily sensations as being produced by an external agency'. Unfortunately, he did not precisely distinguish between influenced (F6) and alienated (e.g. F8) somatic sensations; however, it will be assumed that for Fish both forms of experience would be acceptable as being of the first rank.

In describing this phenomenon, Mellor also did not make it clear if the resulting bodily sensations, despite the external influence, were still being experienced by the subject as his own, or were now experienced as being not his own, that is, as completely foreign sensations. Thus, Mellor's definition of the phenomenon stated that the subject is 'a passive ... and reluctant recipient of bodily sensations imposed upon him by some external agency', and it is stressed that the perception is simultaneously experienced as being both a bodily change and externally controlled. Since he went on to concede that such bodily sensations might be due either to actually present abnormal physical sensations or to haptic, thermic or kinaesthetic hallucinations, Mellor appeared to be quite open to the experiential possibilities of influenced (F6) as well as positively alienated somatic sensations (F8).

Although they included experiences of influence of actual somatic sensations (F6) among their FRSs, Taylor and Heiser failed explicitly to mention that positive alienation in this area (F8) could also occur; however, on the basis of their *influenced* versus *alienated* dichotomy for related phenomena, it can be assumed that they would affirm this possibility for somatic sensations. In defining other hallucinations and delusional elaboration, Wing and colleagues (pp. 166 and 212) apparently differentiated between haptic hallucinations, (something seems to touch him but when he looks nobody is there), and the possibility of delusional elaboration of this hallucinatory experience. For example, such secondary elaboration could take either the form of an experience of influenced (F6-like) or of positively alienated bodily sensations (F8-like), a fact not specifically stated in the glossary definition.

The sense deception continuum

In his classical papers on sense deceptions (*Trugwahrnehmungen*), Jaspers (1911; 1912b) stressed the distinction between true hallucinations and pseudo-hallucinations; his essential criteria were that the latter lacked concrete reality or substantiality (*Leibhaftigkeit*) and occurred within the patient's head or mind, whereas the former were perceptions without an object being experienced substantially in objective space. Schneider (1971) continued to conceptualize his first rank sense deceptions, formally at least, as Jasperian true hallucinations; however, his concrete examples of audible thoughts appeared to be more like Jasperian pseudo-hallucinations. At any rate, the Jasperian position at the present time is not followed by most German-speaking psychiatrists (e.g. Bleuler, 1972), the tendency now being to make the presence of insight (pseudo-hallucination) or its lack (true hallucination), the main criterion of differentiation. Recently, there has also been some non-German criticism of Jaspers' point of view (e.g. Fish, 1962; 1967; Hare, 1973) as well as some more positive renewed interest (e.g. Sedman, 1966a; 1966b).

Audible thoughts or gedankenlautwerden (Table II): In his description of phonemes, Fish (1962, pp. 35–6) apparently favoured a continuum view that ranged from the clarity of ordinary voices to the voices heard in the mind, the latter being called pseudo-hallucinatory. Indeed, Fish (1967, pp. 19–20), although clearly aware of the Jasperian distinction on sense deceptions, maintained (Fish, 1962, pp. 35–6) that 'the pseudo-hallucination is purely of academic interest and has no prognostic or diagnostic value in schizophrenia'. One wonders why Fish (1969) felt it necessary to point out that for the diagnosis of acute schizophrenia 'one should always get the patient to give examples of his hallucinatory experiences and to explain the origin of his voices. It is particularly important to be sure that the patient is not merely describing very vivid auditory imagery'. Moreover, in describing *Gedankenlautwerden* in acute schizophrenia, Fish (1962, p. 24) said: 'the subjects can hear their thoughts being spoken aloud as they think, and the voice which speaks their thoughts may come from inside (F11b) or outside (F12b) the head'. In contrast to Fish, Mellor clearly defined this phenomenon in the Jasperian sense of true hallucinations (F12b), that is, audible thoughts were sharply separated from inner voices, the latter 'usually (being) forms of imagery, including pseudo-hallucinations'.

Taylor and Heiser agreed on this point for in their terminology audible thoughts are considered to be so-called 'complete auditory hallucinations', that is, 'clearly audible voices coming from outside (F12b) the patient's head'; thus, the latter are distinct from what they called non-schizophrenic auditory hallucinations, which are experienced 'as coming from inside the head (inner voices)'. On the other hand, Wing and colleagues (p. 161) subsumed *Gedanken-lautwerden* under *thought broadcasting* or *thought sharing*, as if audible thoughts were a primitive stage of thought broadcast. Their formal definition clearly stated that the subject's 'own thoughts seem to sound aloud in his head almost as though someone standing nearby could hear them'. Obviously, such a description implies a Jasperian pseudo-hallucination (F11b). In addition, for these workers (Wing *et al*; p. 162) *thought echo* (experiences his own thoughts as repeated or echoed, not just spoken aloud in his head) and *thought commentary* (experiences alien thoughts in his head that are in association with his own, or comment on his own) were apparently regarded as variants of *Gedanken-lautwerden*.

Voices arguing and voices commenting (Table II): Fish's (1967; p. 23) continuum position on phonemes (covering F11ab and F12ab), including voices arguing or discussing and commenting, has already been considered under audible thoughts. For Mellor, voices arguing or commenting were 'hallucinatory voices', his examples amply demonstrating that concrete voices with no actual source of origin in objective space in the Jasperian sense (F12a) were meant to be sharply distinguished from inner voices.

Taylor and Heiser also used their concept of complete auditory hallucinations, as defined above, for these voices (F12a), clearly separating them from their non-schizophrenic auditory hallucinations. Taking a broad stand on the matter, Wing and associates (p. 164) gave instructions that not only true hallucinations (F12a) but also pseudo-hallucinations (F11a) should be included when rating positively for such phenomena.

Comment

On examining the writings of important Anglo-American investigators of FRSs (Fish, 1962; 1967; 1969; Mellor, 1970; Taylor and Heiser, 1971; Wing *et al*, 1974), it can be said that the boundaries of these phenomena are often viewed quite differently, sometimes being defined in wider and sometimes in narrower terms. At the risk of oversimplification, it seems that the clinician's main options in judging the presence or absence of FRSs boil down to the following dichotomies of narrow (= a) versus wide (= b) concepts of such symptoms:

1. (a) Are only experiences of positive alienation (F8) of thought (thought insertion), of impulses, of volitional acts, of feelings and of somatic sensations to be considered of the first rank? (b) Or should experiences of influence (F6) in these areas also be rated positively?
2. (a) Is thought broadcasting as a negative-passive alienated experience of thought (F10) only first rank when the thoughts leaving the patient's head are actually also shared with others? (b) Or does it suffice for a first rank rating that the thoughts must only diffuse out, sharing being immaterial?
3. (a) Should the experience of thoughts ceasing in the patient's head because of an external agency in the sense of a negative-active experience of alienated thought (F9) be considered as constituting thought withdrawal of the first rank? (b) Or should so-called pure thought block, when clearly present as an experience, and not just as an objective sign, also be acceptable?
4. (a) Are voices arguing or discussing, voices commenting and audible thoughts only first rank when they are Jasperian true hallucinations (F12ab)? (b) Or should pseudo-hallucinatory experiences (F11ab) also be rated as having first rank quality?
5. (a) Should one define the first rank symptom of delusional perception (F3) very strictly? (b) Or should the frequently occurring delusional notion linked to a perception (F2) also be acceptable as being a first rank phenomenon?

Whether wider or narrower views are considered acceptable remains purely an arbitrary matter. However, the simple realization that such different interpretations are possible and actually do exist, is of no little importance. Thus, until a more generally binding agreement can be hopefully attained, two things seem essential and should be demanded of all clinicians: 1. an unmistakably clear statement of their own personal first rank boundary critieria, and 2. a similar statement of the nosological bias they personally attach to these phenomena.

This second point is particularly relevant when one recalls that, for example, Kraepelin (1913), Leonhard (1968) and Berner (1977) in Europe, as well as some modern American researchers (e.g. Winokur *et al*, 1969; Taylor and Abrams, 1973; Luria and McHugh, 1974), do not automatically give a schizophrenic weighting to first rank or first rank-like phenomena appearing in functional psychosis, especially in the presence of strong affective clinical features. This seems, then, to be in contrast to the usual bias influencing the clinical practice of German Schneiderians (Koehler *et al*, 1977).

References

BERNER, P. (1977) *Psychiatrische Systematik. Ein Lehrbuch*. Bern: Hans Huber.
—— & NASKE, R. (1973) Wahn. In *Lexikon der Psychiatrie* (ed. C. Müller). Berlin: Springer.
BLEULER, E. (1972) *Lehrbuch der Psychiatrie*. 12th edition (ed. M. Bleuler). Berlin: Springer.
CONRAD, K. (1957) *Die beginnnende Schizophrenie*. Stuttgart: Thieme.
FISH, F. (1960) A review of *Die beginnende Schizophrenie. Journal of Mental Science*, **106,** 34–54.
—— (1961) A neurophysiological theory of schizophrenia. *Journal of Mental Science*, **107,** 828–839.
—— (1962) *Schizophrenia*. Bristol; J. Wright & Sons.
—— (1967) *Clinical Psychopathology*. Bristol: J. Wright & Sons.

—— (1969) The diagnosis of acute schizophrenia. Instructions on the use of the acute schizophrenic diagnostic checklist (ASDC). *Psychiatric Quarterly*, **43**, 35–45.

HARE, E. H. (1973) A short note on pseudo-hallucinations. *British Journal of Psychiatry*, **122**, 469–476.

JANZARIK, W. (1959) *Dynamische Grundkonstellationen in endogenen Psychosen*. Monographien aus dem Gesamtgebiete der Neurologie und Psychiatrie, Heft 96. Berlin: Springer.

—— (1968) *Schizophrene Verläufe*. Monographien aus dem Gesamtgebiete der Neurologie und Psychiatrie, Heft 126. Berlin: Springer.

JASPERS, K. (1911) Zur Analyse der Trugwahrnehmungen (Leibhaftigkeit und Realitätsurteil). In *Gesammelte Schriften zur Psychopatholgie* (1963) by K. Jaspers. Berlin: Springer.

—— (1912a) The phenomenological approach in psychopathology. Transl. (1968) in *British Journal of Psychiatry*, **114**, 1313–1323.

—— (1912b) Die Trugwahrnehmungen. In *Gesammelte Schriften zur Psychopatholgie* (1963) by K. Jaspers. Berlin: Springer.

—— (1962) *General Psychopathology*. Engl. translation. Manchester: Manchester University Press.

—— (1965) *Allgemeine Psychopathologie*. 8th edition. Berlin: Springer.

KISKER, K. P. (1960) *Der Erlebniswandel des Schizophrenen*. Monographien aus dem Gesamtgebiete der Neurologie und Psychiatrie, Heft 89. Berlin: Springer.

KOEHLER, K. (1976) Delusional perception and delusional notion linked to a perception. *Psychiatria Clinica*, **9**, 45–58.

—— (1977) Symptome ersten Ranges: Sind sie wirklich so verstaubt? *Fortschritte der Neurologie und Psychiatrie*, **45**, 405–411.

—— & WITTER, H. (1976) Kritische Anmerkungen über die Gedankeneingebung. *Archiv für Psychiatrie und Nervenkrankheiten*, **221**, 369–382.

—— GUTH, W. & GRIMM, G. (1977) First rank symptoms of schizophrenia in Schneider-oriented German centers. *Archives of General Psychiatry*, **34**, 810–813.

KRAEPELIN, E. (1913) *Psychiatrie. Band III. Klinische Psychiatrie. II Teil*. Leipzig: J. A. Barth.

LEONHARD, K. (1968) *Aufteilung der endogenen psychosen*. Berlin: Akademie.

LURIA, R. & McHUGH, P. R. (1974) Reliability and clinical utility of the 'Wing' Present State Examination. *Archives of General Psychiatry*, **30**, 866–871.

MATUSSEK, P. (1952) Unterschungen über die Wahnwahrnehmung. 1. Mitteilung. *Archiv für Psychiatrie und Nervenkrankheiten*, **189**, 279–319.

—— (1953) Untersuchungen über die Wahnwahrnehmung. 2. Mitteilung. *Schweizer Archiv für Psychiatrie und Neurologie*, **71**, 189–210.

MELLOR, C. S. (1970) First rank symptoms of schizophrenia. *British Journal of Psychiatry*, **117**, 15–23.

SCHNEIDER, K. (1959) *Clinical Psychopathology*. Engl. translation. New York: Grune & Stratton.

—— (1971) *Klinische Psychopathologie*. 9th edition. Stuttgart: Thieme.

SEDMAN, G. (1966a) A comparative study of pseudo-hallucinations, imagery and true hallucinations. *British Journal of Psychiatry*, **112**, 9–17.

—— (1966b) A phenomenological study of pseudo-hallucinations and related experiences. *Acta Psychiatrica Scandinavica*, **42**, 35–70.

STRAUSS, J. S. (1969) Hallucinations and delusions as points on continua function. *Archives of General Psychiatry*, **21**, 581–586.

TAYLOR, M. A. & HEISER, J. F. (1971) Phenomenology: an alternative approach to diagnosis of mental disease. *Comprehensive Psychiatry*, **12**, 480–486.

—— & ABRAMS, R. (1973) The phenomenology of mania. *Archives of General Psychiatry*, **29**, 520–522.

WING, J. K., COOPER, J. E. & SARTORIUS, N. (1974) *Measurement and Classification of Psychiatric Symptoms. An Instruction Manual for the PSE and Catego Program*. Cambridge University Press.

WINOKUR, G., CLAYTON, P. & REICH, T. (1969) *Manic-depressive Illness*. St. Louis: C. V. Mosby.

14 The present status of first rank symptoms

C. S. MELLOR

Kurt Schneider asserted that certain symptoms, which he termed 'first rank', invariably distinguished between schizophrenia and manic-depressive psychosis. This assertion, which has attracted considerable critical attention during the past ten years, will be examined in the light of these recent investigations.

Schneider claimed that if a first rank symptom is present and an organic psychosyndrome has been excluded then the diagnosis of schizophrenia should always be made in preference to cyclothymia (Schneider, 1959). However, the diagnosis of schizophrenia does not rest solely upon these symptoms, but can be made if characteristic groups of other disorders of experience (second rank symptoms), or disorders of expression (third rank symptoms) are found. His statements that first rank symptoms have no theoretical value, and that there are probably other symptoms which discriminate as well but occur too infrequently to be of use, reflect Schneider's pragmatic approach to diagnosis.

There are four questions that require an answer if we are to assess the clinical value of first rank symptoms. Do they occur frequently enough to be useful? Do they distinguish between schizophrenia and affective disorder? How are they elicited? What are they?

First let us examine Schneider's contention that first rank symptoms occur frequently enough to be diagnostically useful. Their frequency in patients with a diagnosis of schizophrenia ranges from 72 per cent, found by Mellor (1970) and by Huber, an associate of Schneider (Koehler *et al*, 1977), to 28 per cent (Taylor, 1972). The reasons for this variation have not been adequately examined, and it is not known whether they can be attributed to the examiners, the patient samples, or the alternative criteria used to make the diagnosis of schizophrenia. Generalizing from the published data, about half of the patients with a diagnosis of schizophrenia appear to have identifiable first rank symptoms.

The second question, which has exercised the majority of investigators, is whether this diagnostic primacy of first rank symptoms leads to patients with affective disorders being erroneously diagnosed as schizophrenic? Taylor and Abrams (1973; 1975) reported the presence of first rank symptoms in 12 per cent of patients in one study of mania and 8 per cent in another. Carpenter *et al* (1973) found that 23 per cent of the patients with affective psychosis and 9 per cent of the patients with neurotic and character disorders had first rank symptoms. Wing and Nixon (1975), reporting on the International Pilot Study of Schizophrenia, noted that 13 per cent of patients with mania, 4 per cent with depressive disorders and 2 per cent with neuroses had first rank symptoms of schizophrenia. But this study did, overall, give weight to the diagnostic value of these symptoms.

Investigations using research criteria for the diagnosis of affective disorder, such as those by Koehler and Seminario (1978) and Brockington *et al* (1978) have demonstrated that first rank symptoms occur in about 15 per cent of patients with 'research diagnosable affective disorders'. These research criteria were largely based upon symptomatology, but others (Kendell *et al* (1979) and Bland and Orn (1979)) have employed criteria based upon outcome, and have shown that first rank symptoms have a poor predictive value for the various states that are assumed to be a consequence of schizophrenia.

In a somewhat different approach to outcome, the hospital records of a group of patients originally diagnosed as having schizophrenia, because they had first rank symptoms, were examined eight years later to see if the diagnosis at subsequent hospital contacts had changed (Mellor *et al*, 1981). Such a change had occurred in 12 per cent of patients, the majority of whom had the one first rank symptom, 'voices discussion', at the inception admission.

The conclusions to be drawn from these investigations are that first rank symptoms are strongly associated with schizophrenia, but have been reported in other conditions, particularly mania. Thus Schneider's belief that first rank symptoms invariably distinguish schizophrenia from cyclothymia appears to be discredited.

Turning to the third question, Schneider stated that the phenomenological method as described by Karl Jaspers is used to elicit and identify first rank symptoms. Jaspers adapted the method developed by the phenomenological philosophers to the clinical interview (Jaspers, 1912). The procedure will not be described here, but as it is ignored in most investigators' reports, certain points need to be made for the purpose of this comment.

The practice of the phenomenological method requires a conversation between the interviewer and patient in which the patient is encouraged to turn an inner eye upon his experiences and under the guidance of the interviewer explore and describe them. These descriptions together with any relevant observational data are used by the interviewer to recreate the patient's experiences in his own mind. It is from the examiner's re-creation of the patient's experiences that the phenomena are described and identified.

Practitioners of this method usually have to undertake a painstaking and protracted interview before they can be assured of the presence, or absence, of first rank symptoms. It is questionable whether the structure imposed upon the research interviews used to identify first rank symptoms can accommodate the phenomenological method. Investigations based upon the retrospective identification of these symptoms in case notes are of doubtful value, unless the original interviewers' approaches are known.

The final question—'What are the first rank symptoms?'—is not so straightforward as it first appears. **Koehler** (**1979**), who has examined this question in some detail, remarked that Schneider was uncharacteristically vague when it came to describing these symptoms. Most of them, Koehler observes, can be considered for descriptive purposes to lie on a continuum. The hallucinatory phenomena, for example, range from imagery, through pseudo-hallucinations to hallucinations proper. He describes similar continua for the various forms of ego disorders and for delusional percepts. One end of the continuum represents phenomena that may be found in some normal subjects and certainly in patients with neuroses and personality disorders, whilst the other represents a rigorous definition of what in my view are true first rank symptoms. This distinction may not be made if the patient's initial description is not subject to a phenomenological examination.

In conclusion, Schneider's claims about first rank symptoms find only limited support from the more recent literature. However, as these studies rarely acknowledge the problems of defining and eliciting these symptoms, their conclusions should not be unreservedly accepted. Therefore, those who find first rank symptoms to be of clinical value need not yet abandon them. The choice of a particular diagnostic schema for schizophrenia will be determined by its usefulness until some external validating criterion for this disorder is discovered.

References

BLAND, R. C. & ORN, H. (1979) Schizophrenia: diagnostic criteria and outcome. *British Journal of Psychiatry*, **134**, 34–38.

BROCKINGTON, I. F., KENDELL, R. E. & LEFF, J. P. (1978) Definitions of schizophrenia: concordance and prediction of outcome. *Psychological Medicine*, **8**, 387–398.

CARPENTER, W. T., STRAUSS, J. S. & MULEH, S. (1973) Are there pathognomonic symptoms of schizophrenia? *Archives of General Psychiatry*, **28**, 847–852.

JASPERS, K. (1912) The phenomenological approach in psychopathology. Transl. in *British Journal of Psychiatry*, 1968, **114**, 1313–1323.

KENDELL, R. E., BROCKINGTON, I. F. & LEFF, J. P. (1979) Prognostic implications of six alternative definitions of schizophrenia. *Archives of General Psychiatry*, **36**, 25–31.

KOEHLER, K. (1979) First-rank symptoms of schizophrenia: questions concerning clinical boundaries. *British Journal of Psychiatry*, **134**, 236–248.

—— GUTH, W. & GRIMM, G. (1977) First-rank symptoms of schizophrenia in Schneider-oriented German centres. *Archives of General Psychiatry*, **34**, 810–813.

—— & SEMINARIO, I. (1978) 'First-rank' schizophrenia and research diagnosable schizophrenic and affective illness. *Comprehensive Psychiatry*, **19**, 401–407.

MELLOR, C. S. (1970) First-rank symptoms of schizophrenia. *British Journal of Psychiatry*, **117**, 15–23.

—— SIMS, A. C. P. & COPE, R. V. (1981) Change of diagnosis in schizophrenia and first-rank symptoms: An eight year follow-up. *Comprehensive Psychiatry*, **22**, 184–188.

SCHNEIDER, K. (1959) *Clinical Psychopathology*. Engl. Transl. New York: Grune and Stratton.

TAYLOR, M. A. (1972) Schneiderian first rank symptoms and clinical prognostic features in schizophrenia. *Archives of General Psychiatry*, **26**, 64–67.

—— & ABRAMS, R. (1973) The phenomenology of mania. *Archives of General Psychiatry*, **29**, 520–522.

—— —— (1975) Acute mania: clinical and genetic study of responders and non-responders to treatments. *Archives of General Psychiatry*, **32**, 863–865.

WING, J. & NIXON, J. (1975) Discriminating symptoms in schizophrenia. *Archives of General Psychiatry*, **32**, 853–859.

15 Temporal disorientation in chronic schizophrenia: The implications of an 'organic' psychological impairment for the concept of 'functional' psychosis

T. J. CROW

Background

In the course of a survey of in-patients suffering from long-standing schizophrenic illnesses, Crow and Mitchell (1975) were impressed by the frequency with which such subjects believed their age to be a figure widely different from the true one. They systematically investigated the subjective ages of a group of 237 patients with chronic schizophrenia in the wards of four mental hospitals in Scotland and found that approximately 25 per cent of them believed themselves to be five or more years younger than they really were (Fig. 1). Twelve per cent of this population believed they were within five years of their age on admission, although on average they were 28 years older than this. This figure was significantly ($P < 0.001$) greater than would be expected if the subjects were merely guessing their age. Five per cent of the sample thought their age was within one year of their age on admission.

Although neither Crow and Mitchell nor other authors were aware of a literature, there had been earlier reports of similar findings. Thus Lanzkron and Wolfson (1958) described a 'perceptual distortion of temporal orientation' in 50 chronic schizophrenic patients, and Dahl (1958) replicated the finding in a population of 500 institutionalized patients and claimed that this 'singular distortion of temporal orientation' occurred only in schizophrenia. Ehrenteil and Jenney (1960) found that a number of hospitalized schizophrenic patients gave ages younger than their true age and asked, 'Does time stand still for some psychotics?' Michelson (1968), also apparently unaware of previous reports, described systematic errors made by 62 patients in estimating their ages over a six-year period.

Prevalence

Stevens *et al* (1978) surveyed the population of patients with a diagnosis of schizophrenia in Shenley Hospital in North-West London and found that age disorientation (defined as a five-year discrepancy between true and subjective age) was present in 25 per cent of this sample, a figure closely similar to that reported in the less representative Scottish sample of Crow and Mitchell

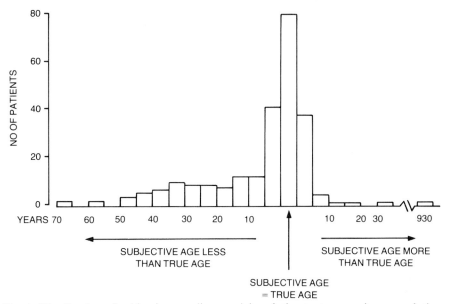

Fig. 1. Distribution of subjective age (in years) in relation to true age in a population of 237 chronic schizophrenic patients in Scottish mental hopsitals. Sixty (25.3%) patients believed themselves to be five or more years younger than they were (from Crow and Mitchell, 1975).

(1975) and that found by Smith and Oswald (1976) in patients in the Harlem Valley Psychiatric Center in New York. Stevens *et al* (1978) found further that when age-matched with schizophrenic patients without age disorientation, those with this feature were younger at first admission and had a longer duration of stay. It was suggested that age disorientation was a feature of a type of schizophrenic illness with early onset and poor prognosis.

The nature of the cognitive deficit

The question arises as to whether age disorientation is an isolated psychopathological curiosity or part of a more general impairment of temporal orientation. Crow and Stevens (1978) found that patients with age disorientation (n = 77) were much less likely than those without age disorientation (n = 227) to be able to give correct answers to simple questions about dates and the passage of time (e.g. their date of birth, the present year and the duration of their hospital stay). The age disorientated systematically underestimated the present year and their duration of hospital stay: the errors made by individual patients in estimating these figures were consistent with their concept of their own age (Figs. 2 and 3).

Thus age disorientation is part of a constellation of defects of temporal orientation. For these patients 'time stands still'. However, in some patients an incorrect appreciation of their own age co-exists with correct awareness of the present year, and between these patients and those for whom subjective

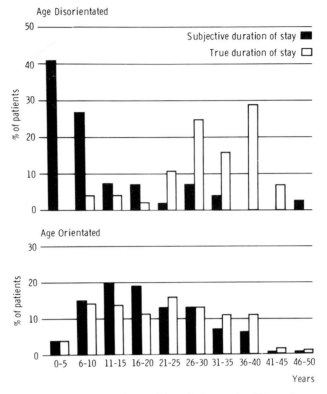

Fig. 2. Subjective and true durations of hospital stay in 299 patients with chronic schizophrenia in Shenley Hospital subdivided according to whether (above) or not (below) they showed age disorientation (from Crow and Stevens, 1978).

time stands still there appears to be a continuum of increasing temporal disorientation. It was suggested that this dimension was a correlate of intellectual impairment.

A comparison between age disorientated and age orientated patients for past physical treatments revealed that the former were slightly, but not significantly, less likely than the latter to have received electroconvulsive therapy, insulin coma therapies, or a combination of the two, or to have been subjected to leucotomy (Table I). Thus age disorientation is not attributable to these physical treatments.

Liddle and Crow (1984) investigated the question of whether age disorientation is associated with wider impairments of intellect in a group of patients selected from a population of 510 cases satisfying the St. Louis criteria for a diagnosis of probable schizophrenia. Twenty-one patients who stated their age to be within five years of their age on admission were matched for age, sex and duration of hospital stay with a group of 21 patients without age disorientation selected from the same population. The age disorientated patients demonstrated substantial impairments on tests of orientation and general knowledge, associational learning, the 'famous personality' test (of remote memory), tests of vocabulary and aphasia, Raven's matrices, the

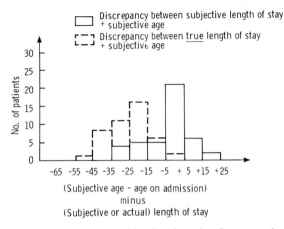

Total No. of patients (true age 5 years more
than subjective age) who gave an estimate
of their length of stay = 44

Fig. 3. The discrepancy between subjective length of stay and subjective age is much less than between true length of stay and subjective age in 44 schizophrenic patients with age disorientation (from Crow and Stevens, 1978).

TABLE I

Past physical treatments in relation to age disorientation

	Age orientated n = 222		Age disorientated n = 88	
ECT	96	(43%)	35	(40%)
Insulin coma	80	(40%)	27	(31%)
Insulin coma and ECT	48	(22%)	16	(18%)
Leucotomy	22	(10%)	6	(7%)

digit-symbol substitution test and the mental test score. It was concluded that age disorientation is a marker for a form of chronic schizophrenia characterized by a severe wide-ranging impairment of intellect (a 'global' intellectual deterioration). The findings on the 'famous personality' test and Peabody vocabulary test did not exclude the possibility that such an impairment arises at a time preceding the onset of illness.

Comment

The phenomenon of age disorientation challenges the conventional psychopathological distinction between the 'organic' and the 'functional' psychoses. Temporal disorientation, the hallmark of the organic psychoses, occurs in a substantial proportion (approximately 25 per cent of three separate populations) of hospitalized patients with chronic schizophrenia. When present and severe (i.e. in those cases where subjective age is close to age on admission) it forms part of a global impairment of intellectual function which cannot readily be distinguished from dementia. This finding is at odds with the concept of schizophrenia and its historical origin (Crow and Johnstone, 1980).

Kraepelin and Bleuler apparently believed that true intellectual impairment does not occur: thus Bleuler (1950) stated that 'in contrast to the organic psychoses, we find in schizophrenia . . . that sensation, memory, consciousness and motility are not directly disturbed (p. 55) and 'memory as such does not suffer in this disease' (p. 59). Kraepelin (1919) thought that intellectual functions (orientation, consciousness and memory—p. 17) were unimpaired, but made an exception for some chronic states (Kraepelin (1919)—p. 190 and pp. 197–198). Thus, in his chapter on terminal states, Kraepelin comments on states of 'simple weak mindedness' that 'a distinct weakness of judgement appears . . . although a considerable residuum of knowledge formerly acquired may come to the surface, yet the patients have lost the capacity of making use of it . . . The patients therefore lose a great part of their knowledge: they become impoverished in thought, monotonous in their mental activities.' These statements might be interpreted as compatible with a degree of intellectual and memory impairment but earlier in the same section Kraepelin states: 'The weakness lies . . . specially in the domain of emotion and volition: to a less degree judgement and still less memory are involved. After the disappearance of the more marked morbid symptoms the patients seem to be clear about time, place and person . . .' (p. 189). Later, in a section on 'drivelling dementia', Kraepelin writes (p. 197) of a 'general decay of mental efficiency' but 'the really characteristic disorder, however, in this form is incoherence of the train of thought' and while 'the patients are often not clear about their position and their surroundings' they 'often answer simple questions quite correctly' (p. 198). Thus it appears that while Bleuler viewed the psychopathological changes as quite distinct from those of the organic dementias, Kraepelin acknowledged features in the defect states compatible with true intellectual impairment but strove to explain them in other ways. Neither Kraepelin nor Bleuler noted the phenomenon of age disorientation.

Some psychometric studies have addressed the issue of the nature of the intellectual impairment in chronic schizophrenia. Klonoff *et al* (1970) applied the Halstead-Reitan test battery to a group of chronic schizophrenics and concluded that 'the test results certainly appear to indicate the presence of organic deficits in these patients.' In a review of psychological test findings Heaton *et al* (1978) concluded that groups of chronic or process schizophrenics 'may look organic on neuropsychological tests because a significant proportion of such patients are organic.' Some studies provide evidence that these intellectual impairments occur with progression of the disease, an issue not resolved by examination of the pattern of deficits in a severely age disorientated group (Liddle and Crow, 1984). In an important study of 101 schizophrenic patients, 99 hospitalized non-schizophrenic psychiatric patients and 50 normal controls, Garside (1969) was able to compare performance on the Wechsler-Bellevue scales with the school grading examination results these subjects had obtained years earlier. Schizophrenic patients showed significant intellectual deterioration by comparison with the other groups, this deterioration being greatest in those diagnosed as hebephrenic and least in those diagnosed as suffering from paranoid schizophrenia.

The first CT scan study of patients with chronic schizophrenia (Johnstone *et al*, 1976; 1978) included small groups of chronic schizophrenic patients with and without age disorientation. Lateral ventricular area was found to be larger in patients with schizophrenia than in age-matched controls and larger, but not significantly so, in patients with, by comparison with those without, age disorientation. This and some later studies (e.g. Donnelly *et al*, 1980; Golden *et al*, 1980) have found ventricular enlargement to be related to intellectual impairment. These findings are consistent with the view (Crow, 1980) that intellectual impairment is a component of the type II syndrome of negative symptoms (equivalent to the 'defect' state) which is conjectured to be the result of structural brain changes. A recent post-mortem study (Brown *et al*, 1985) yields evidence that such changes are taking place in the temporal lobe. By comparison with patients with affective disorders, patients with schizophrenia had increased cross-sectional area of the temporal horn of the lateral ventricle and diminished thickness of the para-hippocampal gyrus, although it could not be determined from case records whether these changes were specifically associated with intellectual impairment.

Whatever its cerebral basis, the presence of age disorientation in chronic schizophrenic patients establishes that a significant proportion of these patients have psychological deficits which are 'organic' in type according to conventional criteria. The psychopathological distinction between the functional and organic psychoses is less easily maintained than is sometimes thought to be the case.

References

BLEULER, E. (1950) *Dementia Praecox or the Group of Schizophrenias* (trans. J. Zinkin). New York: International Universities Press.

BROWN, R., COLTER, N., CORSELLIS, J. A. N., CROW, T. J., FRITH, C. D., JAGOE, R., JOHNSTONE, E. C. & MARSH, L. (1985) Brain weight and parahippocampal gyrus thickness are decreased and temporal horn area is increased in schizophrenia by comparison with affective disorders. *Archives of General Psychiatry* (in press).

CROW, T. J. (1980) Molecular pathology of schizophrenia: more than one disease process? *British Medical Journal*, **280**, 66–68.

—— & MITCHELL, W. S. (1975) Subjective age in chronic schizophrenia: evidence for a sub-group of patients with defective learning capacity? *British Journal of Psychiatry*, **126**, 360–363.

—— & JOHNSTONE, E. C. (1980) Dementia praecox and schizophrenia: was Bleuler wrong? *Journal of the Royal College of Physicians*, **14**, 238–240.

—— & STEVENS, M. (1978) Age disorientation in chronic schizophrenia: the nature of the cognitive deficit. *British Journal of Psychiatry*, **133**, 137–142.

DAHL, M. (1958) A singular distortion of temporal orientation. *American Journal of Psychiatry*, **115**, 146–149.

DONNELLY, E. F., WEINBERGER, D. R., WALDMAN, I. N. & WYATT, R. J. (1980) Cognitive impairment associated with morphological brain abnormalities on computed tomography in chronic schizophrenic patients. *Journal of Nervous and Mental Disease*, **168**, 305–308.

EHRENTEIL, O. F. & JENNEY, P. B. (1960) Does time stand still for some psychotics? *Archives of General Psychiatry*, **3**, 1–3.

GARSIDE, R. F. (1969) *The Relationship between Schizophrenia and Intelligence*. Ph.D. thesis, University of Newcastle upon Tyne.

GOLDEN, C. J., MOSES, J. A., ZELAZOWSKI, R., GRABER, B., ZATZ, L. M., HORVATH, T. B. & BERGER, P. A. (1980) Cerebral ventricular size and neuropsychological impairment in young chronic schizophrenics. *Archives of General Psychiatry*, **37**, 619–623.

HEATON, R. K., BAADE, L. E. & JOHNSON, K. L. (1978) Neuropsychological test results associated with psychiatric disorders in adults. *Psychological Bulletin*, **85**, 141–162.

JOHNSTONE, E. C., CROW, T. J., FRITH, C. D., HUSBAND, J. & KREEL, L. (1976). Cerebral ventricular size and cognitive impairment in chronic schizophrenia. *Lancet, ii,* 924–927.

——— ——— ——— STEVENS, M., KREEL, L. & HUSBAND, J. (1978 The dementia of dementia praecox. *Acta Psychiatrica Scandinavia,* **57,** 305–324.

KLONOFF, H., FIBIGER, H. C. & HUTTON, G. H. (1970) Neuropsychological problems in chronic schizophrenia. *Journal of Nervous and Mental Disease,* **150,** 291–300.

KRAEPELIN, E. (1919) *Dementia Praecox and Paraphrenia* (translated by R. M. Barclay and G. M. Robertson). New York: R. E. Krieger.

LANZKRON, J. & WOLFSON, W. (1958) Prognostic value of perceptual distortion of temporal orientation in chronic schizophrenics. *American Journal of Psychiatry,* **114,** 744–746.

LIDDLE, P. & CROW, T. J. (1984) Age disorientation in chronic schizophrenia is associated with global intellectual impairment. *British Journal of Psychiatry,* **144,** 193–199.

MICHELSON, N. (1968) A note on age confusion in psychosis. *Psychiatric Quarterly,* **42,** 331–338.

SMITH, J. M. & OSWALD, W. T. (1976) Subjective age in chronic schizophrenia. *British Journal of Psychiatry,* **128,** 100.

STEVENS, M., CROW, T. J., BOWMAN, M. J. & COLES, E. C. (1978) Age disorientation in schizophrenia: a constant prevalence of 25% in a chronic mental hospital population? *British Journal of Psychiatry,* **133,** 130–136.

16 Paranoia revisited

ALISTAIR MUNRO

The ICD-9 classificatory system (WHO, 1978) defines paranoia (297.1) as 'a rare chronic psychosis in which logically constructed systematized delusions have developed gradually without concomitant hallucinations or the schizophrenic type of disordered thinking. The delusions are mostly of grandeur ... persecution or somatic abnormality.' The ICD-9 makes no comment about causation, whereas Kraepelin, influenced by contemporary French views (Hoenig, 1981) proposed that paranoia arose from 'understandable' personality features. Both describe paranoia as an encapsulated, monosymptomatic psychosis.

DSM-III's definition (American Psychiatric Association, 1980) is similar, but one diagnostic criterion insists on 'a chronic and stable persecutory delusional system of at least six months' duration'. Fish (1974) pointed out that English-speaking psychiatrists often err in equating 'paranoia' with 'persecution' or 'angry suspiciousness', whereas it simply denotes a delusional state. Kendler (1980a) has argued cogently that DSM-III's insistence on a specific delusional content is of questionable validity.

The subtypes of paranoia

The definitive article on the history of paranoia is that by Lewis (1970), who notes that Kahlbaum (1863) presaged its modern description by Kraepelin. The latter, who observed a mere 19 cases (Fried and Agassi, 1976), regarded paranoia as a distinct illness and did not insist on persecutory ideas or delusions. He described three subtypes (Day and Semrad, 1978); these were *erotomania* (de Clérambault, 1942; Seeman, 1978; Lovett Doust and Christie, 1978; Enoch and Trethowan, 1979), *paranoid jealousy* (Enoch and Trethowan, 1979; Seeman, 1979), and *megalomania*. Kraepelin also mentioned a possible hypochondriacal form, but did not himself see a convincing case of this type, which is now known as *monosymptomatic hypochondriacal psychosis* (MHP), and which does appear to be a subtype of paranoia. Megalomanic paranoia remains a shadowy concept, though grandiosity is a common background factor in paranoia (Swanson *et al*, 1970). On the other hand, erotomania, paranoid jealousy and MHP are well-documented, and apparently not nearly so rare as alleged.

Anger and querulousness are common in paranoia (Munro, 1980) and Sim (1981) describes 'litigious paranoia', in which individuals angrily pursue an unreasonable and unending quest for restitution. Winokur (1977) includes litigious cases within paranoid illness (which he renames 'delusional disorder') along with hypochondriacal, erotic, grandiose and persecutory forms.

The diagnosis of paranoia in clinical practice

Kraepelin's views on paranoia were considerably disputed (Fish, 1962), and some of his diagnoses called in question by Kolle (1931). Authorities insisted on the excessive rarity of 'paranoia vera' (Kolle, 1957), and some declared the illness did not exist at all (Gregory and Smeltzer, 1977). More recently, Slater and Roth (1969) allowed the existence of paranoia and enumerated varieties with delusions of persecution, jealousy, grandeur, disfigurement or of emitting an odour. Recent evidence supports paranoia as an acceptable diagnosis (Johanson, 1964; Kendler, 1980b), yet the *British Medical Journal* (Leading Article, 1980) said that 'Paranoia is no longer a fashionable term'. The following reasons are suggested for this controversy:

1. Kraepelin's few cases and the doubt later cast on them have left a shadow.
2. It is often forgotten that erotomania, pathological jealousy, MHP, megalomania and litigiousness can be included in the diagnosis of paranoia, as well as delusions of persecution. When considered as separate entities, this fragments the overall concept of paranoia.
3. The smallness of case-series may be misleading and MHP recently proves to be much commoner than appreciated (Munro, 1980).
4. The literature is careless in its use of terms like paranoia, paranoiac and paranoid; an extreme of loose definition is reached in the work of Meissner (1978).
5. Terms like 'erotomania' and 'paranoid jealousy' are often used to describe symptoms in cases of varying aetiology, only some of which are paranoiac. Delusions of infestation constitute one form of MHP, but Skott (1978) has shown that similar cases can arise in depressive illness, schizophrenia, organic brain disorder, personality disorder and mental subnormality. Although paranoia can occur in a setting of personality disorder or minor brain damage, primary cases should be distinguished from others due to affective illness (Fry, 1978), cerebral atherosclerosis (Turgiyev, 1978) or psychopathy (Pechernikova, 1979). Deafness (Cooper, 1976) or psychosocial stressors like immigration (Binder and Simoes, 1978) and social isolation (Hitch and Rack, 1980) seem to occur in both primary and secondary cases.
6. Many authors fail to differentiate between neurotic and psychotic disorders with rather similar complaints; for example, dysmorphophobia should be, by definition, a non-psychotic illness (Braddock, 1982), but is often used to describe delusions of misshapenness (Hay, 1970). Also, if 'paranoid' really means 'delusional', then a paranoid personality disorder is a contradiction in terms, and it would be better to rename it as perhaps the 'oversensitive' personality disorder (Leonhard, 1976). More care in diagnosis and nomenclature could greatly clarify the definition and classification of paranoid disorders.
7. Paranoia does not usually degenerate into more severe illnesses, but it is chronic, has been incurable, and has thus not been an attractive illness

to treat. Psychopathological explanations have been attempted (Freud, 1958; Chalus, 1977), but have not led to effective therapy. Nowadays, MHP is seen to respond well to pimozide (Munro, 1980; Reilly, 1977; Freeman, 1979) and possibly to depot neuroleptics, and there is early evidence that pathological jealousy may also improve with pimozide (Dorian, 1979; Pollock, 1982). The therapeutic picture in paranoia may well be improving.

Paranoia and the paranoid spectrum

A longstanding view, not supported by much actual proof, proposes that paranoia and paranoid schizophrenia are the opposite ends of a continuous spectrum (Day and Semrad, 1978; Anderson and Trethowan, 1973; Cameron, 1974; Hamilton, 1978). In a minority of cases, paranoia is known to degenerate towards paraphrenia or paranoid schizophrenia (Kolle, 1931; Swanson *et al*, 1970; Munro and Pollock, 1981). A simple diagnostic schema of the paranoid spectrum is proposed in Fig. 1.

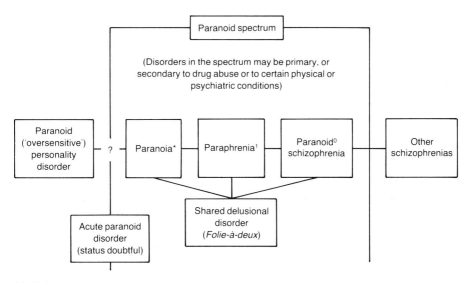

* Including:—erotomania, paranoid jealousy, monosymptomatic hypochondriacal psychosis, delusional grandiosity and litigious paranoia.

[1] Also known as paranoid state, paranoid psychosis, senile paraphrenia, involutional paraphrenia, etc. Not included in DSM-III.

[0] Not included as a paranoid disorder in DSM-III.

Fig. 1. The paranoid spectrum (hypothesized).

Kendler (1980b) believes that only the 10 to 20 per cent of paranoia cases which degenerate belong to the spectrum, the remainder forming a separate diagnostic category. To support this, Kendler and Hays (1981) and Watt *et al* (1980) report that there are relatively few cases of schizophrenia in the families of paranoid patients. A relatively weak genetic loading would probably tend to place a case on the paranoia end of the spectrum, while a stronger loading would place it nearer the schizophrenic extreme. The weakest loading might lead to the development of a 'paranoid' personality disorder, but this condition's link with the spectrum is dubious.

Extreme cases of encapsulated, non-degenerative paranoia on one hand, and of paranoid schizophrenia with incoherence, hallucinations and bizarre delusions on the other, are easily distinguished from each other. However, there are intermediate cases which Kraepelin, adapting a term of Kahlbaum, named paraphrenia. Later, it was decided that paraphrenia could not be differentiated from paranoid schizophrenia (Lange, 1926), but many psychiatrists continue to utilize this intermediate category, regrading paraphrenia to paranoid schizophrenia much as hypomania to mania. Paraphrenia is in ICD-9 (297.2), but not in DSM-III.

Secondary paranoid conditions occur at any point in the spectrum. A head-injury can produce oversensitive personality features; chronic alcoholism may precipitate pathological jealousy; old age may be associated with the onset of paraphrenia, and amphetamine intoxication can induce an illness identical to paranoid schizophrenia (Connell, 1958). Interestingly, it has been found that MHP cases can respond to pimozide even when an element of affective disorder, organic brain disorder or personality disorder is present (Munro, 1980).

Should paranoia be re-named?

To reduce confusion in nomenclature, Kendler (1980b) has suggested that paranoia be re-named 'simple delusional disorder' (SDD), and he suggests the following criteria for the illness: (1) onset before age 60; (2) non-bizarre delusions and/or persistent, pervasive ideas of reference, which have been present for at least two weeks; (3) absence of persistent hallucinations; (4) full affective syndrome absent when the patient is delusional; (5) no schizophrenic symptoms, such as prominent thought disorder, etc.; and (6) no acute or chronic brain disorder.

If MHP can be accepted as one stereotype of paranoia, some of these factors do not hold. For example, cases with an onset well after 60 have been reported (Riding and Munro, 1975; Munro, 1978); in the early recovery phase patients may show secondary affective symptoms requiring an antidepressant (Riding and Munro, 1975); some patients with MHP appear to be hallucinated as, for example, when they graphically describe the non-existent 'stench' they claim to emit; the illogic in relation to the delusion resembles thought disorder and, even if encapsulated, it dominates the patient's behaviour; and as has been remarked (Munro, 1980), a modicum of organic brain disorder is present in some cases. If treatment with pimozide benefits primary and some secondary cases of paranoia, too fine a diagnostic differentiation should be avoided. My findings with MHP bias me against Kendler's term of simple delusional disorder.

Too much can be made of the paranoid spectrum concept and of whether illnesses on it are discrete or form a continuum, but it seems a useful classificatory concept. It is interesting that pimozide, which appears to be uniquely therapeutic in paranoia-type illnesses, is apparently non-unique in the treatment of paraphrenia and paranoid schizophrenia, suggesting a shift in the biochemical basis of the disorders as one moves across the spectrum.

If paranoia is a worthwhile diagnostic category, it requires a name. I suggest that 'paranoia' remains as good a term as any.

Conditions related to paranoia

Folie-à-deux has often been reported in association with paranoid illnesses (Enoch and Trethowan, 1979; Munro, 1980; Skott, 1978). DSM-III, renaming it 'shared paranoid disorder' (297.30), insists that it meets the criteria for paranoid disorder, and defines it as a delusional illness, arising from close contact with a person who has established persecutory delusions. The insistence on persecution is unnecessary, and many victims of *folie-à-deux* are highly impressionable rather than deluded; when separated from the truly deluded individual, they frequently lose their strange beliefs spontaneously. *Folie-à-deux* should be regarded in a threefold way: (1) as an associated phenomenon of paranoid disorder; (2) as a neurotic or personality-determined disorder, caused by prolonged contact with an individual suffering from delusions; and (3) in some cases, especially where the primary and secondary cases share a common hereditary background, as a true delusional illness, shaped by the illness in the primary case.

DSM-III also describes acute paranoid disorder (298.30), an illness of less than six months' duration mostly seen in immigrants, refugees and others who have undergone severe environmental disruption. The onset is relatively sudden and the condition rarely becomes chronic. This last point makes it unlikely to be true paranoia, which is always described as chronic and, as Kraepelin believed, paranoia's onset is more usually a gradual one. Acute paranoid disorder is in fact more likely to be a form of psychogenic psychosis (Faergeman, 1963; McCabe, 1975) or, if very shortlived, possibly an hysterical psychosis in which ideas of persecution happen to be prominent.

Comment

If paranoia were as rare as has been claimed, or as untreatable as it used to be, we could afford to go on neglecting it. However, if its varied presentations are appreciated, it is not so rare, and some of its forms are now amenable to treatment. The condition is prolonged and anguishing, and suicide may sometimes occur (Bebbington, 1976), so that its diagnosis and treatment are not merely matters of academic interest. In addition, since paranoia is a circumscribed and definable disorder, it can be viewed as a kind of naturally occurring model psychosis, and theories of aetiology and treatment may be tested against it. It has been suggested that a relatively specific neurochemical disorder is responsible for MHP and other forms of paranoia (Munro, 1980), with fascinating possibilities for investigation and intervention. Whatever names we give it and its subtypes, it should be emphasized that these illnesses are real, may not be rare, and present a challenge to our diagnostic and therapeutic skills.

Appendix

Working definitions for paranoia and related conditions

Paranoid disorder should be a generic term for delusional illnesses occurring in clear consciousness and not primarily due to underlying physical disorder, depressive illness or organic brain disorder. This would include, among others:

    1. *Paranoia:* a permanent and unshakeable delusional system, accompanied by preservation of clear and orderly thinking, volition and behaviour in the rest of the personality. There are several characteristic subtypes:

    (a) *Erotomania* in which the individual has the fixed, erroneous delusion that another person has sexual feelings towards him or her;

    (b) *Pathological jealousy* where the individual has the fixed, erroneous delusion belief that the sexual partner is unfaithful;

    (c) *Monosymptomatic hypochondriacal psychosis* (*MHP*) in which there is a single, sustained hypochondriacal delusion;

    (d) *Litigious paranoia* in which there is an endless, delusional quest for restitution of a real or imagined wrong;

    (e) *Megalomania* in which there is a delusional preoccupation with one's imagined power, importance or wealth, usually associated with a sense of grandiosity (Kaplan *et al*, 1980).

    2. *Secondary paranoid disorder:* a psychotic illness presenting predominantly with delusional symptoms, which appears to result from an underlying physical disorder or another psychiatric illness.

    3. *Folie-à-deux* (*shared delusional disorder*)*:* for definition see above.

References

AMERICAN PSYCHIATRIC ASSOCIATION (1980) *Diagnostic and Statistical Manual of Mental Disorders* (*DSM III*). Washington: APA.

ANDERSON, E. W. & TRETHOWAN, W. H. (1973) *Psychiatry, 3rd Edition*. London: Baillière, Tindall.

BEBBINGTON, P. E. (1976) Monosymptomatic hypochondriasis, abnormal behaviour and suicide. *British Journal of Psychiatry*, **128**, 475–478.

BRADDOCK, L. E. (1982) Dysmorphophobia in adolescence. *British Journal of Psychiatry*, **140**, 199–201.

BINDER, V. & SIMOES, M. (1978) Social psychiatry of migrant workers. *Fortschritte der Neurologie und Psychiatrie*, **46**, 342–359.

CAMERON, N. A. (1974) Paranoid conditions and paranoia. In *American Handbook of Psychiatry, 2nd Edition*, (eds. S. Arieti *et al*). New York: Basic Books.

CHALUS, G. A. (1977) An evaluation of the validity of the Freudian theory of paranoia. *Journal of Homosexuality*, **3**, 171–188.

CONNELL, P. H. (1958) *Amphetamine Psychoses*. Maudsley Monograph No 5. London: Chapman and Hall.

COOPER, A. F. (1976) Paranoid illness from deafness. *British Journal of Psychiatry*, **129**, 216–226.

DAY, M. & SEMRAD, E. V. (1978) Paranoia and paranoid states. In *The Harvard Guide to Modern Psychiatry*, (ed. A. M. Nicholi). Cambridge, Mass; Belknap Press.

DE CLÉRAMBAULT, G. G. (1942) *Les Psychoses Passionelles. Oeuvre Psychiatrique*. Paris: Presses Universitaires.

DORIAN, B. J. (1979) Successful outcome of treatment of a case of delusional jealousy with pimozide. *Canadian Journal of Psychiatry*, **24**, 377.

ENOCH, M. D. & TRETHOWAN, W. H. (1979) *Uncommon Psychiatric Syndromes, 2nd Edition*. Bristol: John Wright.

FAERGEMAN, P. M. (1963) *Psychogenic Psychoses*. London: Butterworth.

FISH, F. J. (1962) *Schizophrenia*. Bristol: John Wright.

—— (1974) *Clinical Psychopathology*, (ed. M. Hamilton). Bristol; John Wright.

FREEMAN, H. L. (1979) Pimozide as a neuroleptic. *British Journal of Psychiatry*, **135**, 82–83.

FREUD, S. (1958) The case of Schreber. In *Complete Works, Vol. 12*, (ed. J. Strachey). London: Hogarth Press.

FRIED, Y. & AGASSI, J. (1976) *Paranoia: A Study in Diagnosis*. Boston: D. Reidel.

FRY, W. F. (1978) Paranoid episodes in manic-depressive psychosis. *American Journal of Psychiatry*, **135**, 974–976.

GREGORY, I. & SMELTZER, D. J. (1977) *Psychiatry*. Boston: Little, Brown.

HAMILTON, M. (1978) Paranoid states. *British Journal of Hospital Medicine*, **20**, 545–548.

HAY, G. G. (1970) Dysmorphophobia. *British Journal of Psychiatry*, **116**, 399–406.

HITCH, P. J. & RACK, P. H. (1980) Mental illness among Polish and Russian refugees in Bradford. *British Journal of Psychiatry*, **137**, 206–211.

HOENIG, J. (1981) Psychiatric nosology. *Canadian Journal of Psychiatry*, **26**, 85.

JOHANSON, E. (1964) Mild paranoia. *Acta Psychiatrica Scandinavica*, **40**, Supplement 177.

KAHLBAUM, K. (1863) *Die Gruppirung der psychischen Krankheiten*. Danzig: Kafemann.

KAPLAN, H. I., FREEDMAN, A. M. & SADOCK, B, J. (1980) *Comprehensive Textbook of Psychiatry, 3rd Edition*. Baltimore: Williams and Wilkins.

KENDLER, K. S. (1980a) Are there delusions specific for paranoid disorders vs schizophrenia? *Schizophrenia Bulletin*, **6**, 1–3.

—— (1980b) The nosologic validity of paranoia (simple delusional disorder). *Archives of General Psychiatry*, **37**, 699–706.

—— & HAYS, P. (1981) Paranoid psychosis (delusional disorder) and schizophrenia. *Archives of General Psychiatry*, **38**, 547–554.

KOLLE, K. (1931) *Die Primäre Verrücktheit: psychopathologische, klinische und genealogische Untersuchungen*. Leipzig: Thieme.

—— (1957) *Der Wahnkranke in Lichte alter und neuer Psychopathologie*. Stuttgart: Thieme.

KRAEPELIN, E. (1976) *Manic Depressive Insanity and Paranoia*. (Transl. R. M. Barclay, ed. G. M. Robertson). Edinburgh: Livingstone, 1921. New York: Arno Press.

LANGE, J. (1926) *Die Paranoiafrage*. Berlin: Springer.

LEADING ARTICLE (1980) Paranoia and immigrants. *British Medical Journal*, **281**, 1513–1514.

LEONHARD, K. (1976) Paranoia and related states. In *Encyclopaedic Handbook of Medical Psychology*, (ed. S. Krauss). London: Butterworth.

LEWIS, A. (1970) Paranoia and paranoid: a historical perspective. *Psychological Medicine*, **1**, 2–12.

LOVETT DOUST, J. W. & CHRISTIE, H. (1978) The pathology of love: Some clinical variants of De Clérambault's syndrome. *Social Science and Medicine*, **12**, 99–106.

McCABE, M. S. (1975) Reactive psychoses: A clinical and genetic investigation. *Acta Psychiatrica Scandinavica, Supplement 259*.

MEISSNER, W. W. (1978) *The Paranoid Process*. New York: Jason Aronson.

MUNRO, A. (1980) Monosymptomatic hypochondriacal psychosis. *British Journal of Hospital Medicine*, **24**, 34–38.

—— (1978) Monosymptomatic hypochrondriacal psychosis manifesting as delusions of parasitosis. *Archives of Dermatology*, **114**, 940–943.

—— & POLLOCK, B. G. (1981) Monosymptomatic psychoses which progress to schizophrenia. *Journal of Clinical Psychiatry*, **42**, 474–476.

PECHERNIKOVA, T. P. (1979) Paranoiac states in the development of psychopathy. *Zhornale Neuropatologi, Psikhiatri, IM S.S. Korsakova*, **79**, 1578–1582.

POLLOCK, B. G. (1982) Successful treatment of pathological jealousy with pimozide. *Canadian Journal of Psychiatry*, **27**, 86–87.

REILLY, T. M. (1977) Monosymptomatic hypochondriacal psychosis: presentation and treatment. *Proceedings of the Royal Society of Medicine*, **70**, Supplement 10, 39–42.

RIDING, J. & MUNRO, A. (1975) Pimozide in the treatment of monosymptomatic hypochondriacal psychosis. *Acta Psychiatrica Scandinavica*, **52**, 23–30.

SEEMAN, M. V. (1978) Delusional loving. *Archives of General Psychiatry*, **35**, 1265–1267.

—— (1979) Pathological jealousy. *Psychiatry*, **42**, 351–361.

SIM, M. (1981) *Guide to Psychiatry, 4th Edition*. London: Churchill Livingstone.

SKOTT, A. (1978) *Delusions of Infestation*. Reports from the Psychiatric Research Centre. St Jörgen's Hospital, University of Göteborg, Sweden.

SLATER, E. & ROTH, M. (1969) *Clinical Psychiatry, 3rd Edition*. London: Baillière, Tindall and Cassell.

SWANSON, D. W., BOHNERT, P. J. & SMITH, J. A. (1970) *The Paranoid*. Boston: Little, Brown.

TURGIYEV, S. B. (1978) The clinical picture of hallucinatory paranoid psychoses in cerebral atherosclerosis. *Zhornale Neuropatologi, Psikhiatri, IM S.S. Korsakova*, **78**, 421–426.

WATT, J. A. G., HALL, D. J., OLLEY, P. C. *et al* (1980) Paranoid states of middle life. Familial occurrence and relationship to schizophrenia. *Acta Psychiatrica Scandinavica*, **61**, 413–426.

WINOKUR, G. (1977) Delusional disorder (paranoia). *Comprehensive Psychiatry*, **18**, 511–521.

WORLD HEALTH ORGANIZATION (1978) *International Classification of Disease, 9th Edition (ICD 9)*. Section V, Classification of Mental Disorders. Geneva: WHO.

17 The syndrome of Capgras

JOHN TODD, KENNETH DEWHURST and GEOFFREY WALLIS

In 1923 Capgras and Reboul-Lachaux presented to the Société Clinique de Médecine Mentale the case of a woman suffering from a chronic paranoid psychosis who asserted that her husband, her children and a host of other people had been replaced by impersonating doubles. The descriptive term used by Capgras and Reboul-Lachaux, namely *l'illusion des sosies*, (the illusion of doubles) was subsequently adopted by other psychiatrists, until in 1929 Lévy-Valensi suggested the title 'the syndrome of Capgras' in acknowledgement of Capgras' outstanding contributions to our knowledge of this psychiatric entity. Although Capgras thoroughly deserved such recognition, Magnan (1893) and Janet (1903) had anticipated him in describing typical cases of the syndrome. Moreover, Bessière had in 1913 reported the case of a mentally disturbed woman who expressed the belief that another woman with an astonishing resemblance to her had taken advantage of this to perpetrate all kinds of misdeeds; and that a second woman who closely resembled the patient's mother had likewise impersonated the latter, with the same motive. Cases of this nature are important variants of the classic Capgras' syndrome.

Capgras' syndrome has to be distinguished from other disorders of recognition. Vié (1930) distinguished between this syndrome, which involves the perception of non-existent differences, and the disorder of recognition whereby people are mistakenly recognized as a result of the perception of non-existent resemblances. In rare cases, a mentally disturbed patient may affirm that a persecutor torments him or her by assuming the guise of persons the patient encounters in everyday life such as a postman, milkman, bus-conductor or doctor—a disorder of recognition that Courbon and Fail (1927) named the 'illusion of Frégoli' after the famous Italian actor and mimic, Leopoldo Frégoli (Critchley, 1979). Another disorder of recognition from which Capgras' syndrome needs to be distinguished is the very rare 'illusion of intermetamorphosis' (Courbon and Tusques, 1932) in which the patient believes that persons with whom he or she is acquainted have the power to change themselves into one another at will.

The syndrome of Capgras is rare (Nilsson and Perris, 1971; Christodoulou, 1977; Enoch and Trethowan, 1979). Women are afflicted by it more often than men (Vogel, 1974; Christodoulou, 1977). Patients exhibiting it tend to have a clear sensorium (Vogel, 1974; Enoch and Trethowan, 1979). The associated psychosis is most frequently paranoid schizophrenia, and less often a paraphrenic, schizoaffective, affective or organic psychosis (Merrin and

Silberfarb, 1976). It is exceptional for there to be only one impostor or double; more often, the supposed substitutes are multiple, the number often increasing with the passage of time (Cenac-Thaly *et al*, 1962). The Capgras delusion may be short-lived, recurrent, or of long duration.

Cargnello and Della Beffa (1955) discuss the use of the terms *alter* for the original and *alius* for the impersonating double of the original, and record the case of a schizophrenic woman, aged 32 years, who not only falsely affirmed that her mother was dead, but also that a woman, supposedly impersonating her dead mother, was a *reincarnation* of the latter. Capgras' syndrome has been reported in combination with the illusion of Frégoli (Cenac-Thaly *et al*, 1962; Bland, 1971) and also in association with a *folie à deux* psychosis (Bankier, 1966), with de Clérambault's syndrome (Sims and White, 1973), with a schizophreniform psychosis in an XYY male (Faber and Abrams, 1975), and with pseudohypoparathyroidism (Hay *et al*, 1974). The syndrome has been reviewed in detail by Cenac-Thaly *et al* (1962), Merrin and Silberfarb (1976), Arieti and Brody (1974) and Enoch and Trethowan (1979).

The essence of Capgras' syndrome is the delusion held by an individual that one or more persons have been replaced by impostors with a close resemblance to the originals. It is no longer tenable to limit the Capgras delusion to instances in which a prototype has been replaced by an *exact* double, as favoured by Enoch and Trethowan (1979), for the patient often uses the terms 'impostor' or 'impersonator' rather than double (Vogel, 1974) and often discerns minor physical differences distinguishing the prototype from the impostor (Derombies, 1935; Brochado, 1936; Todd, 1957; Merrin and Silberfarb, 1976). The differences perceived by the patient between the prototype and impostor are sometimes of a surprising nature. Davidson's patient (1941) claimed that the woman posing as his wife had differently formed sexual organs from the original. Even if the patient perceives no physical difference between original and substitute, he or she may complain of significant differences of personality distinguishing the two (Derombies, 1935).

The perceptual aspect of Capgras' syndrome merits attention, in that the patient who perceives the supposed imposter in the guise of an exact double of the original can be presumed to have a delusional perception, whereas the patient who perceives non-existent physical differences between the original and the impostor can be presumed to have an illusory perception. Since the patient's belief that the original has been replaced by a substitute is maintained even when the prototype (the object-stimulus) is no longer present, the belief is in the nature of a *delusion* and not merely a delusional perception or illusion. An interesting variant of Capgras' syndrome is the case of the patient who, in addition to expressing the typical Capgras delusion respecting other people, insists that she herself has been impersonated by a double (Capgras and Reboul-Lachaux, 1923; Depouy and Montassut, 1924; Bouvier, 1926; Larrivé and Jasienski, 1931). In such a case, the impersonator of the patient is, of course, never actually perceived.

The state of mind which is probably a prerequisite for the advent of the Capgras delusion is one of intense suspiciousness, the importance of which was initially stressed by Capgras and Reboul-Lachaux (1923) who referred to their patient's 'paranoiac disposition'. This factor has been subsequently stressed by Bankier (1966), Enoch and Trethowan (1979) and others. For instance, Merrin and Silberfarb (1976) have referred to 'a setting of increased vigilance and suspicion' as being a hindrance to the patient's ability to recognize a familiar person, and Christodoulou (1977) has referred, in his study of 11 cases displaying Capgras' syndrome, to the fact that '... the clinical picture of almost all patients was dominated by a marked paranoid component'. Such a mood doubtless paves the way for the emergence of the Capgras delusion and of certain paranoid delusions often associated with it, namely that attempts have been made, or will be made, to poison the patient (Lévy-Valensi, 1929; MacCallum, 1973; Vogel, 1974; and others) and that the missing originals have been kidnapped, imprisoned or murdered (Capgras and Reboul-Lachaux, 1923; Bouvier, 1926; Ball and Kidson, 1968; Vogel, 1974; and others).

Another state of mind that has been closely linked with the Capgras delusion is depersonalization-derealization (Capgras and Reboul-Lachaux, 1923; Frey *et al*, 1956; Todd, 1957; Nilsson and Perris, 1971; Christodoulou, 1977). A feeling of unreality can be expected to facilitate the advent of the Capgras delusion, as the following statements by depersonalized-derealized patients will show: 'Friends and relatives are like strangers, just names to me' and 'Everything looks strange, like painted, not natural...' (Mayer-Gross, 1935). This latter quotation is of particular interest because patients affected by the Capgras delusion sometimes assert that the impostors are wearing wigs (Todd, 1957), are wearing masks, resemble wax models (MacCullum, 1973), or have been changed by plastic surgery (Bland, 1971). It seems likely that in all these cases the patient's impression of artificiality stems from a state of derealization. The symptom known as *jamais vu* is probably a variant of derealization, and in some cases its presence in mild form may facilitate the development of the Capgras delusion. Derealization would appear to be the basis of the suggestion made by Capgras and Reboul-Lachaux (1923) that the idea of an impersonating double arises in the patient's mind as the result of incomplete recognition of objects engendered by simultaneous feelings of familiarity and of strangeness. Merrin and Silberfarb (1976) in their paper on 'The Capgras Phenomenon' saw a connection between depersonalization-derealization and Capgras' syndrome, for they wrote: '... a number of cases began with diffuse feelings of unreality or depersonalization, followed by indiscriminate misidentification and finally by the establishment of the Capgras delusion.' Furthermore, it may be significant that both Capgras' syndrome and depersonalization-derealization occur more often in women: 46 out of 66 depersonalized patients in the group collected by Shorvon (1946) were female. However, depersonalization-derealization cannot *by itself* explain the development of Capgras' syndrome because patients afflicted by feelings of depersonalization or derealization have insight and appreciate the illusory nature of the phenomenon (Shorvon, 1946), whereas patients with the Capgras delusion are without such insight.

There are grounds for believing that certain other psychological factors may have a part to play in the aetiology of Capgras' syndrome. Derombies (1935) attached great importance to the affective state of the patient and expressed the opinion that Capgras' syndrome resulted from a simultaneous intellectual recognition and affectively engendered non-recognition. In some cases patients may gain relief from the disturbing effect on their minds of ambivalent emotions through the medium of the Capgras delusion (Karkalas and Nicotra, 1969).

Usually, such ambivalent emotions are dealt with by saddling the impostor with the faults (often magnified) of the original, and deifying the original by an exaggeration of his good qualities. In this way, a Hyde impostor and a Jekyll original are created (Davidson, 1941; Stern and MacNaughton, 1945). Much less frequently, the impostor or double is cast as a person superior to the original (Larrivé and Jasienski, 1931; Todd, 1957). The case of Larrivé and Jasienski is of particular interest, in that their patient appeared to make use of her Capgras delusions to satisfy the needs of wish-fulfilment and also to give expression to her ideas of grandeur. She claimed that her poorly endowed, sexually inadequate, splay-handed lover had a rich and virile rival with a close resemblance to her lover in appearance except that he had the small hands and feet of the aristocrat. Moreover, she herself had a double whom she suspected was a grand lady of some kind such as an Italian princess. In the case of those patients who exhibit Capgras' syndrome, but who also complain that they themselves are being impersonated by impostors or doubles, the general rule is usually followed in that their impersonators tend to be morally inferior to themselves (Bouvier, 1926; Depouy and Montassut, 1924). Derombies (1935) drew attention to the psychological advantage of such a mechanism: 'When the patients, as we shall see can be the case, create a double of themselves, the latter give expression to their repressed desires.' Depouy and Montassut (1924) published the details of a case which appeared to illustrate the defensive use of the Capgras delusion as well as being a means of vicariously airing repressed desires. They argued that their hallucinating patient's claim that it was the doubles of her neighbours and friends, not the originals, who were denigrating and insulting her gave the Capgras delusion a protective role. Her delusional conviction of having been impersonated by a double leading a voluptuous life also had an exonerating and protective role as she could console herself with the thought that it was not she, but her double, who was being criticized.

Although the Capgras delusion can be used as a mental mechanism to afford the subject a respite from distressing ambivalent feelings, to argue that ambivalency is the basis of the psychopathology of the condition (Enoch and Trethowan, 1979) is perhaps to over-emphasize its role. It is not difficult to accept that a person can have ambivalent feelings about someone to whom he or she is linked by close emotional bonds, such as a husband or daughter, but it is not easy to accept that ambivalent feelings of any strength can exist in respect of mere acquaintances or inanimate objects, of little significance to the patient. Examples of persons towards whom Capgras delusion patients were unlikely to have had strong emotional links, but whom the patient claimed to have been replaced by doubles, include the commissioner and the prefect of police (Capgras and Reboul-Lachaux, 1923), a maid-servant (Halberstadt, 1923) and a group of neighbours (Minns, 1970). MacCallum (1973) cited the case of a woman who, prior to claiming that he was impersonating the real Dr MacCallum, had insisted that the hospital and the staff were exact replicas of what she had known them to be. The patient of Delay *et al* (1952) was convinced that she had been transferred from one room to another while she was asleep, the second room being a reproduction of the first. Bouvier (1926), Brochado (1936) and Christodoulou (1977) likewise reported patients who displayed Capgras' syndrome respecting persons and also expressed the delusion that inanimate objects had been replaced by replicas. Brochado (1936) and Frey *et al* (1956) were sufficiently impressed with the involvement of inanimate objects in Capgras' syndrome to refer respectively to 'an illusion of doubles of things' and 'doubles of objects'. It is therefore evident that some of these Capgras patients become obsessed with ideas of doubles and replicas and that inanimate objects and persons, not intimately connected with the patient, may figure in the Capgras delusion.

The minor differences between prototype and impersonator so often perceived by Capgras' syndrome patients are doubtless produced by the process known as secondary rationalization.

An interesting complication stemming from the Capgras delusion that a husband or paramour has been replaced by a double is that the wife or mistress may come to the conclusion that she has committed innocent adultery, as Alcmene did with Jupiter, impersonator of Amphitryon (Alcmene's husband), in the Greek myth. The term 'Alcmene Complex' (Disertori and Piazza, 1967) is perhaps best used broadly to cover all the sexual difficulties which can face a woman troubled by the Capgras delusion respecting her sexual partner (Vogel, 1974; Christodoulou, 1977). Derombies (1935) and Cenac-Thaly *et al* (1962) cited instances in which patients affirmed that they had had a child sired by a man posing as their husband. Not surprisingly, a woman may avoid the embraces of the impostor (Vogel, 1974; Christodoulou, 1977). Difficulties may also arise in respect of the male partner. Lansky (1974) described a case in which a husband developed feelings of guilt in regard to his wife, because he had 'committed adultery with the doubles, and would be found out'.

The notion that a reversion to primitive modes of thought (*une mentalité prélogique*) may have a part to play in Capgras' syndrome was first advanced by Halberstadt (1923). Stern and MacNaughton (1945), in giving some support to Halberstadt's ideas, quote the anthropologist Lévy-Brühl (1922) as follows: '... in the conception of the primitive mentality, objects, persons, phenomena can be themselves, and at the same time something else.' There is an abundance of evidence that man has been preoccupied with the idea of doubles since time immemorial. According to Crawley (1908–1926) the Nágas, Andamanese, East Indian islanders, Karo Bataks and many other primitive tribes believe that their souls or ghosts take the form of a material replica of the person as he was in life. The religious philosophy of the archaic but advanced culture of the ancient Egyptians was much concerned with the notion of a soul-double. Mackenzie (1913) furnished a wealth of information about the *ka* or spirit (invisible double) envisaged by the Egyptians. He refers to the *ka* as follows: 'During life the human *ka* existed in the human body. It was sustained by the doubles of everything its owner ate or drank, and it continued to require sustenance after the death of its host.' In regard to the idea of impersonation, Crawley states: 'In the Dutch East Indies it is commonly believed that male and female spirits, *nita*, can assume the form and personality of lovers and friends. A man or woman keeping an assignation in the forest is liable to be duped in this way. A person who has intercourse with a *nita* dies in a few days.' Crawley further points out that the Bahar Islanders believe that a male *suwanggi* is able to take the shape of a young woman's husband and cause her to conceive. Tymms (1949) examined the mythological origins of the double theme. He refers to myths and legends whose central motif is impersonation by doubles, such as the Amphitryon-Jupiter-Alcmene myth (Greek), the Nala and Damayanti myth (Indian) and the monkish anthology of the Emperor Jovinian (British). European folklore is richly endowed with accounts of the hallucinatory double, *Doppelgänger* or wraith, it being a tenet of such folklore that to see one's own wraith is an omen of impending death (Todd and Dewhurst, 1962). In modern times, the idea of doubles and impersonators is doubtless kept alive by the natural occurrence of identical twins, by romantic fiction such as Stevenson's *Dr Jekyll and Mr Hyde* and Dostoevsky's *The Double* and by the doubling of actors by, for instance, acrobats or virtuoso pianists.

The possible role of organic disease of the brain in producing a state of mind favourable to the development of the Capgras delusion has been much discussed during the last decade (MacCallum, 1973; Merrin and Silberfarb, 1976; Enoch and Trethowan, 1979; and others). Weston and Whitlock (1971) and Hayman and Abrams (1977) have considered the relationship of prosopagnosia to Capgras' syndrome. However, prosopagnosia must be shown to be present by satisfactory tests before a cause and effect relationship between the two conditions can be seriously considered. Weston and Whitlock conceded that in the case of their Capgras syndrome patient, they were unable to elicit satisfactory evidence of prosopagnosia. In the two cases cited by Hayman and Abrams no specific tests to demonstrate the presence of prosopagnosia were performed. Moreover, neither case showed the presence of a visual field defect, which was present in 38 out of 42 cases of prosopagnosia studied by Meadows (1974). Prosopagnosia is not a severe impediment to recognition of members of the family, because the patient recognizes them on hearing their voices.

In regard to the role of organic factors in Capgras' syndrome, there would appear to be no reason to disagree with the observation of Christodoulou (1977) that: 'In certain cases it is doubtful whether the syndrome would have become manifest if this organic component had not existed.' It is noteworthy that organic cerebral disease was present in two of the three cases recorded in this paper. The 'dissolution of the nervous system produced by organic cerebral disease' (Jackson, 1884) may well bring about a reduction of cognitive efficiency, an impairment of judgement and a phylogenetic regression to less sophisticated modes of thought, features which could be expected to favour the development of the Capgras delusion. Nevertheless, such a dissolution of the nervous system must evidently not be severe to be compatible with Capgras' syndrome because a clear sensorium is the rule in patients displaying it. Furthermore, Derombies (1935) has pointed out that a fair degree of intellectual integrity would appear to be necessary for the syndrome's appearance. However, the role of organic disease in the production of the Capgras delusion should not be over-estimated as in the majority of the published cases the patients have not shown evidence of organic cerebral disease and have presented as functional psychoses (Enoch and Trethowan, 1979).

Merrin and Silberfarb (1976) drew attention to the possibility that patients displaying Capgras' syndrome may in some cases have failed to make allowance for changes which occur in the appearance of relatives and acquaintances as the result of the passage of time and the ageing process. Leonhard (cited by Hamilton, 1974) took a similar view, suggesting that a factor in the psychopathology of the Capgras syndrome is 'excessive concretization of memory images' and the patient's consequent tendency to fasten on to minor discrepancies between the memory image and the current perception. This phenomenon does seem to have had a part to play, as an initiating factor, in cases in which the patient and her relative or relatives have met after a period of separation (Bouvier, 1926; Stern and MacNaughton, 1945; Christodoulou, 1977). Moreover, patients with Capgras' syndrome sometimes produce 'then' and 'now' photographs, in an attempt to justify their contention that an impostor has taken the place of the originals (Bland, 1971; Lansky, 1974; Merrin and Silberfarb, 1976). Haslam (1973) recorded a case in which 'concrete thinking' had appeared to play a significant part in the causation of the patient's Capgras delusion. She had failed to appreciate the true nature of the changes exhibited by her fiancé (which were due to his having developed schizophrenia), and this doubtless initiated her delusional idea that he had been replaced by an impostor.

The factor precipitating the Capgras delusion may be subtle, a point well illustrated by a patient of Minns (1970), whose delusion that her mother was an impostor was inaugurated by an incident in which the mother had hesitated a little before answering 'Yes' when asked by a caller if she were 'Mrs W'.

Treatment: It is generally agreed that in cases of Capgras' syndrome it is the related psychosis which needs to be treated. However, interestingly, the Capgras delusions of the patient of Delay *et al* (1952) were selectively removed by a lobotomy, her other psychiatric symptoms showing only modest improvement.

Conclusion: All the factors discussed in this paper may well play an important part in the aetiology of Capgras' syndrome. However, the essential precursor of Capgras' syndrome, in our view, is a mind impregnated with morbid suspiciousness. A *paranoid interpretation* by the patient of the strange appearance of a relative—which in fact is due to a derealized state, or to a period of separation—may well subsequently result in the advent of the Capgras delusion.

References

Arieti, S. & Brody, E. B. (1974) *American Handbook of Psychiatry*, 2nd Edit. Vol. 3, 712–714. New York: Basic Books.

Ball, J. R. R. & Kidson, M. A. (1968) The Capgras syndrome? A rarity. *Australian and New Zealand Journal of Psychiatry*, **2**, 44–45.

Bankier, R. G. (1966) Capgras syndrome: The illusion of doubles. *Canadian Psychiatric Association Journal*, **2**, 426–429.

Bessière, A. C. R. (1913) *Paranoia et Psychose Periodique*. Paris: Thèse de Paris.

Bland R. C. (1971) Capgras syndrome: a case report. *Canadian Psychiatric Association Journal*, **16**, 369–371.

Bouvier, M. (1926) *Le Syndrome 'Illusion des Sosies'*. Paris: Thèse de Paris.

Brochado, A. (1936) Le syndrome de Capgras. *Annales Médico-psychologiques*, **94**, 706–717.

Capgras, J. & Reboul-Lachaux, J. (1923) Illusion des sosies dans un déliré systématisé chronique. *Bulletin de la Société Clinique de Médecine Mentale*, **2**, 6–16.

—— & Carrette, P. (1924) Illusion des sosies et complex d'Oedipe. *Annales Médico-psychologiques*, **82**, 48.

Cargnello, D. & Della Beffa, A. (1955) L'illusione del Sosia. *Archivio Di Psicologia Neurologia E Psichiatria*, **2**, 173–201.

Cenac-Thaly, H., Frelot, C., Guinard, M., Tricot, J. C. & Lacour, M. A. (1962) L'illusion des sosies. *Annales Médico-psychologiques*, **120**, 481–494.

CHRISTODOULOU, G. N. (1977) The syndrome of Capgras. *British Journal of Psychiatry*, **130**, 556–564.

COURBON, P. & FAIL, G. (1972) Illusion de frégoli. *Bulletin de la Société Clinique de Médecine Mentale*, **15**, 121–124.

—— & TUSQUES, J. (1932) Illusions d'intermétamorphose et de charme. *Annales Médico-psychologiques*, **90**, 401–405.

CRAWLEY, A. E. (1908–1926) Doubles. In *Hastings' Encyclopaedia of Religion and Ethics*, Vol. 4, 835–860. Edinburgh: T. and T. Clark.

CRITCHLEY, M. (1979) In *The Divine Banquet of the Brain*. New York: Raven Press.

DAVIDSON, G. M. (1941) The syndrome of Capgras. *Psychiatric Quarterly*, **15**, 513–521.

DELAY, J., PERRIER, F. & SCHMITZ, B. (1952) Action de diverses thérapeutiques de choc sur un syndrome d'illusion de sosies. *Annales Médico-psychologiques*, **110**, 235–238.

DEPOUY, R. & MONTASSUT, M. (1924) Un cas de syndrome des sosies chez une délirante par interprétations des troubles psycho-sensoriels. *Annales Médico-psychologiques*, **82**, 341–345.

DEROMBIES, M. (1935) *L'Illusion de Sosies, Forme Particulière de la Méconnaisance Systhématique*. Paris: Thèse de Paris.

DISERTORI, B. & PIAZZA, M. (1967) La sindrome de Capgras o illusione dei sosia: il complisso d'Alcmena. *Giornale di Psichiatria e di Neuropatologia*, **95**, 175–183.

ENOCH, M. D. & TRETHOWAN, W. H. (1979) The Capgras syndrome. In *Uncommon Psychiatric Syndromes*. Bristol: John Wright.

FABER, R. & ABRAMS, R. (1975) Schizophrenia in a 47, XYY male. *British Journal of Psychiatry*, **127**, 401–403.

FREY, M., MAUREL, H. & SPIELMANN, J. P. (1956) Sur une observation d'illusion de sosie. *Annales Médico-psychologiques*, **114**, 891–896.

HALBERSTADT, G. (1923) Syndrome d'illusion des sosies. *Journal de Psychologie Normale et Pathologique*, **20**, 728–733.

HASLAM, M. T. (1973) A case of Capgras syndrome. *American Journal of Psychiatry*, **130**, 493–494.

HAY, G. C., JOLLEY, D. J. & JONES, R. G. (1974) A case of the Capgras syndrome in association with pseudohypoparathyroidism. *Acta Psychiatrica Scandinavica*, **50**, 73–77.

HAYMAN, M. A. & ABRAMS, R. (1977) Capgras syndrome and cerebral dysfunction. *British Journal of Psychiatry*, **130**, 68–71.

JACKSON, J. H. (1884) Croonian Lectures on Evolution and Dissolution of the Nervous System. In *Selected Writings of John Hughlings Jackson*. (ed. J. Taylor, 1958). London: Staples Press.

JANET, P. (1903) In *Les Obsessions et la Psychasthénie*. Paris: Alcan.

KARKALAS, Y. & NICOTRA, M. (1969) The Capgras syndrome: a rare psychiatric condition. *Rhode Island Medical Journal*, **52**, 452–454.

LANSKY, M. R. (1974) Delusions in a patient with Capgras' syndrome. *Bulletin of the Menninger Clinic*, **38**, 360–364.

LARRIVÉ, E. & JASIENSKI, H. J. (1931) L'Illusion des sosies. *Annales Médico-psychologiques*, **89**, 501–507.

LEONHARD, K. (1974) In *Fish's Clinical Psychopathology* (ed. M. Hamilton). Bristol: John Wright.

LÉVY-BRUHL (1922) In *La Mentalité Primitive*. Paris: Alcan.

LÉVY-VALENSI, J. (1929) L'illusion des sosies. *Gazette des Hôpitaux*, **55**, 10th July, 1001–1003.

MACCALLUM, W. A. G. (1973) Capgras symptoms with an organic basis. *British Journal of Psychiatry*, **123**, 639–642.

MACKENZIE, D. A. (1913) In *Egyptian Myth and Legend*. London: Gresham.

MAGNAN, V. (1893) In *Leçons Cliniques sur les Maladies Mentales*. Paris: Bataille.

MAYER-GROSS, W. (1935) On depersonalization. *British Journal of Medical Psychology*, **15**, 103–122.

MEADOWS, J. C. (1974) The anatomical basis of prosopagnosia. *Journal of Neurology, Neurosurgery and Psychiatry*, **37**, 489–501.

MERRIN, E. L. & SILBERFARB, P. M. (1976) The Capgras phenomenon. *Archives of General Psychiatry*, **33**, 965–968.

MINNS, R. A. J. (1970) A case of Capgras' syndrome. *The Medical Journal of Australia*, **2**, 239.

NILSSON, R. & PERRIS, C. (1971) The Capgras syndrome: a case report. *Acta Psychiatrica, Scandinavica Supplementum*, **222**, 53–58.

SHORVON, H. J. (1946) The depersonalization syndrome. *Proceedings of the Royal Society of Medicine*, **39**, 779–792.

SIMS, A. & WHITE, A. (1973) Co-existence of the Capgras and de Clérambault syndromes: A case history. *British Journal of Psychiatry*, **123**, 635–637.

STERN, K. & MACNAUGHTON, D. (1945) Capgras syndrome. A peculiar illusionary phenomenon, considered with special reference to the Rorschach findings. *Psychiatric Quarterly*, **19**, 139–163.

TODD, J. (1957) The syndrome of Capgras. *Psychiatric Quarterly*, **31**, 250–265.

—— & Dewhurst, K. (1962) The significance of the Doppelgänger (hallucinatory double) in folk-lore and neuro-psychiatry. *The Practitioner*, **188,** 377–382.

Tymms, R. (1949) In *Doubles in Literary Psychology*. Cambridge: Bowes and Bowes.

Vié, J. (1930) Un trouble de l'identification des personnes: l'illusion des sosies. *Annales Médico-Psychologiques*, **88,** 214–237.

Vogel, B. F. (1974) The Capgras syndrome and its psychopathology. *American Journal of Psychiatry*, **131,** 922–924.

Weston, M. J. & Whitlock, F. A. (1971) The Capgras syndrome following head injury. *British Journal of Psychiatry*, **119,** 25–31.

18 Feigned psychosis—A review of the simulation of mental illness

G. G. HAY

The recent trial of Peter Sutcliffe (*Lancet*, 1981) focused attention on the possibility of the purposive feigning of mental illness. Opportunity was taken to review those patients admitted to a large department of psychiatry over a 12-year period who were thought to be simulating. The patients concerned appeared at the time to be deliberately pretending to a schizophrenic psychosis. Other patients with so-called hysterical psychosis or Ganser states were excluded from the study. The literature on simulation was well reviewed by Anderson *et al* (1959). They mentioned in particular, Jung's classic essay (1903) in which several points were made which have since been repeated by other workers. Jung stressed the rarity of simulation in civilian practice, that it occurred in patients with pre-existing personality disorders and that confessions of simulation should be received with caution.

More recently there have been relatively few papers dealing with this topic. Waschspress *et al* (1953) described three cases in an army general hospital and one of these patients became overtly schizophrenic. Schneck (1970) draws attention to a novel by Andreyev (*The Dilemma*, 1902), in which a doctor who deliberately set out to feign madness ended up with the realization that he was indeed ill. He thought that he simulated, but was really insane. Schneck refers to this mechanism as pseudo-malingering and looks on it as the prodroma of a genuine psychosis—a temporary ego supporting device.

Ritson and Forrest (1970) described 12 patients who 'played schizophrenia'. Three had had a previous schizophrenic episode but, having learnt their lines, decided to prolong their hospital stay purposely. The remainder, suffering from personality problems or disorder, often in the setting of intolerable social stress, 'played psychotic' for various reasons. Ritson and Forrest emphasized the absence of a praecox feeling in the latter patients, the hysterical display of the symptoms and the fact that their peer group saw through them. Berney (1973), in a review of simulated illness, again makes the point that malingering may be a 'last ditch attempt' to ward off the further disintegration of a genuine psychosis. Cheng and Hummel (1978) presented two cases of a 'mental Münchausen syndrome', one of whom repeatedly simulated an acute psychotic state. Finally, Pope *et al* (1982) identified a cohort of 9 patients with factitious psychosis from among 219 patients consecutively admitted for psychotic disorder. They conducted a four- to seven-year follow-up and stated that none of their patients went on to develop a typical psychotic disorder. However, there was a high psychiatric morbidity and poor social outcome due to the severity of the underlying personality disorder, and in that regard Pope *et al* felt that 'acting crazy may bode more ill than being "crazy"'.

The Department of Psychiatry at the University Hospital of South Manchester admits from a catchment area of approximately 200,000, and opened a full service to that area in 1972. The in-patient case register for the years 1972–1982 was searched for patients for whom the discharge diagnosis was simulation, and those patients who had been thought to be feigning psychosis were included in the study. The consultants working in the Department were also personally contacted for the names of such patients. This last is usually a highly unreliable procedure, but as such patients tend to be well remembered, it was thought worthwhile.

Follow-up was either by personal contact if the patient still lived in the area or by postal enquiry if they moved away. One out-patient was also included for the purposes of the discussion.

In total, six patients were found who satisfied the above criteria: five in-patients and the one out-patient. Four of the in-patients were followed up personally and the fifth by postal enquiry. The out-patient was also personally contacted. The length of the follow-up period varied from three months to ten years.

The diagnosis in all but one of the patients had been changed to that of a genuine schizophrenic illness, with which the author was in complete agreement. The one patient (P.W.) for whom the diagnosis remained uncertain, is mentioned in more detail in the case summaries.

Illustrative case summaries

Case 1: M.A., female, was aged 24 when she first presented in 1973 following an overdose. She gave a history of recurrent overdoses and wrist slashing attempts since 1969, and on admission stated she was controlled by her dead sister who kept telling her to take her own life. Her family history was negative.

She was found to be carrying a list of Schneider's first rank symptoms (Schneider, 1959) in her handbag; she behaved bizarrely, picking imaginary objects out of the waste paper basket and opening imaginary doors in the waiting room. She admitted to visual hallucinations and offered four of the first rank symptoms on her list, but her mental state reverted to normal after two days. When she was presented at a case conference, the consensus view was that she had been simulating schizophrenia but suffered from a gross personality disorder; however, the consultant in charge dissented from that general view, feeling she was genuinely psychotic.

On follow-up this turned out to be the case. She was re-admitted in 1975, mute, catatonic, grossly thought disordered, and the diagnosis was changed to that of a schizophrenic illness. She has been followed up regularly since and now presents the picture of a mild schizophrenic defect state; she takes regular depot medication but still complains of auditory hallucinations, hearing her dead sister's voice. She is a day patient.

Case 2: G.W., a married woman of 24 with one child, was referred to the out-patient department in 1982, complaining of life-long feelings of inferiority and sensitivity to criticism. Mental state examination at that time was normal, family history negative. It was thought the diagnosis was that of a mild sensitive personality disorder, but with some attention-seeking traits. Arrangements were made to give her a short course of out-patient psychotherapy; she made a positive transference with the therapist concerned and became upset when he moved to another hospital. He started to receive bizarre letters from her containing indecipherable astrological diagrams and declaring her love for him. She was therefore reviewed in the out-patients by another psychiatrist who could still find no evidence of formal mental illness. It was noticed that some of her 'crazy' letters were enclosed with completely normal covering letters and her husband stated that her behaviour at home was unremarkable. She admitted that she was trying to be of interest to the first psychiatrist and desperately wanted to contact him. The formulation at this time was that of deliberate attention-seeking behaviour with feigned madness; she was also seen by a consultant from another department who thought the diagnosis was that of gross hysterical behaviour.

However, her letters became more bizarre and she sent some to the editors of various women's magazines and also to Buckingham Palace. Some three months after she was first seen she suddenly left home, arrived in another city grossly thought disordered and clearly genuinely psychotic. At the time of writing she is an in-patient with a firm diagnosis of paranoid schizophrenia.

Case 3: P.W., who was a single girl of 23 and a student, was brought to the Casualty Department by the police in 1977 having been found sitting on her doorstep, wrapped in a blanket. She expressed ideas of a plot against her directed at making her fail her examinations. She stated she could not understand the meaning of words and could hear voices; over the following days, she admitted she had been fabricating madness: 'You mustn't think I planned it in cold blood; I half convinced myself I am so confused, I don't know truth from lies any more.' She gave a long history of pathological lying from the age of 10. For example, she had told her school friends that she was going blind and later invented for her fellow students a county background, all of which was quite untrue. Shortly before admission, she had bandaged her head and told a reporter that she had been beaten up on her way back to her digs.

The police had questioned her and she fabricated the details of this story. There was a family history of her mother having had a nervous breakdown when she was pregnant with the patient, but no details were available of the diagnosis of that illness, if indeed it had occurred.

The discharge diagnosis was of personality disorder (pseudologica phantastica) with the simulation of psychosis. She then moved to another part of the country and had further psychiatric contact. Follow-up was carried out by writing to the psychiatrists recently concerned with her care. It was reported in 1982 that the diagnosis was unresolved. Some of the psychiatrists who had seen her since 1977 had said she was definitely schizophrenic, others still thought she was 'shamming mental illness'. However, she was receiving very large doses of major tranquillisers—clopixol 200 mg i.m. weekly; haloperidol 20 mg tds and chlorpromazine 50 mg tds.

Comment

With the exception of Ritson and Forrest's and Pope's papers, the literature on simulation emphasizes its rarity. Ritson and Forrest included patients who had had a definite schizophrenic episode in the past, and not all their patients were followed up. Pope *et al* felt that factitious psychosis was not too uncommon. However, this difference of view may be more apparent than real and may be due to diagnostic differences between the USA and the UK. Case summaries were not included in their paper, but four of their patients were noted to be drug or alcohol abusers, and it may well be that in this country for these patients the diagnosis of simulated psychosis would not have been made.

Simulated psychosis is frequently suspected by nursing and junior medical staff, but experienced clinicians are much more reluctant to consider it. In the present study, the incidence was only of five patients out of all new admissions in the period under review, a number approximating 12,000, and as has been shown on follow-up, four became schizophrenic in time.

The incidence in forensic practice is higher. Mather, in his large series of 320 murderers, had three who feigned psychosis and remained sane after a 10-year follow-up, an incidence of 0.01 per cent. Similarly, it is not uncommon in forensic work to see patients who, having been definitely psychotic, on recovery claim that they had only been 'acting insane'.

The results of this study emphasize the point that even those patients who were thought to be simulating on their initial admission, became overtly schizophrenic with the passage of time. In this regard the possibility of pseudo-malingering as mentioned in the literature, seems as useful a concept as that of pseudoneurotic schizophrenia. The one out-patient (G.W.)—Case 2, mentioned above—illustrated a not unusual onset of psychosis, with early pathoplastic colouring dominating the picture until unequivocal psychotic symptoms developed.

Similarly, Case 3 (P.W.) had an extremely deviant premorbid personality characterized by years of pathological and gross attention-seeking behaviour. At the beginning of the illness it was these traits, highlighted and released by a possible early process, which dominated the clinical picture. Although, to date, a firm diagnosis of schizophrenia has not been made, the patient is receiving huge doses of major tranquillisers.

Usually the simulation of schizophrenia is simply the prodromal phase of genuine illness, albeit occurring on the basis of a markedly abnormal personality. It is argued here that, in ordinary clinical practice the diagnosis of simulation should be made with great caution unless an individual patient has a very clear-cut and obvious motivation. The majority of such patients will be suffering from the early stages of a genuine psychosis and should be managed accordingly.

References

ANDERSON, E. W., TRETHOWAN, W. H. & KENNA, J. C. (1959) An experimental investigation of simulation and pseudo-dementia. *Acta Psychiatrica et Neurologica Scandinavica Supplementum*, **132**, 34.

BERNEY, T. P. (1973) A review of simulated illness. *South African Medical Journal*, **47**, 1429–1434.

CHENG, L. & HUMMEL, L. (1978) The Münchausen syndrome as a psychiatric condition. *British Journal of Psychiatry*, **133**, 20–21.

JUNG, C. G. (1903) On simulated insanity. In *Collected Works of C. G. Jung, Vol I*. 1957. London: Routledge and Kegan Paul.

LANCET (1981) Sutcliffe and after. *Lancet, i*, 1241.

MATHER, N. J. DE V. (1982) Personal communication.

POPE, H. G., JONAS, J. M. & JONES, B. (1982) Factitious psychosis: Phenomenology, family history and long term outcome of nine patients. *American Journal of Psychiatry*, **139**, 1480–1483.

RITSON, B. & FORREST, A. (1970) The simulation of psychosis: a contemporary presentation. *British Journal of Medical Psychology*, **43**, 31–37.

SCHNECK, J. N. (1970) Pseudo malingering and Leonid Andreyev's *The Dilemma*. *Psychiatric Quarterly*, **44**, 49–54.

SCHNEIDER, K. (1959) *Clinical Psychopathology* (trans. M. W. Hamilton). New York: Grune and Stratton.

WASCHSPRESS, M., BERENBERG, A. N. & JACOBSON, A. (1953) Simulation of psychosis: A report of three cases. *Psychiatric Quarterly*, **27**, 463–473.

PROPERTY OF
RIVERWOOD COMMUNITY MENTAL HEALTH

III. Organic aspects

19 Organic aspects of schizophrenia: Overview

DONALD ECCLESTON

Over the past decade the concept of schizophrenia as an 'organic' illness in the broadest sense has hardened. This period has seen the expansion of techniques for the investigation of brain structure and function. Computerized axial tomography (CAT) and nuclear magnetic resonance (NMR) scans as well as the enormous potential in the recently developed positron emission tomography (PET) scan are beginning to pose as well as clarify hypotheses. We are now at a stage of intense speculation as to the cause of schizophrenia or 'the schizophrenias', as they may well turn out to be. This summary proposes to look at some of the recent findings and hypotheses and to try to relate some of the issues which seem, superficially at least, to be disparate, as well as to indulge in some speculative thinking.

There are a number of neuronal systems in the brain which profoundly influence broad areas of cerebral functioning. Their neurotransmitters are the biogenic amines and of these the dopamine system is anatomically well recognized and many areas of its function known. The dopamine theory of schizophrenia postulates dopaminergic overactivity in this disease since its treatment is by neuroleptic drugs whose pharmacological profile prominently features dopamine receptor blockade (**Van Praag**, **1977**). In addition, schizophrenia-like syndromes can be produced in normal subjects by large quantities of amphetamine, a drug which releases dopamine and produces an apparent overactivity in that system. The place of dopamine in the symptomatology of schizophrenia has been incorporated in the work of a number of groups.

In a signal paper on the subject the Northwick Park Group (Johnstone et al, 1978) examined the cognitive function, ventricular size (by CAT scan) and symptomatology in a group of chronic schizophrenic subjects. Enlarged ventricles appear to be associated with both intellectual impairment and negative symptoms of the illness as exemplified by emotional blunting, poverty of thoughts and loss of drive. This led to the postulation of two syndromes in schizophrenia: the first characterized by positive symptoms (Schneiderian, e.g. delusions, hallucinations and thought disorder) mediated by dopaminergic factors termed Type I schizophrenia, and the second by negative symptoms (The Kraepelinian Syndrome) as Type II schizophrenia mediated by an organic, possibly encephalitic, process (Crow, 1980). Variants of the dopaminergic theory were proposed by **Mackay** (**1980**) and **Ashcroft et al** (**1981**). The former suggested that schizophrenia was essentially characterized by dopaminergic underactivity (which is exemplified in the negative aspects of this illness) occasionally flaring into overactivity under the influence of stress which produces transient dopaminergic overactivity and the positive phenomena. **Ashcroft** *et al* (**1981**) suggested a range of function of the dopaminergic system which, when exceeded, gave positive symptoms and when activity fell below the normal range gave the negative symptoms. Interestingly, in addition, they also suggested that, in schizophrenia, there was a more restricted range of dopaminergic activity before symptoms develop compared with normals, such that symptoms could more easily develop in schizophrenia for given dopaminergic activity.

The formal division of schizophrenia into two syndromes is difficult to sustain from the literature. Kraepelin clearly believed in the organic nature of the illness (**Hoenig, 1983**), anticipating a specific anatomical pathology. The clinical course he saw as variable but probably without '*restitutio ad integrum*'; in other words the inevitable presence of the defect state. The first rank symptoms described by Schneider were regarded as secondary by Bleuler; they are not disease specific and moreover are variable in their occurrence depending on the energy with which they are sought (Mellor, 1970). They are also variable in their presence taking a longitudinal view of the illness and may be precipitated by stress. These Schneiderian phenomena although having diagnostic value may be the manifest ephemera of neuronal disorganization. The case for two syndromes appears to be weakened by a more recent paper (Owens *et al*, 1985) which failed to confirm the connection between ventricular enlargement and negative symptoms.

It is likely that the human brain has a limited number of expressions of disorganized cerebral functioning. Dementing processes from many causes have very similar symptomatic expression. Schizophrenia-like syndromes of the positive type may be produced by processes such as temporal lobe epilepsy (Perez and Trimble, 1980) of limbic lobe pathology (Davison and Bagley, 1969) and drug-induced schizophreniform psychosis. A possible explanation is that the disease process in schizophrenia produces an inability to handle information. In acute schizophrenia information generated both from external (perceptual) and internal (correlative) sources may be sufficient to overwhelm the integrative mechanisms and Schneiderian symptoms appear. Similarly, stress later in the illness may produce the same effect. This information-integrative processing may be under the control of the dopaminergic system. A reduction of information flow through inhibition of dopamine by neuroleptic drugs reduces the tendency to positive symptoms and also protects against stress-induced release into psychotic symptoms (Leff and Vaughn, 1980). Similarly, an increase in information flow resulting from drug-induced dopaminergic overactivity could produce a similar picture. This would, of course, mean that in schizophrenia there would be no abnormality detected in the dopaminergic system and that the organizational problems of schizophrenia were related to a system as yet unidentified.

It is similarly difficult to find strong neurochemical evidence for the dopamine hypothesis. From post-mortem studies the most consistent finding appears to be an increase in dopamine receptors in the striatum which may not be related to neuroleptic usage (Owen *et al*, 1978). The advent of techniques which have revealed a formidable array of neuropeptide transmitters in brain has once again rejuvenated the hope of providing the specific biochemical abnormality in the illness. Marked changes have been demonstrated in cholecystokinin-like and somatostatin-like immunoreactivity in the limbic lobe in schizophrenia associated with negative symptoms (Ferrier *et al*, 1983). Whether these changes in both dopamine receptors and neuropeptides are phenomena developing as the result of specific neuronal degeneration or secondary to changed patterns of neurotransmission with the change in neuronal usage, reflected in transmitter content and receptor sensitivity, one cannot yet tell.

The most important point concerning cerebral atrophy is that it is not universal: in patients with severe and chronic illness it may not be present (Owens *et al*, 1985). It is also seen in patients with affective disorders (Rieder *et al*, 1983) who incidentally also exhibit cognitive impairment (Eccleston and Fairbairn, 1984; Owens *et al*, 1985). The paper by Reveley *et al* (1984) may give a key to solve the problem; they studied a group of schizophrenics of twin births and found no evidence of ventricular enlargement in twins with a strong family history for schizophrenia. CAT scan changes were, however, detected in those twins without a family history which might be attributable to obstetric complications. Their work supports the theory that given a genetic multifactorial inheritance where environmental influences form a potential determinant for the illness then: 'It is possible that those with a significant genetic predisposition require little else to become psychotic, that others with less genetic liability become psychotic only after additional environmental influence; and that some people develop a psychosis secondary to environmental influence alone' (Reveley *et al*, 1984).

As an addendum to CAT scan change in both schizophrenia and affective illness one should consider the question of plasticity in the adult brain. In this respect there are interesting observations in the relationship between brain size and learning. Bottijer and Arnold (1984) describe a series of observations on song birds. In the Zebra finch and canaries where the males sing and the females do not there is a larger brain area devoted to song control in the male. DeVoogd and Nottebohm (1981) demonstrated that the length and distribution of dendrites of a certain neuronal type were greater in the male than female in those areas which gave a greater potential for new synaptic connections. What is perhaps more significant is the association between the size of relevant nuclei throughout the season. Zebra finches differ from canaries in that they learn their song as juveniles and repeat it throughout the subsequent breeding seasons without elaboration. By contrast canaries relearn a substantial part of the song each breeding season, in the interim forgetting about two thirds of the 'syllables'. Zebra finches have no volume change in the relevant nuclei, whilst in canaries the volume increases and decreases in parallel with the learning and forgetting process. Indeed a correlation has been reported between vocal virtuosity and the volume of the song control nuclei, the more 'syllables' in the song repertoire being reflected in the nuclear size. Although this is a very specific example of volume change in brain related to learning songs in birds there is no reason to suppose other learned phenomena are not linked with neuronal elaboration. It is not without the bounds of possibility that in the psychoses, where thinking in terms of concept formation, exploratory ideas and stereotyped thoughts are aberrant, that these cognitive processes are not conducive to new dendritic expansion or synapse formation. Indeed, loss of such connections may be observed as a decrease in brain volume. As mentioned below, there is strong suggestive evidence in schizophrenia on PET scanning that total neuronal metabolism is reduced.

There are perhaps lessons to be learned from other diseases whose manifestations resemble schizophrenia. Our attention has been drawn to such similarities by Flor Henry (1976) in temporal lobe epilepsy (TLE). Perez and Trimble (1980) showed that of patients developing a psychosis associated with epilepsy, about 50 per cent can be diagnosed on the Present State Examination as suffering from nuclear schizophrenia. Of these, 90 per cent have a temporal lobe lesion which is usually in the dominant hemisphere. Bernandi *et al* (1984) have investigated such cases using the PET scan and have shown that patients with epileptic psychosis exhibited maximal *decrease* of metabolism on the left side of the brain. Similar PET scan studies by Di Lisi *et al* (1983) demonstrated such a reduction in metabolism on the left side. TLE subjects with psychosis do, however, differ from other schizophrenics by their preservation of affect (Lishman, 1978).

The Aberdeen study (Besson *et al*, 1984) using nuclear magnetic resonance (NMR) has also investigated schizophrenic subjects. The spin lattice relaxation time (T_1) measured during NMR imaging is a sensitive indicator of pathogenic processes. The Aberdeen group, with admittedly a small number of patients, suggested that lesions in the left frontal lobe are associated with positive symptomatology. Perhaps the additional lesion in the frontal lobe in schizophrenia is responsible for the noted differences in affect and personality between this group and those with TLE.

There has been considerable interest in laterality and schizophrenia because of the presumed left hemisphere dysfunction in the illness (Flor Henry, 1969). The data on handedness has yielded conflicting results which may be methodological in origin (Taylor *et al*, 1980). In the Nithsdale study which had the advantage of testing virtually all known schizophrenics in a defined area, McCreadie *et al* (1982) found differences between those in hospital and those in the community. The hospitalized patients were more likely to be those with negative symptoms and also had relatively more non-dextrals. They postulated that this group had more cerebral insults which had shifted natural dextrals to non-dextrality. They also noted a higher incidence of tardive dyskinesia amongst the non-dextrals of this group suggesting brain damage, a fact sustained by the NMR findings of Besson *et al* (1984) of T_1 changes in the basal ganglia in a group with tardive dyskinesia.

In schizophrenia without cerebral damage there might be an excess of strongly right-handed subjects. Boklage (1977) presents the theory that, as in aphasia, the manifestations of cerebral dysfunction are more apparent in those with strong left cerebral dominance and not as intense in those in which cerebral dominance is not complete. The latter group would be expected to have less severe symptoms of schizophrenia. Strongly dextral individuals would be more susceptible to the lasting effects of schizophrenic disorganization. Differences in handedness patterns might then be due to inadvertent selection of the two postulated schizophrenic populations.

In summary, schizophrenics whose left-handedness is likely to be due to brain damage would present a severe group and more likely to have a bad prognosis associated with premorbid schizoid traits and cognitive change.

Those with less dextral tendency in the group with a strong family history would be less severe and be found more in the community.

The pattern is therefore emerging of an inherited tendency to schizophrenia which becomes manifest under environmental influence and particularly organic pathology sustained at birth. There has however, been speculation as to the organic nature of the cerebral insult and a school of thought which postulates a viral aetiology (Torrey, 1973). On this theme, **Hare** (**1983**) in his eloquent and well-researched paper concluded that there was a total increase in the incidence of schizophrenia in the 19th century which, some 200 years ago, was a rare disease. He dismissed with the benefit of hindsight the arguments made at the time: of increased recognition of the illness and accumulation of patients in the asylum as being cogent, but not accounting for the facts. He postulated a 'slow epidemic' due to an environmental factor, possibly a virus, which has decreased in virulence, reflected in a decrease in severity (Ødegård, 1967), in the 20th century.

Hare and Price (1968) drew attention to the excess of winter births for patients suffering from schizophrenia. This, being the season of high incidence of viral infections, leads to the simplest hypothesis (**Machón** *et al*, **1983**) which is that some forms of schizophrenia are due to perinatal viral brain damage; their studies in Denmark strongly support this. They found that urban (also associated with a high risk of viral infection) winter-born children of schizophrenics had a three-fold likelihood for schizophrenia compared with similar genetically high risk progeny born at other times of the year in non-urban settings. It is suggested that similar seasonal factors may operate on neonates not genetically predisposed. Kinney and Jacobsen (1978), for example, found that patients with neither a family history for the illness nor a history of perinatal brain damage were more likely to be born in the winter months and the conclusion could be that viral infection increases risk for schizophrenia both in high and low risk subjects. Direct evidence in terms of the infection itself is at present missing.

Crow (**1984**) has looked in considerable detail at the viral hypothesis of Torrey (1973). In his initial article (Crow, 1983) on the possible viral aetiology of schizophrenia he examines the person to person transmission. He considered that the impetus for this enquiry was, in his eyes, the anomalies in the genetic evidence and in particular the lack of complete concordance in monozygotic twin pairs. He suggested that both genetic predisposition and exposure to an infective agent, presumably viral, are necessary for the development of the illness. In a major critique of this paper (Murray and Reveley, 1983a & b) vigorously opposed the hypothesis and re-examined the interpretation of the twin study data. They concluded that in both family and twin studies the greater proportion of the variance in the liability to schizophrenia is genetically determined (Gottesman and Shields, 1982). It should also be pointed out that from their own work on potential brain damage, monozygotic twins discordant for schizophrenia are likely not to be a homogeneous group, some being genetically predisposed, some not. On the question of seasonality they point out that many polygenic disorders show seasonal enhancement. They do, however, concede that some cases of schizophrenia could be accounted for by perinatal infection.

In **Crow**'s recent exposition (**1984**), there is a shift of position. This paper·

postulated a gene / virus interaction and rules out horizontal transmission (contagion). He suggested that a virus, possibly a retrovirus, becomes incorporated in the genetic machinery as a 'pro virus'. This could be passed from one generation to the next in classical Mendelian fashion, but which could be expressed as virus particles at a later stage in the life of the affected individual. All this is interesting and possible; certainly there could be two mechanisms whereby genes could cause a sequence of events the end product of which is the appearance of schizophrenia. All or part of the virus genome could be introduced into the DNA sequence to give a new gene responsible directly or indirectly for schizophrenia or be similarly introduced to provide a promoter which would then allow derepression of genes present in the chromosome whose expression in that cell is otherwise 'forbidden'. This initiation concept does not require expression as complete virus within the cell since the products of the genes themselves begin the process which results in schizophrenia. Indeed, it is more often the case that production of complete viral particles causes cell death. It is not clear from his paper whether Crow believes that a virus causes the cell death which is seen as the loss of brain substance found on CAT scans. Fortunately the viral hypothesis generates experiments which could identify viral sequences in DNA. Virus sequences associated with schizophrenia could be located using complementary DNA probes. There would, however, have to be a good guess as to which virus was involved and Crow's suggestion of a retrovirus is reasonable.

He also ingeniously incorporates the laterality findings in the hypothesis, suggesting the retrovirus has a particular affinity for a growth factor which would determine developmental asymmetry. A search for evidence of periventricular viral damage, presumably perinatally, in a carefully conducted study reported by Johnstone (1985) using the NMR has failed to find evidence of damage from such attack in schizophrenic subjects, anomalies which, when first seen in schizophrenic subjects suspected of being viral, were found with similar frequency in controls which probably rules out their pathological origin. The theory becomes more global, accounting also for manic-depressive psychosis which shows similar patterns to schizophrenia in season of onset and season of birth. Other factors could account for the season of onset and season of birth findings. There are biological rhythms of annual duration which could be light entrained which determine, for example, variation in sex drive in the schizophrenic group and hence season of conception. However, this is purely hypothetical and does not account for the effect of these rhythms on the fertility of control populations. Even acknowledging the canon of parsimony, it is difficult at this point of our knowledge of gene/virus interaction to accept the theory. It seems to be elaborate and over-inclusive (in relation to manic-depressive illness) and at present to have no direct experimental evidence to justify it. Like Reveley *et al* (1984), I feel there are potentially many causes of schizophrenia which can act as the environmental factor in truly genetically predisposed individuals.

In summary, the symptoms of schizophrenia are likely to arise from a number of causes and to some extent are able to be controlled by regulation of dopaminergic activity. There seems to be little doubt as to the genetic basis for the potential disorder but this tendency may be more frequently realized as a result of cerebral organic change occurring probably at the time of birth. Such changes are likely to be sited in the dominant temporal lobe and may include the frontal lobe. This pathology is probably the reason for CAT scan change in a group of schizophrenics who may well be more likely to become chronic and remain in psychiatric hospitals. Handedness changes may also reflect subgroups. Although encephalitic change may produce a similar clinical picture to schizophrenia and the evidence for a viral origin of the disorder is an exciting prospect, it does not seem that at our present state of knowledge it is warranted to postulate a gene-viral interaction.

References

ASHCROFT, G. W., BLACKWOOD, G. W., BESSON, J. A. O., PALOMO, T. & WARING, H. L. (1981) Positive and negative schizophrenic symptoms and the role of dopamine. *British Journal of Psychiatry*, **138**, 268–272.

BERNARDI, S., GALLHOFER, B., TRIMBLE, M. R., FRACKOWIAK, R. S. J., WISE, R. J. S. & JONES, T. (1984) An inter-ictal study of partial epilepsy using oxygen-15 inhalation technique and positron emission tomography, with special reference to psychosis. In *Current Problems in Epilepsy*, Vol. 1, (ed. M. Baldy-Moulinier). London: John Libbey.

BESSON, J. A. O., CORRIGAN, F. M., FOREMAN, E. I., ASHCROFT, G. W. & SMITH, F. W. (1984) T_1 changes in schizophrenic disorders measured by proton NMR. *Proceedings Society of Magnetic Resonance in Medicine*. 13th–17th August, 1984, New York, New York.

BOKLAGE, C. E. (1977) Schizophrenia, brain asymmetry development and twinning: cellular relationship with etiological and possibly prognostic implications. *Biological Psychiatry*, **12**, 19–35.

BOTTIJER, S. W. & ARNOLD, A. P. (1984) Hormones and structural plasticity in the adult brain. *Trends in Neurosciences*, **7**(5), 168–171.

CROW, T. J. (1980) Molecular pathology of schizophrenia: more than one disease process? *British Medical Journal*, *i*, 66–68.

—— (1983) Is schizophrenia an infectious disease? *Lancet*, *i*, 173–175.

—— (1984) A re-evaluation of the viral hypothesis: Is psychosis the result of retroviral integration at a site close to the cerebral dominance gene? *British Journal of Psychiatry*, **145**, 243–253.

DAVISON, K. & BAGLEY, C. R. (1969) Schizophrenia-like psychoses associated with organic disorders of the central nervous system: A review of the literature. In *Current Problems in Neuropsychiatry* (ed. R. N. Herrington). *British Journal of Psychiatry*, Special Publication No. 4. Ashford, Kent: Headley Brothers.

DEVOOGD, T. J. & NOTTEBOHM, F. (1981) Gonadal hormones induce dentritic growth in the adult avian brain. *Science*, **214**, 202–204.

DI LISI, L. E., BUCHSBAUM, M. S., IRVING, C. A., DOWLING, S., JOHNSON, J., HOLCOMB, H. H., KESSLER, R. & BORONOW, J. (1983) Clinical correlates of PET in schizophrenia. *New Research Abstracts*, American Psychiatric Association Annual Meeting, May 1983 (NR49).

ECCLESTON, D. & FAIRBAIRN, A. F. (1984) Is there a dementia associated with the major psychoses? In *Interdisciplinary Topics in Gerontology*, Vol. 20. Basel: Karger.

FERRIER, I. N., ROBERTS, G. W., CROW, T. J., JOHNSTONE, E. C., OWENS, D. G. C., LEE, Y. C., O'SHAUGHNESSY, D., ADRIAN, T. E., POLAK, J. M. & BLOOM, S. R. (1983) Reduced cholecystokinin-like somatostatin-like immunoreactivity in limbic lobe is associated with negative symptoms in schizophrenia. *Life Sciences*, **33**, 475–482.

FLOR HENRY, P. (1969) Psychosis and temporal lobe epilepsy. *Epilepsia*, **10**, 363–395.

—— (1976) Lateralized temporal-limbic dysfunction and psychopathology. *Annals of the New York Academy of Science*, **280**, 777–795.

GOTTESMAN, I. I. & SHIELDS, J. (1982) *Schizophrenia: The Epigenetic Puzzle*. Cambridge University Press.

HARE, E. (1983) Was insanity on the increase? *British Journal of Psychiatry*, **142**, 439–455.

—— & PRICE, J. S. (1968) Mental disorder and season of birth: comparison of psychoses with neurosis. *British Journal of Psychiatry*, **115**, 533–540.

HOENIG, J. (1983) The concept of schizophrenia: Kraepelin-Bleuler-Schneider. *British Journal of Psychiatry*, **142**, 547–556.

JOHNSTONE, E. C. (1985) NMR studies and its potential for studies in psychiatry: New brain imaging techniques and their relevance for psychopharmacology. In *New Brain Imaging Techniques and Psychopharmacology* (ed. M. R. Trimble). Oxford University Press.

—— CROW, T. J., FRITH, C. D., STEVENS, M., KREEL, L. & HUSBAND, J. (1978) The dementia of dementia praecox. *Acta Psychiatrica Scandinavica*, **57**, 305–324.

KINNEY, D. K. & JACOBSEN, B. (1978) Environmental factors in schizophrenia: New adoption study evidence. In *The Nature of Schizophrenia* (eds. L. C. Wynne, R. Cromwell and S. Matthysse). New York: Wiley.

LEFF, J. & VAUGHN, C. (1980) The interaction of life events and relatives' expressed emotion in schizophrenia and depressive neurosis. *British Journal of Psychiatry*, **136**, 146–153.

LISHMAN, W. A. (1978) *Organic Psychiatry*. Oxford: Blackwells.

McCREADIE, R. G., CRORIE, J., BARRON, E. T. & WINSLOW, G. S. (1982) The Nithsdale schizophrenia survey: III. Handedness and tardive dyskinesia. *British Journal of Psychiatry*, **140**, 591–594.

MACKAY, A. V. P. (1980) Positive and negative schizophrenic symptoms and the role of dopamine. *British Journal of Psychiatry*, **137**, 379–386.

MACHÓN, R. A., MEDNICK, S. A. & SCHULSINGER, F. (1983) The interaction of seasonality, place of birth, genetic risk and subsequent schizophrenia in a high risk sample. *British Journal of Psychiatry*, **143**, 383–388.

MELLOR, C. S. (1970) First-rank symptoms of schizophrenia. *British Journal of Psychiatry*, **117**, 15–23.

MURRAY, R. M. & REVELEY, A. M. (1983a) Schizophrenia as an infection. *Lancet*, i, 583.

—— —— (1983b) Genetics of schizophrenia. *Lancet*, i, 1159–1160.

ØDEGÅRD, O. (1967) Changes in the prognosis of functional psychoses since the days of Kraepelin. *British Journal of Psychiatry*, **113**, 813–822.

OWEN, F., CROSS, A. J., CROW, T. J., LONGDEN, A., POULTER, M. & RILEY, G. J. (1978) Increased dopamine receptor sensitivity in schizophrenia. *Lancet*, ii, 223–225.

OWENS, D. G. C., JOHNSTONE, E. C., CROW, T. J., FRITH, C. D., JAGOE, J. R. & KREEL, L. (1985) Lateral ventricular size in schizophrenia: Relationship to the disease process and its clinical manifestations. *Psychological Medicine*, **15**, 27–41.

PEREZ, M. M. & TRIMBLE, M. R. (1980) Epileptic psychosis—diagnostic comparison with process schizophrenia. *British Journal of Psychiatry*, **137**, 245–249.

REVELEY, A. M., REVELEY, M. A. & MURRAY, R. M. (1984) Cerebral ventricular enlargement in non-genetic schizophrenia: a controlled twin study. *British Journal of Psychiatry*, **144**, 89–93.

RIEDER, R. O., MANN, L. S., WEINBERGER, D. R., van KAMMEN, D. P. & POST, R. M. (1983) Computed tomographic scans in patients with schizophrenia, schizoaffective and bipolar affective disorder. *Archives of General Psychiatry*, **40**, 735–739.

TAYLOR, P. J., DALTON, R. & FLEMINGER, J. J. (1980) Handedness in schizophrenia. *British Journal of Psychiatry*, **136**, 375–383.

TORREY, E. F. (1973) Slow and latent viruses in schizophrenia. *Lancet*, ii, 22–24.

van PRAAG, H. M. (1977) The significance of dopamine for the mode of action of neuroleptics and the pathogenesis of schizophrenia. *British Journal of Psychiatry*, **130**, 463–474.

20 The significance of dopamine for the mode of action of neuroleptics and the pathogenesis of schizophrenia

H. M. van PRAAG

For many years, well into the sixties, research into the biological determinants of schizophrenic psychoses suffered from a dearth of more or less well-founded and testable working hypotheses. Without much system, efforts were made to find abnormal metabolites in a wide variety of body fluids. Strange people, strange substances: not a very powerful research strategy. Recently, however, it has become apparent that neuroleptics could serve as the pacemakers of biological psychosis research (Matthijsse, 1973; Snyder *et al*, 1974; van Praag, 1975), much as the antidepressants are the pacemakers of biological depression research (van Praag, 1976). I shall briefly discuss the arguments which have led to this conclusion.

Neuroleptics and central catecholamine metabolism

All known neuroleptics exert an influence on the central catecholamine (CA) metabolism; they do this in two different ways (reviews by Andén *et al*, 1970; Nybäck and Sedvall, 1970; O'Keefe *et al*, 1970; Randrup and Munkvad, 1970; Westerink and Korf, 1975; Seeman and Lee, 1975; Wiesel and Sedvall, 1975; Iversen, 1975; van Praag, 1976).

Neuroleptics of the receptor-blocking type

The first group, the so-called neuroleptics of the receptor-blocking type, comprises the phenothiazines (e.g. chlorpromazine; Largactil) and the butyrophenones (e.g. haloperidol; Serenace) as well as chemically related groups of thioxanthenes (e.g. clopenthixol; Sordinol) and of diphenylbutylpiperidines (pimozide; Orap). In animals given such a compound the concentration of CA metabolites in the brain increases, whereas that of CA proper remains unchanged. This suggests an increased degradation of CA in combination with increased CA synthesis, which compensates for the loss of CA. In other words: it indicates an increased CA turnover. With the aid of isotope kinetics (administration of radioactive CA precursors) and by the method of synthesis inhibition (with subsequent determination of the rate of disappearance of the amine), this hypothesis has been verified and confirmed.

Functionally, an increased turnover can have two entirely different implications: increased transmission activity in CA-ergic synapses or, alternatively, transmission block in CA-ergic synapses. The latter process leads to an increased impulse flow in the presynaptic element and, probably via this way, to increased CA synthesis. A logical inference is that a compensatory mechanism is involved which aims at breaking the block.

In the case of the above-mentioned neuroleptics, the increased turnover is presumably secondary to transmission block. This presumption is based on the following arguments:

1. At the behaviour level, neuroleptics antagonize symptoms of CA-ergic hyperactivity, e.g. the motor hyperactivity provoked by amphetamines.
2. Neuroleptics cause reduction of motor activity. Motor hypoactivity is a constant symptom when CA-ergic activity is suppressed, e.g. by inhibition of CA synthesis or via destruction of CA-ergic neuronal systems.
3. Neuroleptics inhibit adenylcyclase, an enzyme involved in the synthesis of cyclic AMP. This compound is needed for activation of postsynaptic CA receptors, and inhibition of its synthesis indicates or leads to reduced transmission activity.

Receptors are probably located at two sites in a CA-ergic synapse: not only in the postsynaptic but also in the presynaptic membrane. The former bring the postsynaptic element to a state of excitation. The task of the latter is believed to be regulation of the rate of CA synthesis, guided by the amount of CA available in the synaptic cleft. Neuroleptics are presumed to block both receptor types. Block of the postsynaptic receptors inhibits transmission, while block of the presynaptic receptors is believed to contribute to the increased turnover of transmitter substance due to abolition of the feedback inhibition.

Another important point is that the extent to which neuroleptics of this type block dopamine (DA) and noradrenaline (NA) receptors varies from one compound to the other; and that the classification of neuroleptics on the basis of this ratio is completely at odds with their classification according to chemical structure.

Finally, there are indications that these neuroleptics inhibit the release of DA in the synaptic cleft which is normally effected by excitation of the axon. This mechanism, like that of receptor block, leads to diminished transmission activity.

Neuroleptics of the store-depleting type

Neuroleptics of this second type interfere with the uptake of CA into the stores (synaptic vesicles), causing these compounds to accumulate in the cytoplasm where they are degraded by monoamine oxidase (MAO), so that their concentration decreases. Neuroleptics of this category include reserpine (Serpasil), which depletes the DA, NA and serotonin (5-HT) stores, and the indole derivative oxypertine (Opertil), which shows some predilection for NA stores.

Conclusions

Neuroleptics differ widely in chemical structure, but show unmistakable similarities in their net effect on the central CA metabolism. Neuroleptics of the phenothiazine and the butyrophenone type are believed to block presynaptic and postsynaptic CA receptors, and possibly also the release of DA in the synaptic cleft following nerve stimulation. The ratio between DA receptor-blocking and NA receptor-blocking capacity differs from one neuroleptic to the next. Reserpine and oxypertine interfere with the storage of CA in the intraneuronal stores, causing the CA degradation to increase and their concentration to decrease.

Neuroleptics reduce transmission in DA-ergic and NA-ergic neurons, but to different extents and via different mechanisms. This seems to be a group characteristic.

Research strategy

Neuroleptics are compounds of diverse chemical structure, but they show two similarities.

In biochemical terms: they reduce transmission in CA-ergic systems either by inhibition of postsynaptic receptors or by reduction of the amount of transmitter available. In psychopathological terms: they alleviate motor unrest, anxiety and psychotic disorders of thinking and experiencing.

These data logically prompt a number of closely interrelated questions: (1) Do neuroleptics also reduce transmission in human central CA-ergic neurons? (2) If so, is there a correlation between this effect and (a) the therapeutic and (b) the extrapyramidal (side) effects of neuroleptics? (3) Is the ratio between DA receptor-blocking and NA receptor-blocking capacity predictive of the therapeutic action profile of a neuroleptic? In this respect I note that their chemical structure is of little assistance. (4) Is the activity in central CA-ergic neurons increased in (schizophrenic) psychoses?

In the past few years these questions have provided us with a research strategy in the biological study of psychotic disorders (van Praag, 1967; 1975).

Do neuroleptics reduce human central DA-ergic transmission?

This question has two components: (1) are there indications that neuroleptics of the phenothiazine and the butyrophenone type increase the human central DA turnover; and, if so, (2) is this associated, as it is in test animals, with decreased activity in the postsynaptic DA receptors?

Conclusion

Studies have shown that neuroleptics of the phenothiazine and the butyrophenone type increase the human central DA turnover. Since in addition they increase the prolactin concentration in blood and CSF, this effect is probably based on inhibited transmission in DA-ergic neurons, and *not* on increased DA-ergic transmission.

The increased DA turnover in the CNS (viewed as an index of the inhibition of transmission in DA-ergic systems) shows a significant correlation with the therapeutic effect of neuroleptics and with the occurrence of parkinson-like symptoms. Moreover, patients with a low pretherapeutic DA turnover proved to be particularly susceptible to these side effects. These are strong, direct indications that the clinical effects of neuroleptics are indeed correlated with changes in DA-ergic transmission.

Finally I mention here an argument of a different order. If the therapeutic efficacy of a neuroleptic and a CA-ergic block are related, the profile of clinical (side) effects of a neuroleptic can be expected to be influenced by the ratio between DA-receptor block and NA-receptor block. There is suggestive evidence that this expectation is correct. This statement is based so far on no more than two experiments (van Praag *et al*, 1975). The conclusions from these experiments should therefore be regarded as tentative. They are: (1) the ability of a neuroleptic to induce inertia increases with its ability to block DA receptors; (2) its antipsychotic effect diminishes as its ability to block DA receptors diminishes; (3) its sedative effect increases as its ability to block NA receptors increases.

These findings indicate that the mechanism by which a neuroleptic influences central CA is predictive of the pattern of its clinical effects; and as such these findings support the hypothesis that therapeutic efficacy of neuroleptics and suppression of central CA-ergic activity are related.

The DA metabolism in acute schizophrenic psychoses

Neuroleptics—a group of compounds heterogeneous in terms of chemical structure—all have the ability to suppress transmission in central DA-ergic neurons. Non-neuroleptic phenothiazines differ from their therapeutically active counterparts by lack of DA-antagonistic potency (Matthijsse, 1973). This observation warrants the question whether hyperactivity in central DA-ergic systems is or can be involved in syndromes which show a favourable response to neuroleptics, such as psychoses.

An increased DA turnover can exist in psychoses, but this phenomenon seems less dependent on the factor aetiology of the psychosis or the presence of 'true' psychotic symptoms (delusion and hallucination) than on the presence or absence of motor unrest.

In a group of acute schizophrenics, Post *et al* (1975) also found a normal HVA response to probenecid. Bowers (1974) and Kirstein *et al* (1976) reported decreased post-probenecid HVA values in one study, and increased values in another. The variability of their results likewise raises the suspicion that the disorders of the DA metabolism are not so much related to the syndrome schizophrenia or the disease entity schizophrenia as to a particular component (or to a particular subgroup, as yet unidentified in psychopathological terms). The serum prolactin level, a peripheral indicator of central DA-ergic activity, is normal in schizophrenic patients (Meltzer *et al*, 1975).

In all, there are no indications that hyperactivity in DA-ergic systems plays a decisive role in the pathogenesis of acute schizophrenic psychoses.

Comment

DA and clinical effects of neuroleptics

Neuroleptics are substances of diverse chemical structure which nevertheless have two similarities in common: they reduce transmission in central CA-ergic systems and they have a therapeutic effect on psychoses. This warrants the question whether these two characteristics of neuroleptics are correlated. Such a correlation is indeed plausible, at least so far as disturbed DA-ergic transmission is concerned:

(1) Neuroleptics of the receptor-blocking type increase the probenecid-induced accumulation of HVA in lumbar CSF—a phenomenon accepted as an indicator of increased DA turnover in the CNS.

(2) Since these compounds increase the prolactin concentration in blood and CSF, the increased DA turnover is probably secondary to *inhibition* of transmission, and not an expression of *increased* transmission activity.

(3) A positive correlation exists between the degree of increase in DA turnover during neuroleptic medication and the strength of the therapeutic effect; this is an indication that the two factors are correlated. There is likewise a positive correlation between the increase in DA turnover and the occurrence of hypokinetic-rigid symptoms. Moreover, the risk of these side effects occurring is greater at a low than at a high pretherapeutic DA turnover. This fact also indicates that DA turnover and neuroleptic parkinsonism are indeed related.

(4) There are indications that the ratio DA-ergic : NA-ergic transmission inhibition exerts an influence on the clinical action profile of a neuroleptic. Such a correlation would be unlikely if suppression of CA-ergic activity had nothing to do with the clinical effects of neuroleptics.

Neuroleptics of the receptor-blocking type block not only DA-ergic but also NA-ergic transmission. The significance of this fact for their clinical effects is not entirely understood. There are indications that propranolol, a β-blocker which centrally blocks postsynaptic NA receptors but leaves DA receptors uninfluenced, can have a therapeutic effect on schizophrenic psychoses (Atsmon *et al*, 1971; 1972; Steiner *et al*, 1973; Yorkston *et al*, 1974), although this work still needs confirmation in a controlled trial. In view of this, there are sound reasons for further investigation of the NA-ergic system in its relation to the clinical effects of neuroleptics.

DA and the pathogenesis of schizophrenic psychoses

If transmission inhibition in DA neurons and antipsychotic effects of neuroleptics are related, then it is an obvious inference that increased transmission activity in DA neurons may play a role in the pathogenesis of (schizophrenic) psychoses. There are only indirect arguments in favour of this hypothesis. Drugs which can be expected to increase activity in DA-ergic systems, particularly amphetamines and 1-DOPA, are psychosis-provoking and intensify schizophrenic symptoms (Snyder, 1973; Randrup and Munkvad, 1972; Munkvad *et al*, 1975). Compounds which inhibit synthesis of DA (and NA) potentiate the therapeutic effect of neuroleptics (Carlsson *et al*, 1972; 1973). However, there are no direct arguments to support the above hypothesis: the central DA turnover can be increased in schizophrenic (and other) psychoses, but this corresponds with increased motor activity rather than with the presence of prototypical psychotic symptoms such as delusion and hallucination. The normal serum prolactin level, too, is no indication of increased central DA activity.

A possible explanation of the negativity of these findings is that the HVA concentration in CSF reflects mainly the DA metabolism in the nigrostriatal DA system, whereas serum prolactin is a function of the DA activity in the tubero-infundibular DA system. There are no methods for obtaining information on the human limbic DA system, and it may be precisely this system that is involved in the pathogenesis of psychotic symptoms.

Moreover, it is, of course, to be borne in mind that the mechanism of action of a therapeutically active drug does not necessarily coincide with or is located near the substrate of the symptoms controlled with the aid of this drug. Example: anticholinergic drugs are effective antiparkinson drugs; yet it is not the cholinergic but the DA-ergic system which plays the principal role in many cases of parkinson's disease.

References

ANDÉN, N. E., BUTCHER, S. G., CORRODI, H., FUXE, K. & UNGERSTEDT, U. (1970) Receptor activity and turnover of dopamine and noradrenaline after neuroleptics. *Journal of Pharmacology*, **11**, 303–314.

ATSMON, A., BLUM, I., MAOZ, B., STEINER, M., ZIEGELMAN, G. & WIJSENBEEK, H. (1971) The short-term effects of adrenergic blocking agents in a small group of psychotic patients: preliminary clinical observations. *Psychiatria Neurologia Neurochirurgia*, **74**, 251–258.

—— —— STEINER, M., LATZ, A. & WIJSENBEEK, H. (1972) Further studies with propranolol in psychotic patients. *Psychopharmacologia*, **27**, 249–254.

BOWERS, M. B. Jr. (1974) Central dopamine turnover in schizophrenic syndromes. *Archives of General Psychiatry*, **31**, 50–54.

CARLSSON, A., PERSSON, T., ROOS, B.-E. & WÅLINDER, J. (1972) Potentiation of phenothiazines by α-methyl-tyrosine in treatment of chronic schizophrenia. *Journal of Neural Transmission*, **33**, 83–90.

—— ROOS, B.-E., WÅLINDER, J. & SKOTT, A. (1973) Further studies on the mechanism of antipsychotic action: potentiation by α-methyl-tyrosine of thioridazine effects in chronic schizophrenia. *Journal of Neural Transmission*, **34**, 125–132.

IVERSEN, L. L. (1975) Dopamine receptors in the brain. *Science*, **188**, 1084–1089.

KIRSTEIN, L., BOWERS, M. & HENNINGER, G. (1976) CSF amine metabolites, clinical symptoms and body movement in psychiatric patients. *Biological Psychiatry*, **11(4)**, 421–434.

MATTHIJSSE, S. (1973) Antipsychotic drug actions: a clue to the neuropathology of schizophrenia? *Federation Proceedings*, **32**, 200–205.

MELTZER, H., SACHAR, E. J. & FRANTZ, A. G. (1975) Serum prolactin levels in unmedicated schizophrenic patients. *Archives of General Psychiatry*, **31**, 564–569.

MUNKVAD, I., FOG, R. & RANDRUP, A. (1975) Amphetamine psychosis: A useful model of schizophrenia? In *On the Origin of Schizophrenic Psychoses* (ed. H. M. van Praag). Amsterdam: De Erven Bohn, B.V.

NYBÄCK, H. & SEDVALL, G. (1970) Further studies on the accumulation and disappearance of catecholamines formed from $-^{14}C$ in mouse brain. Effect of some phenothiazine analogues. *European Journal of Pharmacology*, **10**, 193–205.

O'KEEFE, R., SHARMAN, D. F. & VOGT, M. (1970) Effect of drugs used in psychoses on cerebral dopamime metabolism. *British Journal of Pharmacology*, **38**, 287–304.

POST, R. M., FINK, E., CARPENTER, W. T. & GOODWIN, F. K. (1975) Cerebrospinal fluid amine metabolites in acute schizophrenia. *Archives of General Psychiatry*, **32**, 1063–1069.

RANDRUP, A. & MUNKVAD, I. (1970) Biochemical anatomical and psychological investigations of stereotyped behavior induced by amphetamines. In *Amphetamines and Related Compounds* (eds. E. Costa and S. Garattini), pp. 695–713. New York: Raven Press.

—— —— (1972) Evidence indicating an association between schizophrenia and dopaminergic hyperactivity in the brain. *Orthomolecular Psychiatry*, **1**, 2–27.

SEEMAN, P. & LEE, T. (1975) Antipsychotic drugs: direct correlation between clinical potency and presynaptic action on dopamine neurons. *Science*, **188**, 121, 7–9.

SNYDER, S. H. (1973) Amphetamine psychosis: a 'model' schizophrenia mediated by catecholamines. *American Journal of Psychiatry*, **130**, 61–66.

—— BANERJEE, S. P., YAMAMURA, H. I. & GREENBERG, D. (1974) Drugs, neurotransmitters and schizophrenia. *Science*, **184,** 1243–1253.

STEINER, M., LATZ, A., BLUM, I., ATSMON, A. & WIJSENBEEK, H. (1973) Propranolol versus chlorpromazine in the treatment of psychoses associated with child-bearing. *Psychiatria Neurologia Neurochirurgia*, 421–426.

VAN PRAAG, H. M. (1967) The possible significance of cerebral dopamine for neurology and psychiatry. *Psychiatria Neurologia Neurochirurgia*, **70,** 361–379.

—— (1975) Neuroleptics as a guideline to biological research in psychotic disorders. *Comprehensive Psychiatry*, **16,** 7–22.

—— DOLS, L. C. W. & SCHUT, T. (1975) Biochemical versus psychopathological action profile of neuroleptics: A comparative study of chlorpromazine and oxypertine in acute psychotic disorders. *Comprehensive Psychiatry*, **16,** 255–263.

—— (1976) *Depression and Schizophrenia: A contribution on their Chemical Pathology.* New York: Spectrum Publications.

WESTERINK, B. H. C. & KORF, J. (1975) Influence of drugs on striatal and limbic homovanillic acid concentration in the rat brain. *European Journal of Pharmacology*, **33,** 31–40.

WIESEL, F. A. & SEDVALL, G. (1975) Effect of antipsychotic drugs on homovanillic acid levels in striatum and olfactory tubercle of the rat. *European Journal of Pharmacology*, **30,** 364–367.

YORKSTON, N. J., ZAKI, S. A., MALIK, M. K. U., MORRISON, R. C. & HAVARD, C. W. H. (1974) Propranolol in the control of schizophrenic symptoms. *British Medical Journal*, *iv*, 633–635.

21   Positive and negative schizophrenic symptoms and the role of dopamine: A debate

1. A. V. P. Mackay

In a recent review Dr Tim Crow seeks to draw a clear neurobiological distinction between the acute and chronic schizophrenias (Crow, 1980).

Kraepelin succeeded in isolating a number of symptoms which were present in psychiatric disorders with very poor prognosis. The psychoses characterized by the presence of these symptoms were subsumed by Kraepelin under Morel's term *dementia praecox*. A firm nosological category was thus established, the essential characteristics of which were also identified by Bleuler with his introduction of the more convenient neologism 'schizophrenia' (Kraepelin, 1913; Bleuler, 1911). Certain phenomena, many of which are now known as negative symptoms, were identified as fundamental characteristics of the disease. Fifty years later Kurt Schneider advocated an arbitrary checklist of first rank schizophrenic symptoms which he felt to be pathognomonic of schizophrenia and which rapidly gained favour because they were 'positive' and therefore more definable and reliably rateable.

For laudable reasons of phenomenological conformity the Schneiderian and similar checklists have been widely adopted by neuropharmacologists both as entry criteria for therapeutic trials and as target symptoms for the evaluation of neuroleptic drugs. However it has never been demonstrated that the positive phenomena of Schneider either more accurately describe or delineate the original disease. Reliability is of course an important property of any research instrument, but when sight of validity is lost then the way is open for serious misinterpretation (**Kety, 1980**).

Kraepelin and Bleuler recognized most of Schneider's first rank phenomena as superficial and variable accompaniments of schizophrenia, and indeed most contemporary research has shown that the presence of positive symptomatology is a singularly weak prognostic indicator. It is perhaps unfortunate that most modern biological attention has been attracted to an arbitrary set of clinical phenomena which stand in no established relationship to the defining characteristics by which the disease was originally categorized. Moreover it is ironic that, in his belief in a metabolic aetiology, Kraepelin placed great store by chronicity and irreversible deterioration—features which most clinicians still feel are central to any valid definition of schizophrenia, but which correlate so poorly with positive symptoms.

The most widely held neurochemical hypothesis for schizophrenia suggests that the disease is associated with relative overactivity of central dopamine (DA) systems. The roots of this hypothesis lie in observations that neuroleptic drugs, all of which inhibit DA transmission, effectively dispel florid positive symptoms whether they are naturally occurring or chemically-induced. It seems to be a strange turn of events that neurochemical thinking about schizophrenia has been governed by an inference from acute pharmacological effects on a set of symptoms whose relationship to Kraepelin's disease is questionable.

Florid symptoms frequently occur in the setting of schizophrenic illness, often appearing intermittently at times of stress. The backdrop to these florid episodes has become known as the defect state and this is the usual setting for maintenance neuroleptic medication which, in many cases, will reduce the frequency of florid punctuations. Although therapeutic in that sense, neuroleptics are in no sense therapeutic for negative symptoms, nor have they been shown to exert any favourable influence on the long-term course of the disease. Neuroleptic drugs not only appear impotent against Kraepelinian characteristics but there are many who believe that aspects of the defect state are in fact made worse by such medication (Sutter *et al*, 1966; Andrews, 1973).

TABLE I

	Classical schizophrenia (Kraepelin/Bleuler)	Acute non-affective psychosis (Schneider)
Clinical phenomena	Fundamental symptoms: mostly negative, the defect state, simple schizophrenia ± accessory symptoms	First-rank florid symptomatology
Diagnosis	Difficult on cross-section	Easy on cross-section, reliable
Time-course and pattern	Chronic (by definition), no *restitutio ad integrum*	Acute breakdown, sometimes in the setting of the defect state
Outcome prediction	Strong (by definition)	Weak
Response to neuroleptics	Poor (made worse?)	Good
CSF [HVA]	Reduced	?
Post-mortem bio-chemistry	Raised dopamine concentrations. Increased number of dopamine receptors	?
Brain structure	Dilated cerebral ventricles (CAT scan)	?
Intellectual and behavioural performance	Impaired	?
Crow classification	Type II	Type I
Dopaminergic status	Underactive?	Overactive?

These observations are, I think, of crucial importance to neurochemical hypotheses of schizophrenic illness, and in the accompanying Table, I have tried to summarize several related issues.

In a timely attempt to resolve some inconsistencies in current thinking, Crow has designated a Type I and a Type II schizophrenia to describe acute (Schneiderian) and chronic (Kraepelinian) syndromes respectively (Crow,

1980). Under the characteristics of the acute (Type I) illness he rightly lists features such as response to neuroleptics, postulated DA overactivity, etc, and also an increase in the number of DA receptors in post-mortem (PM) schizophrenic brain tissue. This latter finding he sees compatible with the DA hypothesis in that he takes DA receptor proliferation to signify synaptic overactivity.

I would like to suggest a different interpretation of how these and other recent PM findings stand in relation to the DA hypothesis and to classical schizophrenia. Our own PM results are in broad agreement with those of Crow and his colleagues, including the finding that not only is there an increase in the DA receptor population but also in the DA concentration in certain discrete areas of the schizophrenic brain (Bird *et al*, 1979; Mackay *et al*, 1980). In our series these abnormalities are particularly marked in cases where the onset of illness was before the age of twenty-five. Although the elimination of chronic neuroleptic treatment as a cause for these abnormalities is not possible in our series, the Northwick Park series included a small number of apparently drug-free cases and in them the DA receptor proliferation was still evident (Owen *et al*, 1978). If increased DA receptor number and increased DA concentrations have anything at all to do with schizophrenic illness rather than the sequelae of neuroleptic medication, then it is surely with the classical Kraepelinian disease and not with the acute syndrome. Cases whose brain tissue becomes available for PM neurochemical analysis come mainly from the ranks of chronically debilitated and hospitalized schizophrenics. It is most unusual to acquire tissue from a case of purely Schneiderian symptomatology who died during an acute illness. This means that any PM study involves a schizophrenic population selected, of necessity, for chronic hospitalization and therefore predominantly Kraepelinian characteristics.

If one accepts that increased DA receptor numbers and increased DA concentrations may be associated with classical schizophrenia then any interpretation of the functional significance of these abnormalities must take account of the fact that neuroleptic drugs are, at best, ineffectual at treating the syndrome. The interpretation depends essentially upon whether one considers DA receptor proliferation to be a primary or secondary change. If primary, then synaptic activity would be increased and neuroleptic drugs would be expected to ameliorate the condition. If secondary, then a more primary defect may lie presynaptically—for example a reduced DA turnover leading to presynaptic DA accumulation and compensatory DA receptor proliferation.

In the latter case neuroleptic drugs would be expected to exacerbate the clinical condition and patients might be particularly prone to drug-induced parkinsonism. There is ample evidence both from animal studies and from the study of parkinsonian brains that chronic transmitter starvation at central dopaminergic synapses leads to adaptive proliferation of postsynaptic receptor sites (Schwartz *et al*, 1978; Lee *et al*, 1978). There is also evidence that experimental reduction in impulse traffic in dopaminergic tracts leads to a build up of DA concentrations at dopaminergic axon terminals (Roth *et al*, 1973). Thus both of the only two clear abnormalities to have been identified in PM schizophrenic brain are typical of chronic dopaminergic underactivity.

Although Stein and Wise (1971) had earlier proposed a chronic deficiency in central noradrenergic systems, it was Post and his colleagues who were the first to suggest that the basic schizophrenic defect is associated with reduced DA release (Post *et al*, 1975). This proposal was based on their findings that CSF homovanillic acid (HVA) concentrations were reduced in patients after recovery from acute symptoms and that the group with insidious onset of illness had the lowest HVA levels in the post-acute stage. Their patients were highly selected for Schneiderian features but it is impossible to say what proportion would later proceed to chronic debility. The earlier data of Bowers (1974) showed that low CSF HVA was particularly associated with withdrawn and motivationless schizophrenics, judged to have the poorest prognosis. Bowers felt that there was an inconsistency between his findings and the DA hypothesis but I see no inconsistency, if neuroleptic-sensitive Schneiderian phenomena are merely episodically superimposed upon a basic dopaminergic deficit. A similar conclusion was reached by Chouinard and Jones (1978) and these writers went on logically to suggest the therapeutic use of L-DOPA for the defect state. Although requiring a more complex anatomical model, the simultaneous existence of positive and negative symptoms in the same schizophrenic patient might be analogous to the coexistence of rigidity and bradykinesia with L-DOPA-induced hyperkinesia in the same parkinsonian patient.

The excellent clinical studies of the Northwick Park group with chronic hospitalized schizophrenics, and the work of Weinberger and associates, have shown that an independent objective index of negative symptomatology and poor prognosis might be emerging in the form of cerebral ventricular dilatation as demonstrated by CAT scan (Johnstone *et al*, 1978; Owens and Johnstone, 1980; Weinberger *et al*, 1979). I would certainly agree with Crow that classical schizophrenia is likely to be associated with a rather more widespread and gross morbid process of the brain than has until recently been deemed possible (Crow, 1980).

If a chronic dopaminergic deficit is a feature of this illness then it would be naive and counterproductive to suggest that this is the only, or even the most important abnormality. It would, however, allow of a therapeutic strategy for the crippling defect state which might at least have some ameliorative value. The neurochemical relationship between the chronic defect state and any superimposed florid psychosis is unknown but a parsimonious hypothesis would be that chronic dopaminergic underactivity might switch, perhaps under environmental provocation, to acute dopaminergic overactivity. Such a switch might be mediated by a sudden relative increase in the presynaptic release of DA and the existence of an excessive number of DA receptors would naturally amplify the magnitude of the effect. In the defect state any DA receptor 'supersensitivity' would complicate the use of therapies such as L-DOPA and the situation would be closely analogous to the treatment of parkinson's disease where DA receptor proliferation also occurs, and where excessive use of L-DOPA can rapidly precipitate a neurological syndrome of DA overactivity. In the case of schizophrenia this would be expressed as florid Schneiderian symptoms. However, the cautious titration of L-DOPA or similar agents in the defect state would seem to offer a useful test of the hypothesis.

Whether or not DA has anything important to do with schizophrenic illness, let us try to heed the caution voiced by Professor Kety. To ignore the emphasis placed on negative symptomatology and poor outcome by the men who gave us the diagnostic category is to raise the likelihood of inconsistent and trivial information. Crow and his colleagues seem to be bringing neurobiological research into schizophrenia back to the focus originally seen by Kraepelin.

References

ANDREWS, W. M. (1973) Long-acting tranquillisers and the amotivational syndrome in the treatment of schizophrenics. In *Community Management of the Schizophrenic in Chemical Remission* (ed. E. H. King), 1–4, Exerpta Medica, Amsterdam.

BIRD, E. D., SPOKES, E. G. & IVERSEN, L. L. (1979) Increased dopamine concentration in limbic areas of brain from patients dying with schizophrenia. *Brain*, **102**, 347–360.

BLEULER, E. (1911) *Dementia Praecox or the Group of Schizophrenias.* Translated by H. Zinkin, International Universities Press, 1950, New York.

BOWERS, M. B. (1974) Central dopamine turnover in schizophrenic syndromes. *Archives of General Psychiatry*, **31**, 50–54.

CHOUINARD, G. & JONES, B. D. (1978) Schizophrenia as dopamine-deficiency disease. *Lancet*, *ii*, 99–100.

CROW, T. J. (1980) Molecular pathology of schizophrenia; more than one disease process? *British Medical Journal*, **280**, 66–68.

JOHNSTONE, E. C., CROW, T. J., FRITH, C. D., STEVENS, M., KREEL, L. & HUSBAND, J. (1978) The dementia of dementia praecox. *Acta Psychiatrica Scandinavica*, **57**, 305–324.

KETY, S. (1980) The syndrome of schizophrenia: unresolved questions and opportunities for research. *British Journal of Psychiatry*, **136**, 421–436.

KRAEPELIN, E. (1913) *Dementia Praecox and Paraphrenia.* Translated by R. M. Barclay and G. M. Robertson, E. & S. Livingstone (1919), Edinburgh.

LEE, T., SEEMAN, P., RAJPUT, A., FARLEY, I. J. & HORNYKIEWICZ, O. (1978) Receptor basis for dopaminergic supersensitivity in Parkinson's disease. *Nature*, **273**, 59–61.

MACKAY, A. V. P., BIRD, E. D., IVERSEN, L. L., SPOKES, E. G., CREESE, I. & SNYDER, S. H. (1980) Dopaminergic abnormalities in post mortem schizophrenic brain. In *Long-Term Effects of Neuroleptics, Advances in Biochemical Psychopharmacology*, Vol. 24 (eds. F. Cattabeni, G. Racagni, P. F. Spano & E. Costa). New York: Raven Press.

OWEN, F., CROSS, A. J., CROW, T. J., LONGDEN, A., POULTER, M. & RILEY, G. J. (1978) Increased dopamine receptor sensitivity in schizophrenia. *Lancet*, *ii*, 223–225.

OWENS, D. G. C. & JOHNSTONE, E. C. (1980) The disabilities of chronic schizophrenia—their nature and the factors contributing to their development. *British Journal of Psychiatry*, **136**, 384–385.

POST, R. M., FINK, E., CARPENTER, W. T. & GOODWIN, F. F. (1975) Cerebrospinal fluid amine metabolites in acute schizophrenia. *Archives of General Psychiatry*, **32**, 1063–1069.

ROTH, R. H., WALTERS, J. R. & AGHAJANIAN, G. K. (1973) Effect of impulse flow on the release and synthesis of dopamine in the rat striatum. In *Frontiers in Catecholamine Research*, (eds. E. Usdin and S. H. Snyder), 567–574, Pergamon Press Inc, Oxford.

SCHWARTZ, J. C., COSTENIN, J., MARTRES, M. P., PROTAIS, P. & BAUDRY, M. (1978) Modulation of receptor mechanisms in the CNS: hyper- and hyposensitivity to catecholamines. *Neuropharmacology*, **17**, 665–685.

STEIN, L. & WISE, C. D. (1971) Possible etiology of schizophrenia; progressive damage to the noradrenergic reward system by 6-hydroxydopamine. *Science*, **171**, 1032–1036.

SUTTER, J. M., DEBRIE, M. L. & SCOTTO, J. C. (1966) Recherches sur les effets psychologiques de la fluphenazine dans les psychoses chroniques. *Annales Médico-Psychologiques (Paris)*, **124**, 19–33.

WEINBERGER, D. R., TORREY, E. F., NEOPHYTIDES, A. N. & WYATT, R. J. (1979) Lateral cerebral ventricular enlargement in chronic schizophrenia. *Archives of General Psychiatry*, **36**, 735–739.

2. *T. J. Crow*

Angus Mackay raises a number of points on the progress of recent research on the biological aspects of schizophrenia. In particular the unitary view of the disease process has encountered some problems. In our attempts to formulate a solution of these difficulties there are points of agreement between the concept proposed by Dr Mackay and that advanced in the review (Crow, 1980) to which he refers but there are also differences.

Problems which concern us both are that: (1) Some symptoms (e.g. Schneider's first rank symptoms) which have often been regarded as particularly characteristic of schizophrenia are relatively ineffective predictors of long-term outcome (Brockington *et al*, 1978; Bland and Orn, 1980). This is significant in that poor outcome was the characteristic by which Kraepelin considered that dementia praecox could be distinguished from manic-depressive psychosis. (2) While there is a strong case that the antipsychotic effects of neuroleptic drugs are due to their ability to block dopamine receptors (and suggestive evidence of abnormalities of dopaminergic transmission in some patients) the 'dopamine hypothesis' is of restricted application. For example, it has long been recognized (e.g. Hughes and Little, 1967; Letemendia and Harris, 1967) that neuroleptic drugs are of limited value in many chronic patients, and Kornetsky (1976) demonstrated that such patients are often resistant to the psychosis-exacerbating effects of dexamphetamine which are generally attributed to increased dopamine release.

To account for these findings I proposed that the distinction which is made (e.g. Wing, 1978) between positive and negative symptoms should be regarded as reflecting the presence of two different underlying processes. The positive symptoms (abnormal psychological features such as delusions, hallucinations, and thought disorder) I labelled the Type I syndrome, and the negative symptoms (diminished or absent normal functions such as flattening of affect, poverty of speech and loss of volition) the Type II syndrome. While positive symptoms are frequently observed in acute psychotic episodes and negative symptoms are commoner in chronic schizophrenia, the terminology (for reasons that I will explain) is intended to apply to types of symptoms and not to types of illness.

The importance of this distinction is that the two syndromes predict different things—specifically the presence of the Type I syndrome predicts potential response to neuroleptic drugs, while the presence of the Type II syndrome predicts poor long-term outcome irrespective of drug treatment. Because they appear to represent separate dimensions I suggest the two syndromes are related to distinct pathological processes—a disturbance of dopaminergic transmission being related to the drug responsive (the Type I) syndrome and a quite separate and perhaps encephalitis-like process being associated with the Type II syndrome (Table II).

Mackay also makes use of the distinction between positive and negative symptoms but proposes that rather than reflecting separate dimensions of pathology these can be understood as disturbances along a single continuum, specifically as instabilities in the control of dopaminergic transmission. Thus the primary change in classical (Kraepelinian) schizophrenia according to Mackay is an underactivity of dopaminergic transmission (reflected as negative symptoms) but superimposed on this are episodes of dopaminergic hypersensitivity appearing as positive symptoms. Chouinard and Jones (1978) and Lecrubier *et al* (1980) have also suggested negative schizophrenic symptoms may be related to underactivity of dopaminergic mechanisms.

In favour of this view are the findings that increased tone is common in chronic schizophrenia (Owens and Johnstone, 1981) and appears to be related

TABLE II

	Type I syndrome	Type II syndrome
Symptoms	Positive symptoms (delusions, hallucinations, thought disorder)	Negative symptoms (affective flattening, poverty of speech, loss of volition)
Type of illness in which most commonly seen	Acute schizophrenia	Chronic schizophrenia
Potential for response to neuroleptics	Good	Poor
Presence of intellectual impairment	Absent	Sometimes present
Outcome	Reversible	? Irreversible
Pathological process	Increased dopamine receptors	Cell loss and structural changes in the brain

not to neuroleptic medication but to the presence of negative symptoms, and that some patients with simple schizophrenia have been reported to be improved by the addition of L-DOPA to standard neuroleptic medication (Gerlach and Luhdorf, 1975). However, neither observation is overwhelming. The increase in tone may not reflect decreased dopaminergic activity since these patients do not have the other features of parkinson's disease (and no consistent decrease in dopamine turnover is observed in post-mortem brain in schizophrenia, Owen *et al*, 1978), and it remains to be demonstrated that L-DOPA is doing more than reversing the extrapyramidal effects of neuroleptic drugs. A more serious objection to the view that positive and negative symptoms reflect disturbances in different directions along a dopaminergic continuum is that both sets of symptoms can, and often do, occur in the same patient at the same time. For example, in their recent survey of 510 hospitalized schizophrenic patients Owens and Johnstone (1980) found that at least 40 per cent had significant positive *and* negative symptoms (ratings of 2 or more on the Krawiecka scale).

For these reasons I regard the Type I and Type II syndromes as being independent dimensions reflecting different underlying pathological processes.

This concept was based on the following findings: (1) In patients with acute schizophrenia positive and not negative symptoms respond to neuroleptic medication (Johnstone *et al*, 1978a). (2) In some chronic schizophrenic patients there is CT scan evidence of increased ventricular size (Johnstone *et al*, 1978b) and in these patients increased ventricular size is correlated with intellectual impairment and the presence of negative symptoms. (3) In post-mortem brain there is no increase in dopamine turnover (Owen *et al*, 1978) but dopamine receptors (assessed with butyrophenone-binding techniques) are increased (Owen *et al*, 1978; Lee *et al*, 1978).

However, even if the Type I and Type II syndromes represent different dimensions of pathology it is apparent that they do not constitute separate diseases.

They are often associated together. For example, episodes of the Type I syndrome (positive symptoms) often progress into the Type II syndrome defect state with or without the persistence of positive symptoms; this might be described as classical Kraepelinian schizophrenia. On the other hand either syndrome may occur alone. Thus a pure Type I syndrome may be described as a schizophreniform psychosis or psychogenic or reactive schizophrenia. The Type II syndrome when it occurs without positive symptoms is described as simple schizophrenia. The paranoid/non-paranoid dichotomy can also be related to this concept, paranoid schizophrenia being equivalent to a chronic Type I syndrome, while hebephrenic illnesses include a component of the Type II syndrome.

The distinction between Type I and Type II syndromes explains a number of findings:

(1) Angrist *et al* (1980a) found that exacerbation of symptoms in individual patients by amphetamine predicted good response to neuroleptics, while absence of response to amphetamine predicted poor response. Re-analysis of individual BPRS symptom scores (Angrist *et al*, 1980b) revealed that positive symptoms (the Type I syndrome) were exacerbated by amphetamine and improved by neuroleptics, while negative symptoms (the Type II syndrome) showed little change with either drug.

(2) Weinberger *et al* (1980) found that patients with enlarged ventricles (the Type II syndrome) showed little or no response to neuroleptic drugs while there was a marked decrease in symptom ratings in patients with normal sized ventricles.

(3) Holden *et al* (personal communication) found that intellectual impairment (which is associated with the Type II syndrome) was characteristic of patients who failed to respond to neuroleptic drugs.

(4) In a 30-year follow-up study M. T. Tsuang (1980, unpublished) found that disorientation at the time of first psychotic illness is a predictor of poor long-term outcome. Thus disorientation in the acute illness may be a harbinger of the intellectual impairment of the Type II syndrome.

Most recently Owens and Johnstone (1980) have found that negative symptoms in long-stay patients are strongly correlated with intellectual impairment (the Type II syndrome) and also with neurological signs, but that none of these features is significantly related to positive symptoms (the Type I syndrome).

The hypothesis predicts that changes in dopaminergic mechanisms will be associated with positive symptoms rather than, as suggested by Mackay, with the negative symptoms. To date an increase in numbers of dopamine receptors (assessed by butyrophenone binding, Owen *et al*, 1978; Lee *et al*, 1978) is the only consistent abnormality of dopaminergic transmission detected in post-mortem brain, the increase in dopamine content being inconsistent between areas and unassociated with the increased concentrations of dopamine metabolites which would be predicted if there were overactivity of the presynaptic neurone (Owen *et al*, 1978; Bird *et al*, 1979). On the other hand some patients who appear to have been drug-free for at least a year before death have increased numbers of dopamine receptors (Owen *et al*, 1978); therefore it is possible that this change is associated with the disease process.

The prediction that increased dopamine receptors are related to positive symptoms has been tested in a study of 14 patients whose clinical state had been assessed before death on standardized rating scales by Drs Johnstone, Owens and McCreadie. Number of dopamine receptors assessed as maximum spiroperidol binding was found to be significantly (P <0.01) associated with positive but not negative symptoms (Crow *et al*, 1980).

It is hoped that the separation of two distinct syndromes may lead to further research on the underlying pathological changes. For example, outstanding questions are (i) the site and the nature of the process that leads to cell loss in the Type II syndrome, and (ii) the cause of the increased numbers of dopamine receptors which appear to be associated with the Type I syndrome.

References

ANGRIST, B., ROTROSEN, J. & GERSHON, S. (1980a) Responses to apomorphine, amphetamine and neuroleptics in schizophrenia subjects. *Psychopharmacology*, **67**, 31–38.
—— —— —— (1980b) Differential effects of amphetamine and neuroleptics on negative *vs* positive symptoms in schizophrenia. *Psychopharmacology*, **72**, 17–19.
BIRD, E. D., CROW, T. J., IVERSEN, L. L., LONGDEN, A., MACKAY, A. V. P., RILEY, G. J. & SPOKES, E. C. (1979) Dopamine and homovanillic acid concentrations in the post-mortem brain in schizophrenia. *Journal of Physiology*, **293**, 36–70.
BLAND, R. C. & ORN, H. (1980) Schizophrenia: Schneider's first-rank symptoms and outcome. *British Journal of Psychiatry*, **137**, 63–68.
BROCKINGTON, I. F., KENDELL, R. E. & LEFF, J. P. (1978) Definitions of schizophrenia: concordance and prediction of outcome. *Psychological Medicine* **8**, 387–398.
CHOUINARD, G. & JONES, B. D. (1978) Schizophrenia as dopamine-deficiency disease. *Lancet*, ii, 99–100.
CROW, T. J. (1980) Molecular pathology of schizophrenia: more than one disease process? *British Medical Journal*, **280**, 66–68.
—— OWEN, F., CROSS, A. J., FERRIER, I. N., JOHNSTONE, E. C., McCREADIE, R. G., OWENS, D. G. C. & POULTER, M. (1980) Neurotransmitter enzymes and receptors in post-mortem brain in schizophrenia; evidence that an increase in D2 dopamine receptors is associated with the Type I syndrome. In *Transmitter Biochemistry of Human Brain Tissue*, edited by E. Usdin and P. Riederer. London: Macmillan.
GERLACH, J. & LUHDORF, K. (1975) The effect of L-DOPA on young patients with simple schizophrenia treated with neuroleptic drugs. *Psychopharmacology*, **44**, 105–110.
HUGHES, J. S. & LITTLE, J. C. (1967) An appraisal of the continuing practice of prescribing tranquillizing drugs for long-stay psychiatric patients. *British Journal of Psychiatry*, **113**, 867–873.
KORNETSKY, C. (1976) Hyporesponsivity of chronic schizophrenic patients to dextroamphetamine. *Archives of General Psychiatry*, **33**, 1425–1428.
JOHNSTONE, E. C., CROW, T. J., FRITH, C. D., CARNEY, M. W. P. & PRICE, J. S. (1978a) Mechanism of the antipsychotic effect in the treatment of acute schizophrenia. *Lancet*, i, 848–851.
—— —— —— STEVENS, M., KREEL, L. & HUSBAND, J. (1978b) The dementia of dementia praecox. *Acta Psychiatrica Scandinavica*, **57**, 305–324.
LECRUBIER, Y., PUECH, A. J., WIDLOCHER, D. & SIMON, P. (1980) Schizophrenia: a bipolar dopaminergic hypothesis. Abstract no. 390. Proceedings of the 12th CINP Congress, Göteborg. *Progress in Neuro-psychopharmacology*, supplement.
LEE, T., SEEMAN, P., TOURTELLOTTE, W. W., FARLEY, I. J. & HORNYKIEWICZ, O. (1978) Binding of 3H-apomorphine and 3H-neuroleptics in schizophrenic brains. *Nature*, **274**, 897–900.
LETEMENDIA, F. J. J. & HARRIS, A. D. (1967) Chlorpromazine and the untreated chronic schizophrenic: a long-term trial. *British Journal of Psychiatry*, **113**, 950–958.
OWEN, F., CROSS, A. J., CROW, T. J., LONGDEN, A., POULTER, M. & RILEY, G. J. (1978) Increased dopamine receptor sensitivity in schizophrenia. *Lancet*, ii, 223–225.
OWENS, D. G. C. & JOHNSTONE, E. C. (1980) The disabilities of chronic schizophrenia—their nature and the factors contributing to their development. *British Journal of Psychiatry*, **136**, 384–395.
—— —— (1981) Neurological changes in a population of patients with chronic schizophrenia and their relationship to physical treatments. *Acta Psychiatrica Scandinavica*, Supplement 291, Vol 63, 103–109.

TSUANG, M. T. (1980) Thirty to 40 year follow-up of schizophrenia: outcome and stability of diagnosis. Paper presented to the Schizophrenia Group, The Wellcome Trust, 22 May 1980.
WEINBERGER, D. R., BIGELOW, L. B., KLEINMAN, J. E., KLEIN, S. T., ROSENBLATT, J. E. & WYATT, R. J. (1980) Cerebral ventricular enlargement in chronic schizophrenia associated with poor response to treatment. *Archives of General Psychiatry*, **37**, 11–13.
WING, J. K. (1978) Clinical concepts of schizophrenia. pp 1–30 in *Schizophrenia: Towards a New Synthesis*. Edited by J. K. Wing. London: Academic Press.

3. *G. W. Ashcroft* et al

We somewhat hesitantly enter the discussion regarding the nature of the schizophrenias. The relationship between the acute syndromes with 'positive symptoms' and the chronic 'defect' states is an old subject of debate. Recently the alleged occurrence of a high incidence of neurological abnormalities in the defect states, together with a relative failure to respond to neuroleptic therapy and a high hereditary predisposition, led Kety (**1980**) to suggest that two distinct disease entities were likely to be involved in the acute syndromes and defect states rather than different stages or outcome of a single condition. Dr Tim Crow added observations on ventricular size and cognitive functioning to the list of differences and coined the terms Type I and Type II to label the two conditions.

Two hypotheses were presented by Dr Tim Crow and Dr Angus Mackay relating the pathophysiology of the syndromes to changes in dopaminergic systems. Mackay regards the defect state and positive symptoms as both explicable in terms of changes in dopaminergic activity, whilst Crow regards the syndromes as 'independent dimensions reflecting different underlying pathological processes'. Both seem to regard the pathological basis of the defect state as irreversible, representing widespread but subtle brain damage.

Much of the evidence cited by Crow supporting the argument that different pathological processes underlie Type I and Type II syndromes of schizophrenia does not bear close scrutiny.

Kornetsky (1976) reporting the unremarkable effect of amphetamine on the symptomatology of chronic schizophrenics was clearly referring to Type I syndrome and not the Type II as implied by Crow. Thus Kornetsky stated of his patients 'they all exhibited an active thought disorder, delusional thinking, and in some cases hallucinations were present', and was clearly assessing change in these symptoms. His negative results contradict the unpublished results of Angrist quoted by Crow.

Crow stated 'In some chronic schizophrenic patients there is CT scan evidence of increased ventricular size (Johnstone *et al*, 1978a) and in these patients increased ventricular size is correlated with intellectual impairment and the presence of negative symptoms.' Yet in the results section of the paper, we are told that apart from correlations between some measures of cognitive function and measures of brain size: 'All other comparisons between measures of cerebral size and assessment of cognitive function or mental state were not significant.'

Crow cites the work of Johnstone *et al* (1978b) that 'in patients with acute schizophrenia, positive and not negative symptoms respond to neuroleptic medication.' This controversial finding was inherent in the methods of measurement, as change in the positive symptoms was much more likely to be detected than change in negative symptoms. For example, poverty of speech which made up half of the negative symptoms had a mean pre-treatment score of about 0.8 on a 4 point scale. On this scale (Krawiecka *et al*, 1977), a score of 1 for poverty of speech is given when the 'patient only speaks when spoken to, or tends to give brief replies'. This is contrasted with the mean pre-treatment scores of about 3.8 on a 4 point scale for positive symptoms of delusions and about 3.4 for hallucinations.

Acute syndromes with positive symptoms have a variable outcome and may end in complete remission, in recurrent acute episodes or in progression to a defect state. The defect state may be arrested at any stage and acute exacerbations of positive symptoms may be superimposed on the clinical picture at any stage. Defect states rarely occur without evidence of positive symptoms at some stage in the development of the illness and the concept of simple schizophrenia rarely stands up to careful scrutiny. These clinical observations seem to fit the idea of varying manifestations and outcome of a single process rather better than two different pathological processes. Any hypothesis must also take into account other clinical observations, e.g. the occurrence of Schneiderian first rank symptoms in mania and in organic brain disease and also in drug induced psychosis.

The following model is advanced as a possible alternative to those proposed by Mackay and Crow.

In the normal individual, dopaminergic activity will vary over a certain range which will never exceed the limits consistent with organized non-psychotic functioning. The pathological variations are possible using the two variables of dopaminergic activity and tolerated limits (Fig. 1).

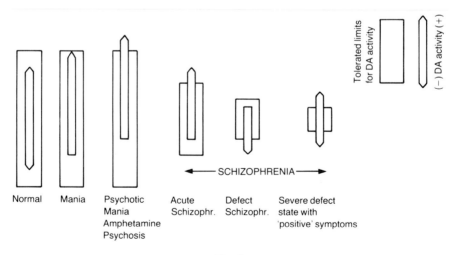

Fig. 1.

On this model the single abnormality distinguishing the acute schizophrenic syndrome and defect states from other states is a constriction of the tolerated range of dopaminergic activity. Thus situations which increase dopaminergic activity, e.g. stress, may result in psychotic symptoms, acute schizophrenic reaction (reactive schizophrenia, Type I schizophrenia).

Further constriction of the range will make attacks of acute symptoms more likely. As the range becomes markedly restricted, dopaminergic activity will fall below the lower limit for normal functioning—this may represent the defect state and in the extreme case there may be no range of dopaminergic activity consistent with normal functioning so that positive and negative symptoms may co-exist at all levels of dopaminergic activity.

Of course this model begs the question as to which neuronal systems are involved in determining the limits of tolerated dopaminergic activity. That these limits exist and show individual variation is demonstrated by the fact that widely different doses of amphetamine are required to precipitate psychotic symptoms in normal individuals.

Constriction of the range might follow selective brain damage as in temporal lobe lesions or Huntington's chorea or some of the cases described by Crow. The possibility, however, exists that there might be two types of constriction— one representing an inherited constriction—the other an acquired constriction.

What practical use is this model? It suggests the possibility that some way might be found to extend the limits of tolerated dopaminergic activity as an alternative to blocking the excess dopaminergic activity in the case of positive symptoms or increasing dopaminergic activity as suggested by Mackay in the defect states.

Since we know little of the factors involved in setting these limits, this may seem like looking for a needle in a haystack. However, we do have animal models which may allow us to study the changes of behaviour under dopaminergic stimulation and these may be used to identify means by which the range of dopaminergic stimulation consistent with the preservation of integrated behaviour patterns, may be extended. If the only justification for presenting another model is that it prevents opinions on schizophrenia from being fixed prematurely, then it may be serving a useful purpose.

References

JOHNSTONE, E. C., CROW, T. J., FRITH, C. D., STEVENS, M., KREEL, L. & HUSBAND, J. (1978a) The dementia of dementia praecox. *Acta Psychiatrica Scandinavica*, **57**, 305–324.
—— —— —— CARNEY, M. W. P. & PRICE, J. S. (1978b) Mechanism of the antipsychotic effect in the treatment of acute schizophrenia. *Lancet, i*, 848–851.
KETY, S. S. (1980) The syndrome of schizophrenia: unresolved questions and opportunities for research. *British Journal of Psychiatry*, **136**, 421–436.
KORNETSKY, C. (1976) Hyporesponsivity of chronic schizophrenic patients to dextroamphetamine. *Archives General Psychiatry*, **33**, 1425–1428.
KRAWIECKA, M., GOLDBERG, D. & VAUGHAN, M. (1977) A standardized psychiatric assessment scale for rating chronic psychotic patients. *Acta Psychiatrica Scandinavica*, **55**, 299–308.

4. T. J. Crow

Presumably one function of an hypothesis is to provoke further thought and observation. Therefore, I welcome the critical comments of Ashcroft and colleagues (**1981**) on my suggestion concerning the relationship between dopaminergic disturbances and the positive and negative symptoms of schizophrenia (Crow, 1980a; **1980b**). However, I think they have misunderstood the proposal and have underestimated some of the relevant evidence.

I believe the evidence for two processes is more compelling than they have conceded and I note that in their own hypothesis they have introduced two factors to account for phenomena that both Mackay (**1980**) and I regard as a problem for the simple dopamine theory.

Ashcroft *et al* liken my concept of two syndromes to the concept of two disease entities (corresponding to acute syndromes and defect states) which they attribute to Kety (**1980**). However, these concepts are by no means identical. The emphasis on *syndromes* rather than disease entities indicates that in many patients both syndromes are present either concurrently or sequentially. At one point in time, only one syndrome may be present as in acute schizophrenia (often equivalent to the Type I syndrome) or the defect state (the Type II syndrome, which can occur in the absence of positive symptoms). On the other hand many patients with the Type I syndrome later acquire the features of the Type II syndrome, and some patients have both from an early stage.

As I suggested in my review (Crow, 1980a), the presence of the Type II syndrome (carefully defined) delimits a group of illnesses of graver prognosis, corresponding more closely to classical or 'Kraepelinian' schizophrenia. The Type II syndrome may occur alone as in simple schizophrenia (an entity whose existence is doubted by Ashcroft *et al*), in the defect state when positive symptoms have disappeared, and sometimes I believe it may precede the onset of positive symptoms—as in the concept of childhood asociality propounded by Quitkin *et al* (1976).

The relationship proposed between the two syndromes is indicated in Fig. 2, together with the correspondence of the three-symptom constellations to various nosological terms of current or recent usage.

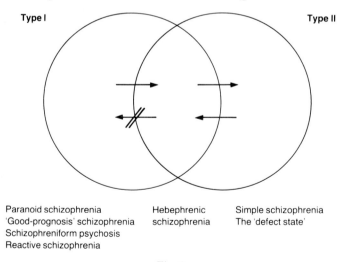

Paranoid schizophrenia
'Good-prognosis' schizophrenia
Schizophreniform psychosis
Reactive schizophrenia

Hebephrenic
schizophrenia

Simple schizophrenia
The 'defect state'

Fig. 2.

Of particular interest are the changes which may occur with the passage of time. Thus patients with the Type I syndrome commonly progress to acquire Type II symptoms and in due course some of these will lose their positive symptoms. Some may re-acquire them, i.e. experience acute exacerbations of psychosis. What I think is unusual, and if it does occur is worthy of note, is that patients with negative symptoms (the Type II syndrome) should lose these symptoms once they are established. According to my hypothesis this is because such symptoms are associated with a structural change in the brain.

Ashcroft *et al* have suggested that the dichotomization of schizophrenic symptoms and their attribution to different pathological processes is less well founded ('does not bear close scrutiny') than I have implied. Perhaps they were misled by the phrase 'This concept was based on ...' which I used to indicate that the concept had arisen from three studies conducted by my colleagues and myself at Northwick Park (Johnstone *et al*, 1976; 1978a; 1978b; Owen *et al*, 1978). The fact that these findings do not by themselves substantiate the hypothesis is neither here nor there. Hypotheses (which may arise from nothing more than speculation) are always at risk of being refuted by further observations. What one should ask is whether the hypothesis generates predictions and can these predictions be verified?

In fact the relationships we observed were not insubstantial and in each case they have been reinforced by later studies:

1. In our study of the two isomers of flupenthixol in the treatment of patients with acute schizophrenia (Johnstone *et al*, 1978b), while it is true that negative symptoms (flattening of affect as well as poverty of speech) were infrequent in this group of patients, it was apparent that when present they responded less well to medication than the positive symptoms. Thus each of the four positive symptoms showed greater change in absolute and percentage terms than the two negative symptoms and for three of the positive symptoms the final ratings on the α-isomer were lower than the final ratings of negative symptoms in the patients in whom these symptoms were present.

   The significance of the study of Angrist *et al* (1980) is that these workers were able to conduct an independent investigation of the non-responsiveness of negative symptoms to drugs acting on dopaminergic mechanisms. Symptoms were divided into positive and negative categories after the original observations had been completed; thus the authors had not anticipated the finding that only positive symptoms would be exacerbated by amphetamine and diminished by neuroleptics.

   Ashcroft *et al* suggest that the findings of Angrist *et al* (which were not available to them) are 'contradicted' by the results of Kornetsky (1976). Kornetsky found that some chronic schizophrenic patients were relatively resistant to amphetamine, a finding which I think is at least consistent with the possibility that such patients are likely to have more negative symptoms than patients with acute schizophrenia, but he did not assess the two groups of symptoms separately. Thus the study of Angrist *et al* is more relevant to the hypothesis, and in the absence of the critical assessments of positive and negative symptoms the Kornetsky study can hardly be used as evidence against it.

2. In our CT studies of ventricular size in chronic schizophrenia (Johnstone *et al*, 1976; 1978a) although the number of patients was not large (13 when those with leucotomies had been excluded) there was a highly significant ($P < 0.01$) relationship between ventricular size and impaired intellectual performance as assessed by the most relevant of the tests that we used—the

Withers and Hinton tests of the sensorium (the findings are given in Table 8 of Johnstone *et al*, 1978a). Other tests employed were repeating digits forward and backwards (neither can be considered incisive tests of intellectual impairment) and a memory-for-faces test devised by Frith (1977). Findings on these tests were in the same direction as the Withers and Hinton finding but did not reach significance (see Table 5 of Johnstone *et al.*(1978a) for differences between groups and Table 6 for relationships between intellectual function as indicated by these tests and other clinical features).

The relationship between ventricular size and intellectual impairment in schizophrenia suggested by this study has been amply confirmed by further work by Donnelly *et al* (1980) using the Halstead-Reitan tests and Golden *et al* (1980) using the Luria-Nebraska test battery, both in chronic institutionalized groups of patients, and in a small group of out-patients by Rieder *et al* (1979).

With respect to the relationship between ventricular size and schizophrenic symptoms the correlation coefficient was -0.24 for positive and 0.38 for negative symptoms (Table 3 of Johnstone *et al*, 1976). Negative symptoms were strongly related to intellectual impairment (Table 6 of Johnstone *et al*, 1978a).

Subsequent studies have confirmed the latter relationship. Thus in the survey by Owens and Johnstone (1980) negative symptoms were strongly related to intellectual impairment ($P < 0.001$) but were not significantly related to positive symptoms. A much larger CT scan study now being analysed will further test the prediction concerning ventricular size and the presence of negative symptoms.

3. In our post-mortem studies (Owen *et al*, 1978) we found dopamine receptors assessed by butyrophenone binding to be increased. According to the hypothesis this change relates to the type I syndrome and our more recent investigations (Crow *et al*, 1981) have shown it to be significantly related to positive but not negative symptoms.

In my discussion with Mackay, I drew attention to other recent findings which are consistent with the view that there are two dimensions of pathology in illnesses commonly described as schizophrenic. What I claim for this hypothesis is that it makes predictions that, at least in principle, are testable. Thus although there may be discussion concerning the ways in which positive and negative symptoms, ventricular size and other structural brain changes, intellectual impairment and even dopamine receptors should be assessed, it is clear that it is in terms of these variables that the hypothesis should be tested.

It is of some interest that the concept advanced by Ashcroft *et al* also includes two variables: (i) tolerated limits of dopaminergic activity; and (ii) the extent to which dopaminergic activity exceeds the upper or lower or both of these limits.

The second variable determines whether positive or negative symptoms are seen, according to whether levels of dopaminergic activity are respectively above or below the 'tolerated limits'. However, even if the level of tolerance (variable i) is reduced to zero it is difficult to see how this concept can explain the simultaneous presence of positive and negative symptoms. Ashcroft and colleagues concede that the concept of tolerated limits is ill-defined in that it 'begs the question as to which neuronal systems are involved'. Since this variable is undefined in terms of any quantity that can be observed (e.g. intellectual impairment or ventricular size) it is difficult to see what testable predictions are generated.

Both Ashcroft and Marsden (*Journal*, March 1981, **138**, 269–70) consider the possibility that increased dopaminergic activity is as relevant to mania as to schizophrenia and Marsden includes also confusional states. This point is well taken. With respect to the confusional states systematic observations are difficult to come by but one might suppose that while behaviour is controlled by neuroleptic drugs (perhaps by dopamine receptor blockade) there may be certain features (e.g. disorientation) which are not improved.

The case of mania is an interesting one and a role for dopaminergic disturbances has been suggested (Randrup *et al*, 1975). However the argument for specific dopaminergic effects in mania is as yet not so compelling as in schizophrenia. For example, whereas it has been clearly demonstrated in schizophrenia that a neuroleptic with weak anti-dopaminergic activity such as promazine is less active than the more potent dopamine antagonist chlorpromazine (Casey *et al*, 1960) this has not yet been demonstrated for mania. Thus while the case for associating dopamine with mania is less convincing than that for the type I syndrome of schizophrenia it cannot be concluded that it will be possible to distinguish mania and schizophrenia on these grounds. Further investigations of this point are required and we will undertake these at Northwick Park.

References

ANGRIST, B. M., ROTROSEN, J. & GERSHON, S. (1980) Differential effects of amphetamine and neuroleptics on negative vs positive symptoms in schizophrenia. *Psychopharmacology*, **72,** 17–19.

ASHCROFT, G. W. *et al* (1981) Positive and negative schizophrenic symptoms and the role of dopamine. *British Journal of Psychiatry*, **138**, 268–269.

CASEY, J. F., BENNETT, I. F., LINDLEY, C. J., HOLLISTER, L. E., GORDON, M. H. & SPRINGER, N. N. (1960) Drug therapy in schizophrenia. A controlled study of the relative effectiveness of chlorpromazine, promazine, phenobarbital and placebo. *Archives of General Psychiatry*, **2,** 210–220.

CROW, T. J. (1980a) Molecular pathology of schizophrenia: more than one disease process? *British Medical Journal*, **280,** 66–68.

—— (1980b) Positive and negative schizophrenic symptoms and the role of dopamine. *British Journal of Psychiatry*, **137,** 383–386.

—— OWEN, F., CROSS, A. J., FERRIER, I. N., JOHNSTONE, E. C., McCREADIE, R. G., OWENS, D. G. C. & POULTER, M. (1981) Neurotransmitter enzymes and receptors in post-mortem brain in schizophrenia: evidence that an increase in D2 receptors is associated with the type I syndrome. In *Transmitter Biochemistry of Human Brain Tissue* (eds. E. Usdin and P. Riederer). London: Macmillan.

DONNELLY, E. F., WEINBERGER, D. R., WALDMAN, I. N. & WYATT, R. J. (1980) Cognitive impairment associated with morphological brain abnormalities on computed tomography in chronic schizophrenic patients. *Journal of Nervous, Mental Disorders*, **168,** 305–308.

FRITH, C. D. (1977) Two kinds of cognitive deficit associated with chronic schizophrenia. *Psychological Medicine*, **7,** 171–173.

GOLDEN, C. J., MOSES, J. A., ZELAKOWSKI, R., GRABER, R., ZATZ, L. M., HORVATH, T. B. & BERGER, P. A. (1980) Cerebral ventricular size and neuropsychological impairment in young chronic schizophrenics. *Archives General Psychiatry*, **37,** 619–623.

JOHNSTONE, E. C., CROW, T. J., FRITH, C. D., HUSBAND, J. & KREEL, L. (1976) Cerebral ventricular size and cognitive impairment in chronic schizophrenia. *Lancet*, ii, 924–926.

—— CROW, T. J., FRITH, C. D., STEVENS, M., KREEL, L. & HUSBAND, J. (1978a) The dementia of dementia praecox. *Acta Psychiatrica Scandinavica*, **57,** 305–324.

—— —— —— Carney, M. W. P. & Price, J. S. (1978b) Mechanism of the antipsychotic effect in the treatment of acute schizophrenia. *Lancet, i*, 848–851.

Kety, S. (1980) The syndrome of schizophrenia: unresolved questions and opportunities for research. *British Journal of Psychiatry*, **136,** 421–436.

Kornetsky, C. (1976) Hyporesponsivity of chronic schizophrenic patients to dextroamphetamine. *Archives of General Psychiatry*, **33,** 1425–1428.

Mackay, A. V. P. (1980) Positive and negative schizophrenic symptoms and the role of dopamine. *British Journal of Psychiatry*, **137,** 379–383.

Owen, F., Cross, A. J., Crow, T. J., Longden, A., Poulter, M. & Riley, G. J. (1978) Increased dopamine receptor sensitivity in schizophrenia. *Lancet, ii*, 223–225.

Owens, D. G. C. & Johnstone, E. C. (1980) The disabilities of chronic schizophrenia—their nature and the factors contributing to their development. *British Journal of Psychiatry*, **136,** 384–395.

Quitkin, F., Rifkin, A. & Klein, D. F. (1976) Neurologic soft signs in schizophrenia and character disorder. *Archives of General Psychiatry*, **33,** 845–853.

Randrup, A., Munkvad, I., Fog, R., Gerlach, J., Molander, L., Kjellberg, B. & Scheel-Kruger, J. (1975) Mania, depression and brain dopamine. In *Current Developments in Psychopharmacology*, Vol. 2 (eds. W. B. Essman and L. Valzelli). New York: Spectrum.

Rieder, R. O., Donnelly, E. F., Herdt, J. R. & Waldman, N. (1979) Sulcal prominence in young chronic schizophrenic patients: CT scan findings associated with impairment on neuropsychological tests. *Psychiatric Research*, **1,** 1–8.

22 Schizophrenia as an infectious disease

E. H. HARE

Attention has recently been given to the idea that a virus infection may be causal for a common type of schizophrenia, and the evidence in support has been summarized by Torrey (1973a), by Torrey and Peterson (1974), and by Kety (1978). Since then, Tyrrell *et al* (1979) have reported a virus-like agent in the cerebrospinal fluid of about one-third of 28 schizophrenic patients, and though their work has yet to be confirmed it provides an opportunity for reconsidering the epidemiological aspects of the viral hypothesis.

Epidemiological studies in schizophrenia are hampered by the subjectivity of diagnosis and by the fact, or the probability, that 'schizophrenia' is an end-state of many disease processes. Nevertheless, there are certain broad patterns of incidence and distribution which perhaps are clear enough to be used for the promotion of causal hypotheses.

One of the more firmly established of such patterns is the excess of winter births in schizophrenics. This can be explained either as due to an abnormal pattern of parental conception or to some seasonally varying factor causing foetal or perinatal damage which increases any genetic risk for schizophrenia. Present evidence seems slightly to favour the damage hypothesis (Kinney and Jacobsen, 1978). Such seasonal damage is as likely to be nutritional or obstetric as due to a virus; but the instance of congenital rubella (Dudgeon, 1973) shows that virus infection can cause the kind of seasonal birth pattern found in schizophrenia. The fact that schizophrenia is equally common in the sexes argues against a causal factor acting during foetal life (Shields and Gottesman, 1977), and this is supported by the evidence that the offspring of schizophrenic fathers are as much at risk of schizophrenia as those of schizophrenic mothers (Kety *et al*, 1975).

The incidence of schizophrenia varies with occupational and social status. If low status were a causal association, then it might well reflect an increased risk for a causal viral infection. But present evidence strongly supports the alternative view that low status is an effect, not a cause, of the illness. Similarly, the high rates of schizophrenia found in some migrant populations are best explained in terms of selection for high genetic risk. Again, the high rate of schizophrenia which has been found to persist in a North-Swedish population is attributed by Böök *et al* (1978) to selection and in-breeding rather than to environmental factors.

Geographical variations in the incidence of a disease are a fruitful source of causal hypotheses; but to an epidemiologist, the rarity of such variations for schizophrenia is both a surprise and a disappointment. The lack of variation might simply reflect an insufficiently sensitive technique, but there is also the possibility that a type of schizophrenia due to a virus began in a particular place, perhaps from a mutation, and has since spread everywhere. This possibility has been framed in the question: is schizophrenia a disease of civilization (Torrey, 1973b)? Insanity was formerly thought to be rare or absent in cultures remote from the industrialized world. More recent observers have found it not uncommon and have concluded that the older opinion was a myth. But in a recent study by Torrey *et al* (1974) in Papua New Guinea, schizophrenia-like states were found to be rare in the remote tribes and commoner in those more in contact with western culture; and indeed, the increase in cases was related to births occurring at the time of the cultural contact. There is a parallel here with general paralysis, which was at first thought to be absent or rare in remote societies, and was later found to be fairly common. The question then arose whether the early observations had been incorrect or whether the societies had acquired the disease through contact with western civilization (Hare, 1959).

The evidence that, within the western world, there have been variations in the incidence and type of schizophrenia over the years is uncertain and conflicting. This is not surprising for an ill-defined disease which was only characterized in the 1880s. But three aspects of the problem may be noted. First, schizophrenia of the Kraepelinian type—that is, a condition with auditory hallucinations, delusions, a chronic course to mental deterioration and an onset typically in early adult life—presents a dramatic picture, and it is therefore curious that there are no descriptions of any such state before the 19th century. Secondly, the alienists of the 19th century were much exercised by the question whether insanity was on the increase. Statistical data in Britain are inadequate to answer this before about 1860, and thereafter interpretations have differed. Third, there is some agreement on changes in the severity and the manifestations of schizophrenia over the past 40 years. The 'profound dementia' which Kraepelin considered the characteristic end-state is rarely seen today; the subtype of catatonia has almost disappeared; and the prognosis, both for clinical and social outcome, has steadily improved.

Explanations are not hard to find. Thus, it may be maintained that schizophrenia has always been as common as now (Altschule, 1976) but was unrecognized as a syndrome before the 19th century—except perhaps by Willis (Cranfield, 1961); or that schizophrenia only became common during the 19th century, and this was due to the social effect of population density (Cooper and Sartorius, 1977); and that the recent changes are either the consequence of better medical treatment, or due to better general health (from improved nutrition, smaller families and fewer infections) leading to increased resistance to diseases of many kinds. But if it were the case that poor-prognosis schizophrenia was rare before the 19th century, became common then and has since been changing in its nature, this could be understood in terms of the explanation proposed by McKeown (1976) and by Fenner (1971) for the variations in incidence and severity of a number of infectious diseases which became common at the time of the Industrial Revolution. Thus (the argument would run), a type of schizophrenia due to an infectious agent became common in the 19th century either because of a mutation or because the high population density in cities facilitated transmission; and now gradually, through increased host resistance or a change in the organism, is becoming less severe.

It may be noticed that, if schizophrenia has always been common, then its persistence in spite of the low fertility of schizophrenics is hard to explain; whereas if it only became common during the last two centuries, this difficulty disappears. Again, if it were the case that severe schizophrenia was formerly rare in non-westernized societies and is only now becoming common, this could be explained in terms of a gradual spread of an infectious type of schizo-phrenia from some centre in the western world; and if this spread is still incomplete, that in turn could explain the better prognosis of schizophrenia which has been found in less developed parts of the world.

There is at present no established evidence for any environmental cause in common schizophrenia; and indeed it is possible that there are no causes of any useful degree of specificity (Boklage, 1977). The viral hypothesis has much explanatory power; but it is one which is likely to seem strange to the clinician and is perhaps essentially less plausible than some competing hypoth-eses. Meanwhile we await the results of further laboratory study.

References

ALTSCHULE, M. (1976) Historical perspective—evolution of the concept of schizophrenia. In *The Biology of the Schizophrenic Process* (ed. S. Wolf and B. Berle). Plenn Press.

BOKLAGE, C. E. (1977) Schizophrenia, brain asymmetry and twinning: cellular relationship with etiological and possibly prognostic implications. *Biological Psychiatry*, **12**, 19–35.

BÖÖK, J. A., WETTERBERG, L., MODRZEWSKA, K. & UNGE, C. (1978) *Clinical Genetics*, **13**, 110.

COOPER, C. & SARTORIUS, N. (1977) Cultural and temporal variations in schizophrenia: a specula-tion on the importance of industrialization. *British Journal of Psychiatry*, **130**, 50–55.

CRANFIELD, P. F. (1961) A seventeenth century view of mental deficiency and schizophrenia. Thomas Willis' 'stupidity or foolishness'. *Bulletin of the History of Medicine*, **35**, 291–316.

DUDGEON, J. A., PECKHAM, C. S., MARSHALL, W. C., SMITHELLS, R. W. & SHEPPARD, S. (1973) National congenital rubella surveillance programme. *Health Trends*, **5**, 75–79.

FENNER, F. (1971) Infectious disease and social change. *Medical Journal of Australia*, **1**, 1043–1047 and 1099–1102.

HARE, E. H. (1959) The origin and spread of dementia paralytica. *Journal of Mental Science*, **105**, 594–626.

KETY, S. S. (1978) Schizophrenia: the challenge and the prospects of biologic research. *Birth Defects: Original Article Series*, Vol. XIV, No. 5. Pp. 5–15 (ed. A. L. Goldstein). New York: Alan Liss.

—— ROSENTHAL, D., WENDER, P. H., SCHULSINGER, F. & JACOBSEN, B. (1975) Mental illness in the biological and adoptive families of adopted individuals who have become schizophrenic. In *Genetic Research in Psychiatry* (ed. R. Fieve, D. Rosenthal, and H. Brill). Baltimore: Johns Hopkins University Press.

KINNEY, D. K. & JACOBSEN, B. (1978) Environmental factors in schizophrenia: new adoption study evidence. In *The Nature of Schizophrenia* (ed. L. C. Wynne, R. L. Cromwell and S. Matthysse). New York: Wiley.

MCKEOWN, T. (1976) *The Role of Medicine: Dream, Mirage or Nemesis*. London: Nuffield Provincial Hospitals Trust.

SHIELDS, J. & GOTTESMAN, I. I. (1977) Obstetric complications and twin studies in schizophrenia: clarifications and affirmations. *Schizophrenia Bulletin*, **3**, 351–354.

TORREY, E. F. (1973a) Slow and latent viruses in schizophrenia. *Lancet*, *ii*, 22–24.

—— (1973b) Is schizophrenia universal? An open question. *Schizophrenia Bulletin*, **7**, 53–59.

—— & PETERSON, M. R. (1974) Schizophrenia and the limbic system. *Lancet*, *ii*, 942–946.

—— TORREY, B. B. & BURTON-BRADLEY, B. G. (1974) The epidemiology of schizophrenia in Papua New Guinea. *American Journal of Psychiatry*, **131**, 567–573.

TYRRELL, D. A. J., CROW, T. J., PARRY, R. P., JOHNSTONE, EVE & FERRIER, I. N. (1979) Possible virus in schizophrenia and some neurological disorders. *Lancet*, *i*, 839–841.

23 The interaction of seasonality, place of birth, genetic risk and subsequent schizophrenia in a high-risk sample

RICARDO A. MACHÓN, SARNOFF A. MEDNICK and FINI SCHULSINGER

Winter births produce a slight excess of individuals later diagnosed as schizophrenic (Barry and Barry, 1961; Hare and Price, 1968). Of particular significance are large population studies (Dalén, 1968; 1975; Ødegård, 1974; Videbech et al, 1974), southern hemisphere studies (Dalén and Roche, in Dalén, 1975; Parker and Neilson, 1976), and equatorial studies (Parker and Balza, 1977), which have all yielded convergent results. This repeated observation has led to the hope that understanding of this relationship might suggest a useful aetiological hypothesis for at least some forms of schizophrenia. In view of the greater prevalence of viral infections during winter (Hope-Simpson, 1981) and other related evidence, some researchers have speculated on the possibility that viral infections are somehow involved in the aetiology of some forms of schizophrenia (Torrey and Peterson, 1976; Torrey, 1980).

An independent body of work has established that genetically transmitted characteristics combine in some way with environmental factors in the development of schizophrenia. This gene-environment interaction has received considerable attention in studies of the pregnancy and delivery of those who later became schizophrenic, and in studies of individuals born to schizophrenic mothers (McNeil and Kaij, 1978). Mednick (1970) has suggested that perinatal difficulties in deliveries involving high-risk children have unique consequences for their nervous system development. Pregnant schizophrenic women have been shown to produce an excess number of still-births and offspring with congenital anomalies (Sobel, 1961; Rieder et al, 1975). These perinatal deaths and anomalies perhaps are the extreme manifestation of a process attacking the high-risk foetus; in less extreme forms this process may result in some nervous system damage which predisposes some high-risk individuals to schizophrenia. Of some significance, in this context, are the results of population studies which indicate that maternal viral infections (Type A influenza) during pregnancy yield a modest excess of congenital anomalies; the most frequent foetal organ system damaged by the viral infection is the central nervous system (Campbell, 1953; Coffey and Jessop, 1959; Saxén et al, 1960).

Based on these bits of evidence, the general hypothesis was entertained that some forms of schizophrenia may result from perinatal viral infections which specifically attack the nervous system of genetically vulnerable foetuses. Some predictions of this general hypothesis were examined in the context of an ongoing, prospective study of Danish children at high-risk for schizophrenia. The Danish high-risk project unfortunately does not have a record of perinatal viral infections. In view of the marked seasonal variation of viral infections (particularly influenza), however, one could safely hypothesize that such infections were more prevalent in the winter and early spring in the years the children were born (Hope-Simpson, 1981). Further, it was assumed that such viral infections were more likely in circumstances which favour the spread of the infection. Pregnant women who work and live in crowded urban conditions, who regularly use mass transportation and mass entertainment and who work in close proximity to others are much more likely to encounter the products of coughs and sneezes. Thus, they are more likely to be exposed to a viral infection while pregnant and/or more likely to transmit it to their newly born children.

The research hypothesis is: genetically vulnerable individuals, born in the winter or early spring months, in an urban area, are more likely to have been damaged by a viral infection and to show the results of these infections in poorer psychological adjustment and a higher likelihood of a schizophrenia diagnosis. In analysis of variance (ANOVA) terminology, a third-order interaction (genetic risk × urban v. non-urban birth place × season of birth) is hypothesized. It must be stressed that all three factors when present *in combination* will be related to later psychological impairment.

The study

Subjects: The sample is drawn from a prospective, longitudinal study begun in Denmark in 1962 by Mednick and Schulsinger (1968). The high-risk (HR) group (at risk for schizophrenia) is composed of 207 offspring of chronic and severely schizophrenic mothers. The low-risk (LR) group comprises 104 children with no known mental illness in their family for two previous generations. Individuals in both groups, normally functioning at the start of the project, had an average age of 15.1 years (range 9–20). The subjects were contacted during 1972–74 and underwent an extended clinical and diagnostic interview. In the HR and LR groups respectively, 173 (83.6 per cent) and 91 (87.5 per cent) completed the full assessment and diagnosis protocol (Schulsinger, 1976).

Measures: Two criterion variables were used: (a) one was the dichotomous diagnosis of schizophrenia and non-schizophrenia. For this purpose, three techniques contributed to the diagnosis of schizophrenia: (1) the current section of the CAPPS (Current and Past Psychopathology Scales) and its corresponding computer-processed programme Diagno II (Endicott and Spitzer, 1972); (2) the PSE (Present State Examination, 9th Edition) and its computer-processed programme CATEGO (Wing *et al*, 1974); (3) a clinical diagnosis based on an extensive interview. A consensus diagnosis, based on agreement of at least two of the three diagnostic methods, became the basis for a diagnosis of schizophrenia.

In view of the relatively small number of subjects, it was decided to use an additional, *continuous* measure of psychopathology, namely (b) level of adjustment or severity of mental illness. For this purpose, the PSE Index of Definition of Syndromes ('Caseness') and CAPPS Severity of Illness (item no. 471) scales were used. The PSE 'Caseness' measure indicates (on a scale of 1–9) the extent to which a subject resembles a hospitalized psychiatric patient. The CAPPS Severity is a rating (on a 1–6 scale) made by the interviewer of the degree of mental illness shown by the subjects. A higher score on both scales reflects greater severity of mental illness. Interrater reliability for the CAPPS Severity of Illness scale is 0.77 (Endicott and Spitzer, 1972). In this study, the PSE 'Caseness' (a computer rating) and CAPPS Severity (rated by trained interviewers) scales correlated 0.70.

Season of birth was defined as winter versus non-winter birth, taking January, February, and March as winter and the rest of the year (April through December) as non-winter months. The first quarter of the year (January– March) was most appropriate for the present purposes; the work of Hope-Simpson (1981) has suggested that these months are dramatically and reliably high viral epidemic months, particularly for influenza. The Hope-Simpson data are from England; Dr Mednick's work with Danish Health statistics indicates that these findings apply equally to Denmark.

Urban births were defined as those occurring in the greater Copenhagen area. Copenhagen was the only Danish city in the late 1940s with a population of approximately one million. The second largest city in Denmark, Aarhus, had only a population of 110,000 (Hammond and Co., Inc., 1949). Births occurring in the remainder of Denmark were therefore considered non-urban.

It is hypothesized that certain pregnancy conditions (genetic risk-urban environment-winter delivery) will increase the probability of outcomes with poor mental health, including schizophrenia.

Schizophrenia/non-schizophrenia analysis: Only the HR group was considered in this analysis since only one LR subject had a diagnosis of schizophrenia. The per cent of consensus-diagnosed schizophrenics in each condition showed that urban births (12 per cent) yielded a marginally higher rate of schizophrenia than the non-urban births (4 per cent) (Fisher's exact probability test, $P < .078$, one-tailed).

As hypothesized, the highest rate of schizophrenia is observed in the high-risk urban-winter births (23.3 per cent). These three factors increase the risk of schizophrenia considerably over the general population base rate of approximately 1 per cent, or the HR base rate of 8.9 per cent. Among the urban births, significantly more schizophrenics result from winter births (23.3 per cent) as opposed to non-winter births (8.4 per cent) (Fisher's exact probability test, $P < .028$, one tailed). It may be worth pointing out that among the urban births, about as many schizophrenics were born in the three winter months (7) as were born in the remaining nine months (8). The differences among the non-urban births are not significant.

Severity of mental illness analyses: As hypothesized, the highest degree of psychopathology was found for the HR urban-winter births.

Analyses were performed using the General Linear Model (GLM) supplied by Statistical Analysis System (SAS Institute Inc., 1979) on both the PSE 'Caseness' score and the CAPPS Severity rating. The GLM programme is appropriate for analyses with unbalanced cell sizes. It uses a regression approach to the analysis of variance.

The hypothesized three-way interaction was significant. As a main effect, high risk status results in more severe psychopathology scores on both dependent measures while urban birth place was significant only for CAPPS Severity rating.

The HR-winter-urban birth group evidenced a higher severity of illness (on both CAPPS Severity and PSE 'Caseness' scales) than all the LR groups (all comparisons $P < .02$), and when compared to the other HR groups, differed only from the HR-winter non-urban group ($P < .03$).

ANOVAs leaving out the schizophrenics: There was concern that the disproportionate number of schizophrenics in the HR-urban non-winter birth condition was accounting entirely for the significant third-order interaction. ANOVAs were performed leaving the schizophrenics out of the analyses. The third-order interaction remained, but it was only marginally significant ($P < .08$). These results suggest that the seasonality-place of birth effect may not simply relate to the diagnosis of schizophrenia but also has relevance to lesser degrees of psychological disturbance.

Comment

Within the context of a high-risk for schizophrenia project, the implications of the viral hypothesis were considered, and some specific predictions were made. In part, the predictions expressed themselves in the form of a third-order ANOVA interaction which was significant. Genetically vulnerable individuals born in winter months (in which there are high frequencies of viral infections) in an urban setting had the highest rates of schizophrenia and the poorest level of psychological adjustment. It is worth emphasizing that the rate of schizophrenia for the genetically vulnerable, winter-urban born reached 23.3 per cent which is considerably above population base rates of schizophrenia (1 per cent), or rates for HR subjects in this population at this time (8.9 per cent). The specific predictions of the viral hypothesis were not rejected. It must be quickly pointed out that these predictions were indirect in the sense that it was not known whether the foetuses or neonates actually suffered a viral attack.

Kinney and Jacobsen (1978), working with a subgroup of Kety and Rosenthal's Danish adoption population, have examined the relationship between season of birth and risk and later schizophrenia. Unfortunately, it is difficult to compare both sets of findings. While the present study's criterion of risk involves having a severely schizophrenic mother, their criteria also included post-natal brain damage. It is also difficult to determine whether the perinatal circumstances surrounding an adoption in some way interacted with the rural-urban or season of birth factors. During the time of these adoptions the adoption agency had a stated policy of attempting to place adoptees at some geographical distance from their biological parents (Mothers Aid Organization for Copenhagen, Copenhagen County and Frederiksborg County, Annual Report for 1946–47). Thus, while Kinney and Jacobsen studied adoptees in the Greater Copenhagen area, it is not clear what proportion were actually born outside of Copenhagen. This would influence the results, since without consideration of place of birth the present study would not have found a seasonality effect.

Plausible alternative explanations

The complexity of the third-order interaction has made it difficult to find alternative explanations of these results. However, some plausible hypotheses will be considered which could explain, in part, the present findings:

1. Procreational patterns by parents of schizophrenics, which might differ from those of the general population, have been proposed as the grounds for the excess of winter schizophrenic births (Huntington, 1938; Hare and Price, 1968; James, 1978). No support for this hypothesis was found. High-risk individuals (27 per cent) did not have significantly more winter births than low-risk individuals (25 per cent).

2. Lewis and Griffin (1981) have devised a correction technique and have shown that the reported excess of winter-born schizophrenics can be explained on the basis of the age-prevalence effect, a methodological artefact. This effect, the authors show, has a negligible influence after age 23. In the present study, the sample of individuals assessed in 1972 had a mean age of 23.7 years and the group diagnosed schizophrenic was somewhat older (mean age of 24.5 years). Thus, these results cannot be explained by the age-prevalence effect.

Watson *et al* (1982) applied the suggested correction technique for the age-prevalence effect and failed to replicate Lewis and Griffin's findings. These authors speculated that the effects of the age-prevalence factor are minimal, at least when severe climates prevail. The source of both the present data (based on a Danish sample) and that of Watson *et al* (based on a Minnesota sample) are similar in that severe winters prevail in these places; Lewis and Griffin's findings are based on data from Missouri, which is affected by a relatively milder climate.

3. It was assumed that an urban environment (interacting with HR and winter birth) favoured the contracting of a viral infection by the mother or infant due to increased likelihood of contact with other people. Other conditions which are associated with urban living, like greater noise, crowding, air pollution, and psychological stress could possibly interact with genetic risk. However, it is not immediately apparent why these urban factors should have a greater influence in January, February, and March. These data do not permit a closer study of the urban–non-urban variable.

4. The assumption was made that a birth occurring during the winter season would increase the likelihood of the foetus or neonate (directly or indirectly through the mother) contracting a viral infection. However other *non-viral* factors, seasonal in nature, could in fact account for the observed seasonality of schizophrenic births (Torrey, 1980). Certain protein deficiencies, commonly occurring during the summer months (the crucial first trimester for the winter births), could be reasonably hypothesized as producing the brain damage which eventually leads to some forms of schizophrenia. In the same manner other nutritional deficiencies (like vitamins C and K) which are more common during the winter have been proposed as explaining the seasonality effect. These alternative, non-viral hypotheses could just as well explain the observed findings, although it is not clear why they would restrict themselves to an urban environment.

5. Carter and Watts (1971) have shown that the relatives of schizophrenics tend to be more resistant to viral infections than people in the general

population. Predictions based on their findings would suggest that the season of birth effect should be more dramatic in the present study's *low-risk* group, where these mothers would be more susceptible to viral infections than their high-risk counterparts. The results are not in agreement with these predictions since the effect was greatest in the high-risk group. It is worth noting that Carter and Watts' data are based on a much broader definition of relative which pools not only mothers (the only relative to form the present investigation's high-risk group) but other family members as well. The results of both studies are therefore not directly comparable. At the same time, one could entertain the hypothesis that the non-schizophrenic relatives of schizophrenics were protected from the illness because of their greater resistance to viral infections. Thus the findings of this study may not be entirely inconsistent with those of Carter and Watts.

6. It was hypothesized that a child born during the winter months was more susceptible to suffering CNS damage due to a viral infection than someone born in a non-winter month. But a majority of this latter group (the non-winter born) also would have passed some earlier stage of foetal development during the high viral infection months. Theoretically, then, they would be just as likely to have been damaged by the viral infection; yet the findings did not support this hypothesis. Why was a viral infection during the winter perinatal period more crucial in terms of predicting schizophrenia than an infection earlier in pregnancy (non-winter birth)? One might speculate that, once born, the infant is no longer protected by the mother's immune system and is therefore more susceptible to the damaging effects of an infection. In addition, infections at earlier stages of pregnancy, particularly the first trimester, are associated with gross congenital malformations (Saxén *et al*, 1960; Torrey and Peterson, 1976). Infections occurring later in pregnancy might be associated with more subtle, and less readily noticeable CNS damage. This in turn might produce effects on behaviour which are delayed until higher level functioning is demanded of the developing individual. Unfortunately, again, the nature of the present data do permit a closer inspection of these and other plausible hypotheses.

In summary, several predictions from a viral hypothesis of the aetiology of schizophrenia have been tested. The results have not disconfirmed the hypothesis. It must be stressed, though, that this investigation represented only an indirect test. It was not known in each individual case whether a perinatal viral infection was contracted. However, the probability of such viral infections are remarkably higher in the months of January, February, and March in Denmark. We are planning a population study to make a more direct test of the viral hypothesis of schizophrenia.

References

BARRY, H. & BARRY, H. (1961) Season of birth. *Archives of General Psychiatry*, **5**, 292–300.

CAMPBELL, W. A. B. (1953) Influenza in early pregnancy: effects on the foetus. *Lancet, i*, 173–174.

CARTER, M. & WATTS, C. A. H. (1971) Possible biological advantages among schizophrenics' relatives. *British Journal of Psychiatry*, **118**, 453–460.

COFFEY, V. P. & JESSOP, W. J. E. (1959) Maternal influenza and congenital deformities: a prospective study. *Lancet, ii*, 935–938.

DALÉN, P. (1968) Month of birth and schizophrenia. *Acta Psychiatrica Scandinavica*, Suppl. **203**, 55–60.

—— (1975) *Season of Birth: A Study of Schizophrenia and Other Mental Disorders*. Amsterdam: North-Holland Publishing Co.

ENDICOTT, J. & SPITZER, R. (1972) Current and past psychopathology scales (CAPPS). *Archives of General Psychiatry*, **27**, 678–687.

HAMMOND, C. S. & CO., INC. (1949) *Hammond's New Liberty World Atlas*. New York: C. S. Hammond & Co., Inc.

HARE, E. H. & PRICE, J. S. (1968) Mental disorder and season of birth: comparison of psychoses with neurosis. *British Journal of Psychiatry*, **115**, 533–540.

HOPE-SIMPSON, R. E. (1981) The role of season in the epidemiology of influenza. *Journal of Hygiene*, **86**, 35–47.

HUNTINGTON, E. (1938) *Season of Birth. Its Relation to Human Abilities*. New York: John Wiley & Sons, Inc.

JAMES, W. H. (1978) Seasonality in schizophrenia. *Lancet*, i, 664.

KINNEY, D. K. & JACOBSEN, B. (1978) Environmental factors in schizophrenia: new adoption study evidence. In *The Nature of Schizophrenia: New Approaches to Research and Treatment* (eds. L. C. Wynne, R. L. Cromwell and S. Matthysse). New York: John Wiley & Sons, Inc.

LEWIS, M. S. & GRIFFIN, P. A. (1981) An explanation of the season of birth effect in schizophrenia and certain other diseases. *Psychological Bulletin*, **89**, 589–596.

McNEIL, T. F. & KAIJ, L. (1978) Obstetric factors in the development of schizophrenia: complications in the births of preschizophrenics and in reproduction by schizophrenic parents. In *The Nature of Schizophrenia: New Approaches to Research and Treatment* (eds. L. C. Wynne, R. L. Cromwell and S. Matthysse). New York: John Wiley & Sons, Inc.

MEDNICK, S. A. (1970) Breakdown in individuals at high risk for schizophrenia: possible predispositional perinatal factors. *Mental Hygiene*, **54**, 50–63.

—— & SCHULSINGER, F. (1968) Some premorbid characteristics related to breakdown in children with schizophrenic mothers. In *The Transmission of Schizophrenia* (eds. D. Rosenthal and S. Kety). London: Pergamon Press.

MOTHER'S AID ORGANIZATION FOR COPENHAGEN, COPENHAGEN COUNTY, AND FREDERIKSBORG COUNTY. Annual Report for 1946–47. Copenhagen, Denmark.

ØDEGÅRD, O. (1974) Season of birth in the general population and in patients with mental disorder in Norway. *British Journal of Psychiatry*, **125**, 397–405.

PARKER, G. & BALZA, B. (1977) Season of birth and schizophrenia: an equatorial study. *Acta Psychiatrica Scandinavica*, **56**, 143–146.

—— & NEILSON, M. (1976) Mental disorder and season of birth: a southern hemisphere study. *British Journal of Psychiatry*, **129**, 355–361.

RIEDER, R. O., ROSENTHAL, D., WENDER, P. & BLUMENTHAL, H. (1975) The offspring of schizophrenics. *Archives of General Psychiatry,*, **32**, 200–211.

SAS INSTITUTE INC. (1979) *SAS User's Guide*, 1979 Edition. Cary, North Carolina: SAS Institute Inc.

SAXÉN, L., HJELT, L., SJOSTEDT, J., E., HAKOSALO, J. & HAKOSALO, H. (1960) Asian influenza during pregnancy and congenital malformations. *Acta Pathologica et Microbiologica Scandinavica*, **49**, 114–126.

SCHULSINGER, F. (1976) A ten-year follow-up of children of schizophrenic mothers: clinical assessment. *Acta Psychiatrica Scandinavica*, **53**, 371–386.

SOBEL, D. E. (1961) Infant mortality and malformations in children of schizophrenic women. *Psychiatric Quarterly*, **35**, 60–65.

TORREY, E. F. (1980) *Schizophrenia and Civilization*. New York: Jason Aronson, Inc.

—— & PETERSON, M. R. (1976) The viral hypothesis of schizophrenia. *Schizophrenia Bulletin*, **2**, 136–146.

VIDEBECH, TH., WEEKE, A. & DUPONT, A. (1974) Endogenous psychoses and season of birth. *Acta Psychiatrica Scandinavica*, **50**, 202–218.

WATSON, C. G., KUCALA, T., ANGULSKI, G. & BRUNN, C. (1982) Season of birth and schizophrenia: a response to the Lewis and Griffin critique. *Journal of Abnormal Psychology*, **91**, 120–125.

WING, J. K., COOPER, J. E. & SARTORIUS, N. (1974) *The Measurement and Classification of Psychiatric Symptoms*. Cambridge: Cambridge University Press.

24 A re-evaluation of the viral hypothesis: Is psychosis the result of retroviral integration at a site close to the cerebral dominance gene?

TIMOTHY J. CROW

The possible aetiologies of schizophrenia are increasingly circumscribed. A genetic component is undoubted, but remains ill-defined in Mendelian terms and cannot account for: (i) the shortfall from 100 per cent in concordance in monozygotic twin pairs, (ii) onset in adult life, and (iii) a continued high prevalence against the selective effects of reduced fertility. To explain these anomalies, a 'gene-environment interaction' is often invoked, but there is a dearth of environmental agents to which an aetiological role can plausibly be attributed. Psychogenic trauma has fallen by the wayside from the failure of its advocates to specify the nature of the trauma or to construct a plausible account of its psychodynamic effects: 'expressed emotion' in relatives is viewed as a predictor of relapse, but is not seriously advanced as an initiator. In a so far unpublished study (CRC Division of Psychiatry) of first episodes of illness, expressed emotion in relatives did not predict relapse when other prognostic factors (length of illness before admission, and drug treatment) were taken into account. Aside from the genetic component, the categories of possible causal agent are reduced to a short-list of three—toxins, infection, and disturbances of immunity. Of these, a toxic factor appears the least likely in view of the wide-spread geographical distribution of the disease. Auto-immunity is frequently mooted, but as with other disorders of immune origin a trigger is required—in several conditions, this is an encounter with an infectious agent (Lewis, 1974). That schizophrenia should be due to an infectious agent is not widely entertained, but the paucity of alternative theories requires that it be considered.

Background to the viral hypothesis

Viral infection as a possible cause of schizophrenic illness was first considered after the 1918 epidemic of influenza. Menninger (1926) reported a series of 175 cases of post-influenzal psychosis, of which 77 received a diagnosis of dementia praecox. Of 50 patients who were followed up, 35 were completely recovered, five improved, five unimproved, and five were worse. Although in some cases the diagnosis at follow-up had been changed to manic-depressive or toxic-infectious psychosis, frequently because recovery had occurred,

Menninger noted that in the original picture there had been 'unmistakable schizophrenic stigmas including intrapsychic ataxia, emotional-ideational splitting, incoherence, stereotypies and other bizarre expressions' and that these symptoms were not conspicuously different from those seen in the usual types of schizophrenic illness. He concluded that the schizophrenic syndrome: (i) was the relatively most frequent post-influenzal psychosis, (ii) occurred with or without predisposition or hereditary taint, and (iii) in most cases terminated in complete recovery. Subsequently, Menninger discussed the implications of these observations for the aetiology of 'acute schizophrenic reactions', which he regarded as of multiple causation. To a question from Adolf Meyer, he replied, 'influenza or other somatic infection is not a cause, but it may be one of the factors involved in the débâcle. I think I said seven years ago that influenza caused psychosis. I have grown older since and I hope, wiser. I have certainly changed my mind' (Menninger, 1928). It was left to Goodall (1932) to formulate the viral hypothesis with precision. In the wake of the encephalitis lethargica epidemic which followed and may well have been related (Ravenholt and Foege, 1982) to the 1918 influenza pandemic, he noted that 'there are observers who consider that there is no essential difference between psychotic disturbances connected with encephalitis (post-encephalitic) and those met with in states covered by the description schizophrenia', and went on to argue that 'epidemic encephalitis, with the somatic disorders which accompany it, may be a virus disease and similarly caused, perhaps, are the schizophrenic states which resemble them . . .'

Goodall (1927) may have been the first to attempt animal transmission experiments in schizophrenia, although no record of the findings survives. His interest in the phenomenological similarities between the psychotic sequelae of encephalitis lethargica and schizophrenia is reflected in contemporary accounts of, e.g. Jelliffe (1927), Hendrick (1928), and McCowan and Cook (1928). The 1918 epidemic of influenza, and possibly therefore the encephalitis lethargica epidemic which followed, was almost certainly due to the 'swine' serotype of influenza A (H_1N_1). Such neuropsychiatric sequelae to influenza no longer occur, although Lloyd Still (1958) described a small group of psychotic illnesses after a later pandemic (due to the H_2N_2 serotype), some of which were confusional and some including olfactory hallucinations.

A number of authors have described illnesses, presumed to be encephalitic, in which schizophrenia-like symptoms were observed. Thus Weinstein *et al* (1955) described six cases of psychosis, four of which followed an upper respiratory tract infection and one infectious mononucleosis. Disorientation, neurological signs, seizures, and CSF changes were observed in various combinations, but catatonic and psychotic symptoms, described by these authors as schizophrenic, were also seen. Sobin and Ozer (1966) reported a somewhat similar series of ten cases of post-infectious psychosis, and stressed that in many, the symptoms could not be distinguished from those of schizophrenia. Such cases with other reports (e.g. Hunter and Jones, 1966; Himmelhoch *et al*, 1970; Misra and Hay, 1971) indicate that schizophrenia-like symptoms are observed in illnesses which for a variety of reasons (e.g. preceding febrile illness, the presence of neurological signs or CSF changes) have been regarded as of viral aetiology, although specific pathogens have not been identified. Schizophrenic symptoms are also described as a manifestation of Vilyuisk encephalitis, an illness attributed to a picornavirus (Lipton *et al*, 1983), seen in the Yakat Republic of the USSR. Recurrent episodes of illness lead to progressive impairments, and there may be neurological signs (e.g. amyotrophy) and a meningoencephalitis, but schizophrenia-like symptoms also occur, which can progress to dementia. Thus, there are precedents for schizophrenic symptoms occurring in association with viral infections of the nervous system.

Some animal viral infections are also of interest. Visna is a slowly progressive neurological disease of sheep in Iceland, caused by a C-type retrovirus which evades the immune response (Petursson *et al*, 1979) to induce a periventricular demyelinating process. The chronicity of the course and the location of the lesions make this model of interest in relation to the psychoses. Of possibly greater relevance, in that the course may be episodic and the agent sometimes enters a latent phase, is the disease borna. This affects horses, sheep, cattle, and possibly deer, and can be transferred to rodents (Narayan *et al*, 1983); it may be caused by an enveloped RNA virus, and the selectivity of the virus for the limbic system is of particular interest.

Epidemiology

(a) Seasonality

Consistent with a viral aetiology for the functional psychoses are observations on seasonal changes. There is an excess of onsets of both mania and schizophrenia in the early summer months (Hare and Walter, 1978) expressed in relation to admissions for other types of illness; the excess probably applies to both first and later episodes.

Even better established with respect to schizophrenia is a season of birth effect—individuals who later develop the disease are more likely (by 4 to 8 per cent) to have been born in the months of winter and early spring than at other times of the year (Torrey *et al*, 1977). Similar effects are seen for mania (Hare and Walter, 1978) as for schizophrenia. A relationship with seasonal temperature at the time of birth has been reported (Hare and Moran, 1980), as also has an association with the incidence of infectious disease in the year preceding birth (Watson *et al*, 1984).

The similarity of the seasonal effects (for date of birth and onset) for the two psychoses is striking. If the finding is not an artefact, it is difficult to avoid the conclusion that the aetiologies of the conditions must be related.

(b) Temporal and geographical variations

It has been generally assumed that the incidence of schizophrenia is uniform with respect to time, and approximately similar in the various populations of the world. Both assumptions have been challenged: **Hare (1983a)** has presented evidence that the incidence of the disease increased in the nineteenth century, and both Hare (1983b) and Torrey (1980) have drawn attention to the relative scarcity before 1800 of case descriptions which with reasonable confidence can be classified as schizophrenia. Although a lifetime prevalence of approximately 8 per 1,000 is reported in many countries, there is evidence for materially higher rates in the north of Sweden (Böök, 1953) in Croatia

(Crocetti *et al*, 1971) and of the west of Ireland (Kelleher *et al*, 1974; Torrey *et al*, 1984). Conversely, it is claimed that the incidence is significantly lower in Papua New Guinea (Torrey *et al*, 1974) and in the eastern islands of Micronesia (Dale, 1981).

With uncertainties of diagnosis and sampling, neither geographical nor temporal variation can be regarded as established. If there are significant variations, this is relevant to a viral aetiology. If on the contrary incidence is truly invariant with respect to time and place this is a singular finding, particularly if the disease is of genetic origin; it suggests that the gene confers significant and universal advantages.

Direct investigation of the viral hypothesis

Three stategies have been adopted in the search for viruses in patients with the disease:

(i) *Serum and CSF antibody titres:* elevated CSF/serum ratios of antibodies to cytomegalovirus were reported in approximately 30 per cent of patients with schizophrenia (Albrecht *et al*, 1980) and an increase in IgM to this virus was detected in 11 per cent of such patients, using an ELISA assay, by comparison with 3 per cent of neurological patients and 3 of 17 patients with bipolar affective illness (Torrey *et al*, 1982). However, this finding has not been consistent in other samples (Torrey *et al*, 1983; Hirsch, 1983) and the meaning of an elevation of IgM in the absence of a change in IgG is obscure. In a comprehensive survey of antibodies in serum to five viruses in a large sample of schizophrenic and other psychiatric patients, King *et al* (1985) found anti-mumps titres significantly reduced in patients with schizophrenia; they argued that impaired immunity to this virus might play a role in aetiology.

(ii) *Cell culture techniques:* in a search for known or unrecognized viruses, cerebrospinal fluid from about one-third of patients with schizophrenia was found to induce a cytopathic effect in human embryonic fibroblast cultures (Crow *et al*, 1979; Tyrrell *et al*, 1979). The effect was not passaged, but was prevented by filters of 50 nm pore size; it was thought that it might reflect the presence of a small RNA virus. Further investigations have shown that the effect is also seen with CSF from some patients with affective disorder and with miscellaneous neurological conditions (Baker *et al*, 1983), and that it is not prevented by protein synthesis inhibition (Taylor and Crow *et al*, 1982). Thus, the effect is unlikely to be due to a replicating virus, but may indicate the release into the CSF by CNS damage of a toxic factor associated with cellular debris.

(iii) *Transmission experiments:* CSF inducing cytopathic effects from patients with schizophrenia was injected intracerebrally into mice and hamsters without significant effects. Marmosets injected with cytopathic CSF from patients with schizophrenia (and also from those with Huntington's chorea) were observed to be significantly less active over a $2\frac{1}{2}$-year period of observation than control-injected animals, and they had an incidence of reproductive anomalies (Baker *et al*, 1983). Examination of the brains of these animals has revealed no evidence of changes in dopamine receptors, gliosis, or the presence of cytomegalovirus. To exclude the possibility that subtle behavioural changes are a manifestation of pathogenic effects (which cannot otherwise be detected) of intracerebral injections of CSF, these experiments are being repeated.

Experiments in which brain tissue obtained at post-mortem and in one case at biopsy was injected intracerebrally into a series of primates (Asher *et al*, 1984) have given negative findings.

While these various approaches to a possible viral aetiology have yielded leads which justify further investigation, none has provided strong evidence for the presence of an infectious agent.

The contagion hypothesis

If schizophrenia is a viral disease, the question must be asked where does the virus come from? That psychosis is sometimes contagious has long been considered (Baillarger, 1857; Hofbauer, 1864; Wollenberg, 1889) although only more recently in a microbial context. It has been argued (Crow, 1981; 1983a) that some findings in family studies are compatible with the notion that in addition to a genetic predisposition, what matters is proximity to an individual who already has the disease:

(i) Concordance rates are higher in dizygotic twins than in their siblings (Fischer, 1973), although these relatives share genes to the same extent; because they are the same age, twins may be in closer contact than siblings.

(ii) Concordance in relatives is greater in same-sex than in opposite-sex pairs (Rosenthal, 1962), but this effect occurs only within the family (i.e. first-degree relatives—Penrose, 1942); again, it may be argued that same sex pairs of relatives are in closer physical proximity.

(iii) In monozygotic twins, the second member of the pair is at increased risk in the first two years after disease onset in the first, and the increase is confined to pairs who are together at this time (Abe, 1969).

(iv) According to Kasanetz (1979), first episodes of psychosis occur more frequently in individuals who live in apartment blocks where there is already an (unrelated) patient with schizophrenia than elsewhere.

These findings have been variously interpreted (Murray and Reveley, 1983a; 1983b; Bryant, 1983; Crow, 1983b). If they are to be taken as evidence for horizontal disease transmission, it must be assumed that this occurs in individuals with a genetic predisposition. Such a gene-infectious agent interaction is not unprecedented; dizygotic-monozygotic twin concordance ratios similar to those in schizophrenia are reported in poliomyelitis and tuberculosis. Harper (1977) has argued that evidence for strict Mendelian transmission, e.g. in Huntington's chorea, does not rule out a role for a virus and the familial occurrence of Jakob-Creutzfeldt disease (Adam *et al*, 1982) requires a direct interaction between an apparently dominant genetic factor and this elusive transmissible agent. In psychosis, Scharfetter (1970) has shown that when cases of *folie à deux* occur in individuals unrelated by blood ties (e.g. spouses), the genetic predisposition is as great in the secondary as in the primary case. Thus, a gene-virus interaction, with horizontal transmission of the latter, could not be ruled out.

A study in pairs of siblings

The contagion (horizontal transmission) hypothesis has been subjected to a further test in pairs of siblings with the disease. The siblings of patients with schizophrenia include individuals at genetic risk, and such individuals are also exposed to someone who already has the disease. The time of onset of illness in pairs of siblings who both have the disease thus provides information on the mode of transmission. In an analysis of five collections of such pairs (Crow and Done, 1985), age of onset has been found strongly correlated (P = 0.68) within pairs, and there is a shift toward earlier age of onset in the younger sibling ($\chi^2 = 42.45$, P < 0.0005).

This observation is susceptible to three explanations: (i) age of onset is genetically determined, but when the disease is seen in an elder sibling, it is detected at an earlier age in a younger sibling (the 'early detection' hypothesis); (ii) the disease is transmitted from one to the other sibling, the age shift being related to the age difference between the siblings at the time of transmission, i.e. from elder to younger or vice versa (the 'contagion' hypothesis); (iii) age of onset is under genetic control, but because pairs are collected at the time of onset of illness in one sibling, an excess of younger siblings with earlier age of onset are included (the 'ascertainment bias' hypothesis).

A decision between these hypotheses can be made by analysing the age shift (to younger age of onset in younger sibling) in relation to whether the disease occurs first in the elder or younger sibling. The 'early detection' and the 'contagion' hypotheses both predict that the age shift will be seen in pairs in which the illness occurs first in the elder sibling. The selection bias hypothesis predicts that the age shift will occur only in the pairs in which the younger sibling is ill first.

The latter is what is observed. Within the set of pairs in which the elder sibling is ill first, age of onset remains highly correlated between members of each pair, but there is no tendency to earlier onset in the younger sibling.

This finding rules out the contagion hypothesis (or at least demonstrates that if contagion does occur, it must be in a proportion of cases so small as not to be detectable in this series of 264 pairs of siblings); it also rules out the early detection theory. Since the data on siblings are more extensive than the series of pairs of monozygotic twins examined by Abe (1969) and the first episodes of illness studied by Kasanetz (1979), and have been collected in circumstances in which possible sources of bias can more readily be examined, it seems that contagion (horizontal transmission) can be excluded as the usual method by which the disease is transmitted. The finding that date of onset of illness in one sibling is independent of date of onset in the other, but that age of onset is highly correlated between siblings, has implications for a role of environmental agents in general. Thus, agents to which both siblings are exposed at a defined point in time (e.g. infective illnesses of childhood, loss of a parent), even though their effects are delayed by many years, appear to be eliminated. If such factors made a significant contribution to onset, a shift to earlier age of onset in pairs in which the elder sibling was ill first would have been observed. From the viewpoint of the viral hypothesis, the findings impose significant constraints and suggest that if viruses play any role, this must be in pre- rather than post-natal life.

A new hypothesis: retroviruses and proto-oncogenes

To accommodate the season of birth effect, a genetic factor, the late age of onset of disease, and a virus which is latent for many years, a hypothesis which is more parsimonious but more restrictive than a gene-virus interaction must be considered. *This is that schizophrenia (and perhaps manic-depressive psychosis) is due to infection with a virus which becomes integrated in the genome, sometimes to be passed from one generation to the next.*

A class of agent with the ability to integrate in the host genome is that of the retroviruses (e.g. Weiss, 1978), which carry the gene for the enzyme reverse transcriptase (Baltimore, 1970; Temin and Mizutani, 1970). This enzyme permits viral RNA to be transcribed into DNA which can then become integrated into the host genome as a 'provirus' (Lwoff, 1965). In early studies, retrovirus-related antigens in chickens (Payne and Chubb, 1968) and tumour-inducing viruses in mice (Bentvelzen and Daams, 1969) had been found to be transmitted in a Mendelian fashion, and inter-species comparisons suggested that exogenously-acquired viral genes have become integrated in the germ-line of some species (Benveniste and Todaro, 1974). In mice germ-line, integration of the Moloney murine leukaemia virus has been reported when infection of the embryo occurs in the pre-implantation stage (Jaenisch, 1976). Thus, exposure to a retrovirus at a critical developmental stage results in host acquisition of a virus which is then passed from one generation to the next as an inherited Mendelian characteristic, but to be expressed as viral particles at a late stage in the life of the affected individual.

According to this hypothesis the element responsible for the disease is acquired either by inheritance from a parent, or as a result of an integration event (assumed to be seasonally influenced) occurring early in ontogeny. Two types of integration event can be envisaged—either that the agent originates from outside the genome (i.e. that horizontal transmission does occur but early in development rather than in postnatal life) or that the agent originates from elsewhere within the genome by transposition. Retroviruses are one member of the class of transposons (mobile genetic elements—Shapiro, 1983). Thus the hypothesis can be more generally stated that *psychosis is due to the expression of a retrovirus or transposon which is integrated at a critical site within the genome either by inheritance or as a result of an integration/transposition (seasonally-influenced) event which occurs early in ontogeny.*

It is of historical interest that a mode of transmission somewhat as suggested above was foreshadowed by Myerson (1925), who in the face of prevailing Weissmanian orthodoxy insisted that in mental illness we are dealing with a toxic environmental influence on the germ-line, this effect being mediated by a mechanism which he referred to as 'blastophoria'.

A prediction of the retrovirus/transposon hypothesis is that evidence for integration/transposition events will be associated with those cases where a family history is absent. Kinney and Jacobsen (1978), in their analysis of the Danish-American adoption study data, found 7 out of 10 of the schizophrenic probands at low 'biological risk' (a category including those without a family history) compared to 5 out of 24 (P <0.02) of those at high 'biological risk' (including those with a family history) were born between January and April. On the retrovirus/transposon hypothesis, the season of birth excess may be taken as an index of the frequency with which integration/transposition in the germ-line occurs—perhaps in between 5 to 10 per cent of cases.

Two problems for the hypothesis are: (i) the low rate of concordance in monozygotic twins. When the provirus is inherited from a parent both twins should be affected, and this would also be expected in at least some cases in which the infection is acquired in utero. Concordance rates of 36 to 58 per cent (Gottesman, 1978) appear too low. (ii) For the effects of genomic integration of a virus to be predictable (i.e. for the disease to breed true), the site of integration should be constant—in particular, the provirus should be integrated in a gene sequence which is expressed in brain. Yet the integration sites of the retroviruses within the genome are random.

A solution of these two problems relates to the role of laterality in psychosis and to the ability of retroviruses to amplify the expression of cellular growth factors, sometimes referred to as 'proto-oncogenes' (e.g. Bishop, 1983) on account of their ability (e.g. when integrated into a retrovirus genome) to induce neoplasia.

Laterality was introduced into discussion of psychosis by Flor-Henry's observations (1969) that in the psychoses associated with temporal-lobe epilepsy, schizophrenic symptoms are more likely to occur with dominant (and affective symptoms perhaps with non-dominant) foci—an observation confirmed by later studies (Taylor, 1975; Lindsay *et al*, 1979). That the functional psychoses themselves are lateralized in the brain has been widely speculated upon, but compelling evidence has been lacking. The notion that a disease (which many suppose to be due to a chemical disturbance) with such global psychological consequences should have an origin confined to one hemisphere has appeared far-fetched. However, two recent post-mortem findings add substance to the concept: (i) Reynolds (1983) found the dopamine content of the amygdala to be elevated in the brains of schizophrenic patients by comparison with controls, but that this change was present in the left but not in the right hemisphere; (ii) in a study of the brains of patients dying in Runwell Hospital over a 26-year period (Brown *et al*, 1985) the parahippocampal gyrus of patients with schizophrenia was significantly thinner than that of the brains of patients with affective disorders ($P < 0.01$), and there was a diagnosis-by-side interaction, the difference between the groups being significantly ($P < 0.02$) greater on the left side.

Boklage (1977) has drawn attention to the relevance of laterality to the rates of concordance in monozygotic twin pairs. In an analysis of the data in the series of twins collected by Gottesman and Shields and by Slater, he found that in 12 pairs concordant for right-handedness, 11 were concordant for schizophrenia, whereas in 16 pairs in which one or both members were not unequivocally right-handed only four pairs were concordant. Boklage argues that while dominance (laterality) is under genetic control, monozygotic twins (perhaps for reasons associated with the twinning process itself) are not always concordant for handedness. If this is the case, the findings suggest: (i) that discordance in monozygotic twins cannot be taken as evidence for an environmental component, i.e. that the genetic component may be greater than is generally assumed, and (ii) that the disease is in some way related to cerebral dominance.

Boklage's conclusions bear a relation to the retroviral hypothesis. He writes that if schizophrenia 'is with rare exception (heritably) cellular in origin, the following considerations are appropriate:

1. Schizophrenic psychosis is clearly not what is inherited; that takes on

average near 30 years to appear, and it is not possible in the majority of cases to say that the individual "was always more or less like that".

2. Therefore, what is inherited or otherwise cellularly imposed before birth is some cellular *anlage*, stable for 20–60 years of growth, with or without intervening development of the *anlage* itself or of identifiable behavioural deviations originating therefrom.

3. That the symptoms of schizophrenia represent lateralized pathology does not prove that the cellular *anlage* is similarly placed. However, it seems fairly safe to defy a simpler explanation . . .'

For the retroviral theory, the term *provirus* can be substituted for cellular *anlage*, but the gist of the conclusions remains. With respect to the strength of the genetic component, Boklage's opinion is close to that of Karlsson (1970a) who drew from a comparison of the rates of schizophrenia in Kallman's genetic studies and those in adopted relatives of schizophrenics the conclusion that environmental factors add little to genes in determining whether or not an individual develops the disease.

The implications of Boklage's analysis depend upon their replicability and the genetics of cerebral dominance, but there are uncertainties in both areas. Luchins *et al* (1980) examined handedness in a series of 14 pairs of monozygotic twins, selected earlier (Pollin and Stabenau, 1968) for discordance for schizophrenia. Only four of the 28 twins were left-handed. At follow-up, four of the 14 pairs had become concordant, but in seven of the remaining ten pairs, both members were right-handed. Thus, in contrast to Boklage's findings, 70 per cent of the two RH pairs remained discordant, and this figure was comparable to the three out of four discordance rate for the 1–2 LH pairs (pairs including a left-hander). Amongst the 1–2 LH pairs, all four of the left-handers, compared to only one of the right-handers, was schizophrenic, and a similar trend toward the left-hander being schizophrenic in discordant pairs was noted in the data analysed by Boklage. Luchins *et al* also noted that while in the seven discordant 2 RH sibships the schizophrenic was lighter at birth in each case, in the three 1–2 LH discordant pairs, the schizophrenic individual was left-handed and heavier at birth (P = 0.008).

On the integrated virus hypothesis, these findings can be explained as follows:

(i) in 2-RH concordant pairs, the virus is inherited as an integrated gene from a parent, or both are infected in utero. The effect of the integrated proviral gene is assumed to be confined to the left hemisphere.

(ii) in 2-RH discordant pairs, the virus is acquired in utero by one member of the pair; the infection could account for low birth weight in this twin. Because they were selected for discordance, the series of Pollin and Stabenau (1968) included an excess of such cases.

(iii) in 1–2 LH discordant pairs, there are two possibilities—either (as suggested by Boklage) the twinning process itself leads to asymmetry of dominance, schizophrenia being associated only with dominance in one hemisphere, or (as suggested by Luchins *et al*, 1980) some factor in one of the twins leads first to the development of left-handedness and later to the onset of a schizophreniform psychosis. In these cases, the illness is less severe.

According to the date of both Boklage and Luchins *et al*, cerebral dominance is relevant to schizophrenia. Although dominance is undoubtedly influenced by genetic factors, there is disagreement concerning the precise mechanism. The simplest hypothesis—and one which accounts for much of the evidence—is, as proposed by Annett (1978, 1981), that a dominantly inherited gene confers a 'shift' to the left hemisphere in most people, and determines that they shall be right-handed. Left-handers (and a proportion of right-handers) are assumed to lack this factor, and in these individuals, handedness is determined by a random process. An interesting fact is that whereas dominance of one hemisphere over the other is common in vertebrates, a systematic deviation to one side may be confined to canaries, some non-human primates (e.g. macaques), and man (Walker, 1980). Perhaps it is an unusual and specific evolutionary development, associated with inter-individual communication.

Of particular relevance to the integrated viral gene hypothesis is that dominance is associated with cerebral asymmetry—in right-handed subjects, auditory cortex and regions within the Sylvian fissure tend to be of greater size in the left hemisphere than the corresponding regions on the right (Galaburda *et al*, 1978). In left-handed subjects, this tendency is less marked and is sometimes reversed, although asymmetries of similar magnitude in the opposite direction are unusual.

The anatomical basis of these asymmetries is obscure—presumably there is differential growth on one side of the brain—but may be critical to an understanding of the functional psychoses. For the reasons already outlined, the agent responsible for psychosis appears in some way to be linked to whatever genetic factor determines the asymmetrical development of the brain. *A hypothesis which relates the retroviral theory to cerebral asymmetries is that the latter depend upon a growth factor for which a retrovirus has a particular affinity.*

Retroviruses have a capacity to incorporate 'oncogenes' which stimulate growth, and when incorporated in a retroviral genome (as viral oncogenes), can induce neoplasia. It is now recognized that such sequences (cellular- or proto-oncogenes) are a component of eukaryotic cells, and probably play a role in normal function, maybe as growth factors. Retroviruses can interact with and incorporate such sequences and, perhaps because when they do so enhanced growth occurs, the interaction is noted sometimes as a pathological effect.

Thus, to account for the site-specific integration of the retrovirus assumed to be responsible for the association of schizophrenia with cerebral dominance, it may be suggested that: *The cerebral asymmetries underlying laterality are established by the trophic effects of a proto-oncogene, and that the retrovirus responsible for psychosis interacts with this cellular oncogene to elicit enhanced activity, which may sometimes be destructive.*

The effects of the interaction could depend upon the stage of development at which enhancement occurs. Thus, increased activity in a period of brain growth might lead to hypertrophy, but at a later stage to inappropriate cellular stimulation and perhaps cell loss. Such differential effects would be relevant to age of onset.

Is there a relationship between manic-depressive psychosis and schizophrenia?

That there is a relationship between major affective disorders and schizophrenia is widely suspected, because intermediate states are encountered and no satisfactory dividing line can be drawn between the two psychoses, (Kendell and Gourlay, 1970). It is also suggested by the similarity of the season of birth and season of onset effects for schizophrenia and mania (Hare and Walter, 1978). However, the inheritance of the two conditions is held to be independent.

A possible relationship is that in successive generations, there is a (small) tendency for manic-depressive psychosis to transmute into schizophrenia. Thus, Rosenthal (1970) summarized the incidence of schizophrenia in a number of studies of the relatives of patients with affective disorder and found an excess in the children (Table I).

TABLE I

Risk of schizophrenia in relatives of manic-depressive probands (From Rosenthal, 1970)

	No. of studies	% ($\pm$S.D.)
Parents	6	0.42 $\pm$ 0.33
Siblings	9	0.79 $\pm$ 0.53
Children	5	2.30 $\pm$ 0.96

Schulz (1940) studied psychoses occurring in the children of two manic-depressive patients, and found 28 per cent to be affective but 12 per cent to have schizophrenic psychoses. In a case register study of parent-child pairs who had both been recorded as being given a diagnosis of psychotic illness, Powell *et al* (1973) found that amongst the children of parents with schizophrenia, nine were recorded as suffering from this disease and none from manic-depressive psychoses, whilst amongst children of parents with the latter disorder, there were ten with manic-depressive disease but 15 with schizophrenia. These authors comment that 'Amongst the children of manic-depressives there are two cases of manic-depression for every three cases of schizophrenia. Yet, from the genetic point of view why should schizophrenia have occurred at all in these families?'

Thus, the form of psychotic disorder may change in succeeding generations; this implies an alteration in the gene, or perhaps its location in the genome. Such an alteration is easier to understand if in the psychoses we are dealing with proto-oncogenes susceptible to alteration by retroviruses or some other type of moveable genetic element (Temin, 1980).

According to this concept, schizophrenia arises in three ways:
(i) by inheritance of the psychosis gene (provirus) from a parent with schizophrenia (or who at least has the predisposing gene); (ii) by inheritance of the psychosis gene (modified in the course of transmission) from a parent with manic-depressive illness (or who has the predisposing gene); (iii) by an integration/transposition event occurring early in ontogeny.

Handedness, psychosis and evolution

Although there may be a relationship between handedness and psychosis, this is not straightforward, since surveys in populations of patients with psychiatric disease do not show striking deviations from the normal population in handedness patterns (Taylor and Dalton *et al*, 1982). Since handedness persists as a genetic polymorphism, there must be advantages and disadvantages associated with the two states (or position on the continuum) of handedness. The development of cerebral asymmetry presumably is in some way associated with the capacity for speech. Left-handers apparently are not disadvantaged in this respect, although they may be with respect to visuospatial abilities (Levy, 1969; Miller, 1971). The fact that not everyone is right-handed suggests there are disadvantages as well as benefits associated with right-handedness. There is also a case for a familial association between creativity and psychosis (Karlsson, 1970b). These associations may all be relevant to the relationship between dominance and psychosis.

Perhaps there is a continuum from a state of cerebral symmetry (which includes most left- and some right-handers) to an extreme of asymmetry associated with right-handedness, so that the point which an individual occupies in this continuum is relevant to the form of the psychosis he develops (but not to the risk of psychosis). Thus, individuals who are more lateralized may have a worse outcome when they develop psychosis; in fact, it is observed that when schizophrenia affects non-righthanded individuals, the illness is less severe (Luchins *et al*, 1979). Conversely, there may be an excess of left-handers amongst bipolar I type patients and particularly amongst their children (Sackheim and Decina, 1983). One possibility is that the psychosis gene persists because it is able to move an individual along the laterality continuum. Thus, human cerebral asymmetry could have arisen because a retrovirus deposits a proto-oncogene in an unusual position amongst genes expressed in the brain. This could have led to adaptive consequences; reduplication of the proto-oncogene (i.e. multiplication of the growth factor effect) by further viral activity might have yielded further gains, but at the cost of maladaptive viral gene expression (e.g. outside the period of cerebral development). According to this concept, psychosis reflects rate of change in the genes (proto-oncogenes) determining laterality, the form of the psychosis being influenced by the number of genes already present. In some such way, the association between cerebral dominance (an apparent genetic polymorphism), the persistence of psychosis, and its relationship to creativity may be explicable.

The action of neuroleptic drugs

A role of retroviruses in the aetiology of the psychoses may be relevant to the question of the mechanism of action of neuroleptic drugs. Thus, repeated doses of haloperidol have been found to delay the onset of disease and to enhance survival in mice infected with the Rauscher murine leukaemia retrovirus (Wunderlich *et al*, 1980), while single doses of reserpine abolish the infectivity of mouse mammary tumour virus, a type B retrovirus (Wunderlich and Zotter, 1982). The mechanism of these actions is not known.

Conclusions

1. A role for genetic predisposition in schizophrenia is established by twin and adoption studies, but the mode of inheritance remains obscure, while the extent of discordance in monozygotic twins, the age of onset, and the persistence of the disease in the face of a decrease in fertility are unexplained.

2. That some viruses can initiate schizophrenia-like illnesses is suggested by observations on the influenza pandemic of 1918, the encephalitis lethargica epidemic, and reports of schizophrenic symptoms occurring in the course of atypical encephalitic illnesses.

3. Schizophrenia could be due to a gene-virus interaction, and the findings of some family studies are consistent with transmission of disease ('contagion') from affected to non-affected individuals. However, a study of age of onset in siblings has established that whereas a shift to earlier age of onset in younger sibling is observed, this is due to an ascertainment bias. When this is taken into account, age of onset in one sibling is strongly correlated with age of onset in the other, but uninfluenced by date of onset. Within the limits of these data, it appears that horizontal transmission does not occur.

4. An alternative hypothesis to the gene-virus interaction is proposed—that the disease results from the integration into the human genome of a retrovirus or transposon which is expressed as disease in adult life. Integration into the germ-line (established for some retroviruses in animal experiments) could account for genetic transmission; also, the theory could explain the problems noted under (1) for the genetic hypothesis, as well as the season of birth effect, and the observation that season of birth clustering is present in cases without a family history.

5. The similarities (particularly with respect to seasonality of birth and onset) between manic-depressive illness and schizophrenia suggest that these illnesses share a common aetiology. There is evidence that manic-depressive illness in one generation is sometimes succeeded by schizophrenia in the next.

6. The association between schizophrenia and the dominant cerebral hemisphere (which may be relevant to the degree of discordance for the disease observed in monozygotic twins) is explained by a postulated interaction between the retrovirus / transposon responsible for the disease and a proto-oncogene which contributes (as a growth factor) to the development of cerebral asymmetry. This cellular proto-oncogene is thus assumed to be a genetic determinant of handedness: according to this theory, it is the human genomic site at which the 'psychosis virus' integrates.

References

ABE, K. (1969) The morbidity rate and environmental influence in monozygotic co-twins of schizophrenics. *British Journal of Psychiatry*, **115**, 519–531.

ADAM, J., CROW, T. J., DUCHEN, L. W., SCARAVILLI, F. & SPOKES, E. (1982) Familial cerebral amyloidosis and spongiform encephalopathy. *Journal of Neurology, Neurosurgery & Psychiatry*, **45**, 37–45.

ALBRECHT, P., TORREY, E. F., BOONE, E., HICKS, J. T. & DANIEL, N. (1980) Raised cytomegalovirus-antibody level in cerebrospinal fluid of schizophrenic patients. *Lancet*, ii, 769–772.

ANNETT, M. (1978) *A Single Gene Explanation of Right and Left Handedness and Brainedness*. Coventry: Lancaster Polytechnic.

—— (1981) The genetics of handedness. *Trends in Neurosciences*, **4**, 256–258.

ASHER, D. M., KAUFMAN, C. A., KLEINMAN, J. E., WEINBERGER, D. R., GIBBS, C. J. & GAJDUSEK, D. C. (1984) Attempts to transmit schizophrenia to animals. Proceedings of the 137th Annual Meeting of the American Psychiatric Association, Los Angeles 5–11th May.

BAILLARGER, L. (1857) Example de contagion d'un délire monomaniaque. *La Moniteur des Hospitaux*, **45**, 353–354.

BAKER, H. F., BLOXHAM, C. A., CROW, T. J., DAVIES, H., FERRIER, I. N., JOHNSTONE, E. C., PARRY, R. P., RIDLEY, R. M., TAYLOR, G. R. & TYRRELL, D. A. J. (1983) The viral hypothesis: some experimental approaches. *Advances in Biological Psychiatry*, **12**, 1–19.

BALTIMORE, D. (1970) RNA-dependent DNA polymerase in virions of RNA tumor viruses. *Nature,* **226,** 1209–1211.

BENTVELZEN, P. & DAAMS, J. H. (1969) Hereditary infections with mammary tumor viruses in mice. *Journal of the National Cancer Institute,* **43,** 1025–1035.

BENVENISTE, R. E. & TODARO, G. J. (1974) Evolution of C-type viral genes: inheritance of exogenously acquired viral genes. *Nature,* **252,** 456–459.

BISHOP, J. M. (1983) Cancer genes come of age. *Cell,* **32,** 1018–1020.

BOKLAGE, C. E. (1977) Schizophrenia, brain asymmetry development and twinning: cellular relationship with etiological and possibly prognostic implications. *Biological Psychiatry,* **12,** 19–35.

BÖÖK, J. A. (1953) A genetic and neuropsychiatric investigation of a North Swedish population. *Acta genetica et statistica Medica,* **4,** 1–100.

BROWN, R., COLTER, N., CORSELLIS, J. A. N., CROW, T. J., FRITH, C. D., JAGOE, R., JOHNSTONE, E. C. & MARSH, L. (1985) Brain weight and parahippocampal gyrus width are reduced and temporal horn area is increased in schizophrenia by comparison with affective disorder. *Archives of General Psychiatry,* in press.

BRYANT, R. C. (1983) Genetics of schizophrenia. *Lancet, i,* 1158–1159.

CROCETTI, G. M., KULCAR, Z., KESIC, B. & LEMKAU, P. V. (1971) Selected aspects of the epidemiology of psychoses in Croatia, Yugoslavia. III The cluster sample and results of the pilot survey. *American Journal of Epidemiology,* **94,** 126–134.

CROW, T. J. (1981) Biological basis of mental disorders: the case for viral aetiology. In *Epidemiological Impact of Psychotropic Drugs,* edited by G. Tognoni, C. Bellantuono and M. H. Lader.. Amsterdam: Elsevier / N. Holland.

—— (1983a) Is schizophrenia an infectious disease? *Lancet, i,* 173–175.

—— (1983b) Schizophrenia as an infection. *Lancet, i,* 819–820.

—— (1984) Integrated viral genes as the cause of schizophrenia: a hypothesis. *Proceedings of the Tenth Annual Conference of the British Association of Psychopharmacology,* Guernsey, April 4th to 8th. Oxford: Oxford University Press.

—— & DONE, D. J. (1985) Age of onset of schizophrenia in siblings: Horizontal or vertical transmission. *Psychiatry Research,* in press.

—— FERRIER, I. N., JOHNSTONE, E. C., MACMILLAN, J. F., OWENS, D. G. C., PARRY, R. P. & TYRRELL, D. A. J. (1979) Characteristics of patients with schizophrenia or neurological disorder and virus-like agent in cerebrospinal fluid. *Lancet, i,* 842–844.

DALE, P. W. (1981) Prevalence of schizophrenia in the Pacific Islands of Micronesia. *Journal of Psychiatric Research,* **16,** 103–111.

FISCHER, M. (1973) Genetic and environmental factors in schizophrenia. *Acta Psychiatrica Scandinavica,* **238,** 1–58.

FLOR-HENRY, P. (1969) Psychosis and temporal lobe epilepsy: a controlled investigation. *Epilepsia,* **10,** 363–395.

GALABURDA, A. M., LE MAY, M., KEMPER, T. L. & GESCHWIND, N. (1978) Right-left asymmetries in the brain. *Science,* **199,** 852–856.

GOODALL, E. (1927) The Eighth Maudsley Lecture: Dealing with some of the work done to elucidate the pathology of the disease falling to be considered under the rubic 'insanity'. *Journal of Mental Science,* **73,** 363–390.

—— (1932) The exciting cause of certain states, at present classified under 'schizophrenia' by psychiatrists, may be infection. *Journal of Mental Science,* **78,** 746–755.

GOTTESMAN, I. I. (1978) Schizophrenia and genetics: Where are we? Are you sure? In: *The Nature of Schizophrenia,* edited by L. C. Wynne, R. L. Cromwell & S. Matthysse. New York: Wiley.

HARE, E. H. & MORAN, P. (1980) A relation between seasonal temperature and the birth rate of schizophrenic patients. *Acta Psychiatrica Scandinavica,* **63,** 396–405.

—— (1983a) Was insanity on the increase? *British Journal of Psychiatry,* **142,** 439–455.

—— (1983b) Epidemiological evidence for a viral factor in the aetiology of the functional psychoses. *Advances in Biological Psychiatry,* **12,** 52–75.

—— & WALTER, S. D. (1978) Seasonal variation in admissions of psychiatric patients and its relation to seasonal variation in their birth. *Journal of Epidemiology and Community Health,* **32,** 47–52.

HARPER, P. S. (1977) Mendelian inheritance or transmissible agent?—the lessons of Kuru and Australia antigen. *Journal of Medical Genetics,* **14,** 389–398.

HENDRICK, I. (1928) Encephalitis lethargica and the interpretation of mental disease. *American Journal of Psychiatry,* **84,** 898–1014.

HIMMELHOCH, J., PINCUS, J., TUCKER, G. & DETRE, T. (1970) Subacute encephalitis: behavioural and neurological aspects. *British Journal of Psychiatry,* **116,** 531–538.

HIRSCH, S. R. (1983) Cytomegalic inclusion virus in schizophrenia c.s.f. Proceedings of VIIth World Congress of Psychiatry, Vienna, June 1983.

HOFBAUER, B. (1864) Infectio psychica. *Osterreichische Medicinische Wochenschrift*, **39.**

HUNTER, R. & JONES, M. (1966) Acute lethargica-type encephalitis. *Lancet, ii*, 1023–1024.

JAENISCH, R. (1976) Germ line integration and Mendelian transmission of the exogenous Moloney leukemia virus. *Proceedings of the National Academy of Science, 73*, 1260–1264.

JELLIFFE, S. E. (1927) The mental pictures in schizophrenia and in epidemic encephalitis. *American Journal of Psychiatry, 6*, 413–465.

KARLSSON, J. L. (1970a) The rate of schizophrenia in foster-reared close relatives of schizophrenic index cases. *Biological Psychiatry, 2*, 285–290.

—— (1970b) Genetic association of giftedness and creativity with schizophrenia. *Hereditas, 66*, 177–181.

KASANETZ, E. F. (1979) Tecnica per investigare il ruolo di fattori ambientale sulla genesi della schizofrenia. *Rivista di Psicologia Analitica, 10*, 193–202.

KELLEHER, M. J., COPELAND, J. R. M. & SMITH, A. J. (1974) High first admission rates for schizophrenia in the West of Ireland. *Psychological Medicine, 4*, 460–462.

KENDELL, R. E. & GOURLAY, J. (1970) The clinical distinction between the affective psychoses and schizophrenia. *British Journal of Psychiatry, 117*, 261–266.

KING, D. J., COOPER, S. J., MARTIN, S. M. *et al* (1985) A survey of serum antibodies to eight common viruses in psychiatric patients. *British Journal of Psychiatry, 147*, 145–149.

KINNEY, D. K. & JACOBSEN, B. (1978) Environmental factors in schizophrenia: New adoption study evidence in *The Nature of Schizophrenia*. Edited by: L. C. Wynne, R. Cromwell & S. Matthysse. New York: Wiley.

LEVY, J. (1969) Possible basis for the evolution of lateral specialisation of the human brain. *Nature, 224*, 614–615.

LEWIS, R. M. (1974) Spontaneous auto-immune diseases of domestic animals. *International Revue of Experimental Pathology, 13*, 55–82.

LINDSAY, J., OUNSTED, C. & RICHARDS, P. (1979) Long-term outcome in children with temporal lobe seizures. III Psychiatric aspects in childhood and adult life. *Developmental Medicine and Childhood Neurology, 21*, 630–636.

LIPTON, H. L., FRIEDMANN, A., SETHI, P. & CROWTHER, J. B. (1983) Characterisation of Vilyuisk virus as a picornavirus. *Journal of Medical Virology, 12*, 195–203.

LLOYD STILL, R. M. (1958) Psychosis following Asian influenza in Barbados. *Lancet, ii*, 21–22.

LUCHINS, D., POLLIN, W. & WYATT, R. J. (1980) Laterality in monozygotic schizophrenic twins: an alternative hypothesis. *Biological Psychiatry, 15*, 87–93.

—— WEINBERGER, D. R. & WYATT, R. J. (1979) Anomalous lateralisation associated with a milder form of schizophrenia. *American Journal of Psychiatry, 136*, 1598–1599.

LWOFF, A. (1965) Interaction among virus, cell and organism. In *Nobel Lectures in Physiology or Medicine 1963–1970*. Amsterdam: Elsevier.

McCOWAN, P. K. & COOK, L. C. (1928) The mental aspect of chronic epidemic encephalitis. *Lancet, i*, 1316.

MENNINGER, K. A. (1928) The schizophrenic syndrome as a product of acute infectious disease. *Archives of Neurology & Psychiatry, 20*, 464–481.

—— (1926) Influenza and schizophrenia. An analysis of post-influenzal 'dementia praecox' as of 1918, and five years later. *American Journal of Psychiatry, 5*, 469–529.

MILLER, E. (1971) Handedness and the pattern of human ability. *British Journal of Psychology, 62*, 111–112.

MISRA, P. C. & HAY, G. G. (1971) Encephalitis presenting as acute schizophrenia. *British Medical Journal, i*, 523–533.

MURRAY, R. M. & REVELEY, A. M. (1983a) Schizophrenia as an infection. *Lancet, i*, 583.

—— (1983b) Genetics of Schizophrenia. *Lancet, i*, 1159–1160.

MYERSON, A. (1925) *The Inheritance of Mental Diseases*. Baltimore: Williams and Wilkins.

NARAYAN, O., HERZOG, S., FRESE, K., SCHEEFERS, H. & ROFT, R. (1983) Behavioural disease in rats caused by immunopathological responses to persistent borna virus in the brain. *Science, 220*, 1401–1402.

PAYNE, L. N. & CHUBB, R. C. (1968) Studies on the nature and genetic control of an antigen in normal chick embryos which reacts in the COFAL test. *Journal of General Virology, 3*, 379–391.

PENROSE, L. S. (1942) Auxiliary genes for determining sex as contributory causes of mental illness. *Journal of Mental Science, 88*, 308–316.

PETURSSON, G., MARTIN, J. R., GEORGSSON, N., NATHANSON, N. & PALSSON, P. A. (1979) Visna, the biology of the agent and the disease. In *Aspects of Slow and Persistent Virus Infections*, edited by D. A. J. Tyrrell. The Hague: Martinus Nijhoff.

POLLIN, W. & STABENAU, J. R. (1968) Biological, psychological and historical differences in a series of monozygotic twins discordant for schizophrenia. *Journal of Psychiatric Research*, **6**, 317–332.

POWELL, A., THOMSON, N., HALL, D. J. & WILSON, L. (1973) Parent-child concordance with respect to sex and diagnosis in schizophrenia and manic-depressive psychosis. *British Journal of Psychiatry*, **123**, 653–658.

RAVENHOLT, R. T. & FOEGE, W. H. (1982) 1918 Influenza, Encephalitis Lethargica, Parkinsonism. *Lancet*, ii, 860–864.

REYNOLDS, G. P. (1983) Increased concentrations and lateral asymmetry of amygdala dopamine in schizophrenia. *Nature*, **305**, 527–529.

ROSENTHAL, D. (1962) Familial concordance by sex with respect to schizophrenia. *Psychological Bulletin*, **59**, 401–421.

—— (1970) *Genetic Theory and Abnormal Behaviour*. New York: McGraw-Hill.

SACKHEIM, H. A. & DECINA, P. (1983) Lateralised neuropsychological abnormalities in bipolar adults and in children of bipolar probands. In *Laterality and Psychopathology*, edited by P. Flor-Henry and J. Gruzelier. Amsterdam: Elsevier.

SCHARFETTER, C. (1970) On the hereditary aspects of symbiontic psychoses. A contribution towards the understanding of the schizophrenia-like psychoses. *Psychiatric Clinics*, **3**, 145–152.

SCHULZ, B. (1940) Erkrandungsalter schizophrenen Eltern und Kinder. *Zeitschrift fur Neurologie und Psychiatrie*, **168**, 709–721.

SHAPIRO, J. A. (1983) *Mobile Genetic Elements*. Orlando: Academic.

SOBIN, A. & OZER, M. N. (1966) Mental disorders in acute encephalitis. *Journal of the Mount Sinai Hospital*, **33**, 73–82.

TAYLOR, D. C. (1975) Factors influencing the occurrence of schizophrenia-like psychosis in patients with temporal lobe epilepsy. *Psychological Medicine*, **5**, 249–254.

TAYLOR, G. R., CROW, T. J., FERRIER, I. N., JOHNSTONE, E. C., PARRY, R. P. & TYRRELL, D. A. J. (1982) Virus-like agent in schizophrenia and some neurological disorders. *Lancet*, ii, 1166–1167.

TAYLOR, P. J., DALTON, R., FLEMINGER, J. J. & LISHMAN, W. A. (1982) Differences between two studies of hand preference in psychiatric patients. *British Journal of Psychiatry*, **140**, 166–173.

TEMIN, H. M. (1980) Origin of retroviruses from cellular moveable genetic elements. *Cell*, **21**, 599–600.

—— & MIZUTANI, S. (1970) RNA-dependent DNA polymerase in virions of Rous sarcoma virus. *Nature*, **226**, 1211–1213.

TORREY, E. F. (1980) *Schizophrenia and Civilization*. New York: Jason Aronson.

—— MCGUIRE, M., O'HARE, A., WALSH, D. & SPELLMAN, M. P. (1984) Endemic psychosis in Western Ireland. *American Journal of Psychiatry*, **141**, 966–970.

—— TORREY, B. B. & PETERSEN, M. R. (1977) Seasonality of schizophrenic births in the United States. *Archives of General Psychiatry*, **34**, 1065–1070.

—— —— & BURTON-BRADLEY, B. G. (1974) The epidemiology of schizophrenia in Papua-New Guinea. *American Journal of Psychiatry*, **131**, 567–573.

—— YOLKEN, R. H. & WINFREY, C. J. (1982) Cytomegalovirus antibody in cerebrospinal fluid of schizophrenic patients detected by enzyme immunoassay. *Science*, **216**, 892–894.

—— & ALBRECHT, A. (1983) Cytomegalovirus as a possible etiological agent in schizophrenia. *Advances in Biological Psychiatry*, **12**, 150–160.

TYRRELL, D. A. J., PARRY, R. P., CROW, T. J., JOHNSTONE, E. C. & FERRIER, I. N. (1979) Possible virus in schizophrenia and some neurological disorders. *Lancet*, i, 839–841.

WALKER, S. F. (1980) Lateralisation of functions in the vertebrate brain: a review. *British Journal of Psychiatry*, **71**, 329–367.

WATSON, C. G., KUCALA, T., TILLESKJOR, C. & JACOBS, L. (1984) Schizophrenic birth seasonality in relation to the incidence of infectious diseases and temperature extremes. *Archives of General Psychiatry*, **41**, 85–90.

WEINSTEIN, E. A., LINN, L. & KAHN, R. L. (1955) Encephalitis with a clinical picture of schizophrenia. *Journal of the Mount Sinai Hospital*, **21**, 341–354.

WEISS, R. A. (1978) Why cell biologists should be aware of genetically transmitted viruses. *National Cancer Institute Monograph*, **48**, 183–189.

WOLLENBERG, R. (1889) Ueber psychische infection. *Archiv für Psychiatrie*, **20**, 62–88.

WUNDERLICH, V. & ZOTTER, S. (1982) Abrogation of infectivity of mouse mammary tumor virus by reserpine. *Experimental Pathology*, **21,** 59–61.

—— FEY, F. & SYDOW, G. (1980) Antiviral effect of haloperidol on Rauscher murine leukemia virus. *Archiv Geschwultsforschung*, **50,** 758–762.

IV. Genetic aspects

25 Genetic aspects of schizophrenia: Overview

**ROBIN M. MURRAY and
ADRIANNE M. REVELEY**

As we have seen, the lineage of the effort to find genetic predispositions runs back through the eugenic thinking of the 1930's and 1920's, with its belief in genes for criminal degeneracy, sexual profligacy, alcoholism, and every other type of activity disapproved of by bourgeois society. It is deeply embedded in today's determinist ideology. Only thus can we account for the extraordinary repetitive perseverance and uncritical nature of research into the genetics of schizophrenia.

[Rose *et al*, 1984]

As the above quote demonstrates, many outside the psychiatric profession, and not a few within it, regard the whole subject of a genetic contribution to schizophrenia as preposterous. But why schizophrenia should arouse such controversy, when disorders of comparably complex causation such as heart disease or diabetes do not, says more about fundamental divisions of attitude towards schizophrenia than it does about the state of the evidence. For those who regard schizophrenia as a reaction to circumstance, evidence for a genetic contribution calls basic tenets into question, while for those who see schizophrenia as an illness, such evidence is a step forward in the search for causation.

This overview will, therefore, not only review what progress those in the field believe has occurred, but also examine the criticisms, since these have at times had very important effects. For example, reviewers both friendly (Rosenthal, 1959) and hostile (Jackson, 1960; Lidz *et al*, 1965) pointed out that the concordance rates in the pre-war twin studies of schizophrenia were much too high. Since the evidence for a genetic contribution had rested largely on these studies, there arose considerable scepticism. In response, more stringent twin studies appeared including both in-patient and out-patient schizophrenics in systematically ascertained series (Kringlen, 1967; Pollin *et al*, 1969; Gottesman and Shields, 1972; Fischer, 1973; Tienari, 1975). These reported lower concordance rates, but nevertheless still demonstrated a disparity between monozygotic (MZ) and dizygotic (DZ) twins.

The adopted-away offspring of schizophrenics were soon shown to have an increased risk of schizophrenia and schizophrenia spectrum disorders (Heston and Denney, 1968; Rosenthal *et al*, 1968), and the biological but not the adoptive relatives of schizophrenic adoptees shown to have increased rates of schizophrenia spectrum disorders (Kety, 1983b). While methodological problems are apparent here also, particularly in the definition of the schizophrenia spectrum, these studies also supported a genetic influence.

A fallow period, particularly marked in Britain, followed the major twin and adoption studies. In 1977 a working party of the Medical Research Council (MRC) complained: 'Since the close of the MRC Psychiatric Genetics Unit on the retirement of Dr Slater there has been little research in psychiatric genetics in this country. While a few individuals continue to work in the field, it attracts few young people.' The 1980s have seen a quickening of interest. New ideas have been incorporated into family, twin, and statistical studies, and we are beginning to move beyond the simple question of 'Genetic influence or not?' to 'What is the nature of the genetic and environmental contributions to aetiology, and how do they interact?'

Family studies using operational definitions

Early studies suggested that the first-degree relatives of schizophrenics have about a 10 per cent risk of also suffering from the disorder; but two recent American studies failed to detect any such familial aggregation. Pope *et al* (1983) found no cases of DSM-III schizophrenia among 199 first-degree relatives, while Abrams and Taylor (1983) reported a morbidity risk of only 1.6 per cent using their own rather idiosyncratic criteria. These small, uncontrolled studies have been extensively criticized (Kendler, 1983a; Weissman *et al*, 1983; Kety, 1983a), particularly for their use of the family history method which relies on information from the proband and therefore underestimates morbidity compared to family studies, where relatives are personally interviewed (Thompson *et al*, 1982).

While these studies attracted more attention than they deserved, more important studies continued to demonstrate a familial clustering of cases. **Tsuang et al (1980)** 'blindly' examined 918 relatives of schizophrenics and controls; the morbidity risks for schizophrenia were 5.5 per cent in the relatives of schizophrenics and 0.6 per cent in the relatives of controls. These differences remained when DSM-III criteria were used (Tsuang, 1985). In a similar study Guze *et al* (1983) found 8.1 per cent of first-degree relatives of schizophrenics were also schizophrenic according to Feighner-like criteria. Thus, studies using operational definitions produce familial rates which are lower than the classical rates, but still significantly raised over general population levels.

Twin studies

Pooling the results from the five twin studies published between 1967 and 1975 yields concordance rates for schizophrenia of 47 per cent for MZ co-twins and 14 per cent for DZ co-twins. Subsequently, Kendler and Robinette (1983) updated the US Army Veteran twin sample. The concordance rates were 30.9 per cent for MZ and 6.5 per cent for DZ twins; this series is selected for health since both twins must have been well enough to be accepted into the Army.

Koskenvuo *et al* (1984) examined psychiatric hospitalization rates of all twins born before 1958 in Finland over a 10-year period. The study design, which necessarily excluded probands admitted to hospital outside the specified period and those chronically hospitalized, selected twins for relatively mild illness. Nevertheless, despite very low pair-wise concordance rates (11 per cent for MZ and 1.8 per cent for DZ twins) the MZ/DZ excess remained. Twin studies continue to attract criticism. Some articles impugn the political morality of twin researchers (Rose *et al*, 1984; Marshall, 1984), while others accuse them of using proband rather than pair-wise rates simply to increase concordance (Marshall and Pettit, 1985). No twin studies so far have set out to use operational definitions of schizophrenia, though McGuffin *et al* (1983) applied a series of such definitions to the twin summaries prepared by Gottesman and Shields (1972). The Research Diagnostic Criteria and the Feighner Criteria produced concordance rates that were comparable to those of the original report.

Crow (1983) pointed out that the concordance rates in schizophrenia are not dissimilar to those in some infectious diseases such as tuberculosis, and argued that an infectious agent might be operating in schizophrenia. However, McGue *et al* (1985) have shown that genetic models fit the family data on schizophrenia but do not do so for tuberculosis. Twin studies alone cannot establish a genetic contribution to schizophrenia even though Kendler (1983b) concludes that the increased MZ/DZ ratio is not the result of any systematic bias. Indeed, there are hints (McGue *et al*, 1983) that an environmental effect specific to twins might operate to lower concordance rates; this could be perinatal morbidity (vide infra).

Adoption studies

Debate about the methodology of the Kety/Rosenthal adoption studies has continued (Lidz and Blatt, 1983; Kety, 1983b; Rose *et al*, 1984), and there have been several independent analyses of the original information. For example, Kendler *et al* (1981) blindly rediagnosed the relatives of the schizophrenic adoptees. They found no increase in paranoid psychosis but they did find an excess of schizotypal personality disorder in the biological relatives. If true, this is a most important finding because previous attempts to find personality abnormalities genetically linked to schizophrenia have not been successful. Since the criteria for schizotypal personality were previously derived from this same sample (Spitzer *et al*, 1979), the above results do not represent a fully independent validation of the criteria. But two other studies have now suggested the schizotypal personality is part of the schizophrenia spectrum (Baron *et al*, 1984; Kendler *et al*, 1984).

Models of genetic transmission and their consequences

Dominant theories

A variety of models of transmission have been proposed, but as yet none has proved satisfactory. Models are important, not only for themselves, but also because of the type of research that they inspire. Among the most influential has been the partial dominance theory which supposes that all homozygotes and a small proportion of heterozygotes will have the illness while the majority of heterozygotes escape. But recent mathematical analyses have demonstrated that single gene models are not compatible with twin and family data (O'Rourke *et al*, 1982; Tsuang *et al*, 1982; McGue *et al*, 1985). Thus despite **Karlsson's** (**1982**) advocacy, it is unlikely that the transmission of schizophrenia is due solely to single locus inheritance. Such a gene may yet be involved in a proportion of cases with non-specific genetic and environmental effects accounting for the remainder (McGuffin, 1984; McGue *et al*, 1985).

If a single gene accounts for a proportion of schizophrenia, it is logical to look for a genetic marker which would identify individuals possessing the gene. For example, McGuffin *et al* (1983) studied 19 marker systems including HLA in 12 families with multiple affected members and failed to find any evidence of linkage. As **Reveley and Reveley** point out in their review later in this volume, enormous effort has gone into the study of platelet monoamine oxidase, much of it under the mistaken impression that it could prove to be a genetic marker. No genetic markers have as yet been identified but now this type of approach to schizophrenia has been revitalized by the dramatic developments in DNA technology.

Polygenic/multifactorial models

These models imply that schizophrenia is caused by the additive effect of a large number of genes plus a variety of environmental influences. They may be simple (Gottesman and Shields, 1972) or more complex, postulating various thresholds of liability beyond which increasingly severe types of schizophrenia become manifest. The threshold models did not initially seem to fit the available data, but McGue *et al* (1985) have produced a modified version which does.

While polygenic/multifactorial models imply that the search for a unique biochemical cause for all schizophrenia is unlikely to be successful, they do allow calculation of the proportion of the aetiology of schizophrenia contributed by genes. Gottesman and Shields (1982) estimate this at 70 per cent while Kendler and Robinette (1983) produce estimates ranging from 71 per cent and 91 per cent. Not only hostile critics (Marshall, 1984) regard such figures as dubious. Edwards (1977) considers such procedures are 'formally irrelevant to the problems presented to relations, to society, and to the scope and nature of future therapy.'

A familial/sporadic distinction

Schizophrenics with a positive family history tend to become ill at an earlier age and to have a more severe form of the illness than those without such a history. Many authors (e.g. Leonhard, 1980) have advocated making a distinction between the two groups. Reveley *et al* (1984) suggest that the familial group have normal sized cerebral ventricles, and they and other researchers report that CT scan abnormalities are more common in the non-familial group (Oxiensterna *et al*, 1984; Turner *et al*, 1986).

Pasamanick and Knobloch (1961) postulated that complications of pregnancy and birth might produce 'a continuum of reproductive casualty' including cerebral palsy, epilepsy, mental deficiency or behaviour disorders. Subsequently, many workers linked birth complications with later schizophrenia (reviewed by Torrey, 1977; Gottesman and Shields, 1977; McNeil and

Kaij, 1978). Reveley *et al* (1984) showed that among normal control twins those with birth complications had bigger ventricles than those without. All their schizophrenic twins with birth complications had relatively large cerebral ventricles and a negative family history. Several other groups have also related perinatal complications to ventricular size in adult schizophrenics (Schulsinger *et al*, 1984; Roberts, 1980; Turner *et al*, 1986).

A familial/sporadic distinction is compatible both with heterogeneity in schizophrenia (i.e. distinct types) or with a multifactorial hypothesis in which genetic and environmental factors act in an additive fashion (Murray *et al*, 1985). Such a distinction may enable researchers to better direct their research efforts and is also of value in genetic counselling, which is difficult in a disorder such as schizophrenia with only a slight increase of cases in relatives (see **Kay**'s review). It is already possible on an empirical basis to suggest to the relatives of sporadic cases with obvious cerebral abnormality that the chance of schizophrenia developing in them or their children is less than in the relatives of schizophrenics without such manifest abnormality (Reveley, 1985).

Conclusion

Prompted by criticism, methodology has now improved and the evidence still points to a genetic contribution to schizophrenia; its significance and mode of transmission remain uncertain, and the search for a genetic marker has been fruitless. Nevertheless, advances in mathematical techniques enable the empirical testing of different models, and researchers can better attempt to tease apart the genetic and environmental components of aetiology. For instance, it is families with several affected members to whom the techniques of molecular genetics are being applied, while the new methods of visualizing the in vivo anatomy of the brain may be particularly valuable in sporadic cases.

References

ABRAMS, R. & TAYLOR, M. A. (1983) The genetics of schizophrenia; A reassessment using modern criteria. *American Journal of Psychiatry*, **140,** 171–175.

BARON, M., GRUEN, R., ASNIS, L. & KANE, J. (1984) Familial relatedness of schizophrenia and schizotypal states. *American Journal of Psychiatry*, **140,** 1437–1444.

CROW, T. J. (1983) Is schizophrenia an infectious disease? *Lancet, i,* 173–175.

EDWARDS, J. (1977) Evidence presented to the MRC Working Party on the Genetics of Psychiatric Disorders, London.

FISCHER, M. (1973) Genetic and environmental factors in schizophrenia. *Acta Psychiatrica Scandinavica,* Suppl. 238.

GOTTESMAN, I. I. & SHIELDS, J. (1972) *Schizophrenia and Genetics: A Twin Vantage Point.* New York and London: Academic Press.

—— —— (1977) Obstetric complications and twin studies of schizophrenia. *Schizophrenia Bulletin,* **3,** 351–354.

—— —— (1982) *Schizophrenia: The Epigenetic Puzzle.* Cambridge: Cambridge University Press.

GUZE, S. B., CLONINGER, C. R., MARTIN, R. L., CLAYTON, P. J. (1983) A follow-up and reliability study of schizophrenia. *Archives of General Psychiatry,* **40,** 1273–1276.

HESTON, I. L. & DENNEY, D. (1968) Interactions between early life experience and biological factors in schizophrenia. In *The Transmission of Schizophrenia* (eds. D. Rosenthal and S. Kety). Oxford: Pergamon.

JACKSON, D. (1960) *The Aetiology of Schizophrenia.* New York: Basic Books.

KARLSSON, J. L. (1982) Family transmission of schizophrenia: A review and synthesis. *British Journal of Psychiatry*, **140**, 600–606.

KENDLER, K. S. (1983a) Heritability of schizophrenia. *American Journal of Psychiatry*, **139**, 1557–1562.

—— (1983b) Overview: A current perspective on twin studies of schizophrenia. *American Journal of Psychiatry*, **140**, 1413–1425.

—— & ROBINETTE, C. D. (1983) Schizophrenia in the National Academy of Sciences National Research Council Twin Registry: A 16-year update. *American Journal of Psychiatry*, **140**, 1551–1563.

—— GRUENBERG, A. M. & STRAUSS, J. S. (1981) An independent analysis of the Copenhagen sample of the Danish adoption study of schizophrenia. I, II, III, *Archives of General Psychiatry*, **38**, 973–987.

—— MASTERSON, C. C., UNGARO, R. & DAVIS, K. L. (1984) A family history study of schizophrenia-related personality disorders. *American Journal of Psychiatry*, **141**, 424–427.

KETY, S. (1983a) Response to Abrams and Taylor. *American Journal of Psychiatry*, **140**, 1111–1112.

—— (1983b) Mental illness in the biological and adoptive relations of schizophrenic adoptees. *American Journal of Psychiatry*, **140**, 720–727.

KOSKENVUO, M., LANGINVAINIO, H., KAPRIO, J., LONNQVIST, J. & TIENARI, P. (1984) Psychiatric hospitalisation in twins. *Acta Genetica Medica Gemellologica*, **33**, 321–332.

KRINGLEN, E. (1967) *Heredity and Environment in the Functional Psychoses.* London: Heinemann Medical.

LEONHARD, K. (1980) Contradictory issues in the origin of schizophrenia. *British Journal of Psychiatry*, **136**, 437–444.

LIDZ, T., FLECK, S. & CORNELISON, A. R. (1965) *Schizophrenia and the Family.* New York: International Universities Press.

—— & BLATT, S. (1983) Critique of the Danish-American adoption studies. *American Journal of Psychiatry*, **140**, 426–435.

MARSHALL, J. R. (1984) The genetics of schizophrenia revisited. *Bulletin of the British Psychological Society*, **37**, 177–181.

—— & PETTIT, A. N. (1985) Discordant concordant rates. *Bulletin of the British Psychological Society*, **38**, 6–9.

McGUE, M., GOTTESMAN, I. I. & RAO, D. C. (1983) The transmission of schizophrenia under a multifactorial threshold model. *American Journal of Human Genetics*, **35**, 1161–1178.

—— —— —— (1985) Resolving genetic models for the transmission of schizophrenia. *Genetic Epidemiology*, in press.

McGUFFIN, P. (1984) *Genetic Markers in Schizophrenia.* PhD Thesis, University of London.

—— FESTENSTEIN, H., MURRAY, R. M. (1983) A family study of HLA antigens and other genetic markers in schizophrenia. *Psychological Medicine*, **13**, 31–43.

McNEIL, T. F. & KAIJ, L. (1978) Obstetric factors in the development of schizophrenia: Complications in the births of preschizophrenics and in reproduction by schizophrenic parents. In *The Nature of Schizophrenia* (eds. L. C. Wynne, R. L. Cromwell and S. Matthysse). New York: J. Wiley.

MEDICAL RESEARCH COUNCIL (1977) *Report of a Working Party on the Genetics of Psychiatric Disorders.* London.

MURRAY, R. M., LEWIS, S. & REVELEY, A. M. (1985) Towards an aetiological classification of schizophrenia. *Lancet*, i, 1023–1026.

O'ROURKE, D. H., GOTTESMAN, I. I., SUAREZ, B. K., RICE, J. & REICH, T. (1982) Refutation of the single locus model in the aetiology of schizophrenia. *American Journal of Human Genetics*, **33**, 630–649.

OXIENSTERNA, G., BERGSTRAND, G., BJERKENSTEDT, L., SEDVALL, G. & WIK, G. (1984) Evidence of disturbed CSF circulation and brain atrophy in cases of schizophrenic psychosis. *British Journal of Psychiatry*, **144**, 654–661.

PASAMANICK, B. & KNOBLOCH, H. (1961) Epidemiological studies on complications of pregnancy and the birth process. In *Prevention of Mental Disorders in Children* (ed. G. Caplan). New York: Basic Books.

POLLIN, W., ALLEN, M. G., HOFFER, A., STABENAU, J. R. & HRUBEC, Z. (1969) Psychopathology in 15,909 pairs of veteran twins. *American Journal of Psychiatry*, **126**, 597–610.

POPE, H. G., JONAS, J., COHEN, B. M. & LIPINSKI, J. F. (1983) Heritability of schizophrenia. *American Journal of Psychiatry*, **140**, 132–133.

REVELEY, A. M., REVELEY, M. A. & MURRAY, R. M. (1984) Cerebral ventricular enlargement of nongenetic schizophrenia: A controlled twin study. *British Journal of Psychiatry*, **144**, 89–93.

—— (1985) Genetic counselling for schizophrenia. *British Journal of Psychiatry*, **147**, 107–112.

ROBERTS, J. (1980) *The Use of the CAT Head Scanner in Psychiatry.* M.Phil Thesis, University of London.

ROSE, S., KAMIN, L. J. & LEWONTIN, R. C. (1984) *Not in Our Genes.* Middlesex: Pelican Books.

ROSENTHAL, D. (1959) Some factors associated with concordance and discordance with respect to schizophrenia in monozygotic twins. *Journal of Nervous and Mental Disease,* **129,** 1–10.

—— WENDER, P. H., KETY, S. S., SCHULSINGER, F., WELNER, J. & OSTERGAARD, L. (1968) Schizophrenics' offspring reared in adoptive homes. In *The Transmission of Schizophrenia* (eds. D. Rosenthal and S. Kety). Oxford: Pergamon.

SCHULSINGER, F., PARNAS, J., PETERSEN, E. T., SCHULSINGER, H., TEASDALE, T. W., MEDNICK, S., MOLLER, L. & SILVERTON, L. (1984) Cerebral ventricular size in the offspring of schizophrenic mothers. *Archives of General Psychiatry,* **41,** 602–606.

SPITZER, R. L., ENDICOTE, J. & GIBBON, M. (1979) Crossing the border into borderline personality and borderline schizophrenia. *Archives of General Psychiatry,* **36,** 17–24.

THOMPSON, W. D., ORVASCHELL, H., PRUSOFF, B. A. *et al* (1982) An evaluation of the family history method for ascertaining psychiatric disorders. *Archives of General Psychiatry,* **39,** 639–642.

TIERNARI, P. (1975) Schizophrenia in Finnish male twins. In *Studies of Schizophrenia* (ed. M. H. Lader). Ashford, Kent: Headley Brothers.

TORREY, E. F. (1977) Birth weights, perinatal insults and HLA types: The return to the original din. *Schizophrenia Bulletin,* **3,** 347–351.

TSUANG, M. (1985) Morbidity risk of DSM-III schizophrenics in relatives of schizophrenics. In *Genetic Aspects of Human Behaviour* (eds. T. Sakai and T. Tsuboi). Igaku-Shoin, Tokyo.

—— WINOKUR, G. & CROWE, R. (1980) Morbidity risks of schizophrenia and affective disorders among first degree relatives with schizophrenia, mania, depression and surgical conditions. *British Journal of Psychiatry,* **137,** 497–504.

—— BUCHER, K. D. & FLEMING, J. A. (1982) Testing the monogenic theory of schizophrenia: An application of segregation analysis to blind family study data. *British Journal of Psychiatry,* **140,** 595–599.

TURNER, S. W., TOONE, B. K. & BRETT-JONES, J. R. (1986) Computerised tomographic scan changes in early schizophrenia. *Psychological Medicine,* in press.

WEISSMAN, M. M., MERIKANGAS, K. R., PAULS, D. L., LECHMAN, J. & GAMMON, G. D. (1983) Heritability of schizophrenia. *American Journal of Psychiatry,* **140,** 131–132.

26 Assessment of familial risks in schizophrenia and their application in genetic counselling

D. W. K. KAY

Although the evidence for genetic factors in schizophrenia is very strong, it is essentially circumstantial; just what is transmitted is mysterious. There is a need for genetic counselling, probably as much to dispel exaggerated fears about heredity as to encourage a rational consideration of the impact of the illness on the family. Admittedly, the public demand for genetic counselling is small, although it may be growing; Reed (1972) stated that less than one per cent of the 3,000 cases seen at the Dight Institute over 20 years were concerned with schizophrenia. Nevertheless, it is probable that much gratuitous and ill-informed advice is given. Several valuable articles on genetic counselling in mental illness have appeared in the last few years (Tsuang, 1978; Kessler, 1980; Targum and Schulz, 1982). Reed (1972) described four particular situations in which genetic counselling may be requested: (1) in adoption cases; (2) in cases of morbid jealousy to prove paternity; (3) to review the desirability of parenthood when one parent is psychotic; and (4) by relatives asking for the evidence for heredity in mental illness and for estimates as to its importance.

For the present purposes, I shall assume that a young couple, one of whom is in remission from a schizophrenic illness, is seeking to make a rational decision about parenthood. The counsellor's role is not to arrive at a decision himself, but to inform, explain, discuss and support. He may need to clear up gross misconceptions about the risks involved, as well as to interpret them in terms of everyday experience. The couple may ask what they can do to reduce the risk, or what is his opinion on the changes in treatment and prognosis which may have occurred by the time the child has grown up. He may have to discuss alternatives to child-bearing, such as adoption, family planning, termination of pregnancy or sterilization, and to deal with the emotional issues (Kallmann, 1956; Rainer, 1975; Kessler, 1980). However, this article is mainly concerned with the evaluation of risks and a review of the factors which may raise or lower them.

General considerations

Mode of transmission and genetic models

Cavalli-Sforza and Feldman (1973) noted that correlations between biological relatives are to be expected, even if there is no genetic variation whatsoever.

In schizophrenia inheritance of the disorder could be due to cultural transmission of behaviour and communication patterns, in the same sort of way that language is handed down. However, adoption studies, which can separate these two modes of inheritance, appear to show that the tendency for schizophrenia to segregate in families is due to the sharing of common genes rather than a common culture (Heston, 1966; Kety *et al*, 1968; Kety, 1983; Rosenthal *et al*, 1968; Rosenthal *et al*, 1971, Wender *et al*, 1974). It seems rational, therefore, to counsel patients and their relatives on the genetic risks but the absence, in schizophrenia, of simple Mendelian dominant or recessive transmission has resulted in the construction of increasingly complex models and the search for genetic markers has, so far, been fruitless (Böök *et al*, 1978; Belmaker, 1984; McGuffin, 1984). Investigation of the genetic control of neurotransmitter enzymes and receptors has, however, made progress (Ciaranello and Boehme, 1982; Shire, 1981; see also **Reveley and Reveley** review).

Techniques of segregation analysis have developed greatly in the past decade, and can now deal with quantitative traits and with mixed monogenic-polygenic models (Elston, 1981). In the single major locus (SML) model the problem is to find the penetrance of the gene in the heterozygous and homozygous states. The model shows that the penetrance will vary depending on the frequency of the schizophrenic gene in the general population. Since this is unknown, a unique solution has been hard to obtain. The main alternative, the multifactorial-polygenic (MFP) model, has been used for the transmission of quantitative traits such as height and IQ, and also for threshold disorders. According to this model, schizophrenia results when a threshold is reached on an underlying, normally-distributed, liability to schizophrenia which is partly genetically and partly non-genetically determined. The risks to relatives are functions of the population prevalence of schizophrenia and the closeness of the biological relationship. However, the position of the threshold on the liability continuum is an unknown parameter.

Matthysse and Kidd (1976) compared the predictions generated by each of these two models with the consensus of risks as reported in the literature; for most classes of relatives the risks were found to be equally well predicted by either model. There seemed, in fact, to be too many solutions, but neither model fitted the observations in MZ twins or in the offspring of two schizophrenic parents. The authors therefore rejected both these models of transmission as being too simplistic. Interestingly, both models predicted that some schizophrenics would be genetically normal. O'Rourke *et al* (1982) compared predictions based on the SML model with the data from each of 15 European and American family and twin studies and also observed the overall fit. They, too, rejected the SML hypothesis.

Modern developments

The more complex models made possible by the new techniques are more realistic and genetic hypotheses and family data can be tested by likelihood methods (Elston, 1981). The value of analysing and reporting data from whole pedigrees and not only from two generation families or as proportions of affected relatives, has been pointed out by Elston and Stewart (1971). Unfortunately, there are obvious difficulties in collecting large pedigrees and in making reliable diagnoses of schizophrenia and its related disorders across several generations.

Path analysis, developed for the study of quantitative traits, can be applied to threshold disorders. Parameters representing cultural inheritance and environmental factors unique to twins can be included (Rao *et al*, 1981). The use, where possible, of MFP models incorporating multiple thresholds (Reich *et al*, 1975) helps to study the genetic relationship between apparently different disorders or different forms of the same disorder. So far, the application of these models to schizophrenia has given negative results (Baron, 1982; Tsuang *et al*, 1983; McGue *et al*, 1983). However, the schizophrenia spectrum (Reich, 1976) seems not to have been studied from this point of view.

Empirical risks and the collection of data

Empirical risks are usually based on pooled data, although the risks of schizo-phrenia in the offspring of a schizophrenic parent do not vary significantly between studies (Kidd and Cavalli-Sforza, 1973); however, they mostly refer to probands suffering from chronic schizophrenia and not from acute or atypical forms of illness. The data on offspring are rather limited compared with the much more extensive data on siblings (see O'Rourke *et al*, 1982), and the rates seem to be a little higher, even after correction for age-distributions. Empirical risks include an unknown component due to non-genetic familial inheritance and to random environmental factors. Naturally, empirical data cannot be found for every family situation, and Morton *et al* (1979) showed that reliance on them could be misleading. However, different genetic models often differed among themselves. In particular, a diagnosis of a milder spectrum disorder in the family could greatly affect the computed risks for a given relative; the importance of collecting complete pedigrees could not be overemphasized.

The risks obtained in family studies are affected by the way in which informa-tion is collected. In the *family history* method, the information about family members is obtained from the proband and usually another relative; hospital records may be consulted. In the *family study* method, so far as possible, every living first-degree relative is personally interviewed and a psychiatric evalua-tion made. The family history method leads to underestimation of rates of psychiatric disorder in relatives (Thompson *et al*, 1982). However, since this method is much cheaper and quicker than the family study method, attempts have been made to improve its reliability and validity (Andreasen *et al*, 1977; Kendler *et al*, 1984).

Empirical risks to offspring of a schizophrenic parent

Risk of schizophrenia

Based on pooled data, the average risk for a child of a schizophrenic parent of developing definite or probable schizophrenia is 12.8 per cent; for definite schizophrenia alone, the risk is 9.4 per cent (McGue *et al*, 1983). The status of the co-parent is not specified. When both parents are schizophrenic, the risk is estimated to be 46.3 per cent, but the number of cases is very small. For comparison, the risks in some other classes of relatives are: for siblings, neither parent schizophrenic, 9.6 per cent; with one parent schizophrenic,

16.7 per cent; with both schizophrenic, 46 per cent; for second-degree relatives (half-sibs, nephews, nieces, grandchildren), 3.0–4.2 per cent; for third-degree relatives (first cousins), 2.4 per cent. Concordance rates in MZ and DZ twins are 46 per cent and 14 per cent respectively. Böök *et al* (1978) studied an isolated community in Sweden where all the known schizophrenics, numbering 214, belonged to three large inter-related pedigrees, and where the psychosis was, presumably, genetically homogeneous. Nevertheless, the risks among the relatives were very similar to those given above; among the children of a schizophrenic parent it was 12 per cent.

Risk of psychopathology of any kind in the offspring of schizophrenics

Recent studies concerned with psychopathology of any kind in the offspring of schizophrenics are summarized in Table I. The risks shown are uncorrected for age. With age correction, the risk for schizophrenia itself falls within the range 8–17 per cent, which corresponds with those in other studies (O'Rourke *et al*, 1982). Two of the studies are unrepresentative in that they concern children put up for adoption, one from the USA (Heston, 1966) the other from Denmark (Rosenthal *et al*, 1971).

The rates for borderline states (column 2, Table I) in different investigations are probably not comparable, but rates in the families of schizophrenics may be compared with the rates in controls. In Schulsinger's (1976) prospective study of high- and low-risk children the unusually large proportion in this category (32 per cent) included 'pseudoneurotic' and 'pseudopsychopathic' disorders, as well as schizoid and paranoid personality, and conditions which showed 'discreet signs of thought disorder, anhedonia and micropsychotic symptoms'. Alcoholism and drug abuse, which were much commoner in the offspring of the schizophrenic mothers, may have contributed to the occurrence of the micropsychotic symptoms. In the Danish adoption study the conditions included under this heading were restricted to borderline schizophrenia and borderline schizophreniform psychosis. As regards the personality disorders (column 3, Table I), Heston (1966) and Bleuler (1974) both found that these disorders were significantly commoner in their schizophrenic than in their control group but neither Schulsinger nor Rosenthal *et al* (1971) demonstrated significant differences. The Danish data of Rosenthal *et al* refer only to disorders falling within the schizophrenic spectrum. The risk of a spectrum disorder (column 4, Table I) in that study was 28 per cent in the schizophrenic and 18 per cent in the control group.

Lowing *et al* (1983) re-examined the original Danish material of Rosenthal *et al* (1971) using DSM-III criteria for diagnosing schizophrenia spectrum disorders in the offspring. They found that the incidence of the schizophrenia spectrum, as defined above (Kendler and Gruenberg, 1984), was still 28 per cent in the adoptees with schizophrenic mothers, but was now only 10 per cent in the control group, and that this difference was significant. In three other studies (Table I) about one quarter of the offspring of schizophrenic parents also suffered from conditions falling into a broad category of schizo-phrenia plus non-neurotic personality disorders (significantly higher than in controls in the two studies where they were available). However, these non-neurotic personality disorders may not be identical with Rosenthal's

TABLE I
Uncorrected risks per cent of various disorders in the offspring of a schizophrenic parent

Author	Diagnosis of ill parent	N	Mean ages in years	Condition in offspring						
				Schizo-phrenia 1	Border-line states 2	Non-neurotic personality disorders 3	Col. 4 (1 + 2 + 3)	Neurotic disorders	Epilepsy Sub-normality Other psychoses	No definite psychiatric diagnosis
Heston (1966)[1]	Mother schizophrenic	47	36	11	—	17	28	28	9	45
	No psychiatric record	50		0	—	4	4	14	0	80
Rosenthal et al (1971)[1]	Either parent schizophrenic	52	33	6	10	12	28	—	1	—
	Not in Psychiatric Register	67		0	6	12	18	—	—	—
Reisby (1967)	Mother chronic schizophrenic	278	37	6	1	3	10	5	2	80
Bleuler (1974)	Either parent schizophrenic	143	38	7	2	16	25	—	2	73
	General population sample	1,077	Not given	1	—	5	6	—	—	92
Schulsinger (1976)[2]	Mother severely schizophrenic	173	23½	9	32	16	57	17	1	22
	Not a psychiatric patient	91		1	4	14	19	36	0	42
Fowler et al (1977)	Either parent chronic schizophrenic	28	>15	4	0	21	25	11	0	64

[1] Child separated from parent early in life.
[2] 'Consensus' diagnoses based on agreement between at least two of the 3 methods used.

spectrum. It is possible that the abnormalities in the Danish co-parents of schizophrenics differ from those occurring in other co-parents in view of their having given up a child for adoption (see Assortative Mating and Table IV).

Schulsinger and Heston disagree about the relative frequency of neurotic disorders in the offspring of schizophrenics and controls, while Heston's findings of a markedly high prevalence of mental deficiency in the former is not borne out in any of the other studies. As regards affective psychoses, these seem to be rare, but the offspring would not yet have passed through the greater part of the risk period for these disorders. It may be noted that in most of the studies the majority of the offspring were reported to be psychiatrically normal.

Factors which may affect the empirical risks

Before he is satisfied that he has assessed the risks to the offspring and the burden incurred by a recurrence of schizophrenia or a related condition as adequately as possible, the counsellor should consider four questions.

Question I: What is the nature of the proband's schizophrenia?

Could the proband's schizophrenia be symptomatic?

Symptomatic schizophrenias may occur during the course of known organic diseases or intoxications, and may be mistaken for schizophrenia at some stage (Davison and Bagley, 1969). The best established examples are the schizophrenia-like states associated with temporal lobe epilepsy, cerebral tumours, encephalitis lethargica and as sequelae of penetrating head injuries; with hereditary disorders such as Huntington's disease, narcolepsy, and porphyria; with Cushing's disease, myxoedema and pernicious anaemia; with the abuse of alcohol, amphetamines, LSD or marihuana (Davison, 1976); with medication with drugs such as L-DOPA and steroids; and possibly with chronic deafness (Cooper *et al*, 1974). Twin studies (Gottesman and Shields, 1972) also suggest that schizophrenia may occur on an organic basis in a person who is not genetically predisposed. It is imperative to recognize symptomatic cases because the expectation of schizophrenia in the relatives is probably no higher than in the general population (1–2 per cent). However, in some drug-induced cases the familial risk may be increased (Propping, 1983).

Could the proband's schizophrenia be sporadic?

There is some evidence to suggest that sporadic (i.e. provisionally non-genetic) cases tend to have larger cerebral ventricles (Reveley *et al*, 1982), more EEG abnormalities (Hays, 1977; Kendler and Hays, 1982b), higher platelet MAO activity (Baron *et al*, 1982, but see also Duncavage *et al*, 1982), more perinatal (McNeil and Kaij, 1978) and postnatal brain damage and a winter birth date (Kinney and Jacobsen, 1978; Shur, 1982), and more neurological soft signs (Quitkin *et al*, 1976), than probands with a family history of schizophrenia. Although the interpretation of these findings is tentative, a combination of them might suggest that the risk of recurrence of the illness was less than the average empirical risk.

Atypical psychoses and schizoaffective psychosis (SAP)

Perhaps, not surprisingly, when probands are selected as having typical illnesses, schizophrenia is found to 'breed true'. However, between unselected pairs of siblings, both hospitalized for psychosis, diagnoses are discordant (i.e. one schizophrenic, one affective) in 30 per cent of the pairs (Tsuang, 1967). Table II (after Ødegård, 1972), shows how the diagnoses in the psychotic relatives varied when probands whose psychoses were not typical were included in a family study. These atypical psychoses have been called acute schizophrenia, reactive schizophrenia, schizophreniform or schizoaffective psychoses, but clinically they are quite similar. Unfortunately, the data on which empirical estimates of recurrence risks for these conditions can be based are scanty (Table III) and it is not clear if any of them form a distinct group. **Karlsson's (1982)** unitary hypothesis overcomes these difficulties by grouping all functional psychoses together. The risk of being hospitalized for psychosis in the close relatives of psychotic patients was estimated to be about 14 per cent. This was about four times the risk for psychosis in the general population of Iceland.

Marked affective features in a schizophrenic illness seem to improve the prognosis but also to increase the familial risk of affective disorder (McCabe *et al*, 1971). Family studies of probands diagnosed as suffering from SAP appeared to confirm this conclusion (Tsuang *et al*, 1977; Mendlewicz, 1976— see Table III) and suggested that SAP is genetically more akin to affective disorder than to schizophrenia. However, using strict criteria for the diagnosis of schizophrenia, affective disorder and SAP, Tsuang (1979) compared the diagnoses in hospitalized pairs of siblings and found that SAP seemed to be divisible into two subtypes, one genetically akin to affective disorder (SAP-A), the other to schizophrenia (SAP-S). Baron *et al* (1982), employing the Research Diagnostic Criteria (Spitzer *et al*, 1975), made a family study of the same three conditions and came to similar conclusions. Scharfetter (1981) found that the relatives of index cases with SAP had a high frequency of functional psychoses of both major types, with a higher proportion of affected relatives than probands with either schizophrenia or affective disorder. Thus SAP appears to be genetically and clinically heterogeneous.

Paranoid psychosis, paranoia and delusional disorder

Paranoia is a chronic form of paranoid psychosis whose relationship to affective disorder on one side and schizophrenia on the other has been ambiguous ever since the time of Kraepelin. In DSM-III paranoid psychosis is distinguished from paranoid schizophrenia by the absence of symptoms such as incoherence, marked thought disorder, prominent hallucinations and bizarre delusions; the essential symptoms are persistent delusions which are not secondary to affective disorder or organic mental disorder. In a series of papers (Kendler, 1980; Kendler and Davis, 1981; Kendler and Hays, 1981; Kendler, 1982) Kendler concluded on demographic and genetic grounds that paranoia, now renamed by Winokur (1977) delusional disorder, is probably a distinct condition. Delusional disorder is found to occur mainly in middle or later

TABLE II

Diagnostic distribution of index patients and their psychotic relatives

Patients with	No. of[1] index patients	No. of psychotic relatives	Diagnosis of psychotic relatives (per cent)			
			Schizo-phrenia	Reactive psychoses	Affective psychoses	Total
Schizophrenia	1,205	656	65	16	19	100
with severe defect at follow-up	233	109	78	7	15	100
with slight defect	654	368	70	16	14	100
without defect	318	179	46	23	31	100
Reactive psychosis	278	82	28	48	24	100
Atypical psychosis	96	39	36	28	36	100
Manic depressive psychosis	99	47	19	11	70	100
All psychoses	1,678	824	57	20	23	100

[1] Number at risk not known.   After Ødegård (1972).

From Kaplan, A. R. (1972) *Genetic Factors in Schizophrenia*. Courtesy of Charles C. Thomas, Publisher, Springfield, Illinois.

TABLE III
Atypical psychoses

Author	Proband's illness	Class relative and no. at risk (BZ)	Relatives with			
			Schizophrenia	Atypical psychosis etc	Affective disorder	Total
			Morbidity risks %			
McCabe et al (1971)[2]	Good prognosis schizophrenia	33[1] sibs	3	6	15	24
McCabe and Strömgren (1975)[3]	Reactive psychoses	67[1] sibs	1.5	12	6	19
Tsuang et al (1976)[4]	'Atypical schizophrenia'	(85)[6] sibs	1	—	7	8.5
	Schizophrenia	(200)[6] sibs	1	—	2	3
	Affective disorder	(325)[6] sibs	0.6	—	8	8
Mendlewicz (1976)[5]	Schizoaffective illness	(45)[6] 1° rel.	11 ± 4	—	36 ± 5	47
	Schizophrenia	(45)[6] 1° rel.	17 ± 2	—	9 ± 4	26
	Bipolar illness	(45)[6] 1° rel.	1.4 ± 1	—	41 ± 4	42.4
	Unipolar illness	(45)[6] 1° rel.	3 ± 2	—	29 ± 6	32

[1] Risk-period 15–60.
[2] See McCabe and Cadoret (1976).
[3] Family histories and review of Central Psychiatry Registry + partial family study. Risk-period 15–60.
[4] Case-record study. Method of calculating risks not stated.
[5] All available relatives personally interviewed without knowledge of diagnosis of proband. Risk-period 15–70. Probands with schizophrenia, bipolar and unipolar illness matched for age/sex with schizoaffective probands.
[6] Refers to number of probands.

adult life, in married or formerly married persons of either sex, more frequently in lower than higher socio-economic groups, and more frequently in immigrants than in the native born; there appears to be little or no genetic relationship to either schizophrenic or affective disorder. These conclusions are tentative but they are supported by Watt *et al* (1980) who used the Aberdeen Case Register and found no genetic connection between schizophrenia and paranoid states of middle life.

In their own study of delusional disorder, Kendler and Hays (1981) found that inferiority feelings were significantly commoner in the relatives of probands with this condition than in relatives of schizophrenic probands. Such premorbid feelings were also found to be more common in the probands with delusional disorder themselves (42 per cent) than in the schizophrenic probands (14 per cent). The patients with delusional disorder seemed to resemble the persons described by Kretschmer (1974) as sensitive personalities, prone to delusions of reference. These findings, if confirmed, have obvious importance for genetic counselling.

DSM-III and other diagnostic systems

The counsellor may be perplexed by the current plethora of systems for diagnosing schizophrenia (Endicott *et al*, 1982)) and may wonder whether the genetic risk is the same for each of them. Studies of the Maudsley series of twins by Gottesman and Shields (1972) and by McGuffin *et al* (1984) suggest that an illness with the largest genetic component may be definable by using criteria which are neither broad nor strict, but intermediate. In studies of families of schizophrenic probands, both Pope *et al* (1982), who used DSM-III criteria for their diagnosis of schizophrenia, and Abrams and Taylor (1983), who used narrowly defined operational research criteria, found very few schizophrenic patients. These studies seemed to suggest that when all other conditions are rigorously excluded by strict criteria, the genetic component in schizophrenia may, after all, be quite small. However, independent analyses of the original interviews from the Danish adoption study of schizophrenia, employing DSM-III definitions of psychiatric disorders to both adoptees and their relatives, confirmed the original conclusions as to the importance of genetic transmission in schizophrenia (Kendler and Gruenberg, 1984). Guze *et al* (1983), in a blind follow-up and family study of schizophrenia, also found that diagnostic criteria very similar to DSM-III identified patients with the same diagnosis after an interval of 6–12 years, and with an increased prevalence of schizophrenia in their first-degree relatives.

Kendler and Gruenberg (1984) and Kendler *et al* (1981, 1984) also found that three diagnoses based on DSM-III criteria appeared to form a 'schizophrenia spectrum': schizophrenia, schizotypal personality disorder and paranoid personality. Schizoaffective disorder, which is not strictly defined in DSM-III, also seemed to belong to the spectrum, but only the schizophrenic subtype, SAP-S (see above). In several reports (cited by Kety, 1983) based on a further analysis of the Danish studies, no association was found between the schizophrenic spectrum and anxiety disorder, major depressive disorder or paranoid psychosis; nor did acute, remitting psychotic illnesses (schizophreniform or atypical psychoses) seem to belong to the spectrum. More studies are needed to clarify these issues, but in the meantime the idea that the schizophrenia spectrum is transmitted genetically and is distinct from other disorders defined in DSM-III seems to be supported.

Question II: What are the special features of the proband's illness?

Severity, course and outcome

The counsellor may be asked if, should a child become ill, the illness will resemble the parent's in its course and severity. Twin studies suggest that risks to relatives may be greater, when the illness is chronic; but good outcome, unfortunately, is not a consistent feature of familial illnesses. Larson and Nyman (1973), for instance, found no difference between the relatives of schizophrenic probands whether the outcome was good or bad. Bleuler (1974) noticed that the course of the schizophrenic illness tended to be more nearly similar between parent and offspring than between unrelated pairs, and that episodic illnesses, when followed by remissions, tended to occur in successive generations.

Reisby (1967) concluded that offspring who developed severe or typical schizophrenia had had more prolonged contact with their psychotic parent than those who developed a milder or less typical form of illness, but Bleuler (1974) found little evidence that this was the important factor. Although many of the children in Bleuler's study suffered greatly in their home environment, this was sometimes due to living with a cruel foster-parent or stepmother and not necessarily with the ill parent.

McCabe *et al* (1971) conducted a blind family study of schizophrenics with good and poor prognosis. They found that the families of probands whose illness had lasted at least two years and who had failed to return to their premorbid level of functioning, contained more schizophrenics, neurotics and ill relatives of any kind, but fewer affective disorders, than the families of probands with good outcome. 'Good prognosis schizophrenia' was defined as an illness of less than six months' duration, without any pre-existing psychiatric illness (other than affective disòrder or good prognosis schizophrenia), and a good premorbid personality (good social functioning). Both types of illness showed characteristic schizophrenic symptoms, but (although not a criterion) all the good prognosis probands also had significant affective symptomatology. The authors point to the overlap between their concept of good prognosis schizophrenia and schizoaffective disorder (see section below).

Age of onset and paranoid subtype

In general, a later age of onset of schizophrenia seems to be associated with lower risks in relatives. However, this statement is tentative; systematic attempts to link age of onset in probands with morbidity risk in relatives have not been carried out. In the extreme case of the schizophrenia-like psychoses of the elderly, the risk is only 3–5 per cent (Kay, 1963). Such cases are almost exclusively paranoid and this subtype is of later onset than the non-paranoid types (Winokur *et al*, 1974; Fowler *et al*, 1974). Onset of schizophrenia in the second half of life may be less unusual than is often supposed.

In a study of a year of birth cohort, Larson and Nyman (1970) found that 32 per cent of their 153 probands had their first overt symptoms of schizophrenia after the age of 40 years. Of all the offspring born to the probands, two-thirds were children of paranoid schizophrenics, whose mean age of onset of illness was 42 years (Larson and Nyman, 1973).

In a study of paranoid and non-paranoid schizophrenics, Fowler *et al* (1974) appeared to confirm the earlier work showing that, in relatives of paranoid probands, the risk of developing any type of schizophrenia is only half the risk in relatives of non-paranoid probands (7 *vs* 14 per cent). The latter were younger than the former, and there was a significant correlation in age at onset between probands and relatives, which is the usual finding, but no correlation as regards subtype, which is unusual. However, the relatives' illnesses in the Fowler study were diagnosed blind, which had not previously been done. Tsuang *et al* (1974) concluded, from the same data, that the observed differences in morbidity risks between relatives of paranoid and non-paranoid schizophrenics is accounted for at least partly by age of onset differences.

Subsequently, Kendler and Davis (1981) pointed to an artefact, due to the way in which risks are corrected for age. When this source of error is avoided, the difference in the schizophrenia risk in the families of paranoid and non-paranoid probands is reduced or abolished (**Tsuang *et al*, 1980**; see Kendler and Davis, 1981 for a full discussion). The question may not be regarded as finally settled.

Premorbid inferiority feelings in schizophrenia

In a study to discover whether the presence of premorbid inferiority feelings defines a distinct subgroup of schizophrenia, Kendler and Hays (1982a) found that 7 per cent of their schizophrenics diagnosed by DSM-III criteria had premorbid inferiority feelings and that the psychosis in these cases was associated with stress at onset, embarrassing physical handicap, less severe thought disorder, and a lower relapse rate than in the remainder. The relatives also tended to suffer from inferiority feelings, while schizophrenia was less common in these families than in the families of schizophrenics lacking premorbid inferiority feelings. These findings, if confirmed, suggest a link with delusional disorder and with the syndrome of the previously mentioned sensitive delusions of reference described by Kretschmer (1974).

Question III: The proband's family

Psychiatric information about the proband's family should be as complete as possible and if spectrum disorders are to be identified the close relatives should be personally interviewed. The health of the proband's family is important for two reasons;

(1) It has been found that the presence of another schizophrenic relative increases the risk from about 10 to 17 per cent (Slater and Cowie, 1971). Ødegård (1972) found that the presence of psychotic uncles or aunts more than doubled the chances of the sibs becoming psychotic. The risks to the patient's offspring may be expected to increase in similar fashion when his sibs who, of course, will be the uncles and aunts of the next generation,

are also schizophrenic. However, a non-schizophrenic psychosis in a sib would not be expected to increase the risk of typical schizophrenia in the proband's children, although it would increase the chances of a psychosis of some kind. The presence of a non-schizophrenic spectrum disorder such as a paranoid personality disorder, in a close relative, would also be expected, on present evidence, to increase the risk to a child.

(2) Risks to the second-degree relatives of a schizophrenic: if neither of the couple are themselves ill but are concerned that a schizophrenic illness in a parent or sib may be passed on to their offspring, they may be advised that the empirical risks in second-degree relatives are only 3–5 per cent. Bleuler (1974) remarked that this low risk offered hope to the children of schizophrenics who, tortured by doubt, sought advice as to whether they should marry and have children of their own.

However, in the given case, what really matters is the genotype of the person with the ill relative (and also of the spouse, see next section) and this should be carefully assessed. For example, how much of the period of risk for schizophrenia has he passed? (The period of greatest risk is completed by the age of 40). Although he is not ill, can a disorder within the schizophrenia spectrum be diagnosed? And if by any chance a schizophrenic sib is the proband's monozygous twin, then the proband's children will run the same risk as if he was schizophrenic (Fischer, 1973).

Question IV: The co-parent and the in-laws; assortative mating

Interest has revived in the health of the spouses of schizophrenics. Now that many patients are being treated outside hospitals, fertile unions between two psychotic or formerly psychotic persons may be becoming more common. The question of marriage between related individuals also arises. In the rare instance of both parents being schizophrenic, the risk to their offspring of developing definite or probable schizophrenia, based on the average of five studies, is between 35 and 58 per cent, at the 99 per cent confidence interval (Gottesman and Shields, 1982). About 30 per cent of the non-psychotic offspring may be abnormal, not necessarily, of course, for genetic reasons, and the remainder are normal. When the schizophrenic parent's co-parent has manic-depressive disorder, schizophrenia and manic-depressive disorder in the offspring are equally frequent; when the co-parent has an atypical psychosis, some of the affected children will resemble one parent and some the other.

What is the effect when one parent has schizophrenia and the other a non-psychotic spectrum disorder? Rosenthal (1974) presented data from the Danish adoption study on the condition of the spouses of psychotic parents who had given up a child for adoption at an early age. Limiting the discussion to the spouses of chronic schizophrenics, only two had 'hard spectrum' diagnoses (borderline or chronic schizophrenia, questionable or definite) but altogether 38 per cent fell into the spectrum as a whole (this category included questionable or definite acute schizophrenia and personality disorders of inadequate, paranoid or schizoid kinds). A further 21 per cent of the spouses suffered from psychopathic disorders. These parents were, of course, unrepresentative, in that they had given up a child for adoption. The spouses of patients admitted to mental hospitals with schizophrenia have been studied by Bleuler (1974),

Fowler and Tsuang (1975) and Fowler *et al* (1977). The results of these and of Rosenthal's study are summarized in Table IV. Combining the data, only 3 per cent of the spouses in the non-adoption studies fell into the schizophrenia spectrum, but 30 per cent had other psychiatric abnormalities, chiefly undiagnosed disorders and alcoholism.

When the diagnoses in the offspring are related to diagnoses in the co-parents, the results are as follows. In the Rosenthal study, when the co-parent had a spectrum diagnosis, the offspring were 3–5 times more likely to have a spectrum diagnosis than when the co-parent had another diagnosis or was normal (the diagnoses were blind). In the study by Fowler *et al* (1977), in which assortative matings were far less frequent than in the Danish study but other diagnoses in the co-parent were common, there was a greater risk of psychiatric disturbance in the offspring when the co-parent was abnormal. The commonest diagnosis in the offspring was definite or suspected antisocial personality, the commonest diagnosis in the co-parent was alcoholism. Fowler and Tsuang (1975) pointed out that having an alcoholic or sociopathic parent has been shown to be one of the strongest predictors of antisocial behaviour for juveniles with such behaviour and there was the possibility that some of the abnormalities in the children of schizophrenics were more likely to be related to the illnesses of the co-parents than to be a schizophrenia spectrum disorder transmitted from the schizophrenic parent.

In a controlled study of psychiatric morbidity among schizophrenic families (Stephens *et al*, 1976), a high risk of personality disorder was found among the male sibs of schizophrenics. Kay *et al* (1976) suggested that this might be connected with the psychopathic abnormalities found in many of the non-psychotic fathers and be unrelated to the schizophrenic trait itself. Rimmer and Jacobsen (1980) did not find a significantly higher rate for antisocial personality in the biological relatives of schizophrenic adoptees than in matched non-schizophrenic adoptees. Since some forms of psychopathic disorder may have a hereditary basis (Schulsinger, 1972; Crowe, 1975), this kind of mating might be called 'cross-assortative', i.e. selective mating between persons of different genotypes but sharing certain social and phenotypical characteristics.

Conclusions

The risks of an offspring of a schizophrenic contracting a definite or probable schizophrenic illness are not more than about 10 per cent, except when other relatives on his or the spouse's side are also schizophrenic. Therefore the counsellor may feel less concerned with the attempt to predict events which may possibly occur in 20–40 years' time, than with the prognosis of his patient's own illness and the likelihood of his being able to shoulder the responsibilities of employment, marriage and childrearing. Childbirth, too, will carry special risks, in the shape of post-partum psychosis and disruption of family life at a critical time. There is, in any case, little information about how patients and their relatives react to genetic counselling. Nevertheless, since many people are aware that mental illness tends to run in families, this aspect should not be avoided but discussed in the context of the illness and its implications for the family now and in the future. The added risk to the child may tilt

TABLE IV

Psychopathology in the spouses of schizophrenics

Author	Schizophrenia (definite or suspected) or schizoid personality N (%)	Alcoholism (definite or suspected) N (%)	Antisocial personality (definite or suspected) N (%)	Feeble-minded N (%)	Other and undiagnosed psychiatric illness and suicide N (%)	Total ill N (%)	Total well N (%)
Bleuler (1974)	4	9	—	7	17[1]	37 (30)	83 (70)
Fowler *et al* (1975)	1	5	2	3	7	18 (37)	31 (63)
Fowler *et al* (1977)	1	6	1	0	5	13 (37)	22 (63)
Total	6 (3)	20 (10)	3 (1.5)	10 (5)	29[1] (14)	68 (33)	136 (67)
Rosenthal (1974)[2] (Adoption Study)	9[3] (37.5)	—	5 (21)	—	8 (33)	22 (92)	2 (8)

[1] Includes three suicides.
[2] Spouses of chronic schizophrenics.
[3] Two in 'hard', seven in 'soft' spectrum.

the balance in favour of caution in regard to childbearing, at least until the potential parent's prognosis has declared itself.

Two particular factors must be assessed: The first factor is the nature of the proband's schizophrenia and its genetic component. Symptomatic schizophrenias must be identified as they usually carry no extra risk. Sporadic cases should be very carefully studied for features to support a diagnosis of non-genetic illness, especially when the pedigree is large and the information complete and reliable. Here, evidence of organic aetiology, or as recently proposed, the presence of a paranoid psychosis or of the Kretschmerian syndrome of sensitive delusions of reference, would suggest that the risk of schizophrenia is low. The finer distinctions from other functional psychoses are less important, since these psychoses carry their own increased risks of recurrence (Kay, 1978). Acute, remitting schizophrenia-like episodes seem to have little genetic relationship with chronic schizophrenia and their nosological status is still uncertain.

The second factor is the contribution which the spouse and his genes will make both to an offspring's welfare and to his constitution. Under the circumstances, the spouse will usually be the one to make final decisions about family matters, and he should be given the opportunity to acquire a firm grasp of the issues. If he or any of his close relatives have had a schizophrenic illness or can be diagnosed as having a disorder within the spectrum, the probability that this will increase the chances of his child becoming ill should be clearly explained.

References

ABRAMS, R. & TAYLOR, M. A. (1983) The genetics of schizophrenia: a reassessment using modern criteria. *American Journal of Psychiatry*, **140,** 171–175.

ANDREASEN, N. C., ENDICOTT, J., SPITZER, R. L. & WINOKUR, G. (1977) The family history method using diagnostic criteria. *Archives of General Psychiatry*, **34,** 1229–1235.

BARON, M. (1982) Genetic models of schizophrenia. *Acta Psychiatrica Scandinavica*, **65,** 263–275.

—— GRUEN, R., ASNIS, L. & KANE, J. (1982) Schizoaffective illness, schizophrenia and affective disorders: morbidity risks and genetic transmission. *Acta Psychiatrica Scandinavica*, **65,** 253–262.

—— LEVITT, M. & PERLMAN, R. (1981) Platelet monoamine oxidase values and genetic heterogeneity in schizophrenia research. *Journal of the American Medical Association*, **246,** 1418–1421.

BELMAKER, R. H. (1984) The lesson of platelet monoamine oxidase. *Psychological Medicine*, **4,** 249–253.

BLEULER, M. (1974) The offspring of schizophrenics. *Schizophrenia Bulletin*, **8,** 93–107.

BÖÖK, J., WETTERBERG, L. & MODRZEWSKA, K. (1978) Schizophrenia in a North Swedish geographical isolate, 1900–1977: Epidemiology, genetics and biochemistry. *Clinical Genetics*, **14,** 373–394.

CADORET, R., FOWLER, R. C., MCCABE, M. S. & WINOKUR, G. (1974) Evidence for heterogeneity in a group of good-prognosis schizophrenics. *Comprehensive Psychiatry*, **15,** 433–450.

CAVALLI-SFORZA, L. L. & FELDMAN, M. W. (1973) Cultural versus biological inheritance: Phenotypic transmission from parents to children (a theory of the effect of parental phenotypes on children's phenotypes). *American Journal of Human Genetics*, **25,** 618–637.

CIARANELLO, R. D. & BOEHME, R. E. (1982) Genetic regulation of neurotransmitter enzymes and receptors: relationship to the inheritance of psychiatric disorders. *Behavior Genetics*, **12,** 11–35.

COOPER, A. F., CURRY, A. R., KAY, D. W. K., GARSIDE, R. F. & ROTH, M. (1974) Hearing loss in paranoid and affective psychoses in the elderly. *Lancet*, ii, 851–854.

—— GARSIDE, R. F. & KAY, D. W. K. (1976) A comparison of deaf and non-deaf patients with paranoid and affective psychoses. *British Journal of Psychiatry*, **129,** 532–538.

CROWE, R. R. (1975) An adoptive study of psychopathy: preliminary results from arrest records and psychiatric and hospital records. In *Genetic Research in Psychiatry* (eds. R. R. Fieve *et al*) Johns Hopkins University Press.

Davison, K. & Bagley, C. R. (1969) Schizophrenia-like psychoses associated with organic disorders of the central nervous system: a review of the literature. In *Current Problems in Neuropsychiatry*. British Journal of Psychiatry, Special Publication No. 4. Royal College of Psychiatrists.

——(1976) Drug-induced psychoses and their relationship to schizophrenia. In *Schizophrenia Today* (eds. A. Kemali, A. Bartholini, D. Richter), Oxford: Pergamon.

Duncavage, M., Luchins, D. J. & Meltzer, H. Y. (1982) Platelet MAO activity and family history of schizophrenia. *Psychiatry Research*, **7**, 47–51.

Elston, R. C. (1981) Segregation analysis. In *Recent Advances in Human Genetics* No. 11 (eds. H. Harris, K. Hirschhorn). London: Plenum Press.

—— & Stewart, J. (1971) A general model for the genetic analysis of pedigree data. *Human Heredity*, **21**, 523–542.

Endicott, J., Nee, J., Fleiss, J., Cohen, J., Williams, J. B. W. & Simon, R. (1982) Diagnostic criteria for schizophrenia: reliabilities and agreement between systems. *Archives of General Psychiatry*, **39**, 884–889.

Fischer, M. (1973) Genetic and environmental factors in schizophrenia. *Acta Psychiatrica Scandinavica*, Supplement 238.

Fowler, R. C., Tsuang, M. T., Cadoret, R. J., Monnelly, E. & McCabe, M. S. (1974) A clinical and family of paranoid and non-paranoid schizophrenics. *British Journal of Psychiatry*, **124**, 346–359.

—— —— (1975) Spouses of schizophrenics: a blind comparative study. *Comprehensive Psychiatry*, **16**, 339–342.

—— —— & Cadoret, R. J. (1977) Psychiatric illness in the offspring of schizophrenics. *Comprehensive Psychiatry*, **18**, 127–134.

Gottesman, I. I. & Shields, J. (1972) *Schizophrenia and Genetics*. London: Academic Press.

—— —— (1982) *Schizophrenia: the Epigenetic Puzzle*. London: Cambridge University Press.

Guze, S. B., Cloninger, R., Martin, R. L. & Clayton, P. J. (1983) A follow up and family study of schizophrenia. *Archives of General Psychiatry*, **40**, 1273–1276.

Hays, P. (1973) Electroencephalographic variants and genetic predisposition to schizophrenia. *Journal of Neurology, Neurosurgery and Psychiatry*, **40**, 753–755.

Heston, L. L. (1966) Psychiatric disorders in foster home reared children of schizophrenic mothers. *British Journal of Psychiatry*, **112**, 819–825.

Kallmann, F. J. (1956) Psychiatric aspects of genetic counselling. *American Journal of Human Genetics*, **8**, 97–101.

Karlsson, J. (1982) Family transmission in schizophrenia: Review and synthesis. *British Journal of Psychiatry*, **140**, 600–606.

Kay, D. W. K. (1963) Late paraphrenia and its bearing on the aetiology of schizophrenia. *Acta Psychiatrica Scandinavica*, **39**, 159–169.

—— Roth, M., Atkinson, M. W., Stephens, D. A. & Garside, R. F. (1976) Genetic hypotheses and environmental factors in the light of psychiatric morbidity in the families of schizophrenics. *British Journal of Psychiatry*, **127**, 109–118.

—— (1978) Assessment of familial risks in the functional psychoses and their application in genetic counselling. *British Journal of Psychiatry*, **133**, 385–403.

Kendler, K. S. (1980) The nosological validity of paranoia (simple delusional disorder): A review. *Archives of General Psychiatry*, **37**, 699–706.

—— (1982) Demography of paranoid psychosis (delusional disorder). A review and comparison with schizophrenia and affective illness. *Archives of General Psychiatry*, **39**, 890–902.

—— & Davis, K. L. (1981) The genetics and biochemistry of paranoid schizophrenia and other paranoid psychoses. *Schizophrenia Bulletin*, **7**, 689–709.

—— & Gruenberg, A. M. (1982) Genetic relationship between paranoid personality disorder and the 'schizophrenic spectrum' disorders. *American Journal of Psychiatry*, **139**, 1185–1186.

—— —— (1984) An independent analysis of the Danish adoption study of schizophrenia. VI. The relationship between psychiatric disorders as defined by DSM-III in the relatives and adoptees. *Archives of General Psychiatry*, **41**, 555–564.

—— —— & Strauss, J. S. (1981) An independent analysis of the Copenhagen sample of the Danish adoption study of schizophrenia. II. The relationship between schizotypal personality disorder and schizophrenia. *Archives of General Psychiatry*, **38**, 982–984.

—— & Hays, P. (1981) Paranoid psychosis (delusional disorder) and schizophrenia. *Archives of General Psychiatry*, **38**, 547–551.

—— —— (1982a) Schizophrenia with premorbid inferiority feelings. *Archives of General Psychiatry*, **39**, 643–647.

—— —— (1982b) Familial and sporadic schizophrenia: a symptomatic, prognostic, and EEG comparison. *American Journal of Psychiatry*, **139**, 1557–1562.

—— MASTERSON, C. C., UNGARO, R. & DAVIS, K. L. (1984) A family history study of schizophrenia-related personality disorders. *American Journal of Psychiatry*, **141**, 424–427.

KESSLER, S. (1980) The genetics of schizophrenia: a review. *Schizophrenia Bulletin*, **6**, 404–416.

KETY, S. S., ROSENTHAL, D., WENDER, P. H. & SCHULSINGER, F. (1968) The types and prevalence of mental illness in the biological and adoptive families of adopted schizophrenics. In *The Transmission of Schizophrenia*. (eds. D. Rosenthal, S. S. Kety). Oxford: Pergamon Press.

—— —— —— —— & JACOBSEN, B. (1978) The biologic and adoptive families of adopted individuals who became schizophrenic: prevalence of mental illness and other characteristics. In *The Nature of Schizophrenia* (eds. L. C. Wynne, R. Cromwell, S. Matthysse). New York: Wiley.

—— (1983) Mental illness in the biological and adoptive relatives of schizophrenic adoptees: findings relevant to genetic and environmental factors in etiology. *American Journal of Psychiatry*, **140**, 720–727.

KIDD, K. K. & CAVALLI-SFORZA, L. L. (1973) An analysis of the genetics of schizophrenia. *Social Biology*, **20**, 254–265.

KINNEY, D. K. & JACOBSEN, B. (1978) Environmental factors in schizophrenia: new adoption study evidence. In *The Nature of Schizophrenia Schizophrenia* (eds. L. C. Wynne, R. Cromwell, S. Mattysse). New York: Wiley.

KRETSCHMER, E. (1974) The sensitive delusion of reference. In *Themes and Variations in European Psychiatry* (eds. S. R. Hirsch, M. Shepherd). Bristol: John Wright.

LARSON, C. A. & NYMAN, G. E. (1970) Age of onset in schizophrenia. *Human Heredity*, **20**, 241–247.

—— —— (1973) Differential fertility in schizophrenia. *Acta Psychiatrica Scandinavica*, **49**, 272–280.

—— —— (1974) Schizophrenia: outcome in a birth year cohort. *Psychiatrica Clinica*, **7**, 50–55.

LOWING, P. A., MIRSKY, A. F. & PEREIRA, R. (1983) The inheritance of schizophrenia spectrum disorders: a reanalysis of the Danish adoptee study data. *American Journal of Psychiatry*, **140**, 1167–1171.

MATTHYSSE, S. W. & KIDD, K. K. (1976) Estimating the genetic contribution to schizophrenia. *American Journal of Psychiatry*, **133**, 185–191.

MCCABE, M. S. (1975) Reactive psychoses: a clinical and genetic investigation. *Acta Psychiatrica Scandinavica*, Supplement 239, 133.

—— & STROMGREN, E. (1975) Reactive psychoses. *Archives of General Psychiatry*, **32**, 447–454.

—— FOWLER, R. C., CADORET, R. J. & WINOKUR, G. (1971) Familial difference in schizophrenia with good and poor prognosis. *Psychological Medicine*, **1**, 326–332.

—— & CADORET, R. J. (1976) Genetics investigations of atypical psychoses. I. Morbidity in parents and siblings. *Comprehensive Psychiatry*, **17**, 347–352.

MCGUE, M., GOTTESMAN, I. I. & RAO, D. C. (1983) The transmission of schizophrenia under a multifactorial threshold model. *American Journal of Human Genetics*, **35**, 1161–1178.

MCGUFFIN, P. (1984) Biological markers and psychosis. *Psychological Medicine*, **14**, 255–258.

MCNEIL, T. F. & KAIJ, L. (1978) Obstetric factors in the development of schizophrenia; complications in the births of preschizophrenics and in reproduction by schizophrenic parents. In *The Nature of Schizophrenia* (eds. L. C. Wynne, R. Cromwell, S. Matthysse). New York: Wiley.

MENDLEWICZ, J. (1976) Genetic studies in schizoaffective illness. In *The Impact of Biology on Modern Psychiatry* (eds. E. S. Gershon, R. H. Belmaker, S. S. Kety, M. Rosenbaum). New York: Plenum Press.

MORTON, J. A., KIDD, K. K., MATTHYSSE, S. W. & RICHARDS, R. I. (1979) Recurrence risks in schizophrenia: are they model dependent? *Behavior Genetics*, **9**, 389–406.

ØDEGÅRD, O. (1963) The psychiatric disease entities in the light of a genetic investigation. *Acta Psychiatrica Scandinavica*, Supplement 169, 94–104.

—— (1972) The multifactorial theory of inheritance in predisposition to schizophrenia. In *Genetic Factors in Schizophrenia* (ed. A. R. Kaplan). Springfield, Illinois: Thomas.

O'ROURKE, D. H., GOTTESMAN, I. I., SUAREZ, B. K., RICE, J. & REICH, T. (1982) Refutation of the general single-locus model for the etiology of schizophrenia. *American Journal of Human Genetics*, **34**, 630–649.

POPE, H. G., JONAS, J. M., COHEN, B. M. & LIPINSKI, J. F. (1982) Failure to find evidence of schizophrenia in first-degree relatives of schizophrenic probands. *American Journal of Psychiatry*, **139**, 826–827.

PROPPING, P. (1983) Genetic disorders presenting as 'schizophrenia'. Karl Bonhoeffer's early view of the psychoses in the light of medical genetics. *Human Genetics*, **65**, 1–10.

QUITKIN, F., RIFKIN, A. & KLEIN, D. F. (1976) Neurological soft signs in schizophrenia and character disorders: Organicity in schizophrenia with premorbid asociality and emotionally unstable character disorder. *Archives of General Psychiatry*, **33**, 845–853.

RAINER, J. D. (1975) Genetic knowledge and heredity counselling: new responsibilities for psychiatry. In *Genetic Research in Psychiatry* (eds. R. R. Fieve, D. Rosenthal, & H. Brill). London: Johns Hopkins University Press.

REED, S. C. (1972) Genetic counselling in schizophrenia. In *Genetics Factors in Schizophrenia* (ed. A. R. Kaplan). Springfield, Illinois: Thomas.

REICH, T., CLONINGER, C. R. & GUZE, S. B. (1975) The multifactorial model of disease transmission: I. Description of the model and its use in psychiatry. *British Journal of Psychiatry*, **127**, 1–10.

REICH, W. (1976) The schizophrenia spectrum: a genetic concept. *Journal of Nervous and Mental Disease*, **162**, 3–12.

REISBY, N. (1967) Psychoses in children of schizophrenic mothers. *Acta Psychiatrica Scandinavica*, **43**, 8–20.

REVELEY, A. M., REVELEY, M. A., CLIFFORD, C. A. & MURRAY, R. M. (1982) Cerebral ventricular size in twins discordant for schizophrenia. *Lancet*, *i*, 540–541.

RIMMER, J. & JACOBSEN, B. (1980) Antisocial personality in the biological relatives of schizophrenics. *Comprehensive Psychiatry*, **21**, 258–262.

ROBINS, L. N. (1966) *Deviant Children Grow Up*. Baltimore; Williams & Williams.

ROSENTHAL, D., WENDER, P. H. & KETY, S. S. (1968) Schizophrenics' offspring reared in adoptive homes. In *The Transmission of Schizophrenia* (eds. D. Rosenthal, S. S. Kety). Oxford; Pergamon Press.

—— —— —— WELNER, J. & SCHULSINGER, F. (1971) The adopted-way offspring of schizophrenics. *American Journal of Psychiatry*, **128**, 397–411.

—— (1974) The concept of subschizophrenic disorders. In *Genetics, Environment and Psychopathology* (eds. S. A. Mednick, F. Schulsinger, F. Higgins, B. Bell). Oxford: North Holland Publ. Co.

—— WENDER, P., KETY, S. S., SCHULSINGER, F., WELNER, J. & REIDER, R. (1975) Parent-child relationships and psychopathological disorder in the child. *Archives of General Psychiatry*, **32**, 466–476.

SCHARFETTER, C. (1981) Subdividing the functional psychoses: a family hereditary approach. *Psychological Medicine*, **11**, 637–640.

SCHULSINGER, F. (1972) Psychopathy: heredity and environment. *International Journal of Mental Health*, **1**, 190–206.

—— (1976) A ten-year follow-up of children of schizophrenic mothers. Clinical assessment. *Acta Psychiatrica Scandinavica*, **53**, 371–386.

SHIRE, J. G. M. (1981) An experimental geneticist looks at catecholamine metabolism. *Clinical Genetics*, **19**, 418–425.

SHUR, E. (1982) Season of birth in high and low genetic risk schizophrenics. *British Journal of Psychiatry*, **140**, 410–415.

SLATER, E. & COWIE, V. (1971) *The Genetics of Mental Disorder*. London: Oxford University Press.

SPITZER, R. L., ENDICOTT, J. & ROBINS, E. (1975) *Research Diagnostic Criteria*. New York, Biometrics Research Division, New York State Psychiatric Institute.

STEPHENS, D. A., ATKINSON, M. A., KAY, D. W. K., ROTH, M. & GARSIDE, R. F. (1976) Psychiatric morbidity in parents and sibs of schizophrenics and non-schizophrenics. *British Journal of Psychiatry*, **127**, 97–108.

TARGUM, S. D. & SCHULZ, S. C. (1982) Clinical applications of psychiatric genetics. *American Journal of Orthopsychiatry*, **52**, 45–59.

THOMPSON, W. D., ORVASCHEL, H., PRUSOFF, B. A. *et al* (1982) An evaluation of the family history method for ascertaining psychiatric disorders. *Archives of General Psychiatry*, **39**, 639–642.

TSUANG, M. T. (1967) A study of pairs of sibs both hospitalised for mental disorder. *British Journal of Psychiatry*, **113**, 283–300.

—— (1978) Genetic counseling for psychiatric patients and their families. *American Journal of Psychiatry*, **135**, 1465–1475.

—— (1979) 'Schizoaffective disorder': dead or alive? *Archives of General Psychiatry*, **36**, 633–634.

—— BUCHER, K. D. & FLEMING, J. A. (1982) Testing the monogenic theory of schizophrenia: An application of segregation analysis to blind family study data. *British Journal of Psychiatry*, **140**, 595–599.

—— —— —— (1983) A search for 'schizophrenia spectrum disorders': An application of multiple threshold model to blind family study data. *British Journal of Psychiatry*, **143**, 572–577.

—— DEMPSEY, G. M., DVOREDSKY, A. & STRUSS, A. (1977) A family history study of schizo-affective disorder. *Biological Psychiatry*, **12**, 331–338.

—— —— & RAUSCHER, F. (1976) A study of 'atypical schizophrenia'. *Archives of General Psychiatry*, **33**, 1157–1160.

—— FOWLER, R. C., CADORET, R. J. & MONNELLEY, E. (1974) Schizophrenia among first-degree relatives of paranoid and non-paranoid schizophrenics. *Comprehensive Psychiatry*, **15,** 295–302.

—— WINOKUR, G. & CROWE, R. R. (1980) Morbidity risks of schizophrenia and affective disorders among first-degree relatives of patients with schizophrenia, mania, depression and surgical conditions. *British Journal of Psychiatry*, **137,** 497–504.

WATT, I. A. G., HALL, D. J., OLLEY, P. C., HUNTER, D. & GARDINER, A. Q. (1980) Paranoid states of middle life. Familial occurrence and relationship to schizophrenia. *Acta Psychiatrica Scandinavica*, **61,** 413–426.

WEINBERGER, D. R., DeLISI, L. E., NEOPHYTIDES, A. N. & WYATT, R. J. (1981) Familial aspects of CT scan abnormalities in chronic schizophrenic patients. *Psychiatry Research*, **4,** 65–71.

WENDER, P. H., ROSENTHAL, D., KETY, S. S., SCHULSINGER, F. & WELNER, J. (1974) Crossfostering: a research strategy for clarifying the role of genetic and experiential factors in the etiology of schizophrenia. *Archives of General Psychiatry*, **30,** 121–128.

WINOKUR, G. (1977) Delusional disorder (paranoia). *Comprehensive Psychiatry*, **18,** 511–521.

—— MORRISON, J., CLANCY, J. & CROWE, R. (1974) Iowa 500: the clinical and genetic distinction of hebephrenic and paranoid schizophrenia. *Journal of Nervous and Mental Disease*, **159,** 12–19.

27 Family transmission of schizophrenia: A review and synthesis

JON L. KARLSSON

Many attempts were made during the first half of this century, especially by investigators in northern Europe, to determine the lifetime risk of schizophrenic illness in different relatives of schizophrenic index cases. Most of the early authors followed the same basic research design, locating mentally ill patients in hospitals and gathering statistics about the relatives through community contacts. Various problems were encountered, such as difficulties in obtaining health information about absent or deceased persons or a need to make questionable age corrections when comparing relatives born in different periods. The exact meaning of the resultant rates of psychosis was also far from clear when different authors used different diagnostic criteria. Distinctions between schizophrenia and other forms of psychosis likewise lacked uniformity.

Zerbin-Rüdin (1972) has published summaries of these older data which must be considered impressive, although the validity of the exact figures remains in dispute. Because of the voluminous material gathered by Kallmann (1953), his figures dominated the outcome, so that the overall values were determined largely by the findings of this one author. As a result of differences in methodology, Zerbin-Rüdin found figures approximately a third lower than those of Kallmann, i.e. in parents of index cases, 6.3 per cent as against Kallmann's 9.2 per cent; in full sibs, 10.4 per cent against 14.3 per cent; and in children, 13.7 per cent against 16.4 per cent. It should be noted that first-degree relatives share one-half of their genes with the index cases, while second-degree relatives share one-fourth and third-degree relatives one-eighth.

Because of the problems inherent in the procedures employed by the early investigators it now seems best to view their results as preliminary, and subject to improvement through application of more precise methods. Little is gained by attempts to reanalyse the records, since the deficiencies in the data collection cannot be corrected. It also appears that there must have been an inclination in these studies to classify all psychosis in close relatives of index cases as schizophrenia, while mental disease in more distant relatives was partitioned into the various categories of psychosis. In general the authors made studies only of relatives, utilizing for comparison data gathered by other investigators on the general population. This appears to be the reason for schizophrenia being reported to be increased 15-fold in first-degree relatives, a much higher figure than that found by investigators who have studied both relatives and the public at large, using the same methods for both. The old family studies helped to pave the way for more definitive investigations, but the figures cannot be viewed as final.

Interrelationships of different psychoses

No discussion of family risks of schizophrenia can have much value without a consideration of the interrelationships between the various psychoses. The original decision to draw a sharp line between schizophrenia and manic-depressive illness, which was made by Kraepelin a century ago, was based mainly on clinical rather than scientific grounds, and its biological validity has always been in question. In practice it is quite common for a patient to be diagnosed manic-depressive during one episode of illness and schizophrenic at another time. A significant family overlap occurs, schizophrenia being increased in kinships with manic-depression and vice versa. Even studies which show an excess of spring births in families with schizophrenia indicate that the same holds for manic-depressive illness (Hare, 1976). Creativity has been related to both the basic forms of psychosis (Karlsson, 1978). Lastly, the same dopamine blocking drugs are effective in both schizophrenic and affective disorders (Wyatt and Torgow, 1977). Since a meaningful biological separation of the major mental disease categories seems impractical, one must consider the possibility that some common factors may be involved in all the functional psychoses.

Tsuang *et al* (1980) have in a recent study reported systematically gathered data which establish that many groups exhibit a preponderance of depressive illnesses, but the rate of schizophrenic diagnoses is indeed higher in first-degree relatives of schizophrenic index cases than in those related to affectively ill persons. Conversely, affective disorders certainly predominate among the relatives of manic or depressed patients, although schizophrenia is also increased. Similar results have been encountered by others, the total rate of psychosis in the close relatives tending to be in the order of 10–20 per cent irrespective of the diagnosis of the index cases, although the type of expression can differ. Such data do not necessarily establish a true biological separation of the various psychoses, rather the trend for similarity within families may reflect the operation of secondary modifying factors.

The most satisfactory way to resolve the dilemma of the genetic overlap between the different psychoses appears to be to postulate that the same fundamental biological substrate may be shared by the various forms. The expression of the principal factors is then modulated by other effects to bring about the final symptom complex, which can vary in different families. With this hypothesis it becomes easy to explain the common findings in the various psychoses as well as their separation from conditions like alcoholism, which is firmly documented (Schulsinger, 1980). Geneticists working in this field have universally encountered problems with the concept of a clear biological distinction between the major psychoses, and detailed clinical studies have failed to support its validity (Kendell and Brockington, 1980).

Distribution of schizophrenia in a Swedish isolate

One of the more recent family studies of schizophrenia deals with a complete survey and a long term follow-up of an isolated population in northern Sweden.

Böök (1953) first published a study of this cohort a quarter-century ago, which was conducted with greater precision than some of the older investigations. The main improvement was in the age correction procedure and in the completeness of ascertainment of the community members, including identification of most instances of overt mental disease. Essentially all functional psychosis seems to have been included under the label schizophrenia, thus leading to figures for the general population three times higher than those reported in older investigations and corresponding to total rates of psychosis in other areas. Recently the findings on the Swedish isolate have been updated to embrace the intervening 25 year period (Böök *et al*, 1978).

The rates found were: parents, 11.3 per cent; full sib, 10.2 per cent; children, 11.6 per cent; general population, 2.7 per cent. The respective rates were about four times as high as the general population, i.e. parents, 4.2; full sib, 3.8; children, 4.3. Several important findings have emerged from this study. The psychosis risks for various relatives are basically similar to those reported in the older investigations. The rates are of the same magnitude in all first-degree relatives, i.e. parents, full sibs, and children of index cases. These rates are, however, increased just four-fold over the rate for the general population. The risk was found to be considerably higher in the sibs if a parent was also affected, a finding which several authors have reported. The material in this study on the offspring of two schizophrenic parents, although too limited to yield significant figures, was in agreement with the best data on such groups, which suggest a risk of approximately 35 per cent (Elsässer *et al*, 1971).

The Swedish study has thus led to rates that can be seen as more precise than the older data, the main limitation being that the samples are rather small because of the elaborate procedure used in this kind of survey, which does not lend itself to a study of large populations.

A North American family study

The largest family study of mental illness carried out in the United States was conducted by the staff of the Dight Institute for Human Genetics at the University of Minnesota by Reed *et al* (1973). After preliminary surveys the authors decided that a meaningful biological distinction could not be made between the different functional psychoses, so that the data dealt with schizophrenia in the broad sense. Extensive pedigree material was gathered around identified index cases, and information was also obtained about the general population of the same region. Age corrections were needed, as the material dealt with groups born in different periods.

The findings for 'corrected' psychosis were: full sib, 24.7 per cent (risk 4.0); children, 26.2 per cent (risk 4.3); nephews/nieces, 14.8 per cent (risk 2.4); and general population, 6.1 per cent (risk 1.0). Although the internal relationships are similar to those reported in the earlier studies, the total psychosis figures are higher, presumably due to a difference in methods.

The authors were impressed with the observation that a somewhat higher risk was observed in the relatives if the study was limited to female index cases, but no other study has confirmed that finding. In general the results are in agreement with other data in this field, with the risk increased four-fold in the first-degree relatives as compared to the population at large.

Psychosis in the Icelandic population

A differently designed investigation, permitting a study of adequate size and bypassing the need for age corrections, has been carried out in Iceland (Karlsson, 1974). The diagnostic criteria in this study are uniform for all classes of relatives, each large group being assessed in terms of its admission rate to the only Icelandic mental hospital with schizophrenia or total functional psychosis, as judged by the staff psychiatrists.

The index cases are psychotic patients born in the interval 1851–1940 who have been treated at least once at the mental hospital in Reykjavik, which serves all of Iceland's 230,000 inhabitants. For the original study random samples of the relatives have been identified and their rates of hospital admission ascertained, expressed in multiples of the general population rate. Three generations of relatives, born 1851–1880, 1881–1910, and 1911–1940 are evaluated separately, with the resultant rates then being combined to obtain overall risks. Such comparative rates can be multiplied by the known risk of mental illness for the Icelandic population to obtain actual rates of psychosis for each group of relatives.

The data show the outcome, giving the risks of mental illness in the relatives when the psychoses are combined. The risks found, as a multiple of the general population (1.0), were: (first-degree relatives)—parents, 3.8; full sib, 3.8; children, 5.0; (second-degree relatives)—uncles/aunts, 2.2; nephews/nieces, 2.3; third-degree relatives, 1.3. A finding of fundamental importance is the approximately four-fold risk in first-degree relatives as compared to the general population while rates in second- and third-degree relatives show lesser increases. The Icelandic investigation shows no difference in risks whether the index cases are male or female. The portion of the data dealing just with those index cases given a specific diagnosis of schizophrenia has been published separately (Karlsson, 1973), the relationships remaining basically similar.

In an attempt to enlarge the total study further a procedure has been developed which is based on estimated figures for all the first-degree relatives that the 1377 available psychotic index cases should possess. This approach is made possible by the existence of published genealogy books which cover in detail one-third of Icelanders. Through these sources a very complete ascertainment can be achieved for a large segment of the potential sample, and multiplication by the appropriate factors leads to the total figures. This method is particularly useful in the case of children of index cases, as it is ordinarily difficult to obtain randomly chosen offspring without some contamination with cases that may have been found only because they were admitted to the mental hospital. Some children of psychotic persons who are free of mental illness are probably missed in community surveys done by geneticists, and this may be the reason why most authors have reported somewhat greater risks in children than in other first-degree relatives. The comparative risks from the study, based on actual counts of hospital treated individuals and estimates of all relatives, are: parents, 3.1; full sib, 4.1; children, 3.7. The risk in children of *propositi* is here no greater than that in sibs.

Since these results are in satisfactory agreement with the older data and at the same time are probably more precise, it seems justifiable to utilize these figures in attempts at deriving a genetic mechanism. Efforts to combine all the data that have been gathered tend to confound the issues and lead to figures that are less reliable than those based on one well designed study of sufficient size.

Analysis of the genetic mechanism

Before it is possible to tackle the question of the precise system of inheritance, it is necessary to discuss the longitudinal distribution of psychosis in kindreds that can be traced for many generations. The most successful study of this type has again depended on the voluminous genealogical data existing in Iceland. One kindred has been encountered which is derived from an ancestral couple born in 1682, all descendants arising in the succeeding three centuries having been identified. Information is available on the occurrence of severe psychosis, affecting approximately one per cent of the members throughout the period covered. There turns out to be an uneven distribution of mental disease between the branches of descendants derived from each of the six children of the original couple. As can be seen in Table I branch A, with

TABLE I

Distribution of mental illness of a kindred descended from a couple born in 1682

Gen.	Branch A		Branch B		Branch C		Branch D		Branch E		Branch F	
	No.	Schiz.	No.	Schiz.	No.	Schiz.	No.	Schiz.	No.	Schiz.	No.	Schiz.
I	1	0	1	0	1	0	1	0	1	0	1	0
II	8	1	7	0	6	0	7	0	5	0	3	0
III	21	1	10	0	23	0	24	1	4	0	11	0
IV	48	1	26	0	39	0	40	1	5	0	21	0
V	128	6	83	1	94	0	95	3	15	0	36	0
VI	359	13	168	4	270	1	213	6	34	0	67	1
Total	565	22	295	5	433	1	380	11	64	0	139	1

565 members in six generations, has 22 instances of documented psychosis while branch C, composed of 433 individuals, shows just one case, in the last generation (Karlsson, 1974). This kind of distribution, also found in other kinships, is inconsistent with polygenic inheritance, which in recent years has been favoured by several investigators, and instead it suggests a system involving no more than one or two genes. Genetic heterogeneity is similarly unlikely in view of these data, as separate disorders would not all be found concentrated in the same branches. It is of interest that the different forms of psychosis show a parallel pattern of fluctuations within the branches of the above kindreds, both schizophrenic and affective disorders being either elevated or reduced in the same segments. Although there exist some reports which claim marginal support for polygenic inheritance (Baron, 1980), the Icelandic longitudinal data are much more convincing, in effect seeming to rule out all mechanisms involving several separate factors.

With the benefit of the above reasoning the family data can now be utilized to narrow further the range of possibilities. Since there is no evidence of sex-linkage, one can focus on dominant versus recessive forms of transmission as the only ordinary systems that remain plausible. Recessive inheritance is improbable in view of the universally high frequency of psychosis or the consistently elevated and essentially equal risk in all first-degree relatives. Furthermore, several families have been described in which psychosis is found to be increased in the relatives of only one of the parents (Karlsson, 1966) while recessive inheritance demands presence of the gene in both. This analysis leaves some form of modified dominant transmission as the most probable mechanism, either dominance with incomplete penetrance or gene modified dominance. The mutant principal gene in such systems must be quite frequent to account for the high rate of psychosis in the general population and the rather modest rise in risk in first-degree relatives as compared to the public at large.

When the data from the various family investigations are expressed in multiples of the general population rates, the constancy of the comparative risks is quite striking. The American, Icelandic, and Swedish studies show 4-fold rates in the first-degree relatives and approximately $2\frac{1}{2}$-fold in the second-degree relatives. All available data which make possible a computation of the comparative risks lead to these same values, which are in agreement with modified dominant inheritance. However, when a conversion is made to total psychosis rates, the final figures depend on the diagnostic criteria, becoming higher as a wider spectrum of disease is included in the schizophrenic category. Consequently one cannot expect here a uniformity in the resultant figures, like that achieved in the comparative rates.

A fairly constant finding of essentially double risk in the sibs of schizophrenics when one parent is affected, as compared to sibs with unaffected parents, has been reported by several investigators. This has led to proposals of a mechanism based on a major gene following a dominant pattern coupled with a separately transmitted recessive gene at a different genetic locus, as this can help account for a $2:1$ ratio between the above groups (Karlsson, 1966; Böök *et al*, 1978). However, the hypothesis creates new problems, particularly the need to explain an extremely high frequency for the second factor. Consequently one wonders whether another gene is really necessary. Besides, increased risk in sibs with affected parents has been encountered in other frequent human conditions, such as diabetes and anxiety neurosis. It seems possible that distortions may sometimes occur in human material for a variety of reasons, leading to an apparent numerical ratio which has no biological meaning.

Since there is doubt about the soundness of postulating a second factor merely to explain the apparent increase in risk among sibs when a parent is affected, the alternative system of just one gene with incomplete penetrance must be given appropriate attention. A frequency of approximately nine per cent for a single major gene and penetrance of one-sixth in heterozygotes in terms of fully expressed psychosis can fairly well account for the observed distribution. With this system the risk is indeed expected to be four times greater in first-degree relatives than in the general population. Since the proposed mutant gene can be received from an affected or definite carrier parent and in some instances from the other parent as well in view of the high gene frequency, the schizophrenic genotype is predicted to occur in over one-half of the first-degree relatives of index cases. It also should exist in about one-sixth of the random population. The occurrence of homozygous individuals cannot be ignored, and the findings on the offspring of two psychotic parents have led to the suggestion that all abnormal homozygotes develop psychosis in addition to the one-sixth of heterozygotes. This is the system proposed originally by Böök (1953), supported by Slater (1958) and more recently adopted by Karlsson (1974). Although Böök *et al* (1978) seem now to have abandoned this mechanism in favour of the two-gene hypothesis proposed earlier by Karlsson (1966), it nevertheless appears to be the best system to account for all the currently available data. The only major problem with this mechanism is the apparent 2:1 ratio discussed above, and acceptable explanations can be developed to explain that finding.

One is thus left with the postulation of a major psychosis gene, existing at a high frequency and leading to mental illness only in a fraction of those who carry it. The agreement of the predictions computed with this hypothesis with the family risks derived in the Icelandic study is evaluated in Table II

TABLE II

Agreement of family psychosis rates derived in the Icelandic study with expectations based on a partially dominant major gene

Relatives	Number	Comparative risk	Psychosis rate %	Dominant hypothesis %
Parents	2,261	3.1	11.2	14.0
Full sibs	5,611	4.1	14.8	14.0
Children	1,507	3.7	13.3	14.0
Uncles/aunts	1,093	2.2	7.9	8.8
Nephews/nieces	1,006	2.3	8.3	8.8
First cousins	2,332	1.3	4.7	6.2
General population	24,171	1.0	3.6	3.6

setting the psychosis risk in the general population at 3.6 per cent in view of the rates reported by Helgason (1964). It is evident that this scheme has considerable merit. The somewhat low rate for parents can be explained by the well established reduced reproductive fitness of schizophrenic persons.

A corollary of the major gene hypothesis for schizophrenia is that one principal metabolic aberration should be associated with psychotic illness. Obviously a disturbance of dopamine metabolism comes to mind, since this chemical has been implicated in both schizophrenic and affective disorders. Other circumstances, both biological and experiential, must be involved in determining the final symptom expression in each individual, the psychosis-prone being subject to personality variation parallel to that observed in other humans.

References

BARON, M. (1980) Schizophrenia on paternal and maternal sides: an analysis of familial factors. *British Journal of Psychiatry*, **137**, 505–509.

Böök, J. A. (1953) A genetic and neuropsychiatric investigation of a North-Swedish population. *Acta Genetica et Statistica Medica*, **4**, 1–100.

—— Wetterberg, L. & Modrzewska, K. (1978) Schizophrenia in a North-Swedish geographical isolate 1900–1977. *Clinical Genetics*, **14**, 373–394.

Elsässer, G., Lehmann, H., Pohlen, M. & Scheid, T. (1971) Nachkommen geisteskranker Elternpaare. *Fortschritte der Neurologie, Psychiatrie und ihrer Grenzgebiete*, **39**, 495–522.

Hare, E. H. (1976) The season of birth of siblings of psychiatric patients. *British Journal of Psychiatry*, **129**, 49–54.

Helgason, T. (1964) Epidemiology of mental disorders in Iceland. *Acta Psychiatrica Scandinavica*, **173**, 1–258.

Kallmann, F. J. (1953) *Heredity in Health and Mental Disorder*. New York: Norton.

Karlsson, J. L. (1966) *The Biologic Basis of Schizophrenia*. Springfield: Thomas.

—— (1973) An Icelandic family study of schizophrenia. *British Journal of Psychiatry*, **123**, 549–554.

—— (1974) Inheritance of schizophrenia. *Acta Psychiatrica Scandinavica*, **247**, 1–116.

—— (1978) *Inheritance of Creative Intelligence*. Chicago: Nelson-Hall.

Kendell, R. E. & Brockington, I. F. (1980) The identification of disease entities and the relationship between schizophrenic and affective psychoses. *British Journal of Psychiatry*, **137**, 324–331.

Reed, S. C., Hartley, C., Anderson, V. E., Phillips, V. P. & Johnson, N. A. (1973) *The Psychoses: Family Studies*. Philadelphia: Saunders.

Schulsinger F. (1980) Biological psychopathology. *Annual Review of Psychology*, **31**, 583–606.

Slater, E. (1958) The monogenic theory of schizophrenia. *Acta Genetica et Statistica Medica*, **8**, 50–56.

Tsuang, M. T., Winokur, G. & Crowe, R. R. (1980) Morbidity risks of schizophrenia and affective disorders among first-degree relatives of patients with schizophrenia, mania, depression and surgical conditions. *British Journal of Psychiatry*, **137**, 497–504.

Wyatt, R. J. & Torgow, J. S. (1977) A comparison of equivalent clinical potencies of neuroleptics as used to treat schizophrenia and affective disorders. *Journal of Psychiatric Research*, **13**, 91–98.

Zerbin-Rüdin, E. (1972) Genetic research and the theory of schizophrenia. *International Journal of Mental Health*, **1**, 42–62.

28 Morbidity risks of schizophrenia and affective disorders among first degree relatives of patients with schizophrenia, mania, depression and surgical conditions

MING T. TSUANG, GEORGE WINOKUR and RAYMOND R. CROWE

This paper reports morbidity risks of schizophrenia and affective disorders among the first degree relatives of probands with schizophrenia, mania, depression and surgical conditions. Some characteristics of the present study are (1) probands were selected according to specified research criteria; (2) personal interviews of the relatives were conducted 30 to 40 years after the proband's admission and therefore most of the relatives had already passed the risk periods for schizophrenia and affective disorders; (3) interviews of the relatives were conducted by trained interviewers using structured interview forms without knowing the probands' diagnoses; and (4) blind and independent diagnostic assessments of the relatives were done by staff psychiatrists after reviewing the completed interview forms. We hope that some biases in estimating familial morbidity risk for schizophrenia and affective disorders can be avoided through the research design of this study.

The study

According to specified diagnostic criteria (Feighner *et al*, 1972; Morrison *et al*, 1972), 200 schizophrenics, 100 manics and 225 depressives were selected from 3,800 consecutive admissions to University of Iowa Psychiatric Hospitals from 1934 to 1944. Also from 3,410 patients with appendicectomy and herniorrhaphy consecutively admitted to the Department of Surgery, University of Iowa Hospitals during a period from 1938 to 1948, a control group of 160 stratified random sample people matched for sex, pay status (private and public) and age range of the psychiatric probands was selected. From 1972 to the end of 1976, we traced these probands concurrently with their first degree relatives. Detail about the follow-up of the probands was reported elsewhere (Tsuang *et al*, 1979). We were able to trace 97 per cent of these probands and the mean ages of those probands who were still living at the time of follow-up ranged from 61 to 72 years. We were able to trace 90 per cent of the total 4,094 relatives ascertained through medical records, telephone and personal interviews. Of those traced, 55 per cent were still living and we were able to interview 1,578 (77 per cent) of those using the Iowa Structured Psychiatric Interview forms (ISPI). Their mean ages ranged from 49.8 to

60.6 years. Since most schizophrenics remained single, their first degree relatives interviewed were mostly sibs and parents; therefore, their mean age was older than those of the relatives of affective disorders and surgical conditions where most were sibs and children. It is important to note that most of the relatives interviewed had passed the risk periods for schizophrenia and affective disorders.

The relatives were personally interviewed by trained interviewers. Data on reliability and validity of the interview forms were presented elsewhere (Tsuang *et al*, 1980). At the time of the interview, a relative might indicate that he or other relatives had been hospitalized in one of the five hospitals in the state. In addition to the information from relatives, our researchers searched through the records of these state mental hospitals to recheck any available records which belonged to any relatives in our study, by cross-checking the names of the relatives studied. We also took the opportunity to look for any records belonging to our study of relatives who were deceased. As mortality rates in schizophrenia and affective disorders were higher than those of the general population (Tsuang and Woolson, 1977), it was important to assess the deceased relatives' psychiatric diagnosis whenever their mental hospital records were available. If a hospital record of a deceased relative was available, a psychiatric resident was asked to complete the same structured interview form using the information from the hospital record. The coding from this 'approximate ISPI' (Iowa Structured Psychiatric Interview) was processed for future data analysis in addition to the personal ISPI from living relatives.

Diagnostic assessment of each relative was systematically made by three staff psychiatrists after reviewing the completed interview forms and any available mental hospital records. The diagnostic assessment of both probands and relatives was done during the same period of time and the psychiatrists were blind to the research diagnoses of the probands and also blind to whether the interview form being assessed was that of a proband or of a relative. The interview form was reviewed by a first psychiatrist (G.W.) who completed a diagnostic assessment form. This was then removed from the interview form and given to a second psychiatrist (R.R.C.) for assessment independently. A third psychiatrist (M.T.T.) then reviewed the two diagnostic assessment forms side by side to make a final diagnosis. If the two independent diagnoses were concordant, the concordant diagnosis became the final diagnosis. However if the independent diagnoses were discordant, blind and independent diagnostic assessment on that particular case was repeated. If it turned out to be still discordant, the third psychiatrist made the final diagnosis by thoroughly reviewing the interview forms, available hospital records, and diagnostic assessment forms.

A: Data derived from 1,578 relatives with personal interview forms

[The authors present data for morbidity risks in first degree relatives of the age adjusted sample. For the personally conducted interviews these figures are: schizophrenia, 3.2 per cent; mania, 1.0 per cent; depression, 0.9 per cent; controls, 0.6 per cent.]

Pairwise comparisons of morbidity risks between each diagnostic group showed that a risk of 3.2 in schizophrenia relatives was significantly higher than those of depressive and control relatives at less than the 5 per cent level. Although 3.2 for schizophrenia relatives was higher than 1.0 for manic relatives, the difference did not reach a conventional statistical significance of 5 per cent level. No significant differences were found between manic and depressive relatives, manic and control relatives and depressive and control relatives.

[The authors present their data for the morbidity risks of affective disorder in the first degree relatives of the four groups. For the personally conducted interviews the risks were: schizophrenia, 7.0 per cent; mania, 13.1 per cent; depression, 12.9 per cent; controls 7.6 per cent.] We can see that the risks were very similar in manic and depressive relatives. The figures were also very similar in schizophrenic and control relatives. Significant differences were found between the relatives of schizophrenics and manics, schizophrenics and depressives and depressives and controls. A significant level of less than 10 per cent was found between manic and control relatives.

The data from this blind family study showed that schizophrenia and affective disorders were different and support heterogeneity of major functional psychosis.

Let us turn to examine heterogeneity within schizophrenia and affective disorders. Traditionally schizophrenia has been divided into paranoid and non-paranoid subtypes. There were 11 schizophrenics among the relatives of schizophrenics. When we divided probands into paranoid and non-paranoid schizophrenia (criteria of Tsuang and Winokur, 1974), 3 schizophrenics were from the relatives of paranoid probands and 8 were from those of non-paranoid probands. The risks of schizophrenia among the relatives of these two groups were the same, 3.2. This finding is different from results of other studies where more cases of schizophrenia were usually found among the relatives of non-paranoid schizophrenics than those of paranoid schizophrenics (Slater and Cowie, 1971). With regard to the subtypes of schizophrenia found among the relatives, all 11 schizophrenics were given a non-paranoid diagnosis. Therefore there is no hint of 'breeding true' according to paranoid and non-paranoid subtypes. It seems that currently available clinical criteria for dividing schizophrenia into paranoid and non-paranoid subtypes are not good enough for studying heterogeneity in schizophrenia. It is worthwhile mentioning that the relatives of schizophreincs were older at the time of the interview and consequently all schizophrenics were chronic cases with undifferentiated clinical features infrequently seen in paranoid schizophrenia.

Now let us examine heterogeneity within affective disorders, using our familial data. All relatives with affective disorders were divided into unipolars and bipolars according to the final diagnosis. [The authors present their data for bipolar affective disorder in the first degree relatives of the four groups. For the personally conducted interviews these were: schizophrenia, 1.8 per cent; mania, 1.9 per cent; depression, 0.9 per cent; controls, 0.3 per cent.] In general, the morbidity risks for bipolars were very low and pairwise comparisons between them were not significant. It is interesting to note that a risk of 1.8 in the relatives of schizophrenics was even higher than 0.9 of the relatives of depressives; and the risk of bipolar illness among schizophrenia relatives was similar to that among manic relatives. Differentiation of schizophrenia and mania may be rather difficult if merely based on blind clinical diagnostic assessment. This point was also illustrated by the figures for schizophrenia among the relatives of patients with schizophrenia and mania; the difference between these two morbidity risks did not reach statistical significance at 5 per cent level.

[The authors present their data for morbidity risk for unipolar affective disorder in the first degree relatives of the four groups. For the personally conducted interviews these were: schizophrenia, 5.1 per cent; mania, 11.3 per cent; depression, 12.0 per cent; controls, 7.3 per cent.] Pairwise comparisons of morbidity risks for unipolars indicate that the depression group can be clearly distinguished from the schizophrenic and control groups. The morbidity risks were about the same for the relatives of mania and depression. With regard to subtype concordance, the 21 affectives found in manic relatives can be divided into 3 bipolars and 18 unipolars; the 44 affectives in depression relatives were divided into 3 bipolars and 41 unipolars. There was no hint of subtype concordance. [The data] suggest that bipolars and unipolars might be different because the morbidity risks for unipolars among schizophrenia and affective relatives were significantly different, but no such differences were found for the risks of bipolars among the relatives of schizophrenia and affective disorders. However, comparisons of the morbidity risks between the relatives of bipolars and unipolars did not show any significant difference. In addition, there was no trend to subtype concordance. Therefore, on the basis of our blind family data, we cannot support a dichotomy of unipolars and bipolars in affective disorders. Of course the division of bipolar and unipolar subtypes cannot be made solely on the basis of familial data. Other variables are also needed. From the finding of the present study, one may infer that current clinical methodology for distinguishing bipolar and unipolar affective disorders may not be good enough for familial and genetic studies of affective disorders.

B: Data derived from 1,648 relatives with personal or approximate interview forms

[The data for schizophrenia risk and affective disorder risk] also show morbidity risks of schizophrenia and affective disorders respectively among the relatives when approximate ISPI's were also used. Comparing the figures we can see that the figures are higher for the relatives of psychiatric probands. As only two records were found among the relatives of controls, the figures for them remained essentially unchanged.

Pairwise comparisons of figures derived from [the additional recorded information] were also done. The trends were very much the same as those of [the personal interviews alone]. The risks of schizophrenia in mania relatives increased from 1.0 to 3.2, and it is now significantly different from that of controls. With regard to subtyping of schizophrenia into paranoid and non-paranoid subtypes, the 20 schizophrenics [included in the additional recorded information] were all classified into non-paranoid, 6 in paranoid families and 14 in non-paranoid families. There is again no evidence of subtype concordance.

[The data for the additional recorded information are presented.] There are remarkable increases of the bipolar figures among the relatives of psychiatric probands when additional records from the deceased were available. Even though the figure was the highest among manic relatives, no statistically significant differences were found between those of the relatives of each psychiatric diagnostic category. However, the figures are all significantly higher than that of control relatives. Although the figures for unipolars derived from additional information become higher among psychiatric relatives the trends of pairwise comparisons within [the data based upon the additional recorded information] remain similar to those presented for [personal information only]. Again, there is no significant difference between those of manic relatives and depressive relatives. It is worthwhile noting that the figures for schizophrenic relatives and control relatives are very similar, which are both remarkably different from that of depressive relatives. For the subtype concordance, there are 9 bipolars and 21 unipolars in manic relatives and 11 bipolars and 55 unipolars in depressive relatives. Again, even when the additional information from medical records was used to increase the morbidity risks, there was no trend to subtype concordance.

Comment

The common clinical practice of making a diagnosis is usually done by a clinician who has all the information available including medical records and family background of the patient. For instance, a clinician examining a depressed patient from a bipolar family may try hard to elicit any previous history of a manic phase. Even if the patient denies or forgets having had manic symptoms, the clinician can make a diagnosis of bipolar affective disorder based on the patient's record, which clearly indicated a previous hospitalization for mania. Likewise, a manic patient from a schizophrenic family may be carefully investigated for the presence of any past or present schizophrenic features; a patient presenting some schizophrenic features from a family loaded with manic-depressive patients may be given a diagnosis of mania, if the record shows that the patient responded very well to lithium during his previous recurrent manic episodes. A distinction between mania and schizophrenia is sometimes difficult, because of the presence of atypical features, and therefore a clinician has to rely on all information and clues to make his own best judgement.

Although there are many benefits in making a diagnosis on a non-blind basis for clinical purposes, the present study was specifically designed to avoid any biases due to non-blind methods. Our morbidity risks may be lower, but at least we know where the bottom lines are, if blind, independent and consensus diagnosis are used. We realized that our figures might be underestimates. However, we were still able to show that morbidity risks of schizophrenia and affective disorders among relatives of schizophrenics, manic-depressives and controls were definitely different. To correct these underestimated figures, without sacrificing the essential feature of the blindness of the probands' research diagnosis, deceased relatives with approximate ISPI's were included for the analyses. The figures obtained from additional information may be overestimated ones since BZ's were compiled from N's representing the numbers of interviewed relatives plus deceased relatives who happened to have hospital records available for approximate ISPI's. We suspect that true figures may lie somewhere between those of personal interview data and personal interview data with additional information from approximate interview forms. Even when additional information from the deceased relatives was added, there was no hint of subtype concordance in terms of paranoid and non-paranoid, or unipolar and bipolar divisions.

It is important that future study of heterogeneity of schizophrenia and affective disorders should be based on subtyping using other biological and psycho-social variables in addition to current criteria based on clinical features.

In conclusion, our data support the distinction between schizophrenia and affective disorders, although the distinction between schizophrenia and mania was not clear cut. Our data could not support familial subtyping of paranoid and non-paranoid schizophrenia or bipolar and unipolar affective disorders. Obviously further analysis should be carried out, if genetic aetiology, modes of transmission and genetic heterogeneity of major psychoses are to be thoroughly studied. Aiming towards these goals, we are now analysing our data including psychiatric disorders other than schizophrenia and affective disorders among the relatives, and using segregation analysis of pedigree data (Elston and Yelverton, 1975; Elston and Sobel, 1979) and multiple thresholds models (Reich *et al*, 1975; Reich *et al*, 1979).

References

ELSTON, R. C. & YELVERTON, K. C. (1975) General models for segregation analysis. *American Journal of Human Genetics*, **27**, 31–45.

—— & SOBEL, E. (1979) Sampling considerations in the gathering and analysis of pedigree data. *American Journal of Human Genetics*, **31**, 62–69.

FEIGHNER, J. P., ROBINS, E., GUZE, S. B., WOODRUFF, R. A., WINOKUR, G. & MUNOZ, R. (1972) Diagnostic criteria for use in psychiatric research. *Archives of General Psychiatry*, **26**, 57–63.

MORRISON, J., CLANCY, J., CROWE, R. & WINOKUR, G. (1972) The Iowa 500: I. Diagnostic validity in mania, depression and schizophrenia. *Archives of General Psychiatry*, **27**, 457–461.

REICH, T., CLONINGER, C. R. & GUZE, S. B. (1975) The multifactorial model of disease transmission: I. Description of the model and its use in psychiatry. *British Journal of Psychiatry*, **127**, 1–10.

—— RICE, J., CLONINGER, C. R., WETTE, R. & JAMES, J. (1979) The use of multiple thresholds and segregation analysis in analyzing the phenotypic heterogeneity of multifactorial traits. *Annals of Human Genetics*, **42**, 371–389.

SLATER, E. & COWIE, V. A. (1971) *The Genetics of Mental Disorders*, pp. 31–32. London: Oxford University Press.

TSUANG, M. T. & WINOKUR, G. (1974) Criteria for subtyping Schizophrenia: Clinical differentiation of hebephrenic and paranoid schizophrenia. *Archives of General Psychiatry*, **31**, 43–47.

—— & WOOLSON, R. F. (1977) Mortality in patients with schizophrenia, mania, depression and surgical conditions: A comparison with general population mortality. *British Journal of Psychiatry*, **130**, 162–166.

—— —— & FLEMING, J. A. (1979) Long-term outcome of major psychoses: I. Schizophrenia and affective disorders compared with psychiatrically symptom-free surgical conditions. *Archives of General Psychiatry*, **39**, 1295–1301.

—— —— & SIMPSON, J. C. (1980) The Iowa structured psychiatric interview: Rationale, reliability, and validity. *Acta Psychiatrica Scandinavica*, Suppl 283, Vol. 62.

29 The search for genetic linkage in schizophrenia

DAVID C. WATT

Enormous industry has been devoted during the last half-century to establishing the genetic contribution to the aetiology of schizophrenia. Demonstration of a familial concentration of the disorder among the blood relatives of schizophrenics is supported by the differential concordance for schizophrenia found between monozygotic and dizygotic twins (Slater and Cowie, 1971; Gottesman and Shields, 1972; Shields, 1978). An alternative explanation offered was that the high familial incidence of schizophrenia was accounted for by the influence of a schizophrenic parent, particularly mother, or a sibling, or by a schizophrenogenic family configuration or pattern of communication. This speculation has been dispelled, however, by the brilliant series of studies which compared the outcome in the offspring of schizophrenics brought up at home with that of those adopted and brought up away from the schizophrenic parent (Heston and Denney, 1968; Kety et al, 1968; Rosenthal, 1970; Rosenthal et al, 1971; Wender et al, 1971; Kety and Matthysse, 1972; Wender et al, 1974).

The several experimental variations (summarized in Shields, 1978) upon this theme have all confirmed that it is the blood relationship with a schizophrenic which is paramount in increasing the probability of schizophrenia, and that those brought up in family proximity with a schizophrenic, but without a blood relationship, show no more risk of schizophrenia than the general population (Rosenthal et al, 1971).

Thus, the contribution of genetics to the aetiology of schizophrenia rests on more secure ground than any other current hypothesis of the cause of schizophrenia. Unfortunately, its mode of operation still eludes us and we do not know the manner of transmission or what it is that is inherited. The position has been clearly stated by Gottesman and Shields (1972), who conclude that the results of family and pedigree studies fit equally well with several possible modes of transmission. The search for genetic linkage offers one possible way of avoiding this impasse.

Mechanism of linkage

Linkage, which has been used mainly for gene mapping, arises from the fact that genes which are adjacent on the same chromosome are more likely to be transmitted together to individuals within a family than if they are widely separated or on different chromosomes. Occasionally genes on the same chromosome are not transmitted together due to an exchange of material between homologous chromosomes at meiosis, referred to as a crossover or recombination. Thus, if in a pair of homologous chromosomes the genes for the characters AB are situated adjacently on one chromosome and for CD on the other, the characters are likely to be transmitted together, i.e. the off-spring will receive either the characters AB or the characters CD, in which case linkage will have occurred. If, however, any offspring show the characters AD or CB a crossover or recombination will have occurred. The requirements for detecting linkage in man are that there should be two specific and readily ascertainable characteristics which are known to segregate in families (Race and Sanger, 1975). The extent to which the two characteristics occur together in families indicates the probability that they are on the same chromosome and linked (i.e. close).

The terms linkage and association may cause confusion. Association refers to the fact that, in a population, two conditions appear together in single persons more often than can be accounted for by chance and a causal connection is presumed. Genes that are linked, however, do not result in association of characters (unless the recombination fraction is very small) nor is a causal connection indicated (Bodmer and Cavalli-Sforza, 1976).

Requirements for studying linkage in schizophrenia

(a) *Markers:* In using linkage to investigate a disease, such as schizophrenia, the disease itself acts as one characteristic and some genetic marker is the other. The marker must be specific, unambiguously shown in those who carry the gene and absent in those who do not. It must be reliably detectable and segregate by understood genetic laws. The most useful substances to act as markers in this way are antigens and enzymes present in blood, and about 30 of these have the required attributes. Turner (1979b) has reviewed the value of many of these substances as markers for psychosis.

A battery of markers distributed on as many chromosomes as possible is desirable, in view of the fact that the number of genes on the 46 chromosomes of a human individual is probably about 100,000 (Bodmer and Cavalli-Sforza, 1976). Many characteristics which do not depend on blood have been consi-dered as markers, such as digital hairiness, hair form, eye-colour (Constan-tinidis, 1958), finger-print (Holt, 1968; Kemali *et al*, 1976), phenothiocarbamide tasting (Constantinidis, 1958), nailfold capillary char-acteristics, handedness (and other forms of laterality, Wexler, 1980), cerebral assymetry (Boklage, 1977; Luchins *et al*, 1979, 1981), pursuit eye movements in tracking a pendulum (Iacono and Lykken, 1979a, 1979b; Brezinová and Kendell, 1977) and albinism (Baron, 1976). Most of these, however, are unreli-able in that there is doubt about their genetic basis or their method of assess-ment. Some require considerable individual expertise and elaborate apparatus. A recent discovery is the polymorphic brain-specific protein labelled Pc 1 Duarte (Comings, 1979). This investigation, however, requires post-mortem brain specimens and is therefore not practical in linkage studies. It can, how-ever, be used in the search for association.

As an entirely new possibility Bodmer (1976) has suggested that the somatic

PROPERTY OF
RIVERWOOD COMMUNITY MENTAL HEALTH

cell hybridization method (Race and Sanger, 1975; Creagen and Ruddle, 1977) could be applied to the study of schizophrenia using markers derived from drug responses.

(b) *Families:* It is most useful to examine families with at least two schizophrenic members. Families with only one affected member yield little information. Families for study should include as many normal members and cover as many generations as possible. Thus larger families are more informative. The probability that a pedigree is showing linkage is obtained by a formula which takes into account the proportion of recombination which has occurred (Morton, 1955).

Linkage study requires expertise beyond that of most psychiatrists, of which the geneticist is the most important source. Some blood characteristics used as markers require the co-operation of a laboratory experienced and of known reliability in the particular test. This necessity has been high-lighted by recent efforts to detect associations between HLA antigens and schizophrenia (reviewed by McGuffin, 1980), and between monoamine oxidase and schizophrenia (Böök *et al*, 1978). Both cases have produced bewilderingly conflicting results which must call in question the reliability of the laboratory procedures adopted.

Special problems in linkage study in schizophrenia

The vital contribution of the psychiatrist to a linkage study has, in its most essential aspect, proved the weakest point. Clinical diagnosis of schizophrenia is so unreliable that it is mandatory to employ more exacting procedures. Of these the use of a standardized, structured diagnostic interview administered blind by more than one experienced assessor is the most valuable.

The difficulty of diagnosis has been compounded by the introduction of the concept of the 'schizophrenia spectrum' (Reich, 1976). That a number of non-schizophrenic psychiatric disorders show a familial concentration in schizophrenic families seems now beyond doubt (Kety *et al*, 1968; Stephens *et al*, 1975). However, which disorders are to be included in the 'spectrum', by what criteria they can be reliably ascertained and what is their relationship to schizophrenia are questions whose answers are obsure at present.

A further difficulty arises from the existence of illness clinically indistinguishable from schizophrenia but having an environmental aetiology; the 'symptomatic' or 'organic', and the 'psychogenic' schizophrenias (Slater and Cowie, 1971). Among organic cases are included those associated with epilepsy; those in the early stages of organic brain disease; Huntington's chorea; cerebral trauma; drugs (Slater and Beard, 1963; Kay, 1963, 1972; Davison and Bagley, 1969; Gelenberg, 1976; Geschwind, 1979). The morbid risk in the relatives of such patients is less than in the relatives of endogenous schizophrenics (Davison and Bagley, 1969; Slater and Cowie, 1971; Kay, 1963, 1972) and on this evidence the genetic predisposition approaches that of the general population. Such cases tend therefore to obscure the existence of linkage. Limiting the families examined to those with more than one schizophrenic member makes it more likely that only cases of genetic aetiology are included. Cases with known organic brain disease should, of course, be excluded.

Finding families, with more than one schizophrenic member, which will be informative in a linkage investigation is difficult. Only 10 per cent of schizophrenics are likely to have first-degree relatives with schizophrenia. Administrative records rarely identify such families, although case-record linkage registers can be helpful in identifying patients with the same surname over a wider area than is covered by one hospital. Families are often scattered and not all members are willing to participate in studies of this kind. A geneticist's experience and expertise is as indispensable in selecting the families as it is in the analysis and interpretation of results.

In the event that there are several schizophrenia loci the possibility arises that each of them may be separately linked to a different marker. Individual families may each therefore show one form of linkage. When results from several families are coalesced, however, the different forms of linkage may obscure one another (Turner and King, 1981).

Diseases in which there is wide variability in the age of onset give rise to doubt as to whether particular individuals possess the gene but have not yet manifested the disease (Morton and Kidd, 1981). This applies strongly to schizophrenia in which the period from 15–45 years is often taken as the limit (for practical purposes) of age of onset, but in which cases with onset outside this wide period, both earlier and later, are believed to occur. Various methods of allowing for the error that this generates have been suggested (Hodge *et al*, 1979; Heimbuch *et al*, 1980), and some of these have been compared in relation to Huntington's chorea by Hodge *et al* (1980) who demonstrate the magnitude of the error in estimating linkage when no allowance is made.

Published studies of genetic linkage in schizophrenia

Four investigations of linkage in schizophrenia have been published. Constantinidis (1958) examined 36 pedigrees which yielded groups of siblings comprising 108 individuals, among whom were 48 schizophrenics. He employed 20 genetic markers for which he tested all individuals. These included sensitivity to phenothiocardamide testing (PTC); hair on the dorsum of the 2nd phalanx of the digits; form, direction of whorl, shade of hair and red hair; ear shape, attachment of lobule and distance from head; eye colour; length of fingers, handedness; tongue curling; ABO, MN and rhesus blood groups. He used the method of sib-pair comparison (Penrose, 1938, 1946), of which he gives a clear exposition, to detect linkage. This method is less powerful than the calculation of lods (logarithm of the odds) (Morton, 1955), which is now used. Constantinidis concludes that he had found probable linkage of schizophrenia with digital hairiness (P <0.1) and form of hair (P <0.1) and possible linkage with eye colour (P < 0.2) and PTC (P < 0.2).

In a single pedigree of 22 individuals Baron (1976) investigated the possibility of linkage and association of albinism with schizophreniform psychosis (as diagnosed by the criteria of Feighner and associates, and Spitzer and associates). Albinism, transmitted by an autosomal recessive gene, showed in 5 individuals in the pedigree, together with schizophreniform psychosis (which was assumed to be transmitted recessively) and one individual showed process schizophrenia without albinism. This was calculated to give odds of 36:1 in favour of linkage. Additionally, the author proposed that albinism is associated with schizophreniform psychosis and aetiologically related because it may lower γ-aminobutyric acid activity and increase dopaminergic activity in the relevant systems of the central nervous system.

Böök *et al* (1978), publishing the results of their genetic investigation of a N. Swedish geographically isolated population of around 6000, selected three major pedigrees, comprising 35 individuals of whom 9 were schizophrenics, for a linkage investigation. They used 30 genetic markers, but only two results have so far been published. There was a significant score for linkage between schizophrenia and low plasma dopamine β-hydroxylase. Group specific antigen showed a possibility of linkage. We await more information on this study.

Turner (1979a) presented 6 pedigrees each containing more than one schizophrenic, giving a total of 65 subjects. Thirty-three (50 per cent) were 'schizophrenic', of whom 27 (42 per cent) were schizophrenic by Feighner's criteria (Feighner *et al*, 1972). Evidence for linkage was found for two markers, HLA and glyoxalase, with 'schizotaxia'. This evidence, although suggestive, has a degree of significance less than that usually accepted as evidence of linkage and requires confirmation. The evidence for glyoxalase was found in two pedigrees only. Turner tentatively suggests that the indication of linkage with HLA provides evidence of inheritance in these schizophrenics with a major locus on chromosome 6. The term 'schizotaxia', proposed by Meehl (1962), embraces three conditions: 1. schizophrenia; 2. schizoid disorders less than schizophrenia; and 3. individuals, phenotypically normal, in whom a 'carrier' state of genetic liability is inferred from the occurrence of a schizophrenic sib and schizophrenic offspring. Besides commenting on the difficulty of diagnosis, for which the adoption of the term schizotaxia is his compromise solution, Turner also draws attention to the fact that his selection of families with such a high concentration of schizophrenia forbids generalization of his findings.

Genetic linkage in other psychiatric conditions

There are a number of studies of linkage with other psychiatric diagnoses than schizophrenia. In affective disorders no settled results have yet appeared. Interest has centred on X-linkage and there have been several studies with positive findings (Reich *et al*, 1969; Winokur and Tanna, 1969; Mendelwicz *et al*, 1971, 1972, 1975, 1979, 1980; Fieve *et al*, 1973, 1975; Turner and King, 1981) but also some negative (Grieff *et al*, 1975; Gershon *et al*, 1979; Leckman *et al*, 1979). Single studies have found positive linkage with group specific component (Tanna *et al*, 1976a, b, c) and haptoglobin (Tanna *et al*, 1979). These results need confirmation.

In Huntington's chorea linkage was reported with haptoglobin (Brackenridge *et al*, 1978) but not confirmed in the study of Hodge *et al* (1980). The latter authors demonstrate that the discrepancy between the two results is probably due to the failure of Brackenridge *et al* to correct sufficiently for the fact that young individuals in their pedigrees who were not showing the disease could not simply be assumed to be unaffected. They recommend that the probability that a proportion of them would show the disease at a later date should be taken into account.

The most spectacular linkage discovery is the demonstration by Davison (1973) that in familial idiopathic severe subnormality (Renpenning's syndrome) twice as many males as females are affected and in 50 out of the 141 families examined all those affected were males. The pattern of inheritance conformed to that of X-linkage in a considerable proportion of these cases. More recent developments have been summarized by Turner and Opitz (1980), who conclude that it is likely that three types of X-linked subnormality can be distinguished, and point out that taken with the discovery in 1967 of a fragile site associated with the X-chromosome in affected males and in their female forebears the possibility arises of detecting female carriers and, by amniocentesis, affected offspring.

References

BARON, M. (1976) Albinism and schizophreniform psychosis: a pedigree study. *American Journal of Psychiatry*, **133**, 1070–1073.

BODMER, W. F. (1976) The HLA system and linkage analysis in cell culture. *Neurosciences Research Progress Bulletin*, **14**, 66–69.

—— & CAVALLI-SFORZA, L. L. (1976) *Genetics, Evolution and Man*. Freeman: San Francisco.

BOKLAGE, C. E. (1977) Schizophrenia, brain asymmetry development and twinning: cellular relationship with etiological and possibly prognostic implications. *Biological Psychiatry*, **12**, 19–35.

BÖÖK, J. A., WETTERBERG, L. & MODRZEWSKA, K. (1978) Schizophrenia in a north Swedish geographical isolate, 1900–1977. Epidemiology, genetics and biochemistry. *Clinical Genetics*, **14**, 373–394.

BRACKENRIDGE, C. J., CASE, J., CHIU, E., PROPERT, D. N., TELTSCHER, B. & WALLACE, D. C. (1978) Linkage study of the loci for Huntington's disease and some common polymorphic markers. *Annals of Human Genetics*, **42**, 203–211.

BREZINOVÁ, V. & KENDELL, R. E. (1977) Smooth pursuit eye movements of schizophrenics and normal people under stress. *British Journal of Psychiatry*, **130**, 59–63.

COMINGS, D. E. (1979) Pc 1 Duarte, a common polymorphism of a human brain protein, and its relationship to depressive disease and multiple sclerosis. *Nature*, **277**, 28–32.

CONSTANTINIDIS, J. K. (1958) Les marqueurs de chromosomes chez les schizophrènes et la recherche du linkage entre ces caractères et la schizophrénie par la méthode de Penrose. *Journal de Génétique Humaine*, **7**, 189–242.

CREAGAN, R. P. & RUDDLE, F. H. (1977) New approaches to human cell mapping by somatic cell genetics. In *Molecular Structure of Human Chromosomes* (ed. J. J. Yunis). New York: Academic Press.

DAVISON, B. C. C. (1973) Familial idiopathic severe subnormality: the question of a contribution by X-linked genes. In *Genetic Studies in Mental Subnormality* (ed. P. S. Benson, B. C. C. Davison, J. D. Studdy and P. N. Swift). British Journal of Psychiatry. Special Publication No 8.

DAVISON, K. & BAGLEY, C. R. (1969) Schizophrenia-like psychoses associated with organic disorders of the central nervous system: a review of the literature. In *Current Problems in Neuropsychiatry* (ed. R. N. Herrington). British Journal of Psychiatry Special Publication No 4. Ashford, Kent: Headley Brothers.

FEIGHNER, J., ROBINS, E., GUZE, S., WOODRUFF, R., WINOKUR, G. & MUNOZ, R. (1972) Diagnostic criteria for use in psychiatric research. *Archives of General Psychiatry*, **26**, 57–63.

FIEVE, R. R., MENDELWICZ, J. & FLEISS, J. L. (1973) Manic-depressive illness: linkage with the Xg blood group. *American Journal of Psychiatry*, **130**, 1355–1359.

—— ROSENTHAL, D. & BRILL, H. (1975) *Genetic Research in Psychiatry*. Johns Hopkins University Press: Baltimore.

GELENBERG, A. J. (1976) The catatonic syndrome. *The Lancet*, June 19, 1339–1341.

GERSHON, E. S., TARGUM, S. D., MATTHYSSE, S. & BUNNEY, W. E. (1979) Color blindness not closely linked to bipolar illness. *Archives of General Psychiatry*, **36**, 1423–1430.

GESCHWIND, N. (editorial) (1979) Behavioural changes in temporal lobe epilepsy. *Psychological Medicine*, **9**, 217–219.

GOTTESMAN, I. I. & SHIELDS, J. (1972) *Schizophrenia and Genetics*. Academic Press: London.

GRIEFF, H. VON, McHUGH, P. R. & STOKES, P. E. (1975) The familial history in 16 males with bipolar manic-depressive illness. In *Genetic Research in Psychiatry* (ed. R. R. Fieve, D. Rosenthal and H. Brill), pp 233–239. Johns Hopkins University Press: Baltimore.

HEIMBUCH, R. C., MATTHYSSE, S. & KIDD, K. K. (1980) Estimating age-of-onset distributions for disorders with variable onset. *American Journal of Human Genetics*, **32**, 565–574.

HESTON, L. L. & DENNEY, D. (1968) Interactions between early life experience and biological factors in schizophrenia. *Journal of Psychiatric Research*, **6** (Supp. 1), 363–376.

HODGE, S. E., MORTON, L. A., TIDEMAN, S., KIDD, K. K. & SPENCE, M. A. (1979) Age-of-onset correction available for linkage analysis (LIPED). *American Journal of Human Genetics*, **31**, 761–762.

—— SPENCE, M. A., CRANDALL, B. F., SPARKES, R. S., SPARKES, M. C., CRIST, M. & TIDEMAN, S. (1980) Huntington's disease: linkage analysis with age-of-onset corrections. *American Journal of Medical Genetics*, **5**, 247–254.

HOLT, S. B. (1968) *The Genetics of Dermal Ridges*. Springfield, Illinois: Thomas, pp 59–63.

IACONO, W. G. & LYKKEN, D. T. (1979a) Eye tracking and psychopathology. *Archives of General Psychiatry*, **36**, 1361–1369.

—— —— (1979b) Comments on 'smooth-pursuit eye movements: a comparison of two measurement techniques' by Lindsay, Holzman, Haberman and Yasillo. *Journal of Abnormal Psychology*, **88**, 6, 678–680.

KAY, D. W. K. (1963) Late paraphrenia and its bearing on the aetiology of schizophrenia. *Acta Psychiatrica Scandinavica*, **39**, 159–169.

—— (1972) Schizophrenia and schizophrenia-like states in the elderly. *British Journal of Hospital Medicine*, October, 369–376.

KEMALI, D., POLANI, N., POLANI, P. E. & AMATI, A. (1976) A dermatoglyphic study of 219 Italian schizophrenic males. *Clinical Genetics*, **9**, 51–60.

KETY, S. S., ROSENTHAL, D., WENDER, P. H. & SCHULSINGER, F. (1968) The types and prevalence of mental illness in the biological and adoptive families of adopted schizophrenics. In *The Transmission of Schizophrenia* (ed. D. Rosenthal and S. S. Kety). Pergamon: Oxford.

—— & MATTHYSSE, S. (1972) Prospects for research on schizophrenia: an overview. *Neurosciences Research Program Bulletin*, **10**, 456–467.

LECKMAN, J. F., GERSHON, E. S., McGINNISS, M. H., TARGUM, S. D. & DIBBLE, E. D. (1979) New data do not suggest linkage between the Xg blood group and bipolar illness. *Archives of General Psychiatry*, **36**, 1435–1441.

LUCHINS, D. J., WEINBERGER, D. R. & WYATT, R. J. (1979) Schizophrenia. Evidence of a subgroup with reversed cerebral asymmetry. *Archives of General Psychiatry*, **36**, 1309–1311.

—— —— TORREY, E. F., JOHNSON, A., ROGENTINE, N. & WYATT, R. J. (1981) HLA-A2 antigen in schizophrenic patients with reversed cerebral asymmetry. *British Journal of Psychiatry*, **138**, 240–243.

McGUFFIN, P. (1980) What have transplant antigens got to do with psychosis? *British Journal of Psychiatry*, **136**, 510–512.

MEEHL, P. E. (1962) Schizotaxia, schizotypia, schizophrenia. *American Psychologist*, **17**, 827–838.

MENDELWICZ, J., FIEVE, R. R. & RAINER, J. D. (1971) Linkage studies in affective disorders. Fifth World Congress of Psychiatry, Mexico City.

—— FLEISS, J. L. & FIEVE, R. R. (1972) Evidence for X-linkage in transmission of manic-depressive illness. *Journal of the American Medical Association*, **222**, 1624–1627.

—— —— —— (1975) Linkage studies in effective disorders: the Xg blood group and manic-depressive illness. In *Genetic Research in Psychiatry* (ed. R. R. Fieve, D. Rosenthal and H. Brill), pp 221–232. Baltimore: Johns Hopkins.

—— LINKOWSKI, P., GUROFF, J. J. & VAN PRAAG, H. M. (1979) Color blindness linkage to bipolar manic-depressive illness. *Archives of General Psychiatry*, **36**, 1442–1447.

—— —— & WILMOTTE, J. (1980) Relationship between schizoaffective illness and affective disorders of schizophrenia. *Journal of Affective Disorders*, **2**, 289–302.

MORTON, L. S. & KIDD, K. K. (1981) The effects of variable age-of-onset and diagnostic criteria on the estimates of linkage. An example using manic depressive illness and colour blindness. *Social Biology*, **27**, 1–10.

MORTON, N. E. (1955) Sequential tests for detection of linkage. *American Journal of Human Genetics*, **8**, 80–96.

PENROSE, L. S. (1938) Genetic linkage in graded human characters. *Annals of Eugenics*, **8**, 233–237.

—— (1946) A further note on the sib-pair linkage method. *Annals of Eugenics*, **13**, 25–29.

RACE, R. R. & SANGER, R. (1975) *Blood Groups in Man* (6th edition). Oxford: Blackwell.

REICH, T., CLAYTON, P. J. & WINOKUR, G. (1969) Family history studies: V. The genetics of mania. *American Journal of Psychiatry*, **125**, 1358–1369.

REICH, W. (1976) The schizophrenia spectrum: a genetic concept. *Journal of Nervous and Mental Disease*, **162**, 3–12.

ROSENTHAL, D. (1970) *Genetic Theory and Abnormal Behaviour*. Maidenhead, Berks: McGraw-Hill. (Series in Psychology).

—— WENDER, P. H., KETY, S. S., WELNER, J. & SCHULSINGER, F. (1971) The adopted away offspring of schizophrenics. *American Journal of Psychiatry*, **128**, 307–311.

SHIELDS, J. (1978) Genetics. In *Schizophrenia: Towards a New Synthesis* (ed. J. K. Wing), pp 53–88. London: Academic Press.

SLATER, E. & BEARD, W. (1963) The schizophrenia-like psychoses of epilepsy: psychiatric aspects. *British Journal of Psychiatry*, **109**, 95–105.

—— & COWIE, V. A. (1971) *The Genetics of Mental Disorders*. Oxford University Press.

STEPHENS, D. A., ATKINSON, M. W., KAY, D. W. K., ROTH, M. & GARSIDE, R. F. (1975) Psychiatric morbidity in parents and sibs of schizophrenics and non-schizophrenics. *British Journal of Psychiatry*, **127**, 97–108.

TANNA, V. L., GO, R. C. P., WINOKUR, G. & ELSTON, R. C. (1976a) Possible linkage between group-specific component (Gc protein) and pure depressive disease. *Acta Psychiatrica Scandinavica*, **55**, 111–115.

—— WINOKUR, G., ELSTON, R. C. & GO, R. C. P. (1976b) A linkage study of pure depressive disease: the use of the sib-pair method. *Biological Psychiatry*, **11**, 767–771.

—— —— —— —— (1976c) A linkage study of depression spectrum disease: the use of the sib-pair method. *Neuropsychobiology*, **2**, 52–62.

—— GO, R. C. P., WINOKUR, G. & ELSTON, R. C. (1979) Possible linkage between α-haptoglobin (Hp) and depression spectrum disease. *Neuropsychobiology*, **5**, 102–113.

TURNER, G. & OPITZ, J. M. (1980) Editorial comment: X-linked mental retardation. *American Journal of Medical Genetics*, **7**, 407–415.

TURNER, W. J. (1979a) Genetic markers for schizotaxia. *Biological Psychiatry*, **14**, 177–206.

—— (1979b) Towards a molecular biology of the psychoses: searches for genetic markers. *Psychiatric Journal of the University of Ottawa*, **3**, 248–255.

—— & KING, S. (1981) Two genetically distinct forms of bipolar affective disorder? *Biological Psychiatry*, **16**, 417–439.

WENDER, P. H., ROSENTHAL, D., KETY, S. S., SCHULSINGER, F. & WENDER, J. (1974) Crossfostering. A research strategy for clarifying the role of genetic and experiential factors in the etiology of schizophrenia. *Archives of General Psychiatry*, **30**, 121–128.

—— —— ZAHN, T. P. & KETY, S. S. (1971) The psychiatric adjustment of the adopting parents of schizophrenics. *American Journal of Psychiatry*, **127**, 1013–1018.

WEXLER, B. E. (1980) Cerebral laterality and psychiatry 1: a review of the literature. *American Journal of Psychiatry*, **137**, 279–291.

WINOKUR, G. & TANNA, V. L. (1969) Possible role of X-linked dominant factor in manic depressive disease. *Diseases of the Nervous System*, **30**, 89–94.

30 Genetics of platelet MAO activity in discordant schizophrenic and normal twins

MICHAEL A. REVELEY, ADRIANNE M. REVELEY, CHRISTINE A. CLIFFORD and ROBIN M. MURRAY

The enzyme monoamine oxidase (MAO) (EC 1.4.3.4.) has been of particular interest to psychiatrists in recent years because of its crucial role in the degradation of biogenic amines. Two forms of MAO, type A and type B, can be distinguished by various inhibitors (Johnston, 1968). Both exist in human brain, but only type B is found in human platelets (Donnelly and Murphy, 1977), where it has the same physicochemical properties and is more accessible for clinical study. A large and contradictory literature (Sandler *et al*, 1981) has developed over the hypothesis that low platelet MAO activity is associated with psychiatric disorder in general, and schizophrenia in particular. It has even been suggested that platelet MAO activity could be a genetic marker for schizophrenia (Wyatt *et al*, 1973).

Several studies based on normal (Nies *et al*, 1973; Winter *et al*, 1978; Hussein *et al*, 1980) and schizophrenic twins (Wyatt *et al*, 1973; Koide *et al*, 1981a; Reveley *et al*, 1981) have demonstrated that platelet MAO activity is under a high degree of genetic control. The precise mechanism of inheritance cannot be determined from twin studies, though the genetic and environmental contributions can be roughly quantified. Because of the apparently unimodal distribution of activity (Murphy *et al*, 1976), lack of an obvious Mendelian gene in family studies (Pandey *et al*, 1979; Propping and Fiedl, 1979) and consistent 'environmental' contribution from twin studies, multifactorial inheritance can be assumed.

It is easy to see how multiple genes could be involved in the final expression of platelet MAO activity. Of course, however many genes are involved, monozygotic (MZ) twins will have them all in common. The environmental influence on the trait, whether resulting from *in vivo* differences in the twins or from variation in the MAO analysis, leads to a lowering of the correlation among MZ twins, and for most twin studies this seems to account for 12–33 per cent of the variation.

In an attempt to determine the genetic contribution to platelet MAO activity on the one hand, and the environmental contribution of the schizophrenic illness and its treatment on the other, we compared a group of MZ twins discordant for schizophrenia and neuroleptic treatment, with age and sex matched control groups of normal MZ twins, normal dizygotic (DZ) twins and normal unrelated singletons. Such comparisons not only provided a control group for mean platelet MAO activity, but also gave an estimate of the environmental contribution to platelet MAO activity under normal conditions with varying genetic identities, from 100 per cent in the MZ twins and an average of 50 per cent in the DZ twins, to 0 per cent in the unrelated individuals.

We also examined the relationship of cerebral ventricular size as measured on computerized axial tomography (CT scan) to platelet MAO activity in the schizophrenic twins and their co-twins. Increased ventricular size has also been associated with schizophrenia (Johnstone *et al*, 1976; Weinberger *et al*, 1979) and shown to be under a high degree of genetic control (Reveley *et al*, 1982). We wished to establish whether the two abnormalities tended to co-vary so that there was a clustering of vulnerability factors in some individuals, or whether they were unrelated.

The study

Twins discordant for schizophrenia from the Maudsley Hospital Twin Register were asked to give blood for platelet MAO determination. Ten pairs agreed to participate. Ten pairs each of MZ and DZ control twins were chosen from the Institute of Psychiatry volunteer twin register to match the schizophrenics for sex and age (within five years) and were also asked to give blood. In addition, blood samples from pairs of unrelated controls, similarly age and sex matched, were collected from volunteer donors at a blood bank. Zygosity of all twins was established by blood groups and direct physical comparison. All twins from schizophrenic and control pairs were personally interviewed by A.R. The format of the SADS-L (Spitzer and Endicott, 1977) was used for the schizophrenics and their co-twins together with case notes and corroborative evidence from relatives. We were thus satisfied that all proband twins met the Research Diagnostic Criteria (Spitzer *et al*, 1975) for schizophrenia, and that none of the co-twins was currently ill or had ever suffered from a schizophrenic or other psychotic illness. We also enquired about birth complications, birthweight, severe head injury and physical illness. CT scans were also obtained on most of the twins, and ventricular size was estimated by a procedure previously described (Reveley *et al*, 1982).

Twenty ml of venous blood was taken by venepuncture and placed into universal containers with 0.5 ml of 5 per cent NaEDTA. A 10 ml aliquot was centrifuged at 320 g for 5 minutes at 20°C to obtain a platelet-rich plasma, which was then spun at 4,300 g for 20 minutes at 20°C. The platelet pellet was resuspended and washed in 1 ml of 0.32 M sucrose, vortex-mixed, and again spun at 4,300 g for 20 minutes at 20°C. The pellet was stored at $-20°C$ until assay, when it was resuspended in 1 ml of 0.32 M sucrose and frozen and thawed once again. All assays were performed in duplicate using tyramine as substrate as described by Reveley *et al* (1980). Platelet MAO was found to be stable for at least one year under these conditions. Duplicate assays on the same patient were accurate within ± 3 per cent. Interassay variation was ± 6 per cent. The assay was performed blind to psychiatric status and zygosity. Our groups contained a mixture of males and females, who have different mean MAO activities, so we analysed our results using non-parametric statistics (Mann Whitney U test and Spearmans rank correlation). However, since the results are quite similar using parametric (2 tailed Students 't' and the twin correlation r) tests, and these are in more common use, we have reported both.

Twins and singletons were matched for age and sex as displayed in Table I. There were no significant differences in mean age among the groups. The

TABLE I
Mean ages and platelet MAO activities of different groups

Group	N	Age mean ± SE	Platelet MAO activity[a] mean ± SE
MZ schizophrenics	10	39.50 ± 3.26	14.86 ± 1.68*†
Non-schizophrenic co-twins	10	39.50 ± 3.26	15.64 ± 2.29
Combined schizophrenics and co-twins	20	39.50 ± 2.24	15.25 ± 1.38**‡
MZ controls	20	40.30 ± 2.70	20.72 ± 1.58
DZ controls	20	41.70 ± 2.91	19.05 ± 1.47
Unrelated singletons	20	38.90 ± 2.59	19.28 ± 1.18
All controls combined	60	40.30 ± 1.56	19.68 ± 0.81

[a] nmole product formed/mg protein/30 min
2-tailed Mann Whitney U test and 2-tailed t-test:
† P <0.05 vs all controls
‡ P <0.01 vs all controls
* P <0.05 vs MZ controls

2-tailed Mann-Whitney U test   2-tailed t-test:
** P <0.002 vs MZ controls   ** P <0.02 vs MZ controls

M : F ratio was 6 : 4. Mean platelet MAO activity was not significantly different among the MZ controls, DZ controls or unrelated singleton controls, and their values were thus combined into one control group.

The mean platelet MAO activity of the schizophrenic twins was not significantly different from that of their co-twins, but this combined 'schizophrenic genotype' group had significantly lower mean platelet MAO activity than either the MZ controls alone or the total group of controls. The schizophrenics alone, without their co-twins, also had significantly lower mean values than MZ controls and all controls (a lowering of 28 per cent and 25 per cent respectively).

Table II shows that the correlation within each of the three control groups decreased in the expected direction MZ twins > DZ twins > unrelated singletons. Thus in our sample, as in others, platelet MAO activity was under a high degree of genetic control. The effects of illness or medication did not reduce the correlation between the schizophrenics and their co-twins. Indeed their correlation was almost exactly the same value as that of the normal MZs.

All but one of the schizophrenics and none of the co-twins were currently taking neuroleptics. In the pair with the lowest platelet MAO activity (schizophrenic = 5.33; co-twin = 2.91; about 25 per cent of mean control activity), the co-twin was taking phenobarbitol and phenytoin (to treat epilepsy resulting from severe birth injury) which are not known to affect platelet MAO activity (Kruk *et al*, 1980). However, if we eliminate this pair and their matched controls from the analysis, the difference was still significant (P <0.05, 75 d.f.). The co-twin's platelet MAO activity remained low (1.57) on reassay with a fresh sample of blood. The platelet MAO activities of their three psychiatrically normal first-degree relatives were also low, at about 60 per cent of the mean control value (father = 12.38; mother = 11.45; brother = 10.51).

There were no significant Pearson product-moment correlations between ventricular size and platelet MAO activity among the schizophrenics (r = 0.01), their co-twins (r = 0.55) or the control twins (r = 0.02).

Comment

Neuroleptic effect

While we found significantly lower mean platelet MAO activity among the MZ twins who had schizophrenia (Table II) compared to controls, there was

TABLE II
Correlation of platelet MAO activity within different groups

Group	N	Spearmans r^*_s	Twin r†
MZ schizophrenics and co-twins	10	0.79 P <0.01	0.79 P <0.01 (F = 8.74)‡
MZ controls	10	0.74 P <0.01	0.80 P <0.01 (F = 8.81)
DZ controls	10	0.26 n.s.	0.35 n.s. (F = 2.08)
Unrelated singletons	10	0.04 n.s.	0.06 n.s. (F = 1.13)

* 1 tailed

† $r = \dfrac{\text{interpair variance} - \text{intrapair variance}}{\text{interpair variance} + \text{intrapair variance}}$

‡ $F = \dfrac{\text{interpair variance}}{\text{intrapair variance}} \dfrac{(n-1 \text{ d.f.})}{(n \text{ d.f.})}$

N = number of pairs

no significant difference between them and their own, non-schizophrenic co-twins. The correlation for these discordant pairs was very similar (0.79) to that found among the normal MZ twins (0.80, Table II). This suggests that the variability of platelet MAO activity was not increased by the neuroleptic agents taken by the schizophrenic twin, or by any factor consequent upon the schizophrenic illness. Thus genetic rather than environmental factors predominate.

Of course, our schizophrenic twins were on various drugs in varying dosages, a situation different from that in a research trial where the drug and its dose are constant; in that case particular neuroleptics may be seen to cause some lowering of activity. Recent controlled studies with haloperidol (De Lisi *et al*, 1981; Chojnacki *et al*, 1981) flupenthixol (Owen *et al*, 1981) and chlorproma-zine (CPZ) (Sahai *et al*, 1981) have found a drop of approximately 20–30 per cent after 2–4 weeks of treatment. However, Owen *et al* (1981) found an inconsistent change in mean platelet MAO activity after 4 weeks of CPZ treatment and earlier studies found either no neuroleptic drug effect (Murphy and Wyatt, 1972; Murphy *et al*, 1974; Mann and Thomas, 1979) or an increase of enzyme activity with neuroleptics (Owen *et al*, 1976). In fact, there was a slightly (14.86 vs 15.64: a 5 per cent difference) lower activity among the schizophrenics compared to their co-twins in the present study, though this was not statistically significant.

Considering the inconsistent findings for antipsychotic agents in general, and the evidence from our study and the family studies discussed below, it seems unlikely that neuroleptic agents are primarily responsible for low platelet MAO activity in schizophrenia.

The genetic contribution to platelet MAO activity

The twin correlation can also be used (Emery, 1976) to give a rough measure of the heritability (h^2), as $h^2 = \frac{r}{R} \times 100$ where r is the correlation and R, the coefficient of relationship. In this case the DZ correlation is effectively doubled since fraternal twins have only half their genes in common. Heritabilities derived from the twin correlations for MZ and DZ twins (80 per cent and 70 per cent respectively) are remarkably similar, and confirm that only 20–30 per cent of the variation in platelet MAO activity is non-genetic. The expected lack of correlation among the unrelated singletons confirms that assay variation has not led to spuriously high correlations between pairs.

Our control twin findings accord well with those from family studies of normal individuals. Pandey *et al* (1979) examined 112 families, finding a uni-modal and normal distribution of activity, supporting multifactorial inheri-tance. Their results using tyramine as substrate, as in this study, were a parent-offspring correlation of 0.27 and a sibling-sibling correlation of 0.32. This is in close agreement with the correlation of 0.35 found among our DZ twins who also share an average of 50 per cent of their genes.

Our results also agree well with previous twin studies (Nies *et al*, 1973; Winter *et al*, 1978; Hussein *et al*, 1980) in which the intraclass correlations vary from 0.76–0.88 in normal MZ and 0.39 to 0.52 in normal DZ twins, varying with the substrate selected. Among discordant schizophrenic twins, Wyatt *et al* (1973) found a Pearson product-moment correlation of 0.67. They assumed lack of drug effect because the mean activities of the schizophrenics and their co-twins were similar, but did not compare variability with normal twin controls. The only other twin study using discordant schizophrenics (Koide *et al*, 1981a) has too small a sample (3 pairs) for meaningful comparison.

A genetic marker?

The high degree of genetic control of platelet MAO activity has led to hopes that it might prove to be a useful genetic marker for schizophrenia. An ideal marker has a known pattern of inheritance and chromosomal location with a number of alleles enabling different populations to be distinguished on this basis. Unfortunately these conditions cannot be fulfilled by the activity of MAO in platelets. The activity of the enzyme is probably affected by many genes, and there is also a great deal of overlap between schizophrenics and controls. So despite a tendency towards lower mean values in the schizophrenics, most schizophrenics do not have low platelet MAO activity. Nevertheless, low platelet MAO activity could be associated with an increased susceptibility to psychiatric problems in general as suggested by Buchsbaum *et al* (1976). Indeed patients with several psychiatric disorders are found to have a tendency toward lowered activity (Sandler *et al*, 1981).

Family studies

As platelet MAO activity seems to be a unimodal polygenic trait, as are height and intelligence, values for the relatives of those with low platelet MAO activity ought to be low but regress to the mean; they will therefore tend to be intermediate between proband values and control mean values. Berrettini *et al* (1980) examined platelet MAO V_{max} and K_m in 29 first degree relatives of 12 schizophrenics with low platelet MAO activity and found this to be the case; the V_{max} of the relatives was intermediate between that of the schizophrenics and the controls. Family studies which have not examined the MAO activities of the schizophrenic probands and which exclude psychiatrically ill relatives (Propping and Friedl, 1979) or which have not specified probands with low MAO activity (Koide *et al*, 1981b; Böök *et al*, 1978) may not be able to detect a mean lowering of activity among the relatives. Only a proportion of the probands could be expected to have low platelet MAO activity; the activity of their relatives will tend towards the normal population mean, and when mixed with the values from relatives of probands without low platelet MAO (who will tend not to have low platelet MAO either), any effect will be so diluted as to be undetectable.

If low platelet MAO activity does increase susceptibility to schizophrenia, then we would expect relatives with low platelet MAO to be at increased risk. No studies have specifically addressed the question by examining both platelet MAO activity and psychiatric status in such relatives. In common with Belmaker *et al* (1977) we did not find an association of low activity with a family history of schizophrenia, but our sample is small and based on twins who may have an increase in environmental vulnerability factors (Reveley *et al*, 1982) precipitating the illness. Baron and Levitt (1980) found lower platelet MAO activity among a larger sample of chronic schizophrenics with a family history of schizophrenia and suggest that low platelet MAO activity is implicated in high genetic load schizophrenia, but whether the affected relatives in their study had particularly low activity, as they should if their illness occurred on this basis, is unknown.

Association with cerebral ventricular size?

Other vulnerability factors have been proposed in association with the development of schizophrenia, such as enlarged cerebral ventricles (Reveley *et al*,

1982). To see if such vulnerability factors tended to cluster in some individuals we examined platelet MAO activity and ventricular size in relation to each other. Among the control twins, as expected, we found no correlation. Neither was there a correlation among the schizophrenic twins, however, though such a relationship might be detectable in a larger group.

Conclusion

The genetic influence on platelet MAO activity is consistent in schizophrenics and controls, and for varying degrees of genetic identity. From the available evidence, it appears that the activity of the enzyme is multifactorial; the result of the action of many genes with many opportunities for environmental variation as well. Any one of the genetic systems involved in the final activity level of the enzyme may prove, in the future, to be more closely implicated in the pathogenesis of psychiatric disorders. Bearing in mind the probable complexity of the systems involved, the finding of even a weak association is an important clue, and deserves continued investigation.

References

BARON, M. & LEVITT, M. (1980) Platelet monoamine oxidase activity; relation to genetic load of schizophrenia. *Psychiatry Research*, **3**, 69–74.

BELMAKER, R. H., GALON, A., PEREZ, L. & EBSTEIN, R. (1977) Platelet MAO in schizophrenics with and without a family history of schizophrenia. *British Journal of Psychiatry*, **131**, 551–552.

BERRETTINI, W. H., BENFIELD, T. C., SCHMIDT, A. O., LADMAN, R. K. & VOGEL, W. H. (1980) Platelet monoamine oxidase in families of chronic schizophrenics. *Schizophrenia Bulletin*, **6**, 235–237.

BÖÖK, J. A., WETTERBERG, L. & MODRZEWSKA, K. (1978) Schizophrenia in a North Swedish geographical isolate, 1900–1977: Epidemiology, genetics and biochemistry. *Clinical Genetics*, **14**, 373–394.

BUCHSBAUM, M. S., COURSEY, R. D. & MURPHY, D. L. (1976) The biochemical high-risk paradigm: behavioural and familial correlates of low platelet monoamine oxidase activity. *Science*, **194**, 339–341.

CHOJNACKI, M., KRALIK, P., ALLEN, R. H., HO, B. T., SCHOOLAR, J. C. & SMITH, R. C. (1981) Neuroleptic-induced decrease in platelet MAO activity of schizophrenic patients. *American Journal of Psychiatry*, **138**, 838–840.

DE LISI, L. E., WISE, C. D., BRIDGE, T. P., ROSENBLATT, J. E., WAGNER, R. L., MORIHISA, J., KARSON, C., POTKIN, S. G. & WYATT, R. J. (1981) A probable neuroleptic effect on platelet monoamine oxidase in chronic schizophrenic patients. *Psychiatry Research*, **4**, 95–107.

DONNELLY, C. H. & MURPHY, D. L. (1977) Substrate and inhibitor related characteristics of human platelet monoamine oxidase. *Biochemical Pharmacology*, **26**, 853–858.

EMERY, A. E. H. (1976) *Methodology in Medical Genetics*, pp. 85–87. Edinburgh: Churchill Livingstone.

HUSSEIN, L., SINDARTO, E. & GOEDDE, H. W. (1980) Twin studies and substrate differences in platelet monoamine oxidase activity. *Human Heredity*, **30**, 65–70.

JOHNSTON, J. P. (1968) Some observations upon a new inhibitor of monoamine oxidase in brain tissue. *Biochemical Pharmacology*, **17**, 1285–1297.

JOHNSTONE, E. C., CROW, T. J., FRITH, C. D., HUSBAND, J. & KREEL, L. (1976) Cerebral ventricular size and cognitive impairment in chronic schizophrenia. *Lancet*, ii, 924–926.

KOIDE, Y., EBERHARD, G., SÄÄF, J., ROSS, S. B., WAHLUND, L-O. & WETTERBERG, L. (1981a) Kinetic aspects of monoamine oxidase activity in twins with psychoses. *Clinical Genetics*, **19**, 395–400.

—— SÄÄF, J., WAHULUND, L-O., ROSS, S. B. & WETTERBERG, L. (1981b) Platelet monoamine oxidase activity in schizophrenic families—kinetic aspects. *Clinical Genetics*, **19**, 405–409.

KRUK, Z. L., MOFFETT, A. & SCOTT, D. F. (1980) Platelet monoamine oxidase activity in epilepsy. *Journal of Neurology, Neurosurgery and Psychiatry*, **43**, 68–70.

MANN, J. & THOMAS, K. M. (1979) Platelet monoamine oxidase activity in schizophrenia: Relationship to disease, treatment, institutionalisation and outcome. *British Journal of Psychiatry*, **134**, 366–371.

MURPHY, D. L., BELMAKER, R. & WYATT, R. J. (1974) Monoamine oxidase in schizophrenia and other behavioural disorders. *Journal of Psychiatric Research*, **11**, 221–248.

—— WRIGHT, C., BUCHSBAUM, M., NICHOLS, A., COSTA, J. L. & WYATT, R. J. (1976) Platelet and plasma amine oxidase activity in 680 normals; sex and age differences and stability over time. *Biochemical Medicine*, **16**, 254–265.

—— & WYATT, R. J. (1972) Reduced monoamine oxidase activity in blood platelets from schizophrenic patients. *Nature*, **238**, 225–226.

NIES, A., ROBINSON, D. S., LAMBORN, K. R. & LAMPERT, R. P. (1973) Genetic control of platelet and plasma monoamine oxidase activity. *Archives of General Psychiatry*, **28**, 834–838.

OWEN, F., BOURNE, R., CROW, T. J., JOHNSTONE, E. C., BAILEY, A. R. & HERSHON, H. I. (1976) Platelet monoamine oxidase in schizophrenia. *Archives of General Psychiatry*, **33**, 1370–1373.

—— —— —— FADHLI, A. A. & JOHNSTONE, E. C. (1981) Platelet monoamine oxidase activity in acute schizophrenia; relationship to symptomatology and neuroleptic medication. *British Journal of Psychiatry*, **139**, 16–22.

PANDEY, G. N., DORUS, E., SHAUGHNESSY, R. & DAVIS, J. M. (1979) Genetic control of platelet monoamine oxidase activity: Studies on normal families. *Life Sciences*, **25**, 1173–1178.

PROPPING, P. & FRIEDL, W. (1979) Platelet monoamine oxidase activity in first degree relatives of schizophrenic patients. *Psychopharmacology*, **65**, 265–272.

REVELEY, A. M., REVELEY, M. A. & MURRAY, R. M. (1981) Effects of neuroleptic drugs on MAO activity. *British Journal of Psychiatry*, **139**, 475–476.

—— —— CLIFFORD, C. A. & MURRAY, R. M. (1982) Cerebral ventricular size in twins discordant for schizophrenia. *Lancet i*, 540–541.

REVELEY, M. A., GURLING, H. M. D., GLASS, I., GLOVER, V. & SANDLER, M. (1980) Platelet γ-aminobutyric acid—aminotransferase and monoamine oxidase in schizophrenia. *Neuropharmacology*, **19**, 1249–1250.

SAHAI, S., ARORA, R. & MELTZER, H. Y. (1981) Effect of chlorpromazine treatment on monoamine oxidase activity in platelets isolated by the Corash method. *Psychiatry Research*, **5**, 111–114.

SANDLER, M., REVELEY, M. A. & GLOVER, V. (1981) Human platelet monoamine oxidase in health and disease: a review. *Journal of Clinical Pathology*, **34**, 292–302.

SPITZER, R. L. & ENDICOTT, J. (1977) *The Schedule for Affective Disorders and Schizophrenia*, Lifetime Version, 3rd Edition. New York: New York State Psychiatric Institute.

—— ENDICOTT, J. & ROBINS, E. (1975) *Research Diagnostic Criteria*, Instrument No. 58. New York: New York State Psychiatric Institute.

WEINBERGER, D. R., TORREY, E. F., NEOPHYTIDES, A. N. & WYATT, R. J. (1979) Lateral cerebral ventricular enlargement in chronic schizophrenia. *Archives of General Psychiatry*, **36**, 735–739.

WINTER, H., HERSCHEL, M., PROPPING, P., FRIEDL, W. & VOGEL, F. (1978) A twin study on three enzymes (DBH, COMT, MAO) of catecholamine metabolism: correlations with MMPI. *Psychopharmacology*, **57**, 63–69.

WYATT, R. J., MURPHY, D. L., BELMAKER, R., COHEN, S., DONNELLY, C. H. & POLLIN, W. (1973) Reduced monoamine oxidase activity in platelets: a possible genetic marker for vulnerability to schizophrenia. *Science*, **179**, 916–918.

31 Genetic markers, biological markers and platelet MAO

**MICHAEL A. REVELEY and
ADRIANNE M. REVELEY**

A wealth of research reports on platelet monoamine oxidase (MAO) in schizophrenia preceded our paper on MAO in discordant schizophrenic twins (**Reveley et al, 1983**), but only a handful of reports have followed it. This is partly because the large number of research projects initiated after the paper by Murphy and Wyatt (1972) on lowered platelet MAO activity in schizophrenia were completed by the late 1970s, but also because the flurry of activity surrounding platelet MAO and schizophrenia seemed directed up a disappointing dead end.

Some of the reasons for the disenchantment with platelet MAO activity as a research tool lie with the enormous expectations aroused by the early reports. Not only was lowered platelet MAO a neat confirmation of the dopamine hypothesis which links symptoms and treatment in a coherent explanation of schizophrenia, but it was also offered as a 'genetic marker' for predisposition to schizophrenia (Wyatt et al, 1974) which would free psychiatrists from the uncertainties of clinical diagnosis. In retrospect, lowered platelet MAO activity seems an unlikely candidate.

The term 'genetic marker' denotes a reliably measured biological characteristic, usually a subtype of an enzyme, or a variation in genomic DNA, with a known Mendelian mode of inheritance and known chromosomal location, and with two or more alternative forms or polymorphisms. Subjects who are of genetic interest will differ with respect to these alternatives. Thus, the polymorphic G8 sequence of chromosome 4 'marks' the region of the Huntington's chorea gene so that the same subtype of G8 runs with Huntington's chorea through given pedigrees (Gusella et al, 1983). The proximity of G8 to the Huntington's gene does not imply any aetiological role for G8 itself, indeed the particular subtype associated with Huntington's will vary from pedigree to pedigree. Lowered platelet MAO activity does not fulfil any of the characteristics of a genetic marker. While the enzyme activity may be under a high degree of genetic control in twin (Nies et al, 1973; Reveley et al, 1983) and family studies, it is likely to be under the influence of several genes and thus not a simple Mendelian trait. There is evidence that it is not 'lower' and 'normal' activities that are possible genetic alternatives—but rather 'normal' and 'raised' platelet MAO activity (Rice et al, 1982).

Research using platelet MAO began before the recent developments in molecular biology. In the 1970s most of the available markers were proteins such as enzymes, blood groups or the like which had two or more structural variations. Examples of such markers include the Rhesus and Duffy blood groups on chromosome 1, the ABO blood group on chromosome 9, colour blindness on the X chromosome and the histocompatibility complex (including histocompatibility antigen (HLA)) on chromosome 6. The HLA/schizophrenia story is well known—and negative—there is little evidence that a gene for schizophrenia is on chromosome 6 (McGuffin *et al*, 1983). Reports linking manic depression with colour blindness, and thus on the X chromosome are similarly under question. Such 'classical' markers cover only about 20 per cent of the human genome (Vogel and Motulsky, 1982).

The number of potential genetic markers has increased dramatically over the past five years, with our ability to detect random and apparently function-less variations in the genetic code itself, which do not necessarily code for proteins. Enzymes are used to split the DNA where it has a particular base-pair sequence, and the resulting fragments may be polymorphic—hence the G8 fragment of chromosome 4, resulting from digestion of chromosome 4 with the *Hin*dIII enzyme. We can go further. We can establish a gene location by linkage analysis with a marker. Linkage analysis is a calculation of the statistical probability that two genes are co-segregating in a series of families, thus indicating that they are physically very close together on a chromosome. The principle of linkage analysis depends on the small number of 'cross-overs' that occur between strands of DNA at meiosis. Thus each unpaired chromo-some in sperm or ova is a composite of the parent's pair of chromosomes. Once a gene location is known, we can go on to characterize the composition of the abnormal gene itself and its protein product. Since each chromosome may contain 6,000 genes (Pembrey, 1983), the number of potential markers is clearly enormous.

Genetic markers do not necessarily have any aetiological relationship to the 'disease gene' under investigation—but only a physical nearness. Some markers, however, may play an aetiological role in disease by themselves confer-ring susceptibility. Thus some autoimmune disorders are associated with parti-cular variants of the major histocompatibility complex (e.g. ankylosing spondylitis and HLA B27). It has been suggested that paranoid schizophrenia is associated in this way with HLA A9, but the evidence is inconclusive. Asso-ciation with traits other than markers may also be used to clarify disease relationships (see below).

Platelet MAO activity could not be a true genetic marker. For a start, the activity level of the enzyme does not have a known Mendelian mode of inheri-tance, but is under the influence of several genes, all of unknown location so far, as well as a number of environmental factors (see below). There are two types of MAO, type A and type B, which were at first distinguished on pharmacological grounds (Johnston, 1968). More recently there is evidence from peptide mapping studies that types A and B represent distinct enzyme molecules (Cawthon and Breakefield, 1979). However, they appear to have different chromosome locations (Breakefield *et al*, 1979). As yet little is known about either form, and whether or not they are polymorphic, although MAO type A has been assigned to the X chromosome (Pintar *et al*, 1981). It is possible that either of these may be closely linked, or associated, with a gene conferring vulnerability for psychiatric disorder and such research will no doubt be possible within the next decade.

Lowered platelet MAO activity might be a biological marker (Rieder and Gershon, 1978). In this case, the term marker loosely refers to a biological characteristic which is associated with the disease process itself, or with vulnerability to it. Ideally such markers are associated with increased risk of the illness itself, are genetically influenced, and represent abnormality whether or not the subject is actually ill or has recovered. Recently, increased cerebral ventricular size has been considered to be as a possible biological marker for schizophrenia, but this appears to be influenced more by environmental than genetic factors (Reveley *et al*, 1984), moreover it is associated with several other psychiatric and neurological disorders.

What of the prospects for lowered platelet MAO as a biological marker for schizophrenia? The first disappointment was that lowered platelet MAO was only found in a proportion of schizophrenics in any study, with substantial overlap between controls and patients; perhaps one third of studies comparing mean enzyme levels in schizophrenics and controls were negative. Secondly, while the negative studies could be explained on the basis of sampling variation (Buchsbaum and Rieder, 1979), an uncomfortable number of factors appeared which, it seemed, could influence MAO activity. Gender, diet, smoking, physical activity, anaemia and the menstrual cycle are all associated with platelet MAO activity changes (for review see Sandler *et al*, 1981). Further, the biological significance of low platelet MAO was questionable, as the degree of lowering was modest (27 per cent on average) while at least an 80 per cent reduction was needed for clinical significance, e.g. when monoamine oxidase inhibitors were used for antidepressant therapy.

Further evidence accumulated on the pitfalls of MAO research. The technique of analysis could substantially influence the results, and as researchers looked beyond schizophrenia to other disorders, it was found to be lowered in manic-depression, alcoholism, and neurological conditions (Sandler *et al*, 1981). Perhaps lowered platelet MAO activity acts as a predisposition to non-specific psychiatric disorder, as Buchsbaum *et al* (1976) have suggested, although even the stylish 'high risk' paradigm does not always confirm an association of psychopathology with lower MAO (Propping and Friedl, 1981). The most serious setback to platelet MAO research came with the finding of no difference in brain MAO between schizophrenics and controls (Schwartz *et al*, 1974; Crow *et al*, 1979; Reveley *et al*, 1981). Though low platelet MAO could be acceptable as a non-specific predisposing factor, and the various extrinsic associations and vagaries of analysis could be accounted for, the activity of MAO in platelets made little sense as a 'window on the brain' if the brain itself did not show the same dysfunction. Workers were quick to accept the brain findings, even though they, too, are open to methodological artefact. For example, all studies of brain MAO have examined activity levels in homogenates of brain tissue from general regions (Crow *et al*, 1979; Schwartz *et al*, 1974; Reveley *et al*, 1981). No study of schizophrenic brain has ever examined glial versus neuronal MAO, nor carefully examined discrete brain regions such as parts of the limbic system, nor selectively examined MAO in the nerve endings of discrete neurotransmitter pathways.

Obvious disappointment with platelet MAO as a biological factor in schizophrenia led workers to a quick acceptance of the idea that neuroleptics were responsible for the lowered activity (Owen *et al*, 1981). There is convincing evidence (De Lisi *et al*, 1981; Chojnacki *et al*, 1981; Owen *et al*, 1981; Sahai *et al*, 1981) that psychotropic drugs can reduce activity by about 25 per cent, roughly the same degree of mean lowering as is found in schizophrenia. However, this does not explain the findings from other disorders such as manic depressive disorder or alcoholism, or the work which shows platelet MAO to be lower in subjects with a presumed genetic vulnerability to psychiatric disorder, or, most importantly, the twin studies (Wyatt *et al*, 1971; Reveley *et al*, 1983). We have already mentioned the work of Buchsbaum *et al* (1976), looking at psychiatric disorder in those with extremes of MAO activity—but what of the families of psychiatric patients?

As we point out in our paper; family studies which have not examined the MAO activities of the schizophrenic probands (Propping and Friedl, 1979), or which have not specified probands with low MAO activity (Koide *et al*, 1981; Böök *et al*, 1978) may not detect lowered activity in the family members. Berrettini *et al* (1980) found platelet MAO in the family members of chronic schizophrenics to be midway between schizophrenics and controls, which is to be expected if platelet MAO activity is predominantly a unimodal polygenic trait. The two studies of monozygotic twins discordant for schizophrenia, our own and that of Wyatt *et al* (1974), suggests that the identical, but well, co-twins of schizophrenics have lower platelet MAO activity than controls. Most importantly, the co-twins of schizophrenics are unmedicated and therefore any lowering of activity cannot be related to neuroleptics in this group.

In our paper we suggested that investigators should examine both platelet MAO activity and psychiatric status in the relatives of schizophrenics whose MAO activity is also known. Such a study has been carried out by Baron *et al* (1984). While they found that low platelet MAO activity distinguished the well from ill relatives within families, the findings are suspect. Not only were many of the relatives and patients receiving neuroleptics, but the assay as described in the paper used C^{14}-benzylamine as substrate for the enzyme, in platelet-rich plasma. Thus the investigators would have measured both platelet MAO, and benzylamine oxidase, distinctly different enzymes (Lewinsohn *et al*, 1978).

In our opinion, research workers were too quick to discard lowered platelet MAO, as they were too eager to take it up. While there is no doubt that lowered MAO activity in platelets has always made nonsense as a genetic marker, it may be a non-specific indicator of psychiatric vulnerability. Even here, its usefulness as a biological marker is limited by activity levels being a final common pathway for many genetic and environmental effects. While much effort has been devoted to the comparison of mean activity levels in patients and controls, few studies have looked at families, which might clarify the genetic influence on MAO activity in health and disease, or studies of general psychiatric populations, which might identify those disorders particularly associated with lowered platelet MAO activity. Future research will no doubt focus on the molecular structures and relationships of the MAO genes themselves. When molecular biologists eventually clarify the chromosomal location and molecular genetics of MAO, there may be a renewed interest in psychiatric studies of this enzyme.

References

BARON, M., LEVITT, M., GRUEN, R., KANE, J. & ASNIS, L. (1984) Platelet monoamine oxidase activity and genetic vulnerability to schizophrenia. *American Journal of Psychiatry*, **141**, 836–842.

BERRETTINI, W. H., BENFIELD, T. C., SCHMIDT, A. O., LADMAN, R. K. & VOGEL, W. H. (1980) Platelet monoamine oxidase in families of chronic schizophrenics. *Schizophrenia Bulletin*, **6**, 235–237.

BÖÖK, J. A., WETTERBERG, L. & MODRZEWSKA, K. (1978) Schizophrenia in a North Swedish geographical isolate, 1900–1977: Epidemiology, genetics and biochemistry. *Clinical Genetics*, **14**, 373–394.

BREAKEFIELD, X. O., CAWTHON, R. M. COSTA, M. R. C., EDELSTEIN, S. B. & HAWKINS, M. (1979) A genetic view of monoamine oxidase. *Society for Neuroscience Symposium*, **4**, 43–66.

BUCHSBAUM, M. S. & RIEDER, R. O. (1979) Biologic heterogeneity and psychiatric research. *Archives of General Psychiatry*, **36**, 1163–1169.

—— COURSEY, R. D. & MURPHY, D. L. (1976) The biochemical high risk paradigm; behavioral and familial correlates of low platelet monoamine oxidase activity. *Science*, **194**, 339–341.

CAWTHON, R. M. & BREAKEFIELD, X. O. (1979) Differences in A and B forms of monoamine oxidase revealed by limited proteolysis and peptide mapping. *Nature*, **281**, 692–694.

CHOJNACKI, M., KRALIK, P., ALLEN, R. H., HO, B. T., SCHOOLAR, J. C. & SMITH, R. C. (1981) Neuroleptic-induced decrease in platelet MAO activity of schizophrenic patients. *American Journal of Psychiatry*, **138**, 838–840.

CROW, T. J., BAKER, H. F., CROSS, A. J., JOSEPH, M. H., LOFTHOUSE, R., LONGDEN, A., OWEN, F., RILEY, G. J., GLOVER, V. & KILLPACK, W. S. (1979) Monoamine mechanisms in chronic schizophrenia: post mortem neurochemical findings. *British Journal of Psychiatry*, **134**, 249–256.

DE LISI, L. E., WISE, C. D., BRIDGE, T. P., ROSENBLATT, J. E., WAGNER, R. L., MORIHISA, J., KARSON, C., POTKIN, S. G. & WYATT, R. J. (1981) A probable neuroleptic effect on platelet monoamine oxidase in chronic schizophrenic patients. *Psychiatry Research*, **4**, 95–107.

GUSELLA, J. F., WEXLER, N. S., CONNEALLY, P. M., NAYLOR, S. L., ANDERSON, M. A., TANZI, R. E., WATKINS, P. C., OTTINA, K., WALLACE, M. R., SAKAGUCHI, A. Y., YOUNG, A. B., SHOULSON, I., BONILLA, E. & MARTIN, J. B. (1983) A polymorphic DNA marker genetically linked to Huntington's disease. *Nature*, **306**, 234–238.

JOHNSTON, J. P. (1968) Some observations upon a new inhibitor of monoamine oxidase in brain tissue. *Biochemical Pharmacology*, **17**, 1285–1297.

KOIDE, Y., SAAF, J., WAHLUND, L.-O., ROOS, S. B. & WETTERBERG, L. (1981) Platelet monoamine oxidase activity in schizophrenic families-kinetic aspects. *Clinical Genetics*, **19**, 405–409.

LEWINSOHN, R., BOHM, K.-H., GLOVER, V. & SANDLER, M. A. (1978) A benzylamine oxidase distinct from monoamine oxidase B—widespread distribution in man and rat. *Biochemical Pharmacology*, **27**, 1857–1863.

McGUFFIN, P., FESTENSTEIN, H. & MURRAY, R. (1983) A family study of HLA antigens and other genetic markers in schizophrenia. *Psychological Medicine*, **13**, 31–43.

MURPHY, D. L. & WYATT, R. J. (1972) Reduced platelet monoamine oxidase activity in blood platelets from schizophrenic patients. *Nature*, **238**, 225–226.

NIES, A., ROBINSON, D. S., LAMBORN, K. R. & LAMPERT, R. P. (1973) Genetic control of platelet and plasma monoamine oxidase activity. *Archives of General Psychiatry*, **28**, 834–838.

OWEN, F., BOURNE, R., CROW, T. J., FADHLI, A. A. & JOHNSTONE, E. C. (1981) Platelet monoamine oxidase activity in acute schizophrenia: relationship to symptomatology and neuroleptic medication. *British Journal of Psychiatry*, **139**, 16–22.

PEMBREY, M. E. (1983) Clinical application of recombinant DNA techniques in families with genetic disease. *British Journal of Hospital Medicine*, **31**, 546–551.

PINTAR, J. E., BARBOSA, J., FRANCKE, U., CASTIGLIONE, C. M., HAWKINS, M. & BREAKEFIELD, X. O. (1981) Gene for monoamine oxidase type A assigned to the human X chromosome. *Journal of Neuroscience*, **1**, 166–175.

PROPPING, P. & FRIEDL, W. (1979) Platelet monoamine oxidase activity in first degree relatives of schizophrenic patients. *Psychopharmacology*, **65**, 265–272.

—— REY, E.-R., FRIEDL, W. & BECKMANN, H. (1981) Platelet monoamine oxidase in healthy subjects: The 'biochemical high-risk paradigm' revised. *Archive fur Psychiatrie und Nervenkrankheiten*, **230**, 209–219.

REVELEY, M. A., GLOVER, V., SANDLER, M. & SPOKES, E. G. (1981) Brain monoamine oxidase activity in schizophrenics and controls. *Archives of General Psychiatry*, **38**, 663–665.

—— REVELEY, A. M., CLIFFORD, C. A. & MURRAY, R. M. (1983) Genetics of platelet MAO activity in discordant schizophrenic and normal twins. *British Journal of Psychiatry*, **142**, 560–565.

REVELEY, A. M., REVELEY, M. A. & MURRAY, R. M. (1984) Cerebral ventricular enlargement in nongenetic schizophrenia: A controlled twin study. *British Journal of Psychiatry*, **144**, 89–93.

RICE, J., McGUFFIN, P. & SHASKAN, E. G. (1982) A commingling analysis of platelet monoamine oxidase activity. *Psychiatry Research*, **7**, 325–335.

RIEDER, R. O. & GERSHON, E. S. (1978) Genetic strategies in biological psychiatry. *Archives of General Psychiatry*, **35**, 866–873.

SAHAI, S., ARORA, R. & MELTZER, H. Y. (1981) Effect of chlorpromazine treatment on monoamine oxidase activity in platelets isolated by the Corash method. *Psychiatry Research*, **5**, 111–114.

SANDLER, M., REVELEY, M. A. & GLOVER, V. (1981) Human platelet monoamine oxidase in health and disease: a review. *Journal of Clinical Pathology*, **34**, 292–302.

SCHWARTZ, M. A., WYATT, R. J., YANG, H. Y. T. & NEFF, N. H. (1974) Multiple forms of brain monoamine oxidase in schizophrenic and normal individuals. *Archives of General Psychiatry*, **31**, 557–560.

VOGEL, F. & MOTULSKY, A. G. (1982) *Human Genetics: Problems and Approaches*. New York: Springer-Verlag.

WYATT, R. J., MURPHY, D. L., BELMAKER, R. H., COHEN, S., DONNELLY, C. H. & POLLIN, W. (1974) Reduced monoamine oxidase activity in platelets: A possible genetic marker for vulnerability to schizophrenia. *Science*, **173**, 916–918.

V. Social aspects

32 Social aspects of schizophrenia: Overview

ANDREW SIMS

The last decade has seen remarkable changes in social aspects of and attitudes towards schizophrenia. Professional opinion concerning the best way to help those with chronic mental illness has been reflected in a change of expectation by the general public. There has been a massive decrease in the resident population of schizophrenic patients in hospital, with schizophrenia representing less than one quarter of admissions to mental hospital (Freeman and Choudhury, 1984), and a proliferation of alternative methods of care within the community. The range of psychopharmacological agents available has increased but so has interest in social methods of management. It is recognized that very few patients now need to be segregated in the 'institution', the large mental hospital, often remote from the centre of population. These hospitals have sometimes been reduced to less than half their resident population of the mid-1950s. Despite the decrease in in-patient numbers and the dramatic lessening in the mean duration of stay, there is still a small accumulation of *new long-stay* patients who tend to be older, socially isolated and occupationally handicapped (Mann and Cree, 1975). The prescribed range of services and facilities in the community is provided by District Health Authorities and Social Service Departments with help from voluntary organizations (Hewett and Ryan, 1975): community psychiatric nursing services (Parnell, 1978), day hospitals and centres, rehabilitation units, hostels and depot injection clinics. This supporting network of social and medical services is essential and early on in the process of emptying the mental hospitals there were instances of patients being discharged from the comfortable security of the old asylum only to be neglected or even exploited in dingy lodging houses or on the benches of railway stations. It was not understood how much disabled people, their relatives and the community at large would suffer if progress towards the new pattern of services was not made in a balanced and comprehensive way (Wing and Olsen, 1979).

Case registers have been used extensively in research. Schizophrenic patients, like most physically ill patients, cannot be relied upon to present for treatment when necessary. There therefore has to be some method of maintaining contact with treatment services for those in the community; a case register has proved useful for this purpose. The profile of treatment services in the community for chronic schizophrenic patients is described by Cheadle *et al* (1978). Contact with psychiatric services in their 12-year follow-up study was maintained by the Salford Case Register; more than two-thirds of the patients had not spent any time in hospital within the previous year. The beneficial effect of neuroleptic medication was demonstrated in that 41 per cent had no psychotic symptoms. Social handicap, such as isolation or unemployment, was usually associated with neurotic and not psychotic symptoms, of which *worrying* was the commonest. Social isolation is a frequent subjective complaint amongst schizophrenic patients in the community; they experience boredom, describe themselves as 'loners' as children and find it difficult to make friends. Others live alone, do not go out or have friends, but do not consider this to be a problem. Most schizophrenic men, even now that living in the community is usual, have never married. More than two-thirds of men and less than one-third of women had never married; for those women who marry divorce is more common than for the general population. In Salford the case register was found to be a valuable way of keeping local psychiatric services in touch with schizophrenic patients who might otherwise have dropped out of treatment.

With the discharge of chronic psychiatric patients from mental hospitals there was an increase in referrals from the police to psychiatric services (Sims and Symonds, 1975); 40 per cent of such referrals were suffering from schizophrenia. These patients tend to live in the inner zone of a big city and to present at city centre police stations. They are more likely to live on their own or in multi-occupied dwellings, to be of low social class or unemployed and to be immigrants especially from Ireland and the West Indies. The behaviour which resulted in referral to psychiatric services by the police was considered to be evidence both of urban disorganization and of lack of facilities for care in the community. The nature of this behaviour was far removed from the ordinary crime; one man, when asked for his fare by a bus conductor, proffered a windscreen wiper and another patient, who was subsequently diagnosed as suffering from paranoid schizophrenia, ran into a police station seeking asylum and claiming that he was being pursued by 10,000 hockey sticks. In general, the type of crime and its motivation are different for schizophrenic patients than others. The 'revolving door' for schizophrenic patients, so eloquently described by Rollin (1965), has continued since the great efflux from the mental hospitals began: soon after discharge from a psychiatric hospital chronic schizophrenic patients may commit a minor offence which, because of their lack of a permanent address, leads to a prison sentence, from which they are soon discharged to be readmitted again to mental hospital following further unacceptable behaviour in a public place. The short interlude between prison and mental hospital may be spent in abject squalor as a vagrant or in a common lodging house. The more recent follow-up study of 120 schizophrenic patients discharged from hospital over a five-year period (**Johnstone et al, 1984**) highlights some more of the negative aspects of community care. Only one patient in six had no significant symptoms and functioned satisfactorily (all the exceptions were female) and more than half showed psychotic features. Although no patients and few relatives sought a return to hospital care, there was a great deal of evidence of severe social disability in terms of dissatisfaction with their accommodation, little attention from medical and social services and a great burden placed upon the relatives.

The current policy of discharging patients from large mental hospitals into the community has the support both of patients and, more surprisingly, their relatives. However, the quality of care in the community is often poor; many patients, although still psychotic, are in contact with no caring agency. Care is not evenly allocated throughout the country, or even within a single city, and the needs of relatives are often unmet. Relatives consider that staff are ill-equipped to deal with those patients in whom recovery is not taking place and there is a need for community services for those patients requiring a high degree of care. Systems of community management need to be developed which take account of schizophrenic morbidity and chronicity, and maintain contact and care whilst disability remains.

Important in helping the relatives of schizophrenics, who had been previously almost as isolated and beleaguered as the patient, has been the founding and development during the 1970s of the National Schizophrenia Fellowship (NSF) (Pyke-Lees, 1980); this voluntary organization met a need because of the lack of community care facilities. The NSF has made a valuable contribution through spreading information (a) to the relatives about the natural history and methods of alleviating the condition and (b) to those in positions of power, about the sufferings of schizophrenic patients and their relatives following return to the community. The NSF has been useful in counteracting the harmful notion harboured by many patients that they are to blame for their child's condition; this was popularized by certain authors during the last twenty years but is happily now less influential.

Relatives of schizophrenics experience numerous difficulties arising from the patient's behaviour and deficiencies in the services provided (Creer and Wing, 1975). Social withdrawal, extreme slowness, suicidal behaviour, embarrassing and occasionally disturbed behaviour are all difficult for relatives to cope with. The effect of family and other social factors and their interaction with biological factors in the aetiology of schizophrenia was summarized by Wing (1975). The effect of stress in the two months prior to onset of illness was investigated as a factor influencing subsequent prognosis in schizophrenic patients diagnosed in the Royal Navy; the more stress to which the patient had been subjected before illness, the better the outcome at follow-up in terms of shorter in-patient stay and higher capacity for subsequent work (Wallis, 1972). Earlier studies on family processes were reviewed by Russell Davis (1978), who summarized the theories used to explain symptoms in terms of interpersonal experience.

Work on Expressed Emotion, considered in detail elsewhere in this publication (see **Leff**'s review), leads to a consideration of the paper by **Cooper and Sartorius (1977)**. This paper speculates on the reasons for the very large difference in prognosis of schizophrenia between Western developed societies and developing countries. For example, at two-year follow-up 58 per cent of patients were free from symptoms in Ibadan, Nigeria as against 8 per cent from Aarhus in Denmark (Leader, 1980). In pre-industrial societies, the social and family structures have an apparently benign effect on patients with schizophrenia; this is lost during and after industrialization. Possible explanations would include the rapid increase in size of towns in industrial communities, decrease of perinatal and infant mortality with the survival of those previously considered vulnerable, and changes in family structure. The effect of this family structure is of particular interest in association with the work on Expressed Emotion. There has recently been a considerable development of interest in the transcultural aspects of psychiatry (Rack, 1982). This has occurred because of the increasingly multicultural nature of society in the United Kingdom and also because of the greater interest in psychiatry and improved services in developing countries. Schizophrenia may be a diagnostic pitfall for doctors working with patients of different culture. Apart from difficulties of language, there are problems in separating delusions from culturally accepted beliefs in magic and superstition. Possession states, acute situationally predisposed psychotic states, and drug-induced psychoses (especially associated with cannabis) may cause diagnostic problems which require the skilful application of descriptive psychopathology as well as knowledge of cultural variation. The cross-cultural study of schizophrenia was reviewed in detail by Jablensky and Sartorius (1975). The prevalence for schizophrenia in widely different populations from different countries is remarkably constant (mean 3.2 per 1,000 population), with the exception of Northern Sweden (high rate of 10.8) and the Hutterite community in the USA (low rate of 1.1). The distribution of different symptoms is extremely variable but the psychopathological descriptions of Kraepelin and Bleuler are found to be universal. The usefulness of schizophrenia as a diagnostic concept (or group of conditions) is confirmed by cross-cultural studies.

Recent research on the social aspects of schizophrenia has given interesting leads for possible future work and also for methods of management. Further work is required on the facilities needed for, and the implications of, community care, on working out the meaning of observations with life events and Expressed Emotion in different cultural settings and especially further studies across at least two different cultures matched as far as possible for other factors. Why is the psychopathology and the incidence of schizophrenia relatively constant, whilst the prognosis is so immensely variable?

The *social* management of schizophrenic patients has attracted considerable emphasis during the last decade. It is recognized that the availability of in-patient care for the acute episode and the appropriate use of neuroleptic drugs is essential; however, there is now much more attention than previously given to counselling the patient, helping and educating the family and on rehabilitation of chronic patients to prevent relapse and minimize disability (Bebbington and Kuipers, 1982).

References

BEBBINGTON, P. & KUIPERS, L. (1982) Social management of schizophrenia. *British Journal of Hospital Medicine*, **28,** 396–403.

CHEADLE, A. J., FREEMAN, H. L. & KORER, J. (1978) Chronic schizophrenic patients in the community. *British Journal of Psychiatry*, **132,** 221–227.

COOPER, J. & SARTORIUS, M. (1977) Cultural and temporal variations in schizophrenia: a speculation on the importance of industrialization. *British Journal of Psychiatry*, **130,** 50–55.

CREER, C. & WING, J. (1975) Living with a schizophrenic patient. *British Journal of Hospital Medicine*, **14,** 73–82.

DAVIS, D. R. (1978) Family process in schizophrenia. *British Journal of Hospital Medicine*, **20,** 524–531.

FREEMAN, H. & CHOUDHURY, M. H. P. (1984) Social characteristics of newly admitted mental hospital patients—a replication study. *Health Trends*, **16,** 55–57.

HEWETT, S. & RYAN, P. (1975) Alternatives to living in psychiatric hospitals—a pilot study. *British Journal of Hospital Medicine*, **14,** 65–70.

JABLENSKY, A. & SARTORIUS, N. (1975) Culture and schizophrenia. *Psychological Medicine*, **5,** 113–124.

JOHNSTONE, E. C., OWENS, D. G. C., GOLD, A., CROW, T. J. & MACMILLAN, J. F. (1984) Schizo-phrenic patients discharged from hospital: a follow-up study. *British Journal of Psychiatry*, **145,** 586–590.

LEADER (1980) Schizophrenia in different cultures. *British Medical Journal*, **280,** 271–272.

MANN, S. & CREE, W. (1975) The 'new long-stay' in mental hospitals. *British Journal of Hospital Medicine*, **14,** 56–63.

PARNELL, J. W. (1978) *Community Psychiatric Nurses*. The Queen's Nursing Institute, London.

PYKE-LEES, P. (1980) The work of the National Schizophrenia Fellowship. In *Coping with Schizophrenia* (ed. H. Rollin). London: Burnett Books.

RACK, P. (1982) *Race, Culture, and Mental Disorder*. London: Tavistock Publications.

ROLLIN, H. R. (1965) Unprosecuted mentally abnormal offenders. *British Medical Journal,* ; 831–835.

SIMS, A. C. P. & SYMONDS, R. L. (1975) Psychiatric referrals from the police. *British Journal of Psychiatry*, **127,** 171–178.

WALLIS, G. G. (1972) Stress as a predictor in schizophrenia. *British Journal of Psychiatry*, **12**(375–384.

WING, J. K. (1975) Epidemiology of schizophrenia. *British Journal of Hospital Medicine*, **8,** 364–367

—— & OLSEN, R. (1979) *Community Care for the Mentally Disabled*. Oxford University Press.

33   Cultural and temporal variations in schizophrenia: A speculation on the importance of industrialization

**JOHN COOPER and
NORMAN SARTORIUS**

The ideas to be discussed resulted from thinking about the following points and questions:

(i) Current concepts of schizophrenia did not develop until the late nineteenth century. We still have little idea of causal mechanisms, and we are still dependent upon description of symptoms and behaviour for diagnosis and assessment; why have these ideas been so late in developing, if they owe nothing to modern laboratory technology?

(ii) Why are good descriptions of what can now be recognized as chronic schizophrenia so scarce in European mediaeval and earlier literature?

(iii) Patients with acute and severe schizophrenic illnesses have been found in every contemporary culture in which they have been properly sought, but why do larger proportions of such patients have a more favourable prognosis in developing countries (rural, non-industrial) than in developed countries (urban, industrial) (e.g. Lambo, 1960, 1965; Rin and Lin, 1962; Raman and Murphy, 1972; Jablensky and Sartorius, 1975).

The general hypothesis

It is suggested that pre-industrial European cultures possessed some social characteristics which are still to be found in contemporary developing cultures and which exert a comparatively beneficial effect upon the course of schizophrenia. These social characteristics were diminished or lost during industrialization, particularly in the nineteenth century in Europe when the increase in population and growth of towns had become pronounced enough to have obvious effects upon the size and structure of communities and families. It is also suggested that industrialization introduces new social effects which increase the likelihood of a poor outcome in patients with schizophrenia.

This general hypothesis rests upon the following three subsidiary hypotheses, each suggesting a separate type of social change resulting from industrialization. These changes are concurrent and tend to reinforce each other in encouraging the development of chronic and incapacitating forms of the schizophrenic illness.

Statement 1: During industrialization and rapid population increase, the increase in size of communities brings together schizophrenics in increasing numbers, resulting in their rejection by their community and a tendency to be gathered together in institutions. This happened on a large scale for the first time in Europe in the nineteenth century and resulted in psychiatrists having to deal with substantial numbers of patients. This made it much easier for common features to be recognized.

Statement 2: Industrialization is accompanied by advances in medical technology which result in decreased mortality rates around birth, and in infancy and childhood. A greater proportion of vulnerable individuals are thus allowed to survive to the age when schizophrenia becomes manifest. In such individuals recovery from the acute illness is less likely and there is an increased risk of chronicity.

Statement 3: A further result of the social changes of industrialization is a series of changes in family size and interpersonal relationships, progressively over several generations, which changes the psychological structure and social reactions of individuals so as to make them less likely to recover from the acute stages of a schizophrenic illness.

The first two of these statements are regarded at this stage as reasonable assumptions whose possible consequences can be examined, although detailed and critical analyses of existing and fresh information will be needed before they can be considered to be firmly established. The third is more tentative, as will be seen from the later discussion. However, all three are presented as adequate for the two main purposes of this paper, which are, first, to put forward ideas which could form the basis of more discrete and testable subsidiary hypotheses, and second, to show that in addition to merely identifying social processes and influences relevant to medical conditions it is necessary to consider how they might interact and reinforce each other in their effects upon communities, upon families and upon individuals.

Hypotheses suggesting non-social reasons for the late recognition of schizophrenia have, of course, been put forward, such as that of a recent viral origin (Torrey and Petersen, 1973), but the discussion in this paper rests upon an assumption that it is more reasonable to examine possible reasons for a delay in its recognition as a clinical syndrome, rather than to assume that a condition as ubiquitous as schizophrenia has only recently arisen.

These hypotheses are not necessarily concerned with the aetiology of schizophrenia; rather they refer to variations in outcome of the illness that appear when it is viewed across cultures and over time.

Comment

For the purposes of this discussion it is assumed that the acute form of schizophrenia has always existed as a comparatively common and serious mental illness in all cultures, and that in a considerable proportion of vulnerable individuals the acute form has a tendency to chronicity which can be minimized but not completely removed by favourable social and inter-personal influences. The term 'schizophrenia' is used to indicate the clinically obvious forms described by Kraepelin and Bleuler, and more recently by Schneider, which are typified by the narrow European concept of the illness (Cooper, 1975).

Some social characteristics of industrial and non-industrial or pre-industrial cultures will now be compared, with a brief contrasting mention of how these characteristics might change or diminish during the process of industrialization.

Family size and social structure

Non-industrial cultures are characterized largely by small towns and villages, whose social structure is typified by small communities which are comparatively self-sufficient. Families are usually large and extended. An individual develops his view of the world and interpersonal relationships in a setting which encourages many important relationships and in which expectations and obligations of social help and support are common and accepted over the whole extended family. This is in contrast to the industrial town cultures in which small communities giving effective support to their members are less frequent, and where personal development usually takes place in small nuclear families with fewer but more focused relationships. Social help and support outside the small nuclear family is often neither expected nor obtained.

Specialization of work roles and social functions

In non-industrial cultures, specialization of work roles is less rigid, and the many different gradations of family and social roles facilitate compensatory changes or substitutions for incapacitated individuals. There are fewer expectations of and less drive towards specialized education or technical training. Improvements in social and financial status are not necessarily expected and are often difficult to achieve; when they do occur they may be independent of each other. In modern industrial cultures there is usually an overt pressure or expectation for individual education and specialization aimed directly at a rise in highly correlated financial and social status. The more tightly the social and work roles are defined, the more likely and more severe will be the punishments and stigmata resulting from deviations from these roles, and the more difficult will be the re-integration of the individual recovering from illness.

Concepts of mental illness

In non-industrial cultures, ideas about the nature of mental illness are poorly differentiated from those about physical illness, and the concepts of both usually overlap with or include religious and magical concepts. When a culture becomes industrial there tends to be an overall fading of supportive and explaining magical and religious systems. The accompanying advances of medical technology lead to the separation of the mentally from the physically ill but yet offer no satisfactory explanation for severe mental illness, thus setting the scene for the rejection and stigmatization of those affected.

Effect of size of community

The small towns and villages of non-industrial cultures will not generate sufficient numbers of schizophrenic patients for them to become a very serious problem, since a few mentally ill persons can be managed on an individual basis. When non-industrial communities become large, those with chronic mental illness tend to gather in small groups, recognized as odd by their peers and living in a social limbo, but yet half accepted. But with the much greater increase in community size which accompanies industrialization the limits of local tolerance and support are exceeded, and the reaction of the community is to attempt to provide a special environment in the form of large institutions. Psychiatrists can then achieve an identity, and have to deal with large numbers of patients over a long enough period of time to be able to recognize common symptoms and develop new ideas about the sub-division of mental illness.

Differential survival effects upon vulnerable individuals

Although acute schizophrenic illnesses may occur in individuals with no known predisposition, a poor recovery from the acute stage is more likely in those who are vulnerable because of some form of 'biological disadvantage' (of either genetic or environmental origin). In non-industrial cultures with poorly developed health services, it is usual to find high foetal wastage, and high perinatal and infant mortality rates. This means that comparatively few vulnerable individuals will survive to the age when schizophrenic illnesses are manifest, and so a smaller proportion of schizophrenic patients may have chronic illnesses. In industrial cultures in which extensive health care systems ensure the survival of many vulnerable individuals, a comparatively larger proportion of these might be expected to develop severe and chronic illnesses. (A relationship between the early detection of minor biological handicaps—the so-called soft neurological signs—and the later development of schizophrenia has been noted by several workers studying schizophrenic twins, but the significance of those findings is not yet clear (Campion and Tucker, 1973; Pollin, 1972; Mosher *et al*, 1971.) The same effective health care systems will also minimize the dangers to life of severe forms of schizophrenia, allowing chronically disabled patients to survive and accumulate.

To summarize these points in terms of contrasting cultural stereotypes, an individual in a non-industrial culture who survives the hazards of a comparatively harsh physical environment, then experiences an interpersonal environment that is characterized by many relationships that are potentially supportive and flexible. There is a comparatively low level of pressure towards differentiation and specialization in work, and social roles are more flexible. There is no intense expectation of social and financial advancement. For a person developing schizophrenia, this environment is more likely to be supportive and tolerant, and there will be little risk of prolonged rejection, isolation, segregation and institutionalization. In an industrial culture, even damaged or specially vulnerable individuals reach the age when schizophrenia becomes manifest, having developed in a setting of small nuclear families where relationships tend to be few and intense. To be mentally ill is to be stigmatized, with attendant dangers of treatment in segregated institutions.

Apart from the very different reactions of the persons and organizations around the patient in these contrasting cultures, different responses in the affected individuals may also be a result of the different cultures in which they grow up. Everyone inevitably absorbs from his social environment a set of attitudes and responses to illness and misfortunes of all kinds, and a set of expectations about the effects of illness and how to cope with them; it is suggested that the individual from the less tightly organized, more flexible and less demanding non-industrial culture will be able to view and experience the novel and often frightening symptoms of the schizophrenic illness with less anxiety and less personal and social disruption than the individual in an industrial setting. For instance, symptoms interpreted as feelings of outside influences and delusions about the activities of malign persons may be less frightening for the individual in a non-industrial culture. He may well have had non-schizophrenic events previously explained and accepted as due to spells or witchcraft, so ideas and experiences of this sort may be familiar and shared with his associates.

It should be noted how the several social mechanisms described can reinforce one another as an industrial change takes place in a culture over several generations. Each generation in turn is subject to more of these changes than its predecessors, and also develops coping mechanisms and expectations about illness that are successively more different from those present at the start of the process of change. Thus the influences reinforce each other in acting upon those with acute schizophrenia so as to increase the probability of severe and prolonged illness. Furthermore, the increasing proportion of vulnerable individuals who survive because of reduced mortality rates means that this self-reinforcing system acts upon a bigger and bigger population of susceptible persons as industrialization proceeds.

The time relationships seem approximately correct, since the peak period of societal change towards industrialization in Western Europe just preceded the development of concepts of schizophrenia and a delay would be expected between the two. The psychiatric landmarks that are usually quoted start with Morel in 1860 and include Kahlbaum (1863), Hecker (1871), Pick (1891), and Sommer (1894) before culminating in Kraepelin's publications from 1896 onwards. In this way, what is now seen as one of the major illnesses of mankind appears to have been recognized over a short period of about fifty years.

This has been essentially a speculative discussion of a hypothesis, or set of related hypotheses, in terms of trends, general tendencies and stereotypes. The changing social system that has been suggested could also be relevant to the medical care and prognosis of other chronic conditions that have social implications (such as senile dementia and mental defect), but schizophrenic patients seem likely to be the group most vulnerable to its effect, in view of their comparative youth at onset, and the non-lethal but potentially chronic nature of the symptoms.

There is a good deal of circumstantial evidence that is consistent with these ideas, and they do not contradict any of the principles or results of accepted treatment. Hare (1974) has speculated that the improvement in the prognosis of schizophrenia noted over the last thirty years or so may be due to an inherent variation in the properties of the schizophrenic disease process, whatever that may turn out to be. This improved prognosis can also be explained on our social hypothesis, but as due to the increasing use of socially orientated and more humane treatment methods, which contrast with the custodial isolation and institutionalization so typical of the first twenty to thirty years of this century; that is, social treatments can be viewed as a purposeful attempt to reverse some of the harmful effects of industrialization.

Having summarized the hypothesis at a level of comparatively abstract concepts and stereotypes, it is worthwhile discussing briefly how these suggestions might be refuted or confirmed. The following studies would be relevant:

(i) *Historical studies:* A historical analysis of time relationships between the development of industrialization, population shifts and changes, the development of institutional care for the mentally ill in Western Europe and the USA, and the recognition of chronic forms of mental illness. (*The Discovery of the Asylum* by Rothman (1971) is a recent example of how interesting a historical analysis in this field can be.)

(ii) *Using existing fairly crude data on contemporary societies:* A number of statistical studies could be done using data from countries or regions of countries where the contemporary prognosis of schizophrenia has been studied. A factor analysis of socio-economic information relevant to the various characteristics and consequences of industrialization discussed above (with special emphasis on statistics of infant mortality and morbidity), should produce factors recognizably relevant to degrees of industrialization.

The hypothesis predicts that factors relevant to the concept of industrialization will be most numerous and clear-cut in those societies or regions which have the worst prognosis for schizophrenia. Comparisons could be made between countries or cultures, and in the case of large countries with very different regions or sub-cultures for which data is available, between different regions of the same country.

(iii) *Using fresh data collected in field studies:* To test the hypothesis discussed here, it would be necessary to do some preliminary work on new ways of describing different types of family size and structure (Fox, 1970). A multidisciplinary effort would be needed, and would probably be welcomed by those sociologists and anthropologists interested in family structure and function; they appear to be increasingly aware of the need for new concepts in this area, and for higher standards of data collection in field studies (Tavuchis, 1970). Particularly relevant to the testing of this hypothesis would be methods of describing families in terms of role flexibility, supportiveness, tolerance of deviance, and other related concepts. When these methods of description have been developed, countries, towns and communities could be chosen that have contrasting positions on the factors and indices of industrialization and institutionalization mentioned above in the statistical studies. The final stage would be the identification in such communities, of families of the various types with and without schizophrenic members, who would then be the subjects for both cross-sectional and longitudinal studies to see if the predicted relationships could be found. These studies would involve detailed interviewing and observation at a personal and family level, and standardized methods of data collection and diagnosis would be needed. Although there are obvious problems in carrying out cross-cultural research, studies such as the International Pilot Study of Schizophrenia (WHO, 1973, 1975, 1976) show that this type of work can be rewarding.

The wide variety of studies contained in this list of examples shows that the inter-disciplinary implications of using abstract concepts such as 'industrialization' and 'institutionalization' are considerable. But unless ideas developed at the level of sociological abstractions are tested in practical field projects involving direct description and observation of people and their interactions, information that is potentially useful for medical and social action is unlikely to result.

This hypothesis is of particular interest to developing countries which are faced with or are striving towards industrialization. If these suggestions can be shown to have any substance, such countries will need to devise ways of avoiding or minimizing the harmful effects of the complex of social influences involved, if they are not to be faced with making special provision of increasing numbers of chronically disabled schizophrenic patients.

References

CAMPION, E. & TUCKER, G. (1973) A note on twin studies: schizophrenia and neurological impairment. *Archives of General Psychiatry*, **29,** 460–463.

COOPER, J. E. (1975) Concepts of schizophrenia in the USA and in Great Britain: a summary of some studies by the US-UK Diagnostic Project. In *Studies of Schizophrenia* (ed. M. H. Lader). *British Journal of Psychiatry* Special Publication No. 10.

FOX, R. (1970) In Chapter 1, *The Family and Its Future* (ed. Elliott, K.). CIBA Foundation symposium report. London: Longmans.

HARE, E. H. (1974) The changing content of psychiatric illness. *Journal of Psychosomatic Research*, **18,** 283–289.

HECKER, E. (1871) Die Hebephrenie: *Virchow Archiv fur Pathologische Anatomie*, **52,** 392–449.

JABLENSKY, A. & SARTORIUS, N. (1975) Culture and schizophrenia. *Psychological Medicine*, **5,** 113–124.

KAHLBAUM, K. L. (1874) *Catatonia*. Translated in 1973. Johns Hopkins University Press.

LAMBO, T. A. (1960) Further neuropsychiatric observations in Nigeria. *British Medical Journal*, *ii*, 1696–1704.

—— (1965) Schizophrenic and borderline states. In *Transcultural Psychiatry* (eds A. V. S. de Renck and R. Porter), pp 62–83. CIBA Foundation Symposium. London: Churchill.

MOREL, B. A. (1860) *Traité des Maladies Mentales*. Paris: Masson.

MOSHER, L. R., POLLIN, W. & STABENAN, J. R. (1971) Identical twins discordant for schizophrenia. *Archives of General Psychiatry*, **24,** 422–437.

PICK, A. (1891) Uber primäre chronische Demenz im jugendlichen Alter. *Prager Medezinische Wochenschrift*, **16,** 312–315.

POLLIN, W. (1972) The pathogenesis of schizophrenia. *Archives of General Psychiatry*, **27,** 29–37.

RAMAN, A. C. & MURPHY, H. B. C. (1972) Failure of traditional prognostic indicators in Afro-Asian psychotics; results of a long-term follow-up study. *Journal of Neurology and Mental Disease*, **154,** 238–247.

RIN, H. & LIN, T. (1962) Mental illness among Formosan aborigines as compared with the Chinese in Taiwan. *Journal of Mental Science*, **108,** 134–136.

ROTHMAN, D. J. (1971) *The Discovery of the Asylum*. Boston, Toronto: Little, Brown.

SOMMER, R. (1894) *Diagnostik der Geisteskrankenheit*. Wein: Urban and Schwarzenburg.

TAVUCHIS, N. (1970) In Chapter 22, *The Family and Its Future* (ed. Elliott, K.). CIBA Foundation symposium report. London: Longmans.

TORREY, E. F. & PETERSON, M. R. (1973) Slow and latent viruses in schizophrenia. *Lancet*, *ii*, 22–24.

WORLD HEALTH ORGANIZATION (1973) *Report of the International Pilot Study of Schizophrenia*. Vol 1. Geneva: WHO.

—— (1975) *Schizophrenia: A Multi-national Study: A Summary of the Initial Evaluation Phase of the International Pilot Study of Schizophrenia*. Geneva: WHO.

—— (1976) *Report of the International Pilot Study of Schizophrenia*. Vol 2. Geneva: WHO.

34 Recent research on relatives' Expressed Emotion

J. LEFF

Since the paper by Leff and Vaughn (1980) was published, the work on Expressed Emotion (EE) has developed in a number of different directions. The paper concluded with a statement that data on life events and relatives' EE needed to be supplemented with material on prophylactic medication for schizophrenia. The required information was collected in the course of a study of social intervention and clarified the relationship among these various factors. Other extensions of the work have been the accumulation of data on relatives' EE in non-schizophrenic conditions other than depressive neurosis, and in schizophrenia across cultures. A further direction has been the successful implementation of trials of social intervention in high EE families of schizophrenic patients. The recent studies in each area will be reviewed in turn.

Life events, relatives' EE and maintenance neuroleptics in schizophrenia

A controlled trial of social intervention in the families of schizophrenic patients containing at least one high EE relative was set up by Leff *et al* (1982). A basic feature of the design was that all patients, whether in the experimental or control groups, should be maintained on neuroleptic drugs. To ensure compliance it was preferred that long-acting preparations should be used, and 21 of the 24 patients received them. By the nine-month follow-up, one patient on oral medication had discontinued her tablets and one patient had stopped receiving injections. Of the remaining 22 patients who received regular maintenance neuroleptics, six had relapsed, all of them still living in high EE homes at follow-up. The relatives of eight of the patients who remained well changed from high to low EE during the follow-up period. Hence, eight patients without relapse were still living in high EE homes nine months after discharge and constituted a comparison group for the relapsed patients. A history of life events in the three months preceding relapse, or the interview in the case of well patients, was obtained using the questionnaire and manual developed by Brown and Birley (1968). Brown's (1974) method of assessing the contextual threat of events was applied by an independent rater. Threat is rated on a four-point scale, a level of four representing a trivial threat or none at all, while a level of one represents the most severe form of threat.

It was found that five (83 per cent) of the six relapsed patients had experienced an independent life event in the three-week period prior to relapse compared with three (38 per cent) of the eight well patients. This is a non-significant difference; however, the exclusion of events with a short-term threat rating of four eliminated one event from the well group. This resulted in the emergence of a significant difference in the proportions of well (25 per cent) and relapsed (83 per cent) patients experiencing a life event in the three weeks before interview or relapse (Leff *et al*, 1983). This finding led to an examination of the threatening nature of the life events recorded in the earlier study by Leff and Vaughn (1980). It was found that all these events were assigned a short-term threat rating of three or more. Hence in the two studies considered, no patient who relapsed had experienced only a trivial or non-threatening event in the preceding three weeks. This suggested that the threatening nature of life events, at least in the short term, is an important aspect of their role in precipitating schizophrenic relapse.

The findings of Leff and Vaughn (1980) suggested that, for schizophrenic patients living with relatives and unprotected by neuroleptic drugs, *either* the acute stress of a life event *or* the chronic stress of exposure to a high EE relative was sufficient to provoke a relapse. Patients on regular medication seem to be protected against one or other stress, but the findings from the later paper suggested that they are still vulnerable to a *combination* of the acute and chronic stresses. Thus medicated patients in high EE homes had a marked concentration of life events preceding a relapse.

This interpretation of the findings from the two studies led to the construction of an explanatory model in which neuroleptic drugs were postulated to raise the threshold for the appearance of schizophrenic symptoms in individuals who were susceptible to the various forms of environmental stress measured. The model predicts that in patients admitted from low EE homes after the occurrence of a life event, the course of the episode of schizophrenia should be shorter than in those admitted from high EE homes. This prediction, which is being tested in a current study, implies that a major determinant of the duration of an episode of schizophrenia is the duration of the environmental stress preceding it.

Relatives' EE in non-schizophrenic conditions

In an earlier study (Vaughn and Leff, 1976) a group of depressed neurotic patients was included with the aim of determining whether high EE attitudes were detectable in the relatives of non-schizophrenic patients, and whether they also bore any relationship to outcome. In the event, the comparison was limited in one direction since only two of the 30 depressed patients lived with parents, whereas half the schizophrenic patients did so. It was possible to compare the spouses of depressed and schizophrenic patients on most of the components of EE. The mean number of critical comments did not differ significantly between these two groups of relatives, showing that critical attitudes could not be ascribed to any genetic link relatives might have with schizophrenic patients. In the schizophrenic samples studied in the Social Psychiatry Unit a cut-off point of seven critical comments had originally been used to assign relatives to high or low EE groups. This was later amended to six, as increasing the power of the index to predict relapse. A cut-off point of six or seven applied to the relatives of depressed neurotic patients failed to discriminate between relapsed and well patients. However, lowering the cut-off point to two critical comments divided the patients into two groups with relapse rates of 67 per cent and 22 per cent. This finding suggested that depressed patients were even more sensitive to criticism than schizophrenic patients. However, this interpretation could only be tentative since the manipulation of the cut-off point had been carried out post hoc. Subsequently the study of depressed neurotic patients has been replicated by Hooley (1984), who found that a cut-off point of two critical comments gave relapse rates of 59 per cent and nil.

Spouses' critical attitudes have also been shown to play a role in the outcome of obesity. Havstad (1979) studied a sample of 28 married women in Los Angeles. The women had each lost at least 15 pounds in weight during the previous year. Their husbands were interviewed and EE ratings made, from which it was calculated that their mean number of critical comments was considerably lower than that of the spouses of depressed patients. However, when the obese women were followed up, the best predictor of relapse (failure to maintain weight loss) was found to be the number of critical comments made by the spouse. Furthermore the best separation between relapsed and non-relapsed women was achieved using a criticism level of 3 or above. With this cut-off point, 72 per cent relapsed in the high criticism group compared with 10 per cent in the low criticism group, a difference significant at the 1 in 100 level. Hence there are considerable similarities between the influence of relatives' critical attitudes on the course of depressive neurosis and on weight maintenance in obese women.

The two key components of EE that are related to the outcome of schizophrenia are critical comments and over-involvement. The studies of depression and obesity have shown that criticism is by no means exclusive to the spouses of schizophrenic patients. However, they have been unable to throw light on over-involvement, which is virtually confined to parents, appearing rarely in spouses. It is only recently that a sample of parents of a diagnostic group other than schizophrenia has been assessed for EE. Szmukler (personal communication) has collected a sample of parents of anorexic patients from London on whom ratings of EE have been made. Using the current cut-off point of three on the six-point scale, 18 per cent of parents of anorexics showed over-involvement compared with 36 per cent of parents of schizophrenics, a non-significant difference. The follow-up of the anorexic patients has still to be completed and will reveal whether parental over-involvement bears any relationship to the outcome of this condition. At this point in time it can be asserted that over-involved attitudes, like criticism, are not confined to the relatives of schizophrenic patients.

Cross-cultural studies of relatives' EE and schizophrenia

The earlier work on EE was conducted within the Social Psychiatry Unit on samples of patients from the London area. Recently, attempts to replicate the findings have been made by researchers in California and in Chandigarh, North India. The Californian study was initiated by Vaughn and her colleagues (1985) and employed the same design and assessment procedures as the

London studies. The mean number of critical comments made by Californian relatives was close to the figure for the relatives in Vaughn and Leff's (1976) study. However, the distribution of the critical comments was quite different, being L-shaped in the London study and approximating to a normal distribution in California. This is reflected in the proportions of relatives making no critical comments; 29 per cent in London and only 4 per cent in California. Furthermore a significantly greater proportion of Californian relatives made six or more critical comments than of London relatives (P <0.05). In all previous studies, the prevalence of hostility has been closely related to the distribution of criticism, and this was so for the Californian relatives. As a consequence, the greater proportion of critical relatives in the Californian sample was paralleled by a significantly higher proportion expressing hostility (28 per cent) than in the London sample (18 per cent, P <0.05). By contrast there was no difference in the proportions of parents rated as over-involved (California, 15 per cent; London, 21 per cent).

As a result of the differences in distribution of EE components, the proportion of Californian relatives assigned to a high EE category, 67 per cent, was significantly (P <0.05) greater than the London figure of 48 per cent. Nevertheless the relapse rates over nine months in high and low EE homes were remarkably similar in the two studies (California, 56 per cent, 17 per cent; London, 50 per cent, 12 per cent), and the relationship between EE and relapse was highly significant (P = 0.015). There was one area in which the Californian data departed from those in the London studies, namely the factors that appeared to protect patients in high EE homes against relapse. In the London samples, maintenance neuroleptics and low face-to-face contact between patient and relative each had an effect in reducing the relapse rate, which summated when they were combined. In the California study no effect on the relapse rate was demonstrable when each factor was considered separately, but a significant reduction occurred when they were present together. Hence the protective effect of these factors appeared to be additive for London patients, but interactive for California patients.

It is reassuring that the findings of the London studies on relatives' EE and schizophrenia have been replicated so closely in California, despite many differences between life on the West Coast of America and that in an inner London suburb. However, the subjects in both sets of studies did speak the same language. A more stringent test of the hypotheses would be replication of the findings across a wider cultural divide and in a different language. This has now been attempted in the context of a study organized by the WHO named the Determinants of Outcome of Severe Mental Disorder. Chandigarh, North India, was chosen as one of the centres in which to conduct a study of relatives' EE and its relationship to the course of schizophrenia in patients making contact with the psychiatric services for the first time.

The first hurdle was to establish whether the techniques of interviewing and rating could be transferred without distortion from English to Hindi. This task was tackled by utilizing a trainee who was bilingual in English and Hindi but who had no field experience of using the techniques in Hindi. It was found that the key components of critical comments and hostility could be transferred with ease from English to Hindi, but that the Hindi-speaking field workers were probably underestimating over-involvement (Wig *et al,*

1986). This, however, was a problem of drift away from established rating conventions rather than the products of distortion across a linguistic frontier. It could be compensated for in data analysis by lowering the threshold for over-involvement.

With this one reservation, the EE ratings of Chandigarh relatives can be compared with those from London. The most striking finding is the contraction of the distribution of critical comments of Indian relatives. A significantly higher proportion (56 per cent, P <0.001) than in the London sample made no critical comments, while only 12 per cent scored six or more, and would be assigned to a high EE category. The highest score was 14, contrasted with 49 in Vaughn and Leff's (1976) sample. This marked difference in distribution is reflected in a much lower mean criticism score for the London relatives. It is surprising, therefore, that the proportion of Chandigarh relatives express-ing hostility, 16 per cent, was very similar to the corresponding London figure of 18 per cent. In fact, that is the only sample of relatives studied in which hostility has been expressed at low levels of criticism. Over-involvement follows the same pattern as criticism and was rated in only 4 per cent of Chandigarh parents, compared with 36 per cent of the London parents of schizophrenics (P <0.001). Even if a lower threshold of two is applied for over-involvement, the proportion of Chandigarh parents rises to only 15 per cent, which still remains significantly (P <0.05) below that for the London parents.

As a consequence of the relative rarity of the key EE components among Chandigarh relatives, the proportion assigned to a high EE category was only 23 per cent, about half the proportion in the London samples and one third of that in the California sample. Nevertheless, relatives' EE was still found to relate significantly to the outcome of schizophrenia among North Indian patients, the relapse rate being 31 per cent in high EE homes and 9 per cent in low EE homes (P = 0.035) (Leff *et al*, 1986).

Trials of social intervention in families of schizophrenic patients

A significant association between relatives' EE and the outcome of schizo-phrenia has now been replicated in three London studies, one Californian study, and one study in Chandigarh. However the consistency of this finding over time and across cultures does not prove that the link is a causal one. High EE attitudes of relatives and relapse of schizophrenia could both be the consequence of some factor in the patients, for example a poor premorbid personality. Numerous statistical analyses have ruled out any of the obvious contenders for such a mediating role, but convincing evidence can only come from an experimental study. The aim would be to intervene in order to alter those features in the social environment which are deemed to be stressful, and to look for a subsequent reduction in the patients' relapse rate. It was the need for experimental evidence for a causal influence of relatives' EE on the course of schizophrenia that spurred Leff and his colleagues (1982) to conduct a trial of social intervention in high EE families.

The trial was based on the standard design for assessing drugs, with randomi-zation to experimental and control groups, but some modifications were dic-tated by the impossibility of providing a placebo for a social treatment. Patients were included in the study if they satisfied the criteria for schizophrenia and were in high face-to-face contact with high EE relatives. All patients were maintained on prophylactic neuroleptic drugs, the majority being prescribed long-acting injections. At the time the trial was started in 1977, there were no published studies indicating that any form of social intervention could successfully alter the family environment of schizophrenic patients. Since then accounts of another three trials have been published (Goldstein *et al*, 1978; Anderson *et al*, 1981; Falloon *et al*, 1982), all conducted in America and all with a similar design. In each, patients have been maintained on neuroleptic drugs and have been randomly assigned to experimental or control groups. The experimental groups have all received a form of social treatment involving family members. Although the theoretical standpoints of the research teams have differed considerably, the techniques of intervention bear a close resemblance to each other across all four studies.

The interventions have started with a programme of education about schizophrenia, which has always been given to relatives, and in some of the studies, to the patients as well. Attempts have been made to improve families' problem-solving ability, particularly by Falloon's group, who taught families a structural approach consisting of six steps. Improving communication was also a specific focus of Falloon's team, and was also addressed by the other researchers, with the exception of Goldstein and his colleagues. The reduction of EE and face-to-face contact were the main targets of Leff's group, but also entered into the programmes of the other three teams. All research groups, with the exception of Goldstein's, made attempts to expand the social networks of patients and their relatives. Goldstein's team focused specifically on lowering relatives' expectations for the patients, and the other three groups also spent some time on this. The content of these four treatment programmes is considered in more detail by Leff (1985), and can be summarized here as follows. The programmes of Leff's team and Anderson's team appear to be most similar, while Falloon's team placed a heavier emphasis on problem-solving and improving communication than the other two. Goldstein's approach stands out as differing most from the others, and it is probably of relevance that his study was the pioneering attempt of the group. The results of a short-term follow-up of up to a year have been published for three of the trials, while Anderson's group has released preliminary findings. The relapse rates for each study are strikingly similar, running at about 50 per cent for the control groups and less than 10 per cent for the experimental groups. This indicates that family treatment can confer a substantial benefit on schizophrenic patients, at least in the short term, provided that they remain on neuroleptic drugs.

To consider the study of Leff *et al* (1982) in more detail, the therapeutic aims of a reduction of EE and/or face-to-face contact were achieved in three-quarters of the families. No patient in these families who remained on neuroleptic medication relapsed during the nine-month follow-up. This finding is interpreted as evidence for a causal influence of relatives' EE on the course of schizophrenia, the issue that this study was designed to clarify.

Conclusions

The research completed since the paper by Leff and Vaughn (1980) was published has established the roles played by independent life events and relatives'

EE in the origin of episodes of schizophrenia. It has been determined that the relationship between EE and the outcome of schizophrenia is not peculiar to the population of one inner London suburb, but holds good across wide cultural divides and linguistic frontiers. It has also become clear that the attitudes represented by EE are shown as commonly by the relatives of depressed patients, anorexic patients and obese women, as by the relatives of schizophrenic patients. We would speculate that EE attitudes probably develop in relatives exposed to any chronic or recurrent condition, be it psychiatric or physical. A series of trials has demonstrated convincingly the therapeutic effectiveness of family treatment in substantially reducing the relapse rate of schizophrenia. It remains for future studies to tease out the elements in the therapeutic programmes that are responsible for their success, and to ensure that they can readily be absorbed into routine clinical procedures.

References

ANDERSON, C. M., HOGARTY, G. & REISS, D. J. (1981) The psychoeducational family treatment of schizophrenia. In *New Developments in Interventions with Families of Schizophrenics* (ed. M. J. Goldstein). San Francisco: Jossey-Bass.

BROWN, G. W. (1974) Meaning, measurement and stress of life-events. In *Stressful Life-Events: Their Nature and Effects* (eds. B. S. Dohrenwend and B. P. Dohrenwend). New York: Wiley.

—— & BIRLEY, J. L. T. (1968) Crises and life changes and the onset of schizophrenia. *Journal of Health and Social Behaviour*, **9**, 203–214.

FALLOON, I. R. H., BOYD, J. L., McGILL, C. W., RAZANI, J., MOSS, H. B. GILDERMAN, A. M. (1982) Family management in the prevention of exacerbations of schizophrenia. *New England Journal of Medicine*, **306**, 1437–1440.

GOLDSTEIN, M. J., RODNICK, E. H., EVANS, J. R., MAY, P. R. A. & STEINBERG, M. R. (1978) Drug and family therapy in the aftercare treatment of acute schizophrenics. *Archives of General Psychiatry*, **35**, 1169–1177.

HAVSTAD, L. F. (1979) *Weight Loss and Weight Loss Maintenance as Aspects of Family Emotional Processes.* Unpublished doctoral dissertation. University of Southern California.

HOOLEY, J. (1984) *Criticism and Depression.* D. Phil Thesis, Oxford.

LEFF, J. (1985) Family treatment of schizophrenia. In *Recent Advances in Clinical Psychiatry*, **5** (ed. K. Granville-Grossman). London: Churchill Livingstone.

—— KUIPERS, L., BERKOWITZ, R., EBERLEIN-FREIS, R. & STURGEON, D. (1982) A controlled trial of intervention in the families of schizophrenic patients. *British Journal of Psychiatry*, **141**, 121–134.

—— —— —— VAUGHN, C. & STURGEON, D. (1983) Life events, relatives' Expressed Emotion and maintenance neuroleptics in schizophrenic relapse. *Psychological Medicine*, **13**, 799–807.

—— WIG, N., GHOSH, A., BEDI, H., MENON, D. K., KUIPERS, L., KORTEN, A., ERNBERG, G., DAY, R., SARTORIUS, N. & JABLENSKY, A. (1986) Influence of relatives' Expressed Emotion on the course of schizophrenia in Chandigarh. *British Journal of Psychiatry*, in press.

—— & VAUGHN, C. (1980) The interaction of life events and relatives' Expressed Emotion in schizophrenia and depressive neurosis. *British Journal of Psychiatry*, **136**, 146–153.

VAUGHN, C. E. & LEFF, J. P. (1976) The influence of family and social factors on the course of psychiatric illness: A comparison of schizophrenic and depressed neurotic patients. *British Journal of Psychiatry*, **129**, 125–137.

—— SNYDER, K. S., JONES, S., FREEMAN, W. B., FALLOON, I. R. H. & LIBERMAN, R. P. (1985) Family factors in schizophrenic relapse: a California replication of the British research on Expressed Emotion. *Archives of General Psychiatry*, in press.

WIG, N. N., MENON, D. K., BEDI, H., GHOSH, A., KUIPERS, L., LEFF, J., KORTEN, A., DAY, R., SARTORIUS, N., ERNBERG, G. & JABLENSKY, A. (1986) The cross-cultural transfer of ratings of relatives' Expressed Emotion. *British Journal of Psychiatry*, in press.

35 Schizophrenic patients discharged from hospital—A follow-up study

EVE C. JOHNSTONE, DAVID G. C. OWENS, AVIVA GOLD, TIMOTHY J. CROW and J. FIONA MACMILLAN

Policies of closure of the mental hospitals and transfer to community services have been advocated for a considerable time (Tooth and Brooke, 1961) and are currently being actively pursued (Department of Health and Social Security, 1981). As part of a study of the contribution of institutionalization to the disabilities of schizophrenia, the total number of patients fulfilling the St Louis (Feighner et al, 1972) criteria for schizophrenia, and discharged from Shenley Hospital in North London between 1970 and 1974 were followed up (Johnstone et al, 1981). The patients were examined in detail and an account of the social circumstances and functioning was obtained from all those who were not in-patients. The study provided an opportunity to examine the success of community care in a group who were discharged at a time when discharge policies were generally less active than at present.

The information was obtained with the interviewer blind to the mental state and historical variables, at an unstructured interview. It was recorded in terms of standardized forms, based on those designed at the Medical Research Council Social Psychiatry Unit at the Institute of Psychiatry, for interviews concerning discharged patients.

The present study reports on 66 patients who had been discharged from Shenley Hospital during the period 1970–1974, who had fulfilled the St Louis criteria for schizophrenia and who were currently living in the community. [Full details of the tracing procedure are given in the original report and also in an earlier report by Johnstone et al (1981).] The social circumstances and functioning of these patients were assessed by interview with the patients and, provided consent was obtained, those (if any) with whom they lived.

Social information was obtained from the patients; no attempt was made to seek an informant in the case of patients who lived alone, in lodgings, private residential accommodation, or group homes. Although some patients did not wish their relatives to be interviewed, information from an informant(s) was obtained in 42 cases and assessed living circumstances, attitudes to these circumstances, recent difficulties, behaviour, social contacts and activities, personal care, occupational activity, medication and compliance with medication, the burden on the family, contact with medical and social agencies and problems for the patient. Seven patients lived alone, 23 with their spouse, 26 with other family members (most commonly parents), seven lived in some form of hostel or residential accommodation, two in lodgings and one in a group home; 53 patients were satisfied with their living circumstances, a further ten thought that there was probably no better alternative; three would have preferred to live in other circumstances, but none wished to return to hospital. Twenty-seven of informants were satisfied with the patient's presence in the home, nine found this arrangement difficult but probably the best alternative; three thought that the patient would be better off elsewhere (not specified, but not hospital) and three thought the patient would be better off in hospital. Sixteen reported no serious problems with the patient's clinical condition, 19 considered there were problems and that the patient had not recovered, while in a further five cases, these problems were felt to be very severe and to require to be dealt with away from the home situation. Two relatives, both of whom were elderly and appeared to be rather overwhelmed by chronic difficulties, could express no specific opinion on this issue. A number of questions dealt with the patients' social functioning and in particular with the number of their social contacts. Frequently, these were few and considered by relatives to be abnormally limited, but because the patients' backgrounds and ages varied, meaningful generalization was difficult.

Personal care was considered either by the account of the relative or the direct observation of the interviewer to be impaired in 25 cases, but the remaining 41 cases achieved a normal standard. With regard to work, 25 were in regular full-time competitive work, two in part-time competitive work, three in sheltered employment, and four attended day centres. Four patients were said to be effective full-time housewives, ten were ineffective housewives, three were retired, and 15 did no work. Forty-two patients had neuroleptic drugs prescribed and were said to take them, seven patients had the drugs prescribed and did not take them, and 17 were not on neuroleptic drugs.

Arbitrary rules (Table I) were adopted for completion of the item concerning the burden for the family.

Thirteen informants reported no items in this area, but 18 gave positive answers to at least three items. In spite of these major difficulties, a number of patients were receiving little attention from the medical or social services; in the year before the interview, 55 patients had not seen a psychiatrist and 51 patients and their families had had no contact with a social worker. During that year, 18 patients had had no contact at all with the medical or social services; nine had seen only community nurses, and 15 saw only their general practitioners. The remainder were involved with psychiatric clinics, social workers, or more than one agency. Brief summaries of the mental condition and social circumstances and functioning were made in each case, on the basis of the interviews with the patient and the informant; using these, patients were classed as having mental states which were: 'clearly morbid' (36 patients); 'doubtfully morbid' (13 patients); and 'not morbid' (17 patients): examples of these classes are given in the Appendix.

The findings as regard the state of morbidity were analysed according to the category of supervision: (i) no medical or social support; (ii) seen only by community nurses; (iii) seen only by general practitioner; (iv) attending clinics and perhaps other agencies; and (v) attending agencies but not a clinic. Negative and positive symptom scores were assessed by the Krawiecka *et al* (1977) scale. Negative symptom scores did not vary between patients in the five categories of supervision, but the positive symptom scores of the patients

TABLE I

Arbitary rules adopted for assessing items concerning burden for the family (42 cases)

Item	Definition used	No (%) of positive replies
Time off work	At least two weeks off work in past year on part of any family member to look after patient.	7(16)
Stopped work to care for patient	Any family member at the time of the interview having ceased paid employment to look after the patient.	7(16)
Emotional illness in family	A family member being affected by emotional illness requiring medical intervention and considered by informant to result from patient's illness.	5(13)
Physical illness in family	A family member being affected by physical illness requiring medical intervention and considered by informant to result from patient's illness.	2(6)
Social restrictions for the family	Definable restrictions in terms of a family member either being unable to go out because of problems in leaving patient without him/her or being unable to have visitors to the home because of patient's attitudes/behaviour.	20(48)
Disruption of family relationships	Circumstance whereby a family member or branch of the family has broken off visits or contact to patient's home because of patient's illness.	15(35)
Financial difficulties	Loss of wage on which family partly depended (either of patient or other family member) because of cessation of work resulting from patient's illness.	8(19)

receiving specialist psychiatric care, the fourth of the above categories, were greater than in patients in the first three categories.

There was considerable overlap between the categories: some minimally ill patients were receiving care from multiple agencies and others who were floridly ill and in circumstances of social distress, were receiving much less or no care at all. Scrutiny of the individual case descriptions suggested that the greatest distress for patients and relatives was found among those receiving no medical or social attention. Although some very disturbed patients were being seen only by community nurses or general practitioners, their condition did not appear to be associated with as much distress or social disorganization as was found in those without care; examples are shown in the Appendix. The degree of attention given by the general practitioners was variable, but in some cases was of a very high order, e.g. one patient was visited at least monthly at home by the general practitioner over a period of years. Thirty-nine informants made some spontaneous comment about problems they saw for the patient. These included concern for the future of the patient after the death of relatives; distress about the patient's evident suffering, dependence, loneliness, apathy and slowness; and fear of relapse or deterioration.

In discussing the difficulties that they thought the patient would experience following the death of relatives, a number of informants strongly stated that they did not think that they had received adequate assistance from the health and social services. They expressed the view that the services were interested in patients when they first became ill, but lost interest as time passed and the patients did not become well. The informants did not think that those concerned realized just how great a burden was being placed upon relatives when such patients were discharged from hospital. They regretted the frequent changes in staff associated with the patient, and would have valued the possibility of contact, albeit occasional over the years, with a constant figure who was familiar with the facts of the patient's case.

Comment

The disabilities of schizophrenic patients discharged into the community have been described before (Cheadle *et al*, 1978; National Schizophrenia Fellowship, 1979; McCreadie, 1982; Wing, 1982) and the problems that may be experienced by their relatives considered (Creer and Wing, 1974; Creer, 1975; Creer *et al*, 1982). Leff and Vaughn (1972) compared clinical and social assessments in 40 schizophrenic patients who were in touch with psychiatric services with those in 27 schizophrenic patients who had not been in contact with such services for one year, although they had been in touch with them before that. Contact with general practitioners was not fully discussed, but some 'out of contact' patients did see their own doctors. Social difficulties were common in both groups, but although details are not given, serious psychotic symptoms are said to have been infrequent. The present study is unusual in that, in addition to considering those patients in touch with the psychiatric services or receiving care from their general practitioners, it examines patients who were part of a defined cohort discharged from hospital but not in contact with the medical or social services at all. This account of the disability among the 120 patients discharged between 1970 and 1974 is not complete, because 15 patients were untraced, nine refused consent, and three would only participate to a limited extent. It is unlikely that these 27 patients were entirely well.

The findings indicate that recovery from schizophrenia may take place even in patients fulfilling the St Louis (Feighner *et al*, 1972) criteria for that diagnosis, which include six months of reduced function as an obligatory feature; 18 per cent of the sample had normal mental states and evidently functioned entirely normally. It is of interest that 11 of the 12 well patients were female—a finding consistent with the report of Watt *et al* (1983) that the outcome of schizophrenia is less adverse in females than in males. This degree of well-being appears to be less than that reported by Leff and Vaughn (1972), but is a good deal higher than the 3 per cent reported by McCreadie (1982). The differences probably reflect the different means of selection of the samples. Nonetheless, 5–9 years after discharge, over 50 per cent of this sample (from which the currently re-admitted had been eliminated) remained clearly psychotic and by all available accounts, many were consistently and severely impaired.

In spite of their disabilities and difficulties, the patients did not want to go back to hospital; perhaps more surprising was the fact that the relatives who described many problems resulting from the patients' illness rarely wished them to return there. Current policies (DHSS, 1975; DHSS, 1981) of discharging patients into the community from large mental hospitals had the general support of both the patients and the relatives with whom this study was concerned. The standard of care in the community revealed by this survey was, however, far from optimal. Causes for concern are the number of psychotic patients in social difficulty who were in touch with no service, the apparent uneven allocation of care, and the number of unmet needs, particularly of relatives. There are many reasons for these problems, including the fact that many patients had moved away from districts where they were known, the nature of the psychiatric problems themselves which had led to impaired judgement, poor co-operation, and the difficulties of the relatives in coming to terms with the prognosis of the illness.

The relatives themselves expressed the view that the staff of the psychiatric services were ill-equipped to deal with patients in whom recovery is not taking place. The chronicity of illness shown here highlights the need for developing community services to take account of the fact that there is a substantial proportion of the schizophrenic population in whom, with available methods of treatment, recovery is not going to take place, and that many of these patients need a high degree of care. In the present sample, as in earlier work (Stevens, 1972), this care was provided by relatives who were in many cases frail, ageing, and coping only with great difficulty.

If policies of transferring as many patients as possible into the community continue, the problems described here will increase, unless systems of care are developed which recognize the severity and chronicity of the abnormalities of many schizophrenic patients and attempt, in the face of the undoubted difficulties, to keep a degree of contact with as many cases as possible until recovery has clearly taken place.

Appendix

Mental states classed as not morbid

Patients 062: No medical or social support. A 28-year-old single woman, who lived with her foster mother between engagements as a highly successful night club dancer in Europe and North Africa. No problems were reported by the patient or her foster mother, who was proud of her exotic and prosperous daughter. Her mental state was normal.

Patient 079: Seen by more than one agency, but not attending a psychiatric clinic. A 38-year-old man, living in lodgings and working regularly as an accounts clerk. He had a fairly active social life, mainly centering upon the church. No difficulties were reported, and at interview his mental state was normal.

Mental states classed as doubtfully morbid

Patient 066: Seen only by community nurses. A 36-year-old single woman, living in a group home and working as a hospital domestic. Her home was well kept and her social presentation good. She had a fairly active social life, centering upon the church. She was preoccupied with religious ideas of an intensity which would be unusual even for someone of her own observant religious background, but otherwise her mental state was normal.

Patient 081: Seen only by general practitioner. A 47-year-old man, living with his wife and baby daughter and working as a booking clerk. There were said to be difficulties at home because of his excessive irritability and anxiety. At interview, he was strikingly anxious, and described a preoccupation with spiritualism, which was not unequivocally delusional.

Mental states classed as clearly morbid

Patient 035: Seen only by community nurses. A 29-year-old single woman, living in a council flat and assisting in her GP's surgery, making coffee, etc. on a voluntary basis. She had a fairly active social life through her church and family, despite by all accounts being continuously floridly psychotic for years. At interview, she scored maximally on delusions and hallucinations, but was socially fairly well preserved.

Patient 036: Seen only by general practitioner. A 57-year-old divorcee, living with her 78-year-old diabetic, chair-bound mother. She worked intermittently in a clerical capacity, but at the time of interview was on sick leave. Her social life was very limited, but her domestic responsibilities would have prevented her from going out much. At interview, the patient was hostile, suspicious, and disorganized in her behaviour. Incoherence of speech was marked, and she scored maximally on delusions.

Patient 071: Attending psychiatric clinic. A 50-year-old man, living with his 71-year-old mother, and attending a day centre for many years. He was described as very dependent upon his mother with regard to most aspects of his life, and had no friends or social contacts. At interview, he was unkempt and rather dirty. He scored maximally on hallucinations and thought disorder; he was probably deluded, but his incoherence was so severe that this could not be clearly determined.

Patient 114: No medical or social support. A 27-year-old woman, living with her 61-year-old widowed father. She did no work and never went out without him. She was verbally and physically aggressive towards him and at times destructive of furnishings. She could make no attempt at personal cleanliness and was at times incontinent. Her father was much troubled by the unsuitability of his dealing with her personal hygiene. At interview, she adopted bizarre postures and her behaviour was very degraded. She showed gross affective incongruity and incoherence of speech, and although she would not discuss them, alluded to delusions and hallucinations.

Patient 120: No medical or social support. A 58-year-old housewife, living with her 59-year-old husband and 22-year-old son. She believed that they were poisoning her. She cooked and shopped for herself alone and would not be in the same room with them. She shouted at night to hallucinations and was abusive to any visitors who called. At interview, she would not reply to any questions. Her dress was bizarre and she was surrounded by items which appeared to have symbolic significance. Affective incongruity was gross and her brief remarks were not entirely coherent.

References

CHEADLE, A. J., FREEMAN, H. L. & KORER, J. (1978) Chronic schizophrenic patients in the community. *British Journal of Psychiatry*, **132,** 221–227.

CREER, C. (1975) Living with schizophrenia. *Social Work Today*, **6,** 2–7.

—— STURT, E. & WYKES, T. (1982) The role of relatives. In *Long-term Community Care Experience in a London Borough* (ed. J. K. Wing). Psychological Medicine Monograph, Supplement 2.

—— & WING, J. K. (1974) *Schizophrenia at Home.* National Schizophrenia Fellowship, 79 Victoria Road, Surbition, Surrey, KT6 4JT.

DEPARTMENT OF HEALTH AND SOCIAL SECURITY (1975) *Better Services for the Mentally Ill.* Cmnd 6233, London: HMSO.

—— (1981) *Care in the Community: A Consultative Document on Moving Resources for Care in England.* London: DHSS.

FEIGHNER, J. P., ROBINS, E., GUZE, S. B., WOODRUFF, A., WINOKUR, G. & MUNOZ, R. (1972) Diagnostic criteria for use in psychiatric research. *Archives of General Psychiatry*, **26,** 57–63.

JOHNSTONE, E. C., OWENS, D. G. C., GOLD, A., CROW, T. J. & MACMILLAN, J. F. (1981) Institutionalisation and the defects of schizophrenia. *British Journal of Psychiatry*, **139,** 195–203.

KRAWIECKA, M., GOLDBERG, D. & VAUGHAN, M. (1977) A standardised psychiatric assessment for rating chronic psychotic patients. *Acta Psychiatrica Scandinavica*, **55,** 299–308.

LEFF, J. P. & VAUGHN, C. (1972) Psychiatric patients in contact and out of contact with services: a clinical and social assessment. In *Evaluating a Community Psychiatric Service* (eds. J. K. Wing & A. M. Hailey). London: Oxford University Press.

McCREADIE, R. G. (1982) The Nithsdale Schizophrenia Survey: I. Psychiatric and social handicaps. *British Journal of Psychiatry*, **140,** 582–586.

NATIONAL SCHIZOPHRENIA FELLOWSHIP (1979) *Home Sweet Nothing: The Plight of Sufferers from Chronic Schizophrenia.* National Schizophrenia Fellowship: 79 Victoria Road, Surbiton, Surrey, KT6 4NS.

STEVENS, B. C. (1972) Dependence of schizophrenic patients on elderly relatives. *Psychological Medicine*, **2,** 17–32.

TOOTH, G. C. & BROOKE, E. M. (1961) Trends in the mental hospital population and their effect on future planning. *Lancet, i,* 710–713.

WATT, D. C., KATZ, K. & SHEPHERD, M. (1983) The natural history of schizophrenia: a 5-year prospective follow-up of a representative sample of schizophrenics by means of a standardized clinical and social assessment. *Psychological Medicine*, **13,** 663–670.

WING, J. K. (1982) Long-term community care; experience in a London borough. *Psychological Medicine*, Monograph Supplement 2.

36 Chronic schizophrenia in the community

HUGH FREEMAN

With the control of infectious diseases, schizophrenia and dementia are now among the major public health problems of developed societies. In the UK, 150,000 people are affected by schizophrenia at any one time, and more of working age (in hospital or disabled in the community) suffer from it than from any other condition (Office of Health Economics, 1979). Since the illness usually begins in adolescence or early adulthood and schizophrenics now have a life expectancy similar to the general population, they may be chronically ill or susceptible to further relapse for up to 50 years. Such lengths of time constitute the real extent of the problem and should govern the pattern of services, for instance in trying to reduce the discontinuities resulting from constant changes of professional staff (Freeman, 1980). No population is known in which schizophrenia does not exist (Smith, 1982), although in the island populations of Micronesia, separated by long sea distances and by race and culture, substantial differences have been reported in prevalence rates (Dale, 1981); various hypotheses can be proposed to explain this, including genetic differences and increasing amounts of grain in the diet (Dohan *et al*, 1983).

Although an association has long been noted between schizophrenia and low social class, it is now generally accepted that this is not causal but the result of social drift (Goldberg and Morrison, 1963). Cooper (1978) describes a pattern in which early timidity and shyness, loss of peer relationships in adolescence, poor school performance and early work record, reduction in social status and migration into a decaying, disorganized urban area occurs in those with an inherent vulnerability, often combined with environmental stress. Their migration takes place along with many others who show reduced economic effectiveness and reduced social network cohesiveness (Levy and Rowitz, 1973). The result is an excess of schizophrenics (as of alcoholics and persons with severe personality disorders) in inner city districts; they are often unmarried and detached from family or other social networks. They represent a considerable problem for mental health services because social isolation and often poverty further increase their demands, and a higher level of service provision is therefore needed in inner city areas, yet the opposite is often the case (Freeman, 1984a). By no means all are socially isolated, but Cooper (1961) found that patients who had been living alone at the time of admission to hospital had a much worse outcome than those from a family setting, perhaps because of lack of social support or perhaps because their illnesses were more severe. Social isolation was originally put forward as an aetiological factor in schizophrenia but is almost certainly a result of the condition (Kohn and Clausen, 1955). There is no evidence that the incidence of schizophrenia differs in socieities with different political or economic systems.

A summary of 15 surveys from 12 countries, dating from 1929 to 1972, showed that one-year prevalence rates of schizophrenia were between 1.5 and 4.2 per 1,000 of the total population, but most were in the range of 2.0 to 3.5 (Cooper, 1978). The reverse of the process of social drift is 'social residue', i.e. that the mentally healthy migrate away from socially and environmentally undesirable areas, leaving behind the relatively incompetent; both processes may operate at the same time and place. Possibly as a result of differential migration, a high rate of schizophrenia has been recorded both for the inner city of Salford, an industrial town in the North of England (Freeman, 1984b), and for rural areas of Ireland. In the former, a study of treated prevalence for 1974, based on the Psychiatric Case Register, gave an annual rate of 4.87 per 1,000 of the total population and a point-prevalence rate of 3.28. The one-day prevalence figure for three rural counties in Ireland was 8.3 per 1,000 of the adult population, compared with 2.36 for the Camberwell area of South London (Walsh *et al*, 1980) and 4.33 for Salford. This Irish excess is particularly high among unmarried males, and may be partly related both to socio-cultural factors in the population and to the high provision of psychiatric beds. In general, there is little reliable evidence of consistent urban–rural differences in the prevalence of schizophrenia (Webb, 1985).

So far as outcome is concerned, the International Pilot Study of Schizophrenia (World Health Organization, 1979) found a marked difference between developed and developing countries—prognosis being more favourable in the latter—although most of the variance could not be related to any known factors, and the difference was mainly in the less severe (or Type 1) cases. This favourable outcome presumably results from the lower social demands and complexity of tasks, together with the support of extended families, to be found in most agrarian societies, but it does not follow that chronic psychosis generally runs a benign course there (Murphy and Raman, 1971). Although both 'labelling' by professional staff or society and institutionalism have been blamed for much of the disability of chronic schizophrenics, Asian villagers who had never been seen by a doctor or entered an institution showed the same degree of social handicaps as patients in Western societies (Westermeyer, 1980). There is now general agreement that schizophrenia emerges as the resultant of an interaction between environmental stress and genetic vulnerability, but 'the alleged stresses all lack specificity and appear to be ubiquitous in the population' (Gottesman and Shields, 1982).

In the UK and other developed countries, the most handicapped schizophrenics are likely to be chronic in-patients, each of their various abnormalities showing a strong correlation with the others, so that only hospital care can cope adequately with the combined degree of disability (Owens and Johnstone, 1980); although these patients represent one end of the spectrum of prognosis, their numbers are significant. In the 1950s and '60s, institutionalism resulting from long stay in mental hospitals was regarded as the major factor causing the deterioration of many chronic schizophrenics, but it is now understood that this is largely the product of the illness itself and may occur in people who have never been admitted to a mental hospital (Johnstone *et al*, 1981).

Wing and Brown (1970) emphasized that although about a third of long-stay patients affected by institutionalism benefited from environmental manipulation, this did not rule out a biological process underlying the deficits found.

Relatives continue to bear the greatest part of the burden of care despite the trend toward smaller families and greater social mobility. Professional help for these patients and their families needs to be on an interdisciplinary basis. Relatives reported that the most frequent behaviour problems in the home were social withdrawal, underactivity, odd ideas and behaviour, depression, and neglect of appearance (Creer and Wing, 1974) and it was surprising that so many families had managed to find a way of coping. Hoenig (1974) found that although over 80 per cent of the families of patients who had been discharged from hospital experienced 'objective burdens' such as loss of earnings and coping with abnormal behaviour, only 24 per cent complained of feeling severely burdened.

Schizophrenia causes special difficulties in the roles of professional staff because of the complexity of its effects; 'chronic schizophrenia' includes syndromes within a wide range of types and severities, consisting of both intrinsic and reactive components (Wing, 1978). As a long-term disease, with most sufferers outside hospital, its management should be the responsibility of the general practitioner (Parkes *et al*, 1962; Freeman, 1968), but this tends not to happen and the concept of the 'primary health care team' remains largely a mythical ideal (Priestley, 1979). Therefore, specialist secondary care workers must often take over continued responsibility, but since no individual is constantly available for the long periods involved, this has to be a team commitment. The psychiatrist generally has the additional function of co-ordinating relevant services and, in this respect, the relatively non-hierarchical nature of the medical role is particularly valuable. Although Priestley found that relatives of schizophrenics are very unlikely to seek help from social services, an experienced social worker with psychiatric knowledge could support and counsel these families, for instance by helping them to develop more effective ways of handling difficult behaviour (Creer, 1978). An informative, non-judgemental and readily available counselling service is one of the overwhelming needs of relatives, but at present social services very rarely provide it (Sturt *et al*, 1982). Partly as a consequence of this, the last 20 years have seen a very rapid growth of community psychiatric nursing in Britain; nurses have the advantage of being both experienced in the management of psychotic behaviour and qualified to administer medication. Where community nursing has been well developed it is a primary source of help for many families, but the provision of this service varies greatly between different districts. A Royal College of Psychiatrists Working Party (1980) recommended that every chronically handicapped patient in the community should have a personal counsellor who could be a doctor, nurse, social worker, or occupational therapist, and that the counsellors should meet regularly in order to review all cases.

A study carried out in Salford into the use of hospital services by chronic schizophrenics, excluding long-stay hospital patients, showed that only 8 out of 102 had made heavy demands during a year, mainly through hospital admission (Freeman *et al*, 1979b). Medium use of services was by prolonged day care, while the great majority were light users, receiving depot injections and out-patient supervision only. Against expectation the use of social services followed the same trend as hospital services, rather than making up for them. The total service use by the 538 schizophrenic patients from the Salford population in 1974 consisted of 78,740 in-patient days (107 admissions); 8,231 day attendances (43 patients), 533 out-patient attendances or domiciliary visits and 17,214 days on the books of social workers (Freeman, 1984b). When these patients were compared to patients with other diagnoses, mean hospital in-patient days per patient were more than three times those for all other diagnoses, while total days for non-schizophrenic patients were much less than those for schizophrenics. However, day attendances for schizophrenics were very much lower than those for the rest, which was surprising in view of the value widely placed on day care for chronic and recurrent schizophrenia. Social work involvement for other diagnoses was more than twice the total for schizophrenics; the latter, however, used less than a fifth the number of out-patient attendances and domiciliary visits, compared with other patients. The conclusion to be drawn is that schizophrenia occupied a central role in the in-patient care of psychiatric disorder in Salford at that time, but made relatively modest demands on other forms of service. Subsequently, however, it made substantial use of the developing community psychiatric nursing service (Wooff *et al*, 1983).

Medication

Whatever the role of social factors such as life events or the emotional atmosphere of the family, antipsychotic drugs remain the foundation of any long-term programme of care for schizophrenics. Medication is still important by the fourth year after an episode of illness, particularly for those who have remained in a steady mental state until then, although the rate of relapse is up to 40 per cent even on uninterrupted treatment (Johnson, 1979). Stopping drugs after two years' remission was followed in the next year by relapse in 68 per cent of one group; the superiority of maintenance treatment over no treatment increased steadily with time, and the view that patients with good prognostic signs do not need prophylactic medication was not supported (Hogarty, 1979). However, the continued supply of medication to the large number of patients outside hospitals causes great problems of management and information. Patients are easily lost from the system of care, and to prevent this from happening, there is a need for some form of continuously updated register, such as the one that has been developed in Salford (Freeman *et al*, 1979a). Alternatives to conventional treatment of schizophrenia have not so far been evaluated (Mosher and Menn, 1978).

Although most schizophrenics require antipsychotic drugs to maintain a state of reasonable mental health, they are generally expected to manage their own treatment, either by taking tablets or by attending for injections. At the beginning of relapse, when insight deteriorates, the patient who is left unsupervised will often stop treatment; relatives may then bear the brunt of a major relapse, unless they can call on professional services and the services respond quickly and appropriately. These activities should receive the highest priority from any community-orientated mental health service and, although in the absence of available services, many families learn to manage unaided, the price is high in terms of burden and distress.

Since antipsychotic drugs appear to reduce the physiological responsiveness of schizophrenics to environmental stimuli, including emotional interactions with relatives, pharmacological effects may differ according to the social environment and the need for long-term treatment might be partly determined by physiological measures of arousal (Leff, 1979). However, this is not yet clinically possible and even in families where expressed emotion is low, medication remains important, not least because of the effects of life events. It is believed that arousal plays a central role in mediating the effects of the social environment to the individual and that both genetic and environmental influences may lead to a chronic state of over-arousal, which can develop into psychosis through such influences as life events or high expressed emotion. There may thus be an inability to screen the stimuli constantly received from the environment and to distinguish those which are relevant (Frith, 1979). One strategy for coping with this situation would be to avoid over-arousal by remaining in a tranquil environment, but this involves social costs such as withdrawal from human contacts, which in its turn may eventually produce harmful effects from lack of stimulation, since schizophrenics have an increased sensitivity to social deprivation (Wing and Brown, 1970). There is evidence that schizophrenics characteristically maintain a greater space between themselves and other people (body-buffer zone) than do non-schizophrenics (Horowitz *et al*, 1964) and this may be another mechanism for reducing the level of internal arousal.

Rehabilitation

The pursuit of unrealistic goals in terms of work and social functioning is unlikely to be successful because of the frequent cognitive defects that make schizophrenic patients abnormally distractible and unable to process information, including language. On the other hand, a simplified environment and freedom from the need for complex decision making can be very helpful. A series of limited objectives need to be defined, together with a programme of specific action to reach them, proceeding by trial and error until an optimum level is obtained; the aims therefore are to prevent relapse and develop any personal assets (Wing, 1978). However, it is far from easy to tread the knife edge between the dangers of social withdrawal and understimulation on the one hand and those of excessive arousal on the other, particularly since many patients have fluctuating insight and are affected periodically by delusions and hallucinations. Behaviour therapy would seem to provide a possibility of improving the quality of life but so far remains at an experimental stage (Jones, 1978). Hemsley (1978) emphasized that operant procedures, applied without understanding patients' basic impairments, may either fail or actually make symptoms worse. However, the response to even the greatest efforts is often disappointing, and it has been said that 'what they want to do they can't, and what they can do they don't want to.'

While the British psychiatric hospital population has fallen considerably in the last 25 years, 'new long-stay' patients continue to accumulate, and most are schizophrenics; Bewley *et al* (1981) pointed out that most of them are not 'new' at all, except in an administrative sense, having long histories of chronic or recurrent illness. In their national sample of this group, Mann and Cree (1976) found that only 15 per cent were suitable to live outside hospital without supervision; 33 per cent needed further hospital care and 20 per cent required a supervised residential setting. In addition to persistent psychiatric problems, these patients showed a characteristic pattern of social disadvantage.

However, the fact that many patients need long-term care does not mean that all of them have to remain in a conventional hospital setting. Wykes (1982) reported the results of a hospital hostel, which was staffed at the level of an acute general hospital unit, although such hospitals are usually very unsuitable for care of the chronically disabled. Compared with conventional wards, the atmosphere was more home-like, active rehabilitation was more possible, patients' social behaviour improved, none of them had to be transferred back to hospital, and relatives were very pleased with the change. Such a unit can cope with episodes of disturbed behaviour which would generally not be tolerated in local authority or voluntary hostels. However, organized programmes of supervised accommodation remain scanty, and the right degree of social pressure for different degrees of vulnerability can only be applied if there is a continuum of residential settings (National Schizophrenia Fellowship, 1979). This would be most effective if facilities and staff for varying degrees of supervision were on a single site; some of this accommodation could be for patients aged over 65. Since hostels are relatively expensive to set up and staff, the group home, with visiting supervision by nurses and social workers, has emerged as a much cheaper alternative (Soni *et al*, 1978). However, all forms of sheltered accommodation, including that provided by patients' families, require day care as an essential complement; in fact better integration of the activities of existing services would lead to all of them working more effectively.

Recent surveys

Using the Salford Psychiatric Case Register as a sampling frame, Cheadle *et al* (1978) surveyed all those people who: (a) were diagnosed as schizophrenic on criteria of symptoms, assessed from case notes and clinical knowledge; (b) were in contact with some part of the psychiatric service during 1974; (c) were not long-stay hospital patients (i.e. over 12 months). Those excluded from the survey were those aged over 65, who had moved away, had doubtful or multiple diagnoses, refused interview or had died. The final sample numbered 190, and they were all examined using the Present State Examination (PSE). The average age of the men was 42.9 and of the women 48.3 and the difference was significant; significantly more men had never married. Of the females, a third had never married, whereas the figure for the female population is Salford over 15 years of age was 23 per cent; however, a quarter of the women had been divorced, compared to 2 per cent of the general female population. There was little difference in the numbers living alone, but rather more men than women were living with their parents. It was satisfying to note that 49 patients (24 men and 25 women) were working at the time they were interviewed. According to the respondents, social isolation was a problem for a quarter of them and this was not confined to those living alone. These people felt that they were cut off from others and could not mix on an equal footing; many felt they had been 'loners' as children. Whether or not they were living alone did not seem to be related to this complaint. On the other hand, many of those who did not complain of social isolation did in fact appear to be isolated; they lived alone, did not go out and had no friends, but did not seem to consider this to be a problem.

Of the PSE results, 157 were suitable for analysis. The 35 syndromes were divided into four groups: schizophrenic and paranoid (S&P); manic and other psychoses (M&O); borderline psychotic (P); and neurotic (N); the group totals for each patient were ranked. At the time of interview, 28 respondents were free of symptoms, and 50 had their symptoms confined to the N group. Thus, 41 per cent were then without any visible signs of psychosis; only eight of these 78 patients were not having some form of antipsychotic drug, so that it is very likely that medication played an important part in this finding. Of the 157 results analysed, some S&P symptoms were shown by 27 patients, some M&O by 70, some P by 31, and 124 had N symptoms; there was no difference between the sexes on any of the four syndrome groups. Who, if anybody, the patients lived with was not associated with their clinical condition, and those who felt socially isolated were significantly more neurotic, but not more psychotic than the rest. The subjects who were working were least ill. Thirty-four patients were not on any treatment and they were not significantly different from the rest, as far as their current clinical condition was concerned; 72 per cent were receiving depot phenothiazines and their general practitioners were prescribing oral medication only for 19 patients. Patients' attitudes towards treatment were mostly positive.

Since the sample had been in contact with some psychiatric service for an average of 12 years and the majority were maintained on depot phenothiazines, it was clear that their handicaps were still moderately severe, and that these could not be attributed to any recent effects of an institution. That it was almost exclusively the neurotic problems which were associated with social handicaps, e.g. isolation and unemployment, was surprising. The socially isolated were more neurotic than the others, as were those who nearly always stayed at home in the evenings. The most prominent symptom was 'worrying', and it was the patients with a predominance of neurotic symptoms, especially 'worrying', who gave the impression that they were most concerned by their handicaps. Thus, while antipsychotic drugs seem to control much of the psychotic symptoms, satisfactory methods of dealing with these patients' neurotic problems still remain to be developed. The low level of psychotic disturbance in this large group of people with a diagnosis of schizophrenia living in the general community should be noted, although it partly reflects the fact that many of the most handicapped remained in hospital as long-stay patients.

The second survey was by **Johnstone *et al* (1984)** in which a cohort of 120 patients, discharged from one mental hospital over a five-year period (1970–74), were followed-up in the community after an interval of five to nine years; 18 per cent had recovered to the extent that they had no significant symptoms, and appeared to function satisfactorily. However, more than 50 per cent had definite psychotic features and severe emotional, social, and financial difficulties were commonplace. Twenty-seven per cent had no contact with medical or social services, a further 14 per cent saw only community nurses, and 24 per cent only their general practitioners. The degree of super-vision was divided into five categories, with considerable overlap between them; some minimally ill patients were receiving care from multiple agencies, while others, who were floridly ill and in circumstances of social distress, had received much less or no care at all. The greatest distress for patients and relatives was found among those receiving no medical or social attention. Although some very disturbed patients were only being seen by community nurses or general practitioners, their condition did not appear to be associated with as much distress or social disorganization as was found in those without any care.

In addition to those patients in touch with the psychiatric services or receiv-ing care from their general practitioners, there were 27 patients who were not in contact with the medical or social services at all; those who were currently readmitted to hospital were excluded from the cohort. Eleven of the 12 well patients were female—a finding consistent with the report of Watt *et al* (1983) that the outcome of schizophrenia is less adverse in females than in males. This degree of well-being in the sample is less than that reported by Leff and Vaughn (1972), but much higher than in the Nithsdale survey (McCreadie, 1982). Although relatives described many problems resulting from the patients' illnesses, they rarely wished them to return to hospital; current policies had general support, but the number of psychotic patients in social difficulty who were not in touch with any service, the apparent uneven allocation of care and the number of unmet needs, particularly of relatives, were causes for concern. The authors (**Johnstone *et al*, 1984**) concluded that the staff of the psychiatric services were ill-equipped to deal with patients in whom re-covery is not taking place. Community-orientated services therefore need to take account of the fact that there is a substantial proportion of the schizophre-nic population in whom, with currently available methods of treatment, reco-very is not going to occur, and that many of these patients need a high degree of care. Often, the responsibility was carried by relatives who were themselves frail, ageing, and coping only with great difficulty. Unless services are de-veloped which recognize the severity and chronicity of the abnormalities of many schizophrenic patients, and attempt to keep a degree of contact with as many cases as possible, the problems revealed in this survey will steadily increase as hospital care diminishes.

A third study (Sturt *et al*, 1982) reported on patients in Camberwell who were continuing in long-term contact with community services, but were not long-stay in-patients, although many would have been so in the past; almost half the total were schizophrenics. The rate of 13.9 per 1,000 population is an underestimate because other people with similar needs must have been present in the community, but not in touch with services. The socio-demo-graphic characteristics of the sample were similar to those of long-stay patients in psychiatric hospitals, i.e. chronically disabled, with a history of inability to reach expected levels of social performance; three-quarters of the subjects had first contacted psychiatric services more than ten years before, and nearly half also had some quite severe physical disability, such as epilepsy, brain damage, or severe sensory deficit. Their commonest behavioural problems were those associated with social withdrawal and socially embarrassing conduct, but over 40 per cent had caring and supportive relatives.

Heredity and environment

In spite of general acceptance of the importance of environmental contributors to the aetiology of schizophrenia, these are difficult to identify; Gottesman and Shields (1982) point out that if such factors cause the illness only in the relatively few individuals who are genetically predisposed, they may have no noticeable effect as independent causes in the population as a whole. They conclude that environmental factors (such as life events) may contribute about 30 per cent to individual differences in the liability to schizophrenia of the general population but will be critical factors to someone who is in the 'neighbourhood' of the threshold, in the distribution of combined liability. Thus, people at the extreme of genetic liability will find almost any environment they experience as stressful enough to cause the illness. These authors' conclusions, from the diathesis-stressor framework, is that 'although the genes may be necessary but not sufficient for causing schizophrenia, the environmental contributors may also be necessary but not sufficient, and yet not specifiable other than on a case-by-case basis.'

References

BEWLEY, T. H., BLAND, M., MECHAN, D. & WALCH, E. (1981) New chronic patients. *British Medical Journal*, **283,** 1161–1164.

CHEADLE, A. J., FREEMAN, H. L. & KORER, J. R. (1978) Chronic schizophrenic patients in the community. *British Journal of Psychiatry*, **132,** 221–227.

COOPER, B. (1961) Social class and prognosis in schizophrenia. *British Journal of Preventive and Social Medicine*, **15,** 17–21.

—— (1978) Epidemiological aspects. In *Schizophrenia Towards a New Synthesis*. London: Academic Press.

CREER, C. (1978) Social work with patients and their families. In *Schizophrenia Towards a New Synthesis*. London: Academic Press.

—— & WING, J. K. (1974) *Schizophrenia at Home*. Surbiton: National Schizophrenia Fellowship.

DALE, P. W. (1981) Prevalence of schizophrenia in the Pacific island populations of Micronesia. *Journal of Psychiatric Research*, **16,** 103–111.

DOHAN, F. C., HARPER, E. H., CLARK, M. H., RODRIGUE, R. & ZIGAN, V. (1983) Where is schizophrenia rare? *Lancet, ii,* 101.

FREEMAN, H. L. (1968) Management of schizophrenia in the community. *British Medical Journal, ii,* 371–373.

—— (1980) Coping with schizophrenia. *British Journal of Hospital Medicine*, **23,** 54–58.

—— (1984a) Mental health in the inner city. *Environment and Planning*, **16,** 115–121.

—— (1984b) *Treated Prevalence of Schizophrenia in Salford County Borough 1974*. Report to the Department of Health and Social Security.

—— CHEADLE, A. J. & KORER, J. R. (1979a) A method for monitoring the treatment of schizophrenics in the community. *British Journal of Psychiatry*, **134,** 412–416.

—— —— —— (1979b) Use of hospital services by chronic schizophrenics in the community. *British Journal of Psychiatry*, **134,** 417–421.

FRITH, C. D. (1979) Consciousness, information processing and schizophrenia. *British Journal of Psychiatry*, **134,** 225–235.

GOLDBERG, E. M. & MORRISON, S. L. (1963) Schizophrenia and social class. *British Journal of Psychiatry*, **109,** 785–802.

GOTTESMAN, I. I. & SHIELDS, J. (1982) *Schizophrenia: The Epigenetic Puzzle*. Cambridge: Cambridge University Press.

HEMSLEY, D. R. (1978) Limitations of operant procedures in the modification of schizophrenic functioning. *Behavior Analysis and Modification*, **2**, 165–173.

HOGARTY, G. E. (1979) Aftercare treatment of schizophrenia. In *Management of Schizophrenia* (ed. H. M. van Praag). Assen: Van Goreum.

HOENIG, J. (1974) The schizophrenic patient at home. *Acta Psychiatrica Scandinavica*, **50**, 297–308.

HOROWITZ, M. J., DUFF, D. F. & STRATTON, L. O. (1964) Body-buffer zone. *Archives of General Psychiatry*, **2**, 651–656.

JOHNSON, D. A. W. (1979) Clinical considerations in the use of depot neuroleptics. In *Management of Schizophrenia* (ed. H. M. van Praag). Assen: Van Goreum.

JOHNSTONE, E. C., OWENS, D. G. C., GOLD, A., CROW, T. J. & MACMILLAN, J. F. (1981) Institutionalisation and the defects of schizophrenics. *British Journal of Psychiatry*, **139**, 195–203.

—— —— —— —— (1984) Schizophrenic patients discharged from hospital—a follow up study. *British Journal of Psychiatry*, **145**, 586–590.

JONES, H. G. (1978) Psychological aspects of treatment of in-patients. In *Schizophrenia Towards a New Synthesis* (ed. J. K. Wing). London: Academic Press.

KOHN, M. L. & CLAUSEN, J. A. (1955) Social isolation and schizophrenia. *American Sociological Review*, **120**, 265–273.

LEFF, J. P. (1979) Psychophysiological monitoring of drug effects in schizophrenia. In *Management of Schizophrenia* (ed. H. M. van Praag). Assen: Van Goreum.

—— & VAUGHN, C. (1972) Psychiatric patients in contact and out of contact with services. In *Evaluating a Community Psychiatric Service* (eds. J. K. Wing and A. M. Hailey). London: Oxford University Press.

LEVY, L. & ROWITZ, L. (1973) *The Ecology of Mental Disorder*. New York: Behavioral Publications.

MANN, S. & CREE, W. (1976) 'New long-stay' psychiatric patients; a national survey of fifteen mental hospitals in England and Wales, 1972–3. *Psychological Medicine*, **6**, 603–616.

McCREADIE, R. G. (1982) The Nithsdale Schizophrenia Survey: I. Psychiatric and social handicaps. *British Journal of Psychiatry*, **140**, 582–586.

MOSHER, L. R. & MENN, A. Z. (1978) Lowered barriers in the community: the Soteria model. In *Alternatives to Mental Hospital Treatment* (eds. L. I. Stein and M. A. Test). New York: Plenum Press.

MURPHY, H. B. M. & RAMAN, A. C. (1971) The chronicity of schizophrenia in indigenous tropical peoples. *British Journal of Psychiatry*, **118**, 489–497.

NATIONAL SCHIZOPHRENIA FELLOWSHIP (1979) *Home Sweet Nothing*. Surbiton: National Schizophrenia Fellowship.

OFFICE OF HEALTH ECONOMICS (1979) *Schizophrenia*. London: Office of Health Economics.

OWENS, D. G. C. & JOHNSTONE, E. C. (1980) The disabilities of chronic schizophrenia—their nature and the factors contributing to their development. *British Journal of Psychiatry*, **136**, 384–395.

PARKES, C. M., BROWN, G. W. & MONCK, E. M. (1962) The general practitioner and the schizophrenic patient. *British Medical Journal*, i, 972–975.

PRIESTLEY, D. (1979) *Tied Together with String*. Surbiton: National Schizophrenia Fellowship.

ROYAL COLLEGE OF PSYCHIATRISTS (1980) *Psychiatric Rehabilitation in the 1980s*. London: Royal College of Psychiatrists.

SONI, S., SONI, S. D. & FREEMAN, H. L. (1978) Group Home for discharged psychiatric hospital patients. *International Journal of Mental Health*, **6**, 66–79.

SMITH, A. C. (1982) *Schizophrenia and Madness*. London: Allen & Unwin.

STURT, E., WYKES, T. & CREER, C. (1982) A survey of long-term users of the community psychiatric services in Camberwell. *Psychological Medicine*, Monograph Supplement 2, 5–55.

WALSH, D, O'HARE, A., BLAKE, B., HALPENNY, J. B. & O'BRIEN, P. F. (1980) The treated prevalence of mental illness in the Republic of Ireland—the Three Country case register study. *Psychological Medicine*, **10**, 465–470.

WATT, D. C., KATZ, K. & SHEPHERD, M. (1983) The natural history of schizophrenia. *Psychological Medicine*, **13**, 663–670.

WEBB, S. D. (1985) Rural-urban differences in mental health. In *Mental Health and the Environment* (ed. H. L. Freeman). London: Churchill Livingstone.

WESTERMEYER, J. (1980) Psychosis in a peasant society: social outcomes. *American Journal of Psychiatry*, **137**, 1390–1394.

WING, J. K. (1978) Clinical concepts of schizophrenia. In *Schizophrenia Towards a New Synthesis*. London and New York: Academic Press.

—— & BROWN, G. W. (1970) *Institutionalism and Schizophrenia*. Cambridge: Cambridge University Press.

WORLD HEALTH ORGANIZATION (1979) *Schizophrenia. An International Follow-up Study*. Chichester: John Wiley.

WOOFF, K., FRYERS, T. & FREEMAN, H. L. (1983) Psychiatric service use in Salford. *British Journal of Psychiatry*, **142,** 588–597.

WYKES, T. (1982) A hostel ward for 'new' long-stay patients: an evaluative study of 'a ward in a house'. *Psychological Medicine*, Monograph Supplement 2, 59–97.

VI. Treatment

37 Treatment in schizophrenia: Overview

HAMISH McCLELLAND

The term dementia praecox is obsolete but Kraepelin anticipated the growing modern view that the illness is an organic brain disorder. However, dementia implies an unchanging or progressive course and schizophrenia viewed over the long-term seems a more complex illness than has been appreciated hitherto. M. Bleuler (1978) maintains that in his lifetime there has been an improvement in the natural history not fully explained by modern treatment and **Hare** (**1983**) believes the disorder to be less frequent and less malignant in its manifestations and outcome now than in the 19th and early 20th centuries. More pertinent to the present day is the evidence from recent long-term studies that the disease process is most active in the first decade or so and thereafter tends to stabilize and even improve (Bleuler, 1974; Huber *et al*, 1980; Pfohl and Winokur, 1982; Bridge *et al*, 1978). Such findings have implications for management in that, in the early active phase, caution should be exercised in implementing forms of employment or social therapy which may lead to excessive pressure on patients' coping abilities.

The overriding problems in the care of schizophrenic patients are the tendency to relapse and the presence of a defect state. The essential vulnerability is that patients function within a narrow range of stimulation: too much leads to over-arousal and relapse and too little enhance withdrawal and defect features. The aim in management therefore is to reduce the patient's tendency to over-arousal with drugs while controlling adverse environmental influences and, for this, the co-operation of the patient and his family through long-term relationships with key therapists is vital.

The recent awareness of a natural tendency to improve has to be balanced by the realization that the overt schizophrenic illness in poor prognosis cases may be part of a complex process which affects the individual from infancy onwards. The chronic patient with persistent psychotic symptoms or a serious defect state has often shown personality, educational and social problems in childhood and adolescence and has had a poor employment and marital record. Schulsinger and his colleagues (1984) have suggested that these difficulties constitute the essence of the genetic component of that form of schizophrenia which is hereditary, the frank manifestation of illness depending on the occurrence of certain environmental (probably organic) stressors. Brain scan studies have demonstrated that one subgroup of schizophrenia has abnormal brain structure at the onset of illness which suggests that organic changes may be present at an even earlier stage. Such findings are reminders that the outcome in a psychiatric illness may be determined, not just by the illness but by pre-morbid characteristics. In such cases one must not expect too much of rehabilitation. Furthermore the premorbid handicaps and persisting illness bring about secondary handicaps arising from the lowered expectancy of the patients and those close to them (Wing and Brown, 1970).

The emphasis in this review in on drug management of the schizophrenic patient. But of considerable and complementary importance are the psychological, social and rehabilitation aspects of care and these are examined elsewhere in this section on treatment.

In acute, or relapsing, schizophrenia controlled trials have consistently shown neuroleptic medication to be superior to placebo. Moreover, neuroleptics add to the effectiveness of other treatments. In maintenance therapy the aim is to reduce the risk of relapse of patients in remission and to control persisting positive symptoms. The value of neuroleptics in reducing relapse rate is unequivocal. Indeed Davis (1975) calculated that summating 24 double-blind studies the chance of there being no drug effect was 10^{-80}. However, the view held during the first two decades after their introduction, that these drugs improved the negative symptoms (or defect state) of schizophrenia, is no longer supported.

The risk of relapse, whether on drugs or placebo, is highest during the first year of follow-up after which it levels off. Roughly one-third of patients on neuroleptics relapse in the first year compared with two-thirds on placebo, and despite the subsequent decline in relapse rates there continues to be a differential between drugs and placebo effect. In **Johnson's (1979)** four-year follow-up study, discontinuation of depot neuroleptics resulted in a relapse rate twice as high as those maintained on medication. As the author points out, maintenance therapy is therefore probably required for a longer period.

Johnson's observation that the outcome did not differ whether medication was stopped by the patients themselves or by the psychiatrists implies that psychiatrists are not good predictors, despite basing their judgement on accepted prognostic signs. This could contradict the finding by Leff and Wing (1971) that psychiatrists predicted a good outcome group who did not relapse even without drug treatment, although this study was over a period of only one year. However, Goldberg *et al* (1977) found, over a two-year period, that their good prognostic group profited from drug treatment particularly as this facilitated the benefits of social therapy.

But it is not justifiable to assume that patients with chronic schizophrenia should remain on chemotherapy indefinitely. If schizophrenia is at its most active in the early years then there may well be a time when medication can be stopped with only a minimal risk of relapse. Unfortunately no clear answer can be given. It is well known that schizophrenics may relapse after many years in remission and much may depend on the patient's environment.

An interesting study by Letemendia and Harris (1967) reported on a group of 28 chronic schizophrenic patients in an isolated hospital annexe untouched by the tide of chemotherapy. The patients were middle aged (mean 53 years) with an average period of hospitalization of 18 years and the introduction of chemotherapy for nine months improved only one patient. However, this is to be balanced by an out-patient study (Cheung, 1981) which showed that, after three to five years in full remission on neuroleptics, schizophrenic patients had a greater risk of relapse if benzodiazepines were substituted for neuroleptics than the control schizophrenic group which remained on neuroleptics.

The value of maintenance therapy in patients living in homes with low Expressed Emotion (EE) has been demonstrated in recent studies (see **Leff**'s review in the section on 'Social Aspects'). The earlier study by Vaughn and Leff (1976) showed that in homes with low EE there was little difference in relapse rates over a nine-month period between those patients on drugs and those who were not; but observations over an extended period of two years (Leff and Vaughn, 1981) showed a widening in relapse rates with those not on drugs having a poorer prognosis. The authors suggest that it is the unpredictable stress of random life events which is likely to cause decompensation in the unmedicated patient, even in those living in low EE homes.

From time to time the benefits of 'drug holidays' are reported together with the claim that the risk of long-term adverse reactions such as tardive dyskinesia (TD) is reduced, but the evidence does not support this claim (Jeste and Wyatt, 1981). Indeed drug holidays may increase the risk of TD by a kindling process while **Johnson (1979)** demonstrated that drug holidays increase the risk of relapse. Furthermore, it is difficult in practice to maintain such regimes for long periods.

Some patients rapidly relapse on reduction of medication and can be considered as having a schizophrenic disorder barely suppressed by neuroleptics. However, it has been suggested that there are some patients who seem to develop a 'super-sensitivity' psychosis which, in severe cases, requires increasing amounts of neuroleptics for control or may only show itself in milder cases on discontinuation of a standard drug regime (Chouinard and Jones, 1980).

An unresolved issue is whether the final outcome of schizophrenia is altered by maintenance regimes. Pritchard (1967) stated that neuroleptics made no difference in the long term but his work was carried out in an era when there was high non-compliance with drug therapy and psychiatrists had not fully appreciated the need for maintenance therapy. Continental psychiatrists such as Bleuler, believe that the ultimate prognosis is better with medication. The writer has seen cases where repeated relapses due to non-compliance can still result in remission with further treatment until the fourth, fifth or sixth decompensation occurs when a serious defect state becomes established for the first time. In the long-term follow-up study by Ciompi (1980) this course and outcome was seen in 12 per cent of the 289 patients. It is reasonable to infer that if maintenance therapy had been taken such an outcome might not have occurred.

Dosage of neuroleptics: In recent years some workers have studied the effects of prescribing below standard dosages. The increased risk of relapse has been accepted but the advantages of reduced adverse effects (including TD) and greater patient co-operation emphasized. Gibson (1980) reported favourably on low dosage fluphenazine decanoate, mainly 12.5 mgs every four weeks, while Kane (1983), using 1/10 (2.5 to 5 mgs) depot fluphenazine dosage, found a 40 per cent relapse rate in the first year compared with 4 per cent relapse for those on standard dosage. But the low dosage patients did better on scales measuring dyskinesia and social adjustment and, if they relapsed, they responded rapidly to increased medication. Low dosage medication is worth further study to identify appropriate patients, but only if there are facilities for frequent and regular monitoring.

There are also claims that very high dosage neuroleptic therapy benefits a minority of treatment-resistant patients. However, McClelland *et al* (1976) found that, while for some patients higher than average dosage was required, no further benefit was obtained from extremely high dosage. Aubree and Lader (1980) concluded that there was a minority of patients who benefited from high doses and pharmacokinetic factors were probably involved. However, unwanted adverse effects, particularly extrapyramidal reactions, were more frequent and severe.

Depot neuroleptic preparations: The introduction of depot neuroleptic medication in the 1960s was a major advance as non-compliance in taking oral drugs was recognized as a major factor in relapse. But it was soon appreciated that depot delivery systems largely depended for their success on a support network of psychiatric community nurses and special clinics. However, a number of studies (Rifkin *et al*, 1977; Hogarty *et al*, 1979; Falloon *et al*, 1978; Schooler *et al*, 1980) have claimed that depot medication does not produce superior results to oral treatment. This is surprising given the non-compliance of many patients, but van Putten (1974) has shown that compliance is not an all or none affair. Many patients on oral medication regulate their dose to bring about a reduction in side-effects and such self-regulation clearly carries a higher risk of relapse.

Some adverse effects of neuroleptic medication

Akinesia: is a subtle side-effect as well as a great mimic. There is retardation of movement with diminished spontaneity, whether physical (slow movements, lack of arm swing) or behavioural (less social activity, speech and gestures), which closely resembles the picture of retarded depression and is one reason why neuroleptics have a reputation for causing depression (van Putten and May, 1978). The clinical picture can also ape the defect state and a Chinese box of features may be observed with akinesia being superimposed on a defect state complicated by the effects of institutionalization.

Tardive dyskinesia: At the turn of the century Kraepelin and Bleuler described abnormal neurological movements in schizophrenic patients and more recent investigators (Owens *et al*, 1982) have reported that dyskinesia occurs in psychosis independently of neuroleptics. However, TD as a clinical syndrome is linked to neuroleptic usage. About 20 per cent of chronic psychotic patients are affected by dyskinesia with some in-patient populations having a reported prevalence rate of up to 50 per cent. Jeste and Wyatt (1981) have argued convincingly that there has been a true increase in prevalence rates in recent years.

Mackay and Shephard (1979) emphasize that tardive dyskinesia is probably a collection of different movement disorders with varying pharmacological origins and that it is unlikely that any one form of management will be effective across the spectrum. Since their article was published there has been no breakthrough in management. Increasing the dosage of neuroleptics is often effective (by causing further blockade of the dopamine supersensitive postsynaptic membrane) but there is the fear that the dyskinesia may eventually escape such constraint. The strategy of acute drug challenge has not been taken up generally because of the poor effectiveness in clinical practice of the drugs claimed to be of benefit. The concept of receptor modification treatment by L-DOPA, based on the accepted but not proven dopamine supersensitivity hypothesis, promised a new approach but has not been developed. Recent claims that sulpiride with its selective D2 receptor action is a prophylactic agent await confirmation.

In the management of tardive dyskinesia the most effective technique is early detection by regular monitoring and reduction of neuroleptic dosage. Treatment of the more severe case may require drugs such as tetrabenazine or a switch to sulpiride or pimozide. Increasing the neuroleptic dosage should only be considered as a last resort.

That *depression* may be caused by neuroleptics is discussed elsewhere in this publication in the section on 'Outcome' (**Johnson, Hirsch** and **Galdi**).

Non-neuroleptic medication: Certain other preparations are claimed to be of value in the treatment of schizophrenia, but none has been shown to be superior to dopamine-blocking drugs.

After more than a decade the role of propranolol remains uncertain. Initially, the drug was used in doses of more than 1 gram a day with encouraging results being claimed in the treatment of acute and chronic schizophrenia. However, recent work using low (Peet *et al*, 1981a) or high dosage (Myers *et al*, 1981) has not found any benefit for chronic schizophrenia. In those trials where propranolol or placebo was added to a neuroleptic regime, it has been suggested that the antischizophrenic effect is indirect, due to a pharmacokinetic interaction, by which propranolol raises the serum levels of chlorpromazine and its active metabolites (Peet *et al*, 1981). However, Yorkston *et al* (1981) found propranolol alone to be almost as effective as chlorpromazine alone in the treatment of acute schizophrenia. A study (Eccleston *et al*, 1986) of patients undergoing an exacerbation of their psychosis found propranolol to be of equal efficacy to thioridazine in controlling positive symptoms.

The position with regard to lithium is of interest. Initially lithium was thought to be of no value in schizophrenia and that it might enhance neurotoxicity. The next step was to accept that excited or affectively-laden patients could benefit, though this raised the possibility that such patients belonged to the manic-depressive category. However, **Delva and Letemendia** (**1982**) showed that lithium has a definite place in the treatment of schizophrenia and that it is not only affective symptoms that respond. A recent controlled study (Zemlan *et al*, 1984) gives further support to the benefits of lithium in patients with strictly defined schizophrenia of whom up to half may benefit. They suggest that lithium response occurs about one week after therapeutic serum levels are established while Alexander and his co-workers (1979) found improvement in the third week of therapy.

The experimental use of endorphin-related agents has given contradictory results while carbamazepine is in the early stages of evaluation.

Antiparkinsonian medication: The routine prescribing of antiparkinsonian drugs has come under severe criticism in the past decade. They may reduce the antipsychotic efficacy of neuroleptics (Singh and Kay, 1975; Johnstone *et al*, 1983), perhaps by reducing neuroleptic serum levels (Gautier *et al*, 1977), and cause sedation and anticholinergic effects which may summate with similar properties in the neuroleptics. On rare occasions such summation brings about a central cholinergic crisis characterized by a florid atropine-type delirious state (McClelland, 1981), but the antiparkinsonian drugs by themselves can produce confusional states (Stephens, 1967). Benzhexol is probably the most toxic of the antiparkinsonian agents. Potamianos and Kellett (1982) have shown that only 2 mgs can cause psychometric impairment in non-psychiatric, non-demented geriatric patients. Younger schizophrenic patients may develop dependence on benzhexol and other antiparkinsonian medication, the drugs being used to produce 'highs' and also toxic psychoses with intense hallucinations (Kaminer *et al*, 1982; Marriott, 1976; Jellinek, 1977; Crawshaw and Mullen, 1984).

The prescribing of a class of drugs which can produce serious problems can only be justified if there are major benefits. Yet there are studies which have found either that antiparkinsonian drugs are unnecessary in a substantial majority of patients (Klett and Caffey, 1972; Orlov *et al*, 1971) or ineffective in the control of extrapyramidal symptoms (Mindham *et al*, 1972). There is also a widespread view that most patients develop tolerance to the neurological side-effects of neuroleptics and therefore antiparkinsonian drugs may only need to be continued for a few months (Dimascio, 1971).

The case for not prescribing this medication on a routine basis would therefore appear strong (Mindham, 1982). However, the issue may not be as clear-cut as is claimed. Many patients do not develop a tolerance to neuroleptic-induced extrapyramidal reactions, particularly those on depot injections (Ching-Piao *et al*, 1974) and two studies (Rifkin *et al*, 1978; Manos *et al*, 1981) found that withdrawal of antiparkinsonian drugs in a chronic schizophrenic population caused a marked increase in parkinsonism.

The contradictory findings between these studies and those quoted earlier may be a consequence of different dosages of neuroleptics (McClelland, 1976). It is also not sufficiently recognized that these drugs alleviate akathisia (van Putten, 1975) and akinesia (Rifkin *et al*, 1975; van Putten and May, 1978). Johnson (1981), in a study of depressive symptoms in schizophrenic patients, found that some patients improved on orphenadrine and in this subgroup muscular weakness and stiffness was associated with their 'depression'.

It is reasonable to conclude that in the early stages of neuroleptic medication a small dose of an antiparkinsonian agent is justifiable as a prophylactic measure but this can usually be stopped within a few months. The elderly are a particularly vulnerable group as they readily develop extrapyramidal reactions to neuroleptics and also are susceptible to cognitive impairment on antiparkinsonian drugs. In many patients who develop parkinsonism after withdrawal of an antiparkinsonian agent the dose of neuroleptic is often too high and may be reduced or another neuroleptic substituted; if necessary, the antiparkinsonian drug will need to be restarted.

Electroconvulsive treatment: The indiscriminate and prolonged use of ECT in schizophrenia continued well into the neuroleptic era. One careful but non-blind trial (May and Tuma, 1965) had shown ECT to be effective in the short term but the subsequent medical and social reaction probably led to underusage. Nevertheless, a recent survey in Ontario (Shugar *et al*, 1984) showed that ECT was used more widely than generally recognized, though there was little uniformity of application with the treatment being given as frequently to patients with negative symptoms as to those with acute and positive symptoms. The authors found evidence that in acute forms of illness the addition of ECT to medication was associated with more rapid discharge.

In recent years, two double-blind studies using simulated and real ECT (Taylor and Fleminger, 1980; Brandon *et al*, 1985) have confirmed that ECT hastens the recovery process in acute or relapsing schizophrenic patients who are also receiving neuroleptics, although the outcome was similar in the two groups four to six months later.

References

ALEXANDER, P. E., VAN KRAMMEN D. P. & BUNNEY, W. E. (1979) Antipsychotic affects of lithium in schizophrenia. *American Journal of Psychiatry*, **136,** 283–287.

AUBREE, J. C. & LADER, M. H. (1980) High and very high dosage antipsychotics: A critical review. *Journal of Clinical Psychiatry*, **41,** 341–350.

BLEULER, M. (1974) The long-term course of the schizophrenic disorders. *Psychological Medicine*, **4,** 244–254.

—— (1978) *The Schizophrenic Disorders.* New Haven: Yale University Press.

BRANDON, S., COWLEY, P., McDONALD, C., NEVILLE, P., PALMER, R. & WELLSTOOD EASON, S. (1985) The Leicester ECT Trial: results in schizophrenia. *British Journal of Psychiatry*, **146,** 177–183.

BRIDGE, T. P., CANNON, H. E. & WYATT, R. J. (1978) Burned-out schizophrenia: Evidence for age effects on schizophrenic symptomatology. *Journal of Gerontology*, **33,** 835–839.

CHEUNG, H. K. (1981) Schizophrenics fully remitted on neuroleptics for 3–5 years—to stop or continue drugs? *British Journal of Psychiatry*, **138,** 490–494.

CHING-PIAO, C., DIMASCIO, A. & COLE, J. O. (1974) Antiparkinson agents and depot pheno-thiazines. *American Journal of Psychiatry*, **131,** 86–90.

CHOUINARD, G. & JONES, B. D. (1980) Neuroleptic-induced supersensitivity psychosis. *American Journal of Psychiatry*, **137,** 16–21.

CIOMPI, L. (1980) Catamnestic long-term study on the course of life and aging of schizophrenics. *Schizophrenia Bulletin*, **6,** 606–618.

CRAWSHAW, J. A. & MULLEN, P. E. (1984) A study of benzhexol abuse. *British Journal of Psychiatry*, **145,** 300–303.

DAVIS, J. M. (1975) Overview: Maintenance of therapy in psychiatry. *American Journal of Psychiatry*, **132,** 1237–1245.

DELVA, J. J. & LETEMENDIA, F. J. J. (1982) Lithium treatment in schizophrenia and schizo-affective disorders. *British Journal of Psychiatry*, **141,** 387–400.

DIMASCIO, A. (1971) Towards a more rational use of antiparkinson drugs in psychiatry. *Drug Therapy*, **1,** 23–29.

ECCLESTON, D., FAIRBAIRN, A. F., HASSANYEH, F., McCLELLAND, H. A. & STEPHENS, D. A. (1986) The effect of propranolol and thioridazine on positive and negative symptoms of schizophrenia. *British Journal of Psychiatry*, in press.

FALLOON, I., WATT, D. C. & SHEPHERD, M. (1978) A comparative controlled trial of pimozide and fluphenazine decanoate in the continuation therapy of schizophrenia. *Psychological Medicine*, **8,** 59–70.

GAUTIER, J., JUS, A., VILLENEURE, A., JUSS, K., PIRES, P. & VILLENEURE, R. (1977) Influences of the antiparkinsonian drug on the plasma level of neuroleptics. *Biological Psychiatry*, **12,** 389–399.

GIBSON, A. C. (1980) Depot fluphenazine and tardive dyskinesia in an out-patient population. In *Tardive Dyskinesia: Research and Treatment* (eds) W. E. Farn, R. C. Smith, J. M. Davis and E. F. Domino). New York: MTP Press.

GOLDBERG, S. C., SCHOOLER, N. R., HOGARTY, G. E. *et al* (1977) Prediction of relapse in schizo-phrenic patients treated by drugs and social therapy. *Archives of General Psychiatry*, **34,** 171–184.

HARE, E. (1983) Was insanity on the increase? *British Journal of Psychiatry*, **142,** 439–455.

HOGARTY, G. E., SCHOOLER, N. R., ULRICH, R., MUSSARE, F., FERRO, P. & HERRON, E. (1979) Fluphenazine and social therapy in the aftercare of schizophrenic patients. *Archives of General Psychiatry*, **36,** 1283–1294.

HUBER, G., GROSS, G., SCHUTTLER, R. & LINZ, M. (1980) Longitudinal studies of schizophrenic patients. *Schizophrenia Bulletin*, **6,** 592–605.

JELLINEK, T. (1977) Mood elevating effects of trihexyphenidyl and biperidin in individuals taking antipsychotic medication. *Diseases of the Nervous System*, **38**, 353–355.

JESTE, D. V. & WYATT, R. J. (1981) Changing epidemiology of tardive dyskinesia: An overview. *American Journal of Psychiatry*, **138**, 297–309.

JOHNSON, D. A. W. (1979) Further observations on the duration of depot neuroleptic maintenance therapy in schizophrenia. *British Journal of Psychiatry*, **135**, 524–530.

—— (1981) Studies of depressive symptoms in schizophrenia. *British Journal of Psychiatry*, **139**, 89–101.

JOHNSTONE, E. C., CROW, T. J., FERRIER, I. N., FRITH, D. C., OWENS, G. C. O., BOURNE, R. C. & GAMBLE, S. G. (1983) Adverse effects of anticholinergic medication on positive schizophrenic symptoms. *Psychological Medicine*, **13**, 513–527.

KAMINER, Y., MUNITZ, H. & WISSENBECK, J. (1982) Trihexyphenidyl (Artane) abuse: euphoriant and anxiolytic. *British Journal of Psychiatry*, **140**, 473–474.

KANE, J. M. (1983) Low dose medication strategies in the maintenance treatment of schizophrenia. *Schizophrenia Bulletin*, **9**, 528–532.

KLETT, C. J. & CAFFEY, E. (1972) Evaluating the long-term need for antiparkinson drugs by chronic schizophrenics. *Archives of General Psychiatry*, **26**, 374–379.

LEFF, J. P. & VAUGHN, C. (1981) The role of maintenance therapy and relatives' expressed emotion in relapse of schizophrenia: A two-year follow-up. *British Journal of Psychiatry*, **139**, 102–104.

—— & WING, J. K. (1971) Trial of maintenance therapy in schizophrenia. *British Medical Journal*, *iii*, 559–604.

LETEMENDIA, F. J. J. & HARRIS, A. D. (1967) Chlorpromazine and the untreated chronic schizophrenic: A long-term trial. *British Journal of Psychiatry*, **113**, 950–958.

McCLELLAND, H. A. (1976) Discussion on assessment of drug-induced extrapyramidal reactions. *British Journal of Clinical Pharmacology*, **3**, Supplement 2, 401–403.

—— FARQUHARSON, R. G., LEYBURN, P. & SCHIFF, A. (1976) Very high dose fluphenazine decanoate: A controlled trial in chronic schizophrenia. *Archives of General Psychiatry*, **33**, 1435–1439.

—— (1981) Psychiatric disorders. In *Textbook of Adverse Drug Reactions* (ed. D. Davies). Oxford: Oxford University Press.

MACKAY, A. V. P. & SHEPPARD, G. P. (1979) Pharmacotherapeutic trials in tardive dyskinesia. *British Journal of Psychiatry*, **135**, 489–499.

MANOS, N., GKIOUZEPAS, J. & LOGOTHETIS, J. (1981) The need for continuous use of antiparkinson medication with chronic schizophrenic patients using long term neuroleptic therapy. *American Journal of Psychiatry*, **138**, 184–188.

MARRIOTT, P. (1976) Dependency on antiparkinsonian drugs. *British Medical Journal*, *i*, 152.

MAY, P. R. A. & TUMA, A. H. (1965) Treatment of schizophrenia: An experimental study of five treatment methods. *British Journal of Psychiatry*, **111**, 503–510.

MINDHAM, R. H. S., GAIND, R. H., ANSTEE, B. H. & RIMMER, L. (1972) Comparison of amantidine, orphenadrine and placebo in the control of phenothiazine induced parkinsonism. *Psychological Medicine*, **2**, 406–413.

—— (1982) Antiparkinson drugs and depot neuroleptics. *British Journal of Psychiatry*, **141**, 211–214.

MOLLER, L. & SILVERTON, L. (1984) Cerebral ventricular size in the offspring of schizophrenic mothers. *Archives of General Psychiatry*, **41**, 602–606.

MYERS, D. H., CAMPBELL, P. L., COCKS, N. M., FLOWERDEW, J. A. & MUIR, A. (1981) A trial of propranolol in chronic schizophrenia. *British Journal of Psychiatry*, **139**, 118–121.

ORLOV, P., KOSPORIAS, G., DIMASCIO, A. & COLE, J. O. (1971) Withdrawal of antiparkinson drugs. *Archives of General Psychiatry*, **25**, 410–412.

OWENS, D. G. C., JOHNSTONE, E. & FIRTH, C. D. (1982) Spontaneous involuntary disorders of movement. *Archives of General Psychiatry*, **39**, 452–461.

PEET, M., MIDDLEMISS, D. N. & YATES, R. A. (1981) Propranolol in schizophrenia: II. Clinical and biochemical aspects of combining propranolol with chlorpromazine. *British Journal of Psychiatry*, **139**, 112–117.

—— BETHELL, M. S., COATES, A., KHAMNEE, A. K., HALL, P., COOPER, S. J., KING, D. J. & YATES, R. A. (1981a) Propranolol in schizophrenia: I. Comparison of propranolol, chlorpromazine and placebo. *British Journal of Psychiatry*, **139**, 105–111.

PFOHL, B. & WINOKUR, G. (1982) *Schizophrenia: Course and Outcome in Schizophrenia as a Brain Disease* (eds. F. A. Henn and H. A. Nashrallah). New York: Oxford University Press.

POTAMIANOS, G. & KELLETT, J. M. (1982) Anticholinergic drugs and memory: the effects of benzhexol on memory in a group of geriatric patients. *British Journal of Psychiatry*, **140**, 470–472.

PRITCHARD, M. (1967) Prognosis of schizophrenia before and after pharmacotherapy. *British Journal of Psychiatry*, **113**, 1345–1359.

RIFKIN, A., QUITKIN, F., RABINER, C. J. & KLEIN, D. F. (1977) Fluphenazine decanoate, fluphenazine hydrochloride given orally, and placebo in remitted schizophrenics. *Archives of General Psychiatry*, **34**, 43–47.

—— —— & KLEIN, D. F. (1975) Akinesia: a poorly recognised drug-induced extrapyramidal behaviour disorder. *Archives of General Psychiatry*, **32**, 672–674.

—— —— KANE, J., STRURE, F. & KLEINE, D. F. (1978) Are prophylactic antiparkinson drugs necessary? *Archives of General Psychiatry*, **35**, 483–489.

SCHOOLER, N. R., LEVINE, J., SEVERE, J. B., BRAUZER, B., DIMASCIO, A., KLERMAN, G. L. & TUASON, V. N. (1980) Prevention of relapse in schizophrenia. *Archives of General Psychiatry*, **37**, 16–24.

SCHULSINGER, F., PARNAS, J., PETERSEN, E. T., SCHULSINGER, H., TEASDALE, T. W., SARNOFF, A., MEDNICK, A., MOLLER, L. & SILVERTON, L. (1984) Cerebral ventricular size in the offspring of schizophrenic mothers. *Archives of General Psychiatry*, **41**, 602–606.

SHUGAR, G., HOFFMAN, B. F. & JOHNSTON, J. D. (1984) Electroconvulsive therapy for schizophrenia in Ontario: A report on therapeutic polymorphism. *Comprehensive Psychiatry*, **25**, 509–520.

SINGH, M. M. & KAY, S. R. (1975) Therapeutic reversal with benztropine in schizophrenics. *Journal of Nervous and Mental Disease*, **160**, 258–266.

STEPHENS, D. A. (1967) Psychotoxic effects of benzhexol hydrochlorine (Artane). *British Journal of Psychiatry*, **113**, 213–218.

TAYLOR, P. J. & FLEMINGER, J. J. (1980) ECT for schizophrenia. *Lancet*, i, 1380–1382.

VAN PUTTEN, T. (1974) Why do schizophrenic patients refuse to take their drugs? *Archives of General Psychiatry*, **31**, 67–72.

—— (1975) The many faces of akathisia. *Comprehensive Psychiatry*, **16**, 43–47.

—— & MAY, P. R. (1978) Akinetic depression in schizophrenia. *Archives of General Psychiatry*, **35**, 1101–1107.

VAUGHN, C. E. & LEFF, J. P. (1976) The influence of family and social factors on the course of psychiatric illness. *British Journal of Psychiatry*, **129**, 125–137.

WING, J. K. & BROWN, G. W. (1970) *Institutionalism and Schizophrenia*. Cambridge: Cambridge University Press.

YORKSTON, N. J., ZAKI, S. A., WELLER, M. P., GRUZELIER, J. H. & HIRSCH, S. R. (1981) DL-propranolol and chlorpromazine following admission for schizophrenia: A controlled comparison. *Acta Psychiatria Scandinavica*, **67**, 13–27.

ZEMLAN, F. B., HIRSCHOWITZ, J., SAUTTER, F. J. & GARVEY, D. L. (1984) Impact of lithium therapy in core psychotic symptoms in schizophrenia. *British Journal of Psychiatry*, **144**, 64–69.

38 Further observations on the duration of depot neuroleptic maintenance therapy in schizophrenia

D. A. W. JOHNSON

It is now the usual practice to prescribe neuroleptic drugs, most commonly in the form of long-acting injections, for long periods following an acute schizophrenic illness. Although it is generally accepted that approximately two-thirds of schizophrenic patients with a second or subsequent illness remain free from relapse with regular maintenance therapy (Leff and Wing, 1971; Hirsch et al, 1973; Hogarty et al, 1974; Johnson, 1976a), there is little information on how long regular medication should be continued with the expectation of therapeutic benefit to the patient. The risk of the unwanted side-effects, i.e. extrapyramidal symptoms (McClelland et al, 1974; Mindham, 1976; Johnson, 1978), tardive dyskinesia (Gibson, 1978) and weight gain (Johnson and Breen, 1979) emphasizes the need to maintain patients on the lowest dose, for the shortest possible time that is compatible with the patient's clinical progress.

A review of discontinuation studies of oral medication by Hogarty et al (1976) suggested that maintenance phenothiazine therapy is required for at least two years, with their own results suggesting a longer period. The samples studied were exclusively chronic patients. The only study on patients treated within the community with long-acting injections suggested the need for continued medication for a minimum of three years following the most recent relapse (Johnson, 1976b).

The need for further information upon which to base guidance for both the likely minimum duration of maintenance therapy, and the possibility of using 'drug holidays' to reduce the risk of long term side-effects, has prompted the author to report an extension of the results of an earlier study (Johnson, 1976b) in addition to a comprehensive follow-up of all schizophrenic patients discontinuing depot injections at his present hospital (University Hospital of South Manchester). The outcome has been further analysed to investigate any differences between the depot injections used.

The study

Two samples have been studied:

Sample 1: This is an extension of an earlier study (Johnson, 1976b) and has been collected over a thirteen-year period.

All patients were diagnosed as suffering from schizophrenia on the basis of Schneiderian first rank symptoms being present at some time during their mental illness, and had experienced two or more acute episodes. All patients were under continuous assessment as part of ongoing research and had been free from clinical relapse for a minimum period of twelve months on regular maintenance therapy with long-acting neuroleptic injections. The decision to discontinue medication was made by the patient alone, or by the patient on the advice of a relative or rarely by another medical practitioner. Following the discontinuance of depot medication, the patients were followed up prospectively for a period of six months, with regular mental state examinations (Johnson, 1976b). Patients were only accepted into the study if they were in a steady mental state at the time of their decision to discontinue depot injections.

A control sample corrected for age, sex and duration of illness, but remaining on regular depot injections, was selected from the same clinic register.

Sample 2: The depot injection clinic of the Department of Psychiatry at UHSM has been functioning for eight years. All patients with the diagnosis of schizophrenia who had been successfully maintained on regular depot injections for a minimum of three months, and who had had their medication subsequently discontinued by the psychiatrist, were surveyed. In each case the diagnosis of schizophrenia had been confirmed by the teaching hospital consultant concerned and was the sole diagnosis throughout treatment.

The history and progress of each patient before discontinuance of medication was from hospital records alone, but progress after discontinuance was determined from records, personal interview, contact with relatives, family doctor or social worker as appropriate. Relapse means a significant deterioration in mental state with the appearance of new symptoms requiring a change of management.

The next patient of the same consultant, of the same sex and similar age on the same depot injection, was selected as a control group for comparison of outcome.

Sample 1: The patients have been divided into three groups. Group A discontinued injections after 12–24 months (mean 19 months) on regular injections free from relapse; Group B after 24–36 months (mean 29 months); Group C after 36–48 months (mean 42 months). Satisfactory controls were found for Groups A and B, but for Group C controls could be matched only for age and sex. A total of 56 patients have been studied, 41 on fluphenazine and 15 on flupenthixol.

The results showed an increased risk of relapse for all groups discontinuing maintenance injections, relative to their controls remaining on regular injections. The difference reaches a level of significance for Groups A and B (P <0.01), but although the same trend continues for Group C, it just fails to reach a level of significance, possibly because of the small numbers involved.

Sixty-eight per cent of patients who relapsed having discontinued medication responded to resumed medication within a six-week period. In the control group, only 40 per cent showed improvement within the same period. Since the effect of medication alone can be judged more accurately when the patient's environment remains unaltered, the relative proportions responding within the same community environment have been analysed. In this comparison,

45 per cent of patients discontinuing injections responded to resumed drugs, compared to 20 per cent of controls who improved with increased medication.

The overall relapse rates of each of the first three months following discontinuation of medication showed that at the end of two months there is a marked trend for the relapse risks of those patients discontinuing medication to have exceeded the risks of those remaining on medication. At the end of three months, the difference in risks was statistically significant.

Within the limitations of the small numbers involved, no differences could be demonstrated between the drugs prescribed (fluphenazine and flupenthixol).

Sample 2: Out of 609 patients maintained on long-acting injections for a minimum period of three months within the community, 123 had their injections discontinued at some time. Thirty-two patients were excluded from the follow-up survey (incomplete records = 9; original diagnosis not schizophrenia = 5; change of diagnosis = 14; died on regular medication = 3; suicide two weeks after discontinuing medication = 1). The remaining 91 patients were followed up either until their next relapse or, if free from relapse, for a maximum period of four years.

All patients had been treated with either flupenthixol decanoate (n = 49) or fluphenazine decanoate (n = 42). The proportion of patients relapsing within the survey period and the distribution of relapse within the first, second, and subsequent two years is shown in Table I. The results for first illness schizophrenia and chronic schizophrenia (second or subsequent illness) are analysed separately. Almost all chronic schizophrenic patients treated within the hospital were prescribed long-acting depot injections (over 90 per cent within any one year analysed), but only 60 per cent of patients with a first illness were prescribed depot injections.

For the chronic schizophrenic patient, the relapse rate was 76 per cent within the first four years following discontinuation of medication. The majority of chronic patients destined to relapse within this period did so within the first year (60 per cent), only a further 11 per cent relapsed in the second year, and 2–4 per cent in the third and fourth years.

The relapse rates for first illness schizophrenia are also shown in Table I. The absolute rate of relapse must be interpreted with caution since, although

TABLE I

Sample 2: Relapse following discontinuance of depot injections and comparison with control group for chronic patients (percentages)

	All patients (n = 91)	1st illness (n = 20)	Chronic (n = 71)	Controls (chronic) (n = 87)
Relapse in 1 year	51	29	60	21
Relapse in 2 years	59	32	71	36
Total relapse (max. 4 years)	66	43	76	43

the majority of first illness schizophrenic patients were prescribed depot injections (60 per cent), it is not a fully comprehensive sample. It is likely that fewer 'good prognosis' patients were included in the sample and the inclusion of these omissions would, in all likelihood, have emphasized the differences of first illness schizophrenia shown, rather than have changed any trend demonstrated. It is clear that the overall prognosis at four years is substantially better for a first illness, with a risk of relapse little more than half that of a chronic illness. There is also an important difference in the intervals before relapse. The majority of relapses take place within the first year (29 per cent), but thereafter, unlike chronic schizophrenia, the relapse rates remain fairly constant (3–6 per cent) over the next three years.

Next, the results were analysed to examine any possible influence that the duration of medication prior to discontinuance could have upon either the ultimate relapse rate or the interval before relapse. For chronic schizophrenia, there was no difference in the expectation of survival at six months, one year or two years after discontinuation. For a first schizophrenic illness, there was a very substantial trend for patients who had received depot maintenance therapy for a minimum of twelve months to have a better survival rate at the end of both the first and second years of follow-up.

The proportion of chronic schizophrenic patients relapsing at the end of each month, for the first three months following discontinuation of medication was also examined. At the end of two months, there was a marked trend for the discontinuance group to have a higher risk of relapse; by the end of the third month this difference was highly significant. There is a trend for patients who have been on regular medication for more than two years to remain well longer for the first four months following discontinuation. However, these differences do not reach levels of statistical significance and the numbers involved are small.

To test the accuracy of the clinician's expectation of prognosis for individual patients, the records were analysed of 39 patients where it was specifically recorded that discontinuance was prescribed in the expectation of a good outcome. Within the limits of the small numbers involved, no trends could be demonstrated that differed from overall results of the chronic schizophrenic sample.

No differences or trends could be detected in patients treated with the two depot drugs used.

Within the control group, four of the selected patients were suffering from a first illness, so only the results of the 87 chronic patients are reported (Table I). All the controls have a minimum two-year follow-up, but only a minority have four years. The total relapse rate at any point sampled is substantially less (35–57 per cent) than the rate for patients discontinuing drugs. The distribution of relapse is also different, with the most important difference occurring within the first twelve months.

Comment

The results of both surveys of chronic schizophrenia clearly demonstrate that the risk of a further relapse following drug discontinuance within a four-year period of a previous relapse is substantially higher than that when remaining on regular drug therapy. The risk of relapse within the first twelve months following discontinuation, when the effect of drug withdrawal is likely to be most obvious, is three times as high as that of controls. Even after an interval of four years off drugs, the risk is twice as high. The importance of maintenance therapy in patients initially controlled by drugs is emphasized by the response to drugs, particularly in the same community environment, within a six-week period.

The distribution of relapse, when it occurs, is also clinically important for both service and research considerations. Without drugs, the greatest risk is within the first twelve months (60 per cent), much less during the second year (11 per cent), and then remains fairly constant at an even lower rate for the next two years (2–3 per cent). In contrast, in both surveys, the risk of relapse for patients remaining on drugs during the first and second years is very little different (15–20 per cent), but again during the third and fourth years is much lower (3–4 per cent). These results confirm earlier observations in a different patient population (Johnson, 1979) which emphasized that the shape of survival curves, even more than absolute relapse rates, demonstrated the therapeutic gain of maintenance therapy. These earlier studies also showed that after two years without relapse, whatever the treatment (depot injections, oral medication or even no medication), the prognosis was substantially improved, with a low rate of overt relapse. This trend is important as it would be illogical to change treatments, even to a theoretically more efficient one, after this period of survival. Equally, unless this trend is taken into consideration in research methodology, results are likely to have an increased risk of false negative results in comparisons between drugs, and give unrealistically high expectations of outcome in prognostic studies. In this particular survey, the postponement of the maximum risk of relapse, in addition to a much lower final relapse rate, would again suggest confirmation of the need for drugs to be continued.

The analysis of duration on drugs before discontinuance, and the outcome both in terms of relapse and distribution of relapse, suggest that there is no significant change of outcome with increasing duration of treatment within the four-year period. This must suggest that drugs are doing no more than suppressing symptoms, and that if drugs given for four years do not alter the relapse pattern for the successive four years, then maintenance is likely to be required for a much longer period. It must not be overlooked that in suppressing primary symptoms, the treatment may be having much wider beneficial effects, in that it may prevent secondary handicaps.

The possibility of using 'drug holidays' to reduce the risk of long-term side-effects has been considered. Overall, the results suggest that as early as two months following drug discontinuation, a trend is developing for patients without drugs to be at a higher risk. At three months, this risk is statistically significant in comparisons with both control groups and an earlier prognostic study (1976a). There is a slight trend for patients who have been on drugs more than two years to have a slightly reduced rate of relapse during the first four months, but this never reaches significant levels and has vanished by the sixth month. It would seem unwise to consider drug holidays of more than three months within the first four years of treatment, and there is no indication that there would be a diminution of the risk of relapse associated with longer drug holidays even after this interval. It would seem unlikely after such a short drug holiday, particularly after an extended period on drugs, that there has been an opportunity for all the pharmacological effects of the drugs to be reversed, since the development of secondary depots may extend the direct exposure of neurological receptors to drug action. However, adequately controlled studies need to be conducted to investigate the possibility.

A consideration of the results of first illness schizophrenia suggests important differences from chronic schizophrenia. The generally accepted better initial prognosis for a first illness is confirmed, but the pattern of relapse shown suggests that relapses continue at a steady rate throughout the second, third and fourth years of follow-up. This must emphasize the need for a fairly lengthy period of follow-up for any study investigating outcome. The longer the duration of the study, the more the relative differences between first illness and chronic schizophrenia may diminish. The exclusion of some good prognosis patients may have led to an overestimation of relapse, but their exclusion would be unlikely to influence the trend in the distribution of relapse. A second potentially important trend that has been demonstrated is for first illness patients prescribed regular medication for a minimum of twelve months to have a better prognosis over a two-year period. However, the number of patients involved was small and again this possibility needs further clarification.

The agreement between the results of the two samples studied is particulary important. In addition to possible differences in the criteria of diagnosis, the decision to discontinue medication was made by the patient in the first sample, and in the second sample substantially by the psychiatrist. It made no difference to the results when a subgroup of patients selected for their anticipated good outcome was analysed separately. This is contrary to some opinions, but the analysis of individual items or symptoms in previous studies has never allowed the author successfully to identify good prognosis patients amongst an epidemiologically based or catchment-area based samples treated within the community. Possibly, this reflects the wide range of dependent variables involved other than drugs.

Perhaps the most important indication that regular medication is required is a consideration of the future treatment of patients discontinued from established maintenance therapy. It is known that 85 per cent of the discontinued group of chronic schizophrenics were subsequently prescribed further maintenance drug therapy, and that this proportion rises to 92 per cent if restricted to those patients with long-term follow-up.

Within the limitations of the assessments made, no differences could be detected between fluphenazine decanoate or flupenthixol decanoate in the control of either acute symptoms or overt relapse.

In the absence of any clear indication that drugs can be discontinued, after even lengthy periods of four years or more, the emphasis must remain on the proper use of the long-acting neuroleptics with minimal doses. Prescriptions should be personalized, and the dose reduced with time, particularly over the first two years. The development of extrapyramidal side-effects should also be treated by dose reduction or prescription modification whenever possible (Johnson, 1977, 1978).

References

GIBSON, A. C. (1978) Depot injections and tardive dyskinesia. *British Journal of Psychiatry*, **132**, 361–365.

HIRSCH, S. R., GAIND, R., RHODE, P. D., STEVENS, B. C. & WING, J. K. (1973) Out-patient maintenance of chronic schizophrenic patients with long acting phenothiazine. *British Medical Journal*, i, 633–637.

HOGARTY, G. E., GOLDBERG, S. C., SCHOOLER, N. R., ULRICH, R. F. AND THE COLLABORATIVE STUDY GROUP (1974) Drug and sociotherapy in the aftercare of schizophrenic patients. *Archives of General Psychiatry*, **31**, 603–608.

—— ULRICH, R., MUSSARE, F. & ARISTIGUETA, N. (1976) Drug discontinuation among long term successfully maintained schizophrenic out-patients. *Diseases of the Nervous System*, **57**, 494–500.

JOHNSON, D. A. W. (1976a) The expectation of outcome from maintenance therapy in chronic schizophrenic patients. *British Journal of Psychiatry*, **128**, 246–250.

—— (1976b) The duration of maintenance therapy in chronic schizophrenia. *Acta Psychiatrica Scandinavia*, **53**, 298–301.

—— (1977) Practical considerations in the use of depot neuroleptics for the treatment of schizophrenia. *British Journal of Hospital Medicine*, **17**, 546–559.

—— (1978) The prevalence and treatment of drug induced extrapyramidal symptoms. *British Journal of Psychiatry*, **132**, 27–30.

—— BREEN, M. (1979) Weight changes with depot neuroleptic maintenance therapy. *Acta Psychiatrica Scandinavica*, **59**, 525–528.

—— (1979) Clinical considerations in the use of depot neuroleptics for the treatment of schizophrenia. In *Management of Schizophrenia: Biological and Sociological Aspects* (Ed. by H. M. van Praag). Utrecht: Van Gorcum.

LEFF, J. P. & WING, J. K. (1971) Trial of maintenance therapy in schizophrenia. *British Medical Journal*, iii, 559–604.

McCLELLAND, H. A., BLESSED, G., BHATE, S., ALI, N. & CLARKE, P. A. (1974) The abrupt withdrawal of antiparkinson drugs in schizophrenic patients. *British Journal of Psychiatry*, **124**, 151–159.

MINDHAM, R. H. S. (1976) Assessment of drug induced extrapyramidal reactions. *British Journal of Clinical Pharmacology*, Supplement 3, 395–400.

39 Lithium treatment in schizophrenia and schizoaffective disorders

N. J. DELVA and F. J. J. LETEMENDIA

The use of lithium in the treatment of schizophrenia was first reported by Cade (1949). In the initial series he treated six patients with dementia praecox, and stated that 'although there was no fundamental improvement in any of them, three who were usually restless, noisy and shouting nonsensical abuse ... lost their excitement and restlessness and became quiet and amenable for the first time in years ... They reverted to their previous state upon cessation of lithium medication.' Since then over twenty clinical studies evaluating the use of lithium in schizophrenia have been published. These are reviewed in Part I below. At least thirty clinical studies have been published on lithium treatment in the group of disorders which includes schizoaffective (SA) illness, atypical manic-depressive illness, mixed psychosis, cycloid psychosis, and schizophreniform psychosis. These disorders are reviewed in Part II; this describes a group rather than a diagnostic category.

I. Lithium treatment in schizophrenia

Four of the 24 articles reviewed were controlled studies. These four, plus 11 uncontrolled studies which gave information about individual patients, are listed in Table I.

It can be seen that approximately half of the schizophrenic patients treated with lithium were reported as showing improvement. In these patients there was no report of clinical deterioration. It might be objected that excited schizophrenics, and schizophrenics with affective overlay are really schizoaffective patients, but even if these patients in the first four reports (Glesinger, Rice, White and Blinder) are excluded from the calculation, 45 out of 111 still show improvement.

This generally favourable therapeutic impression differs from the current view expressed in some widely used textbooks and specialized monographs. In the *Comprehensive Textbook of Psychiatry* (3rd edition—1980), Fieve states that lithium 'seems to be of minimal or no value against agitations of schizophrenic, neurotic, or organic origin. It may, however, be of value in a limited number of schizoaffective psychoses with a moderate to marked elation component. Although it has no effect on schizophrenic hallucinations, delusions, or paranoid thinking, it may remove the affective overlay.' Two articles are reviewed by Watanabe and Ishino in Chapter V of the 1980 *Handbook of Lithium*

TABLE I
Lithium treatment in schizophrenic patients

Author	Year	Diagnosis of patients	Study			Number of patients	Results			
			Criteria	Con-trolled	Blind		Re-covered	Im-proved	Same	Worse
Cade	1949	Dementia praecox	0	0	0	6		3	3	
Glesinger	1954	Excited schizophrenics	0	0	0	39		31	8	
		Hebephrenics	0	0	0	12		9	3	
Rice	1956	Schizophrenia with affective overlay	0	0	0	4	1	2	1	
		Schizophrenia	0	0	0	12		3	9	
White	1966	Schizophrenia with excitement	0	0	0	1			1	
Blinder	1968	Schizophrenia with psychotic excitement	0	0	0	2		2		
Gottfries	1969	Chronic schizophrenia with normal activity level	0		0	10			10	
Sikes	1970	Undifferentiated schizophrenia	0	0	0	1			1	
		Paranoid schizophrenia	0	0	0	3		2	1	
Tupin	1973	Schizophrenia and possible schizophrenia	0	0	0	12		7 (est)	5 (est)	
Small	1975	Catatonic schizophrenia	+	+	+	5		2	3	
		Paranoid schizophrenia	+	+	+	2		1	1	
		Hebephrenic schizophrenia	+	+	+	6		3	3	
Van Putten	1975	Schizophrenia	0	0	0	11		5	6	
Taheri	1976	Chronic schizophrenia	0	0	0	4		4		
Alexander	1979	Schizophrenia	+	+	+	5		2	3	
Glick	1980	Schizophrenia	+	0	0	3		3		
Hirschowitz	1980	Schizophrenia and schizophrenia with depression	+	0	0	19		1	18	
Total (%)						157 (100%)		80 (51%)	76 (48%)	

Criteria not specified 0, specified +.

Therapy, and their conclusion is that 'the effects of lithium in the treatment of schizophrenics are still controversial and further studies are required.' In the same book (Ch. X), Spring writes that 'no research or clinical data support the use of lithium with schizophrenics. In fact, it is possible that lithium worsens schizophrenic symptomatology.' According to Gerbino *et al* in *Psychopharmacology: A Generation of Progress* (1978), 'although some studies have seemed to indicate a therapeutic value for lithium in schizophrenia, other studies have reported conflicting results and have even warned of a possible detrimental effect of lithium in schizophrenic patients ... The most that can be said is that there may be a subgroup of schizophrenics who can benefit from lithium therapy, but that this subgroup, if it does exist, still needs to be defined.' Eight papers, including five on schizoaffective illness, are reviewed in that book. In the *Primer of Lithium Therapy* (1977), Jefferson and Greist state that 'it is generally felt that patients with schizophrenia are unlikely to respond positively to lithium, may deteriorate on lithium, and may be predisposed to developing lithium toxicity.' In their view, whether certain schizophrenic patients might benefit from lithium treatment requires further inquiry.

Controlled studies

Some of the papers included in this section will also be discussed again in Part II because patients of several diagnoses have been mentioned in the one paper.

(a) Shopsin *et al* (1971) published the first controlled study of lithium versus chlorpromazine in acute schizophrenics. The 21 'newly hospitalized acute schizophrenics' were diagnosed by two psychiatrists. Two were suffering their first attack; 19 exhibited an exacerbation of chronic illness. The diagnostic subtypes included chronic undifferentiated type manifesting acute decompensation (9), paranoid type (8), and schizoaffective type (4). Affective symptoms were present in 14 patients. After a placebo baseline of one week, there was a three-week period of active medication (with random allocation to either lithium or chlorpromazine), followed by a second placebo period of seven days. Three to four identical capsules containing 100 mg of chlorpromazine or 250 mg of lithium carbonate were given daily and increased until a therapeutic response or side effects appeared. Maximum dosage was fixed at twelve capsules daily or achievement of 1.5 mEq/l serum lithium. The following measurements were used: Clinical Global Inventory (CGI), Brief Psychiatric Rating Scale (BPRS), Inpatient Multidimensional Psychiatric Scale (IMPS) Structured Clinical Interview (SCI), Nurse's Observation Scale for In-Patient Evaluation (NOSIE) and Self Rating Symptom Scale (SRSS).

This paper shows that although chlorpromazine may well be superior to lithium in the treatment of acute schizophrenia, as it is in acute manic patients who are highly active (Prien *et al*, 1972b), it cannot be concluded that lithium is of no value nor that there is any particular danger of neurotoxicity if lithium is used at the usual prophylactic level. There is little evidence of the alleged neurotoxicity though their experimental design favours its development.

(b) The second controlled study, this time double blind, was reported by Small *et al* (1975). Chronic schizophrenic patients meeting the diagnostic criteria of Feighner *et al* were treated in a cross-over design with lithium or placebo. Of the 22 patients, eight satisfied Feighner's criteria for schizophrenia (except for the criterion, lack of sufficient depressive or manic symptoms for a diagnosis of affective disorder) and affective disorder. All had failed to respond to various repeated treatments. They were stabilized on the optimum dosage of the neuroleptic drug known to give maximal improvement and/or best tolerance. Antiparkinsonian medication was used if necessary. They were then treated during periods of four weeks with lithium (plasma level of 0.6–1.0 mEq/l) or placebo, with three cross-overs. Premature cross-overs (17 cases) were implemented if there was clinical deterioration (11 patients) or toxicity (one patient).

Comparison of the periods on lithium with those on placebo showed a significant superiority for lithium over placebo on all rating scales (BPRS, CGI, NOSIE, and Manic State Rating Scale (MSRS)). Tests designed to show neurotoxicity (Shipley-Hartford Vocabulary Test, Digit Symbol Sub-Test of the Wechsler Adult Intelligence Scale, the Lubin Adjective Checklist, and Trials A and B of the Halstead-Reitan-Wepman Neuropsychological battery) failed to show any evidence of neurotoxicity or impaired mental functioning with lithium.

The conclusion was that 'a trial of lithium combined with psychotropic drugs is warranted in schizophrenic patients who do not respond to major tranquilizing drugs alone.'

(c) Growe *et al* (1979) published a controlled and double-blind study on eight patients with the same design as Small *et al* but using only the Psychotic In-patient Profile (PIP) to evaluate change. Six patients met Research Diagnostic Criteria (RDC) (Spitzer *et al*, 1975) for schizophrenia and two for schizoaffective schizophrenia. Patients were admitted to the study if they 'failed to respond significantly to medication'.

Neuroleptic medication was maintained at constant dosage throughout the trial. Serum lithium levels were maintained between 0.5 and 1.0 mEq/l. The patients were analysed together. Of the eight subscales of the PIP there was statistically significant improvement in only one, psychotic excitement, lithium being superior to placebo. There were trends towards reduced seclusiveness and retardation while patients were on therapeutic levels of lithium. No patient showed serious lithium toxicity.

(d) Alexander *et al* (1979) reported a controlled, double-blind study comparing lithium with placebo in five schizophrenic and eight schizoaffective patients (Research Diagnostic Criteria). Patients were on placebo for one week, lithium for three and finally placebo for two weeks. No other medication was used. Nursing staff rated patients blindly on the Bunney-Hamburg Global Rating Scale. Two of the five schizophrenic and five of the eight schizoaffective patients responded favourably, i.e. a mean rating improvement of at least 1.5 points during the third week on lithium. Four of the responders relapsed within two weeks after lithium withdrawal; one was schizophrenic and three schizoaffective. No patient developed neurotoxicity (serum levels during week three of lithium administration were 0.7 to 1.2 mEq/l, with a mean of 0.9), nor was there aggravation of symptoms with lithium. The responders were analysed as a group, the improvement seen with lithium was modest and in no case was there a complete remission. Responders were similar to non-responders on all other criteria including age of onset, prognostic scales and symptoms of schizophrenia.

The authors concluded that lithium had antipsychotic as well as antimanic and anti-depressant properties. This article was followed by criticism from Gardner and Staton (1979), and also from Solomon (1979), that conclusions based on a group of responders constituted mostly by schizoaffective patients should not lead to conclusions about the response of schizophrenic patients to lithium. In spite of this criticism it remains that two out of five patients with schizophrenia by RDC (by DSM II, one was catatonic, the other paranoid schizophrenic) responded while on lithium, and one of these relapsed within two weeks of withdrawal.

Uncontrolled studies

These will be discussed only when special claims are made, as most have been summarized in the table.

Noack and Trautner (1951) found that 'whilst excited schizophrenics were temporarily quietened, there was no effect on the underlying thought disorder.' Glesinger's (1954) excited schizophrenic and hebephrenic patients responded better to lithium than did his manic depressive or recurrent manic patients. He found that 'all kinds of manifestations were beneficially influenced, from hostility to hypochondria, and from ideas of persecution to obsession. Restlessness, confusion, irrationality, hyperactivity, agitations, hallucinations, delusions, impulsive actions and garrulity were the manifestations most relieved.' Rice (1956) concluded that 'in those patients where the illness has been a mixed psychosis (SA disorder), or where there has been a marked affective element, it is this affective element which has been so noticeably improved.'

Gershon and Yuwiler (1960) gave the first review of the literature. They gathered a total of 269 patients from various papers, including the 73 patients in the papers by Cade, Glesinger and Rice. The remainder of the patients in uncontrolled studies were in papers ·difficult to obtain and hence were excluded from this review. Gershon and Yuwiler's 60 per cent improvement rate for schizophrenia compares with an 84 per cent improvement rate for mania. The improvement in the majority of the schizophrenic patients was 'limited to decreased psychomotor activity and not to improvement of the basic condition.' They add that 'it is very unlikely that lithium treatment has any specific therapeutic effect on the schizophrenic process itself. Certainly, lithium given to chronic, hospitalized schizophrenics with excitement, gross overactivity and/or disturbed behaviour is effective in controlling these symptoms but does not affect the underlying process. In acute schizophrenic excitements, however, lithium administration results in control of the psychomotor overactivity and behavioural disturbances and in addition often produces complete disappearance of all symptoms.'

Blinder (1968) treated two schizophrenic patients with psychomotor excitement and found that the 'thought disorder persisted but without the affective component.' It is not mentioned whether the patients were also receiving neuroleptics. Serry (1969) reported 18 schizophrenic patients treated with lithium. Fifteen were (high) lithium excretors, two intermediate, and one a lithium retainer. Although he did not discuss the therapeutic outcome, he stated:

'lithium excreting schizophrenic patients seem to show no response to lithium'. He discussed the SA patients treated but the reader is left wondering about the three schizophrenic patients in the intermediate and lithium retainer groups. Gottfries (1969) measured movements in the upper and lower limbs to record the activity level in various psychiatric disorders. He separated schizophrenic patients into 'psychosis schizoaffectiva (with disturbed activity level)' and 'psychosis schizophrenia'. The 10 schizophrenic patients had a normal activity level and showed no change with lithium.

Meiers (1970) reported on a group of 19 schizophrenic patients who 'received significant help from adding lithium carbonate to their treatment'. Unfortunately, there is no mention of other patients treated without success. Of the four cases described, two seem to us to be manic depressive, and in another there is no good evidence for a diagnosis of schizophrenia. Sikes and Sikes (1970) reported on 10 patients with 'schizophrenic reactions'. Two of the three patients with paranoid schizophrenia showed a 'very good response' (criteria for improvement are specified). The SA and 'mixed' patients are discussed in Part II. The paranoid subgroup showed the best response to lithium.

Tupin *et al* (1973) reported on the long-term use of lithium in aggressive prisoners. Their 27 patients, already on neuroleptics, included eight with schizophrenia and four with possible schizophrenia. These drugs were not effective in controlling violent behaviour; 'however, for those subjects who were schizophrenic there was some control of the usual schizophrenic symptomatology.' The patients were also on anticonvulsant and antidepressant drugs. Fourteen showed substantial improvement on a global rating scale, seven minimal, and two were not changed or worse (no data on four). Although the schizophrenic patients were not discussed separately, it was stated that psychiatric diagnosis was not related to outcome. Estimates have therefore been made in the entry in Table I.

Cade (1978) stated in a review that 'in some cases of SA illness and so called chronic schizophrenia, lithium may prove dramatically effective ... Those in the latter category have frequently had manic or hypomanic features documented from time to time in their bulky clinical histories.' Van Kammen and De Fraites (1979) discussed four papers already considered in this review, and two papers on SA illness which will be referred to below. They summarize that 'lithium treatment is not as useful in schizophrenia as it is in affective disorders. However, some excited schizoaffective patients have responded well.' They give an example of a schizophrenic patient whose main improvement while on lithium was a reduction in thought disorder, and note that this 'may give evidence for lithium's ability to affect the "schizophrenic" aspects of some patients' illness.'

In summary, the data suggest that between one third and one half of patients with schizophrenia will benefit from lithium. The controlled and double-blind studies by Small *et al* and Alexander *et al* reflect this. Growe *et al* found lithium to be superior to placebo. The only unfavourable controlled study is that of Shopsin *et al*: their main conclusion is that chlorpromazine is superior to lithium in treating acute schizophrenic episodes. Chlorpromazine is either superior or equal to lithium in treating acute manic states. Their claim that lithium is not useful in schizophrenia is unjustified by their observations, and their remarks on neurotoxicity are at variance with the rest of the literature.

II. Lithium treatment in schizoaffective disorders

A difficulty in the review of studies in this category (which will be called SAD for short) is the lack of diagnostic precision. Of the 31 papers, 22 discuss patients called schizoaffective and the remainder deal with 'atypical manic depression', 'manic-depression with schizophrenic characteristics', 'schizophreniform psychosis', 'cycloid psychosis', 'initial diagnosis mania later revealing schizophrenic characteristics', and 'mania with paranoia'. These papers have been taken as a whole to assess the value of lithium in those conditions neither clearly manic-depressive nor clearly schizophrenic. In 19 papers individual patients could be analysed and they are shown in Table II; eight papers were on controlled studies. Eleven papers were not tabulated; these included lithium prophylaxis studies and group comparisons (lithium versus placebo or chlorpromazine). The figures for successful use of lithium in SAD are superior to those for schizophrenia. A major difference is that a proportion of patients, 14 per cent, made a full recovery (as against the absence of full recovery in any of the schizophrenic group), and 73 per cent benefited from lithium treatment. In two studies some patients fared worse on lithium; the composite rate was 7 per cent. In spite of diagnostic difficulties the evidence points to lithium being effective in treating this miscellaneous group of illnesses.

Controlled studies

Schou *et al* (1954) reported on the use of lithium in manic-depressive patients, both typical (30) and atypical (8). The atypical cases had symptoms such as 'delusions without overt relation to the mood, hallucinations of more than episodic character, periods with reticence and contact difficulties, gross hysterical symptoms, etc.' There was not 'any doubt as to the diagnosis of manic-depressive insanity'. Both open and blind evaluations of the effect of lithium were made. The links between the periods of blind investigation and the results are not specified, nor how many patients were investigated blind. A placebo control was used. Of the 30 cases, 12 showed a positive effect, 15 a possible effect and three no effect. Of the eight atypical cases, two showed a positive effect, three a possible effect and three no effect. Thus there is a less satisfactory outcome in the atypical cases.

Johnson *et al* (1968) first reported a controlled evaluation of lithium versus chlorpromazine in manic and SAD states. The design of this study is similar in many respects to that of Shopsin *et al* reported above. The results are not included in the table, because a subsequent paper by Johnson *et al* appears to include all those SAD patients treated with lithium.

It cannot be disputed that chlorpromazine may well be superior to lithium in both acute SAD illness and acute schizophrenia. However, to conclude that lithium is disease specific would be going further than the evidence warrants. The studies of Shopsin *et al*, and Johnson *et al*, are the only ones using a design in which medication is increased until clinical improvement or toxicity occurs. This may well account for their reports of serious toxicity or worsening which are unconfirmed by other workers. Schizophrenic and schizoaffective patients may be more susceptible to toxic manifestations of lithium than acute manic patients (as are non-acute manic patients).

TABLE II

Lithium treatment in schizoaffective and like disorders

Author	Year	Diagnosis of patients	Study			Number of patients	Results			
			Criteria	Controlled	Blind		Recovered	Improved	Same	Worse
Noack	1951	Mania with paranoia	0	0	0	2		2		
Schou	1954	Atypical manic depression	+	+	+/0	8		5	3	
Rice	1956	Mixed psychoses—SA states	0	0	0	5	1	3	1	
White	1966	SA—manic	0	0	0	2		1	1	
		Manic—subsequent schizophrenic reaction	0	0	0	1		1		
Zall	1968	Initial diagnosis manic—later schizophrenic characteristics	0	0	0	10	1	8	1	
Gottfries	1969	SA with disturbed activity	0	0	0	19		16	3	
Forssman	1970	SA	CD	0	0	1	1			
Johnson	1970	SA	+	+	0	11	1	4		6
Aronoff	1970	SA	+	+	+/0	6		4		2
Sikes	1970	SA	0	0	0	4		3	1	
		Mixed schizophrenia	0	0	0	2		1	1	
Martorano	1972	SA	CD	0	0	2	2			
Van Putten	1975	SA	CD	IR	IR	3			3	
Small	1975	SA—excited	+	+	+	3		3	3	
		SA—depressed	+	+	+	4		1		
Reiser	1976	SA	CD	0	0	2	2			
McGennis	1977	SA	CD	0	0	2	2			
Hussain	1978	SA	CD	0	0	3	3			
Brockington	1978	Schizomanic	+	+	0	6	3	2	1	
Alexander	1979	SA—manic	+	+	+	3		3	3	
		SA—depressed	+	+	+	5		2		
Hirschowitz	1980	Schizophreniform psychosis	+	0	0	9	0	7	2	
Total (%)						113 (100%)	16 (14%)	66 (58%)	23 (20%)	8 (7%)

Criteria not specified 0, specified +.
SA—Schizoaffective; CD—Case description; IR—In responders.

Johnson incorporated the above findings into his paper of 1970, and reported on 11 SAD and 19 manic depressive patients. There is little to add here except that the four new cases seem to have fared better than the original seven. His conclusions remain the same as those of the 1968 paper.

Aronoff and Epstein (1970) report on six SAD patients in a paper on manic patients who had a 'poor or irregular response to lithium therapy'. Criteria for SAD diagnosis were 'distinct affective episodes but also disorganization panic, identity fragmentation or looseness of associations'. They acknowledged that some of these patients would be designated atypical manic-depressive illness by others.

Melia (1970) reported a double blind prophylactic study comparing lithium with placebo in 18 patients. Thirteen were typical manic-depressives or recurrent depressives. Five had schizophrenic features, four during the previous history of illness (three manic depressives and one recurrent manic) and one had schizophrenic features during the index admission. In the total of 18 patients, lithium just failed to be significantly superior to placebo $(0.10 > P > 0.05)$ as judged by length of remission. Obviously, the numbers of patients with schizophrenic features are too small to permit any conclusion.

Johnson *et al* (1971) compared lithium and chlorpromazine in the treatment of acute manic and SAD patients. Initially there were 13 SAD patients in the study; 11 remained.

For the authors, 'lithium had a specific impact on the pattern of mania but not that of schizoaffective disorder; chlorpromazine, in contrast, affected the pattern of schizoaffective disorder but not that of the manic disorder.' They concluded that chlorpromazine, but not lithium, produced significant improvement in the SAD patients but that the difference was not significant. Their interpretation of the results plays down the efficacy of lithium in SAD illness. The SAD patients, as has been mentioned, improved on all the scales given in the paper, and on two (TRAM, NOSIE), there was no significant change in either the lithium or chlorpromazine-treated SAD patients. Chlorpromazine may well be superior to lithium in the treatment of such excited patients, but this paper presents evidence that lithium is also effective in treating this group. Although it is stated that 'in a proportion of the SA patients treated with lithium a transient adverse behavioural reaction with impairment of comprehension, fluctuating levels of attention and disorientation occurred' with serum levels of lithium between 1.1 and 1.9 mEq/l, the toxicity described in other papers, using this kind of experimental design, does not appear to have occurred.

Prien *et al* (1972a) compared chlorpromazine with lithium in a controlled, double blind study of 83 SAD patients diagnosed in accordance with DSM-II. The patients were rated on BPRS, IMPS, and PIP scales. Chlorpromazine was found significantly superior to lithium in SAD patients judged highly active on the pre-treatment IMPS. The difference was due almost entirely to the poor clinical response in the lithium carbonate drop-outs. Ten out of 17 patients in the highly-active lithium treated SAD group terminated the study prematurely. These patients were included in the results. When only those patients completing the full three weeks of study were analysed, there was no major difference between treatments.

It was stated that 'lithium carbonate failed to adequately control hostile, excited behaviour in a significant proportion of patients, resulting in their termination from the study.' However, in the mildly active group, lithium and chlorpromazine were equally effective. In each treatment group there 'was significant improvement in both affective and schizophrenic symptomatology over the three-week period. These results are of interest since they raise the possibility that lithium carbonate has neuroleptic properties. This suggests that the popular conception of lithium carbonate as a specific anti-manic agent warrants reconsideration.'

The frequency of toxic confusion with lithium in SAD patients was approximately the same as that in the study on manic patients. In that study (Prien *et al*, 1972b), chlorpromazine was found clearly superior to lithium in treating the highly active manic patient. The difference between the two treatments among mildly active patients was less pronounced, but lithium appeared to be the better treatment.

Prien *et al* (1974) reported on factors associated with treatment success in lithium carbonate prophylaxis in manic-depressive illness. Two hundred and five patients were studied. Six had their diagnosis changed to SAD after entering the study. Patients were randomly assigned to lithium or placebo and the study was double blind. Five of the SAD patients were on lithium. Three relapsed in the first year, as did the one on placebo. This compares to a two-year relapse rate of 47 per cent in the lithium treated and 87 per cent in the placebo-treated manic-depressives. The relapse rate was higher in the SAD group than in the manic-depressive group (three out of five compared to three out of 86). Thus SAD episodes would appear to recur true to type. It cannot be concluded from such a small sample that lithium is less effective in prophylaxis of SAD illness.

The paper by Small *et al* (1975) has been discussed fully in Part I. It is noteworthy that the response of the excited SAD patients was better than that of the depressed ones.

Brockington *et al* (1978) compared lithium with chlorpromazine in the treatment of manic SAD patients. The study was designed to be blind but the investigators were able to guess correctly the medication given. Case notes of newly admitted patients were screened for the concurrent presence of schizophrenic and affective symptoms. The Present State Examination (PSE) (Wing *et al*, 1974) was then administered and patients were included in the study if they presented evidence of a schizophrenia or paranoid psychosis and also mania. Of the 19 patients, 11 completed the study. They were treated with identical capsules containing either 250 mg lithium carbonate or 100 mg chlorpromazine. The dosage was determined by the clinical team in charge of the patient. Benzodiazepines were given if necessary and, if essential, extra known chlorpromazine was given (for the control of severely disturbed behaviour and in the first week only). The BPRS and PSE were used to assess change. Of the six patients treated with lithium, three are shown in the table as recovering. In the text, it is stated that 'two patients made complete recoveries and a third became depressed'. Two were listed in the partial recovery group.

Biederman *et al* (1979) reported on the combined use of lithium carbonate and haloperidol in SAD. The Research Diagnostic Criteria (Spitzer *et al*, 1975) were used to select acutely ill, newly admitted SAD manic patients. They were then subdivided into six categories ranging from manic to schizophrenic; the clinical criteria are given. The two extreme groups were dropped and the remaining four were studied. Haloperidol was prescribed by the clinical psychiatrist to get the best therapeutic result with it. Lithium was given double-blind, with placebo in identical capsules. The double-blind design was effective because the side effects from haloperidol covered any differences. The trial lasted five weeks. The BPRS, MS (manic scale) and GCI (global clinical impression) were used to assess change. Thirty-six patients (18 lithium, 18 on placebo) completed the five weeks. There was a trend for patients on placebo to receive higher doses of haloperidol. A significant improvement was seen by the fifth week in the lithium-treated group as measured by the BPRS. The MS and GCI showed consistently greater improvement in the lithium carbonate group but this failed to reach statistical significance. The benefit of lithium was at least as great at the schizophrenic end of the SAD spectrum (the so-called 'schizophrenic schizoaffectives') as it was at the affective end of the SAD spectrum (the 'affective schizoaffectives'). There was a suggestion that the percentage of total improvement attributable to lithium carbonate might be higher in the schizophrenic SAD patients, who showed significantly less improvement than the affective SAD patients. The investigators could not demonstrate any specificity of lithium carbonate for manic symptoms, although lithium's prevention of the development of a depressive syndrome was statistically significant. BPRS items such as conceptual disorganization and unusual thinking improved more with lithium than with placebo. They concluded: 'our data do not support the clinical impressions of those who report that lithium carbonate ameliorates only the affective component of mixed disorder.'

The study of Alexander *et al* (1979) was reviewed in Part I. By RDC, there were three SAD-manic and five SAD-depressed patients. It will be noted that a greater proportion of the former benefited from lithium, although two of the five SAD-depressed patients responded, and one of these relapsed when it was withdrawn.

Uncontrolled studies

Not all the papers will be discussed. Of the 10 SAD patients treated by Zall *et al* (1968), nine improved and in one case 'both the affective and the schizophrenic components remitted completely. In none of the other nine did the thought disorder improve on lithium alone. However, in eight of the nine the affective component did respond. In six of these eight responders, after a manic-like state cleared on lithium, delusions of persecution and unreasonable hostility emerged and dominated the clinical picture. A phenothiazine additive controlled the emerging paranoid psychosis after increased doses of lithium alone had failed.'

Serry (1969) describes the treatment of 11 SAD patients with lithium. Six of these patients were lithium retainers. Although he stated that the lithium-excreting schizoaffective patient (one patient) showed no response to lithium, he did not state what happened to the intermediate group (four patients). Thus we are unable to analyse this paper. He implied that all the lithium retainers responded. He stated that treatment with lithium alone removed the euphoric affective element, but the patients still showed schizophrenic thought disorder, delusions and hallucinations. The latter symptoms responded to phenothiazines.

Gottfries (1969) measured the arm and leg movements of 19 SAD patients. Although diagnostic criteria are not specified, it is stated that 'only those were included who, besides their base symptoms, also had a disturbed activity level. In these the lithium treatment seemed to normalize the activity level.' Two classes of patients are not presented—schizophrenics with disturbed activity level and SAD patients with normal activity level. Unfortunately, treatment of these groups was not attempted. Their conclusion was that 'patients with psychotic disorders and with a disturbed activity level also seem to benefit from lithium treatment, their activity level being normalized' which might have had more force if some schizophrenic patients with abnormal activity level had been included.

Forssman and Walinder (1970) used a response to lithium to make a diagnosis of manic-depressive illness on the grounds that it is a specific treatment for manic-depressive illness. This is clearly unjustified. Of the two cases they present, we think that one could fairly be called SAD, and that case is included in the table.

Angst *et al* (1970) reported on 250 patients who included 72 SAD patients (WHO 295.7). 'Lithium treatment led to a pronounced and statistically significant reduction in the number of both episodes and hospital admissions. This was demonstrated ... for each of the affective disorders, manic-depressive psychosis, recurrent depressive psychosis, and schizoaffective psychosis ... lithium treatment led to a significant prolongation of the cycles, considerable in manic depressive [61 per cent longer] and recurrent depressives [76 per cent longer] and moderate in schizoaffective psychosis [30 per cent longer].'

Sikes and Sikes (1970) found that 'patients with the highest affective components showed the best results.' Martorano (1972) reported two cases treated with lithium. His point was that less emphasis should be placed on diagnosis than on target symptoms when drug treatment is being considered, and he concluded that lithium can be used effectively 'to treat a specific symptom-complex characterized by mental and physical hyperactivity'. Smulevitch *et al* (1974) reported a study of lithium prophylaxis in 50 affective and 49 SAD patients. Criteria for SAD are provided. The SAD patients did as well as those with manic-depression. They conclude that 'lithium salts are an effective preventive drug in affective and schizoaffective psychoses.' Procci (1976) surveyed 22 papers in which lithium had been used in schizophrenia or SAD. His review found that 87 per cent of 149 manics showed improvement compared with 77 per cent of 94 schizoaffectives. This figure is very close to that found in the present survey, which includes eight papers not available to Procci (i.e. published after his review) and another two papers that were available but were not incorporated. Perris (1978) reported a study on the prophylactic use of lithium in cycloid psychosis. Diagnostic criteria are given. The study was not blind. There was a significant reduction in morbidity in patients who took their lithium regularly.

Comment

Two initial points must be made. First, there is some evidence that it is not only affective symptoms that respond to lithium. This emerges in spite of the prevailing but unjustified notion that if there is a response to lithium, the diagnosis must be manic-depression, which is largely the result of the specificity claimed by Schou (1963), for lithium treatment of affective illness. Second, the schizoaffective category is diagnostically blurred. The choice of the reviewers has been to include the no-man's-land between schizophrenia and the affective illnesses, the marginal psychoses of the two functional psychoses. Having this in mind, the following conclusions emerge.

The patients with SAD show a better response to lithium than the schizophrenic patients. Nevertheless, a surprisingly high proportion (40–55 per cent) of those diagnosed as schizophrenic without affective overlay or excitement also respond. The findings in the studies which specify diagnostic criteria and use double-blind control methods support this proportion, though the numbers involved are small. Toxicity is not a salient feature in most studies. It is only claimed in three studies, all of which use a design favouring its development. As a whole, the evidence indicates that the drug can be used safely at the usual prophylactic level of 0.7–1.2 mEq/l in both categories of patients, at least in the relatively short term.

In those cases in which the diagnosis is clearly schizoaffective, and in the less clearly defined marginal group, the favourable response is even higher (75 per cent and over). It is not helpful to postulate that those who do respond are therefore manic-depressive, because it prejudges the issue and prevents an unbiased examination of the responses. All studies comparing lithium with placebo in both schizophrenia and SAD have shown lithium to be superior. Three of five studies of prophylactic effect of lithium in SAD have shown a significant benefit from lithium. The numbers in the other two studies are too small for analysis.

Two further questions remain. First, although the practical value of lithium treatment in schizophrenia and SAD seems well established, there is no adequate theory to account for its effectiveness. Second, it is not known which symptom or group of symptoms in schizophrenia or SAD are affected by the treatment. There is obvious disagreement as to whether lithium is specific for excitement, over-activity and affective symptoms, or whether it has a broader therapeutic spectrum. Affective symptoms and hyperactivity figure prominently, but a number of careful studies done in recent years (e.g. Small *et al*; Brockington *et al*; Biederman *et al*) have found lithium to be as effective in treating schizophrenic symptoms. Two studies have found that excited or manic SAD patients respond more to lithium than depressed SAD patients.

It is unjustified at the present time to conclude that lithium is a specific treatment. Several studies have challenged the commonly held view that the drug alters only mood or activity. Prien *et al* (1972b) raised the question of lithium having neuroleptic properties. It is well known that neuroleptic drugs may calm a schizophrenic patient and allow him to function, yet fail to rid him of delusions. If lithium has a similar calming effect, the use of the term neuroleptic would be equally justified.

Evidence has been presented that some schizophrenic patients given an initial trial of lithium are then continued on the drug. Others require a neuro-leptic in addition to lithium. In these the issues of potentiation and of cumula-tive toxicity are important, but have received little or no attention. If patients could be treated with a much lower dose of neuroleptic while on lithium, the chances of development of undesirable effects such as tardive dyskinesia might be diminished. On the other hand, the degree of cumulative toxicity of lithium is not yet known. At present, all that can be stated is that the use of lithium in the treatment of patients with schizophrenia or SAD remains empirical.

References

ALEXANDER, P. E., VAN KAMMEN, D. P. & BUNNEY, W. E. (1979) Antipsychotic effects of lithium in schizophrenia. *American Journal of Psychiatry*, **136**, 283–287.

ANGST, J., WEIS, P., GROF, P., BAASTRUP, C. & SCHOU, M. (1970) Lithium prophylaxis in recurrent affective disorders. *British Journal of Psychiatry*, **116**, 604–614.

ARONOFF, M. & EPSTEIN, R. S. (1970) Factors associated with poor response to lithium carbonate: a clinical study. *American Journal of Psychiatry*, **127**, 472–480.

BIEDERMAN, J., LERNER, Y. & BELMAKER, R. H. (1979) Combination of lithium carbonate and haloperidol in schizo-affective disorder. *Archives of General Psychiatry*, **36**, 327–333.

BLINDER, M. G. (1968) Some observations on the use of lithium carbonate. *International Journal of Neuropsychiatry*, **4**, 26–27.

BROCKINGTON, I. F., KENDELL, R. E., KELLETT, J. M., CURRY, S. H. & WAINWRIGHT, S. (1978) Trials of lithium, chlorpromazine and amitriptyline in schizo-affective patients. *British Journal of Psychiatry*, **133**, 162–168.

CADE, J. F. J. (1949) Lithium salts in the treatment of psychotic excitement. *Medical Journal of Australia*, **36**, 2, 349–352.

—— (1978) Lithium—past, present and future. In *Lithium in Medical Practice*, (eds. F. N. Johnson and S. Johnson). Baltimore: University Park Press.

FIEVE, R. R. (1980) Lithium therapy. In *Comprehensive Textbook of Psychiatry III*, (eds. H. Kaplan, A. Freedman and B. Sadock). Baltimore: Williams & Wilkins.

FORSSMAN, H. & WALINDER, J. (1970) Lithium effect as aid in psychiatric diagnostics. *Acta Psychiatrica Scandinavica Supplement*, **219**, 59–66.

GARDNER, R. & STATON, E. D. (1979) Lithium in schizophrenia (letter). *American Journal of Psychiatry*, **136**, 1479–1480.

GERBINO, L., OLESHANSKY, M. & GERSHON, S. (1978) Clinical use and mode of action of lithium. In *Psychopharmacology: A Generation of Progress*, (eds. M. Lipton, A. DiMascio and K. Killam). New York: Raven Press.

GERSHON, S. & YUWILER, A. (1960) Lithium ion: A specific psychopharmacological approach to the treatment of mania. *Journal of Neuropsychiatry*, **1**, 229–241.

GLESINGER, G. (1954) Evaluation of lithium in treatment of psychotic excitement. *Medical Journal of Australia*, **41**, 277–283.

GLICK, I. D. & STEWART, D. (1980) A new drug treatment for premenstrual exacerbation of schizophrenia. *Comprehensive Psychiatry*, **21**, 281–287.

GOTTFRIES, C. G. (1969) The effect of lithium salts on various kinds of psychiatric disorders. *Acta Psychiatrica Scandinavica Supplement*, **203**, 157–167.

GROWE, G. A., CRAYTON, J. W., KLASS, D. B., EVANS, H. & STRIZICH, M. (1979) Lithium in chronic schizophrenia. *American Journal of Psychiatry*, **136**, 454–455.

HIRSCHOWITZ, J., CASPER, R., GARVER, D. L. & CHANG, S. (1980) Lithium response in good prognosis schizophrenia. *American Journal of Psychiatry*, **137**, 916–920.

HUSSAIN, M. F. & GOMMERSALL, J. D. (1978) The use of lithium in the treatment of schizo-affective disorders. In *Lithium in Medical Practice*, (eds. F. N. Johnson and S. Johnson). Baltimore: University Park Press.

JEFFERSON, J. W. & GREIST, J. H. (1977) *Primer of Lithium Therapy*. Baltimore: Williams & Wilkins.

JOHNSON, G., GERSHON, S. & HEKIMIAN, L. J. (1968) Controlled evaluation of lithium and chlor-promazine in the treatment of manic states: an interim report. *Comprehensive Psychiatry*, **9**, 563–573.

—— (1970) Differential response to lithium carbonate in manic depressive and schizo-affective disorders. *Diseases of the Nervous System*, **31**, 613–615.

—— GERSHON, S., BURDOCK, E. I., FLOYD, A. & HEKIMIAN, L. (1971) Comparative effects of lithium and chlorpromazine in the treatment of acute manic states. *British Journal of Psychiatry*, **119**, 267–276.

MARTORANO, J. T. (1972) Target symptoms in lithium carbonate therapy. *Comprehensive Psychiatry*, **13**, 533–537.

MEIERS, R. L. (1970) Lithium carbonate as an adjunct in the treatment of schizophrenia. *Schizophrenia*, **2**, 87–91.

MELIA, P. I. (1970) Prophylactic lithium: a double-blind trial in recurrent affective disorders. *British Journal of Psychiatry*, **116**, 621–624.

McGENNIS, A. J. (1977) Lithium carbonate in schizo-affective states. *British Medical Journal*, ii, 124.

NOACK, C. H. & TRAUTNER, E. M. (1951) The lithium treatment of maniacal psychosis. *Medical Journal of Australia*, **36**, 219–220.

PERRIS, C. (1978) Morbidity suppressive effect of lithium carbonate in cycloid psychosis. *Archives of General Psychiatry*, **35**, 328–331.

PRIEN, R. F., CAFFEY, E. M. & KLETT, C. J. (1972a) A comparison of lithium carbonate and chlorpromazine in the treatment of excited schizo-affectives. *Archives of General Psychiatry*, **27**, 182–189.

—— —— —— (1972b) Comparison of lithium carbonate and chlorpromazine in the treatment of mania. *Archives of General Psychiatry*, **26**, 146–153.

—— —— —— (1974) Factors associated with treatment success in lithium carbonate prophylaxis. *Archives of General Psychiatry*, **31**, 189–192.

—— (1979) Lithium in the treatment of schizophrenia and schizo-affective disorders. *Archives of General Psychiatry*, **36**, 852–853.

PROCCI, W. R. (1976) Schizo-affective psychosis: fact or fiction? *Archives of General Psychiatry*, **33**, 1167–1178.

REISER, D. E. & WILLETT, A. B. (1976) A favorable response to lithium carbonate in a 'schizo-affective' father and son. *American Journal of Psychiatry*, **133**, 824–827.

RICE, D. (1956) The use of lithium salts in the treatment of manic states. *Journal of Mental Science*, **102**, 604–611.

SCHOU, M. (1963) Normothymics, 'mood normalizers'. *British Journal of Psychiatry*, **109**, 803–809.

—— JUEL-NIELSEN, N., STROMGREN, E. & VOLDBY, H. (1954) The treatment of manic psychoses by the administration of lithium salts. *Journal of Neurology, Neurosurgery and Psychiatry*, **17**, 250–260.

SERRY, M. (1969) Lithium retention and response. *The Lancet*, i, 1267–1268.

SHOPSIN, B., KIM, S. S. & GERSHON, S. (1971) A controlled study of lithium vs chlorpromazine in acute schizophrenics. *British Journal of Psychiatry*, **119**, 435–440.

SIKES, J. C. & SIKES, S. C. (1970) Lithium carbonate treatment in psychiatry. *Diseases of the Nervous System*, **31**, 52–55.

SMALL, J. G., KELLAMS, J. J., MILSTEIN, V. & MOORE, J. (1975) A placebo controlled study of lithium combined with neuroleptics in chronic schizophrenic patients. *American Journal of Psychiatry*, **132**, 1315–1317.

SMULEVITCH, A. B., ZAVIDOVSKAYA, G. I., IGONIN, A. L. & MIKHAILOVA, N. M. (1974) The effectiveness of lithium in affective and schizo-affective psychoses. *British Journal of Psychiatry*, **125**, 65–72.

SOLOMON, K. (1979) Lithium in schizophrenia (letter). *American Journal of Psychiatry*, **136**, 1480.

SPITZER, R. L., ENDICOTT, J. & ROBINS, E. (1975) *Research Diagnostic Criteria*, 2nd edition. New York: Biometrics Research, New York State Psychiatric Institute.

SPRING, G. K. (1980) The relative efficacies of lithium and alternative modes of treatment. In *Handbook of Lithium Therapy*, (ed. F. Johnson). Baltimore: University Park Press.

TAHERI, A. (1976) Lithium in schizophrenia. *American Journal of Psychiatry*, **133**, 10, 1208.

TUPIN, J. P., SMITH, D. B, CLANON, T. L., KIM, L. I., NUGENT, A. & GROUPE, A. (1973) The long-term use of lithium in aggressive prisoners. *Comprehensive Psychiatry*, **14**, 311–317.

VAN KAMMEN, D. P. & DE FRAITES, E. G. (1979) Lithium treatment in schizophrenia: a review of treatment and prophylaxis in schizophrenia, schizo-affective disorders, and periodic catatonia. In *Lithium, Controversies and Unresolved Issues*, (eds. T. B. Cooper, S. Gershon, N. S. Kline and M. Schou). Amsterdam: Exerpta Medica.

VAN PUTTEN, T. & SANDERS, D. G. (1975) Lithium in treatment failures. *Journal of Nervous and Mental Disease*, **161**, 255–264.

WATANABE, S. & ISHINO, H. (1980) Special cases of affective disorder and their treatment with lithium. In *Handbook of Lithium Therapy*, (eds. F. Johnson). Baltimore: University Park Press.

WHITE, R. B., SCHLAGENHAUF, G. & TUPIN, J. P. (1966) The treatment of manic depressive states with lithium carbonate. In *Current Psychiatric Therapies*, Vol 6, (ed. J. Wasserman). New York: Grune and Stratton.

WING, J. K., COOPER, J. E. & SARTORIUS, N. (1974) *The Measurement and Classification of Psychiatric Symptoms*. Cambridge: Cambridge University Press.

ZALL, H., PER-OLOF, G. T. & MYERS, J. M. (1968) Lithium carbonate: a clinical study. *American Journal of Psychiatry*, **125,** 549–555.

40 Pharmacotherapeutic trials in tardive dyskinesia

**ANGUS V. P. MACKAY and
GRAHAM P. SHEPPARD**

It is clear that no generally satisfactory treatment has yet been demonstrated for tardive dyskinesia (TD). It is over 20 years since the syndrome was defined (Schonecker, 1957) and although there was reluctant clinical recognition of the syndrome initially, the past decade has seen intense interest in both the aetiology and treatment of TD. Before considering in detail the pharmacological strategies which have been explored in the treatment of TD we will discuss some of the particular problems which face the clinical investigator in both the definition and rating of TD. It is arguable that these problems are as responsible for the current therapeutic failure as our ignorance of the precise underlying pathology. There are probably three major sources of difficulty; nosological issues of diagnostic definition and syndrome delineation; patient variables not directly related to TD but which affect the capacity for change, and environmental variables which may affect the nature and severity of the disorder.

(a) *Nosological issues:* Such questions are familiar to psychiatrists, having been amply rehearsed over disorders such as schizophrenic illness. A lack of generally agreed diagnostic rules and standard rating instruments for TD has undoubtedly helped to create problems such as widely variable prevalence rates, inconsistent drug effects and a confusing array of putative aetiological factors (Gardos *et al*, 1977).

How inclusive should the operational diagnostic criteria be? Most clinicians agree that the cephalic triad of bucco-linguo-masticatory (BLM) movements is of central diagnostic importance but it is not clear whether this must always be present, whether axial and peripheral movements should have diagnostic weight, and if the latter are present alone whether the diagnosis can still apply. Variations in syndrome classification represent a potential source of serious error. We may be crudely labelling one syndrome which is, in fact, a composite of several neurochemically and even phenomenologically distinct syndromes. Attempts have been made to carry out multivariate analyses of abnormal movements in patients receiving chronic neuroleptic medication (Kennedy *et al*, 1971; Crane and Naranjo, 1971; Barnes *et al*, 1979). All seem to agree upon three broad clusters; a parkinsonian syndrome characterized mainly by tremor, a cephalic dyskinesia, and an axial and limb syndrome which may be a mixture of akathisia and true choreiform movements. Even within the cephalic syndrome, Villeneuve and his colleagues (Jus *et al*, 1972) have drawn a distinction between the BLM and the 'rabbit syndrome' which is a high frequency lip movement associated with increased muscle tone and which behaves pharmacologically like parkinson's disease. Lack of distinction between these groups of phenomena can obviously complicate the results of any therapeutic trial in TD.

The precise description of individual dyskinetic phenomena, often idiosyncratic, is frequently neglected in rating scales. Phenomena tend to be forced into global categories which may aid statistical analyses at the expense of attention to detail in both the nature and distribution of abnormal movements. There is ample evidence from animal models that change in the severity of such movements may be accompanied by change in their distribution.

(b) *Patient variables:* Finding appropriate patients for therapeutic experiments in TD is not always easy and several characteristics may have to be attended to and matched in control and treatment groups. These characteristics, additional to the phenomenological issues discussed above, may affect the capacity for response and the clarity of any change. The age of the patient, the degree of institutionalization (tending to encourage behavioural rigidity), quantity and duration of neuroleptic medication, the duration of the TD, the stability of the TD and the presence or absence of dentures can all be expected to affect outcome. There is no evidence that sex or psychiatric diagnosis can influence response (Crane, 1978) but it is probably advisable to control for these variables if possible.

(c) *Environmental variables:* The conditions under which the patient is rated should be standardized and familiar to the patient. Arousal can have unpredictable effects on the severity and distribution of TD; anxiety usually produces an exacerbation but the embarrassment of being watched can make the patient voluntarily inhibit the movements for limited periods. Often such voluntary inhibition is followed by a rebound amplification. Focusing the patient's attention on some standard task (such as a simple manual task or attempts to memorize a picture) usually allows the dyskinesia to emerge fully and reproducibly. The time of day at which assessments are made should be standardized, since, on the basis of an animal model of TD, there may be reason to predict a diurnal fluctuation in dyskinetic phenomena (Weiner *et al*, 1978). Background medication may influence the disorder and should be kept constant if possible. The use of long-acting depot neuroleptics poses a particular problem because constant plasma concentrations cannot be assumed and thus, in theory at least, rating should be carried out at a standardized time relative to injections.

A summary of fairly minimal requirements for any therapeutic trial in TD is given in Table I. A double-blind design is as important in this context as in any other clinical trial in view of both the influence the patient can have on the disorder and the imprecision of the clinical rating methods. Several rating scales are currently available, (for review see Gardos *et al*, 1977), the most popular probably being the Rockland Tardive Dyskinesia Rating Scale (Simpson *et al*, 1976a; Simpson *et al*, 1979) and the Abnormal Involuntary Movements Scale (AIMS, 1976). They include both multi-item ratings and global clinical judgements. The choice of rating scale should be taken in the light of established validity and reliability—the more global and clinical the scale, the more valid (in other words it measures what the clinician believes to be TD), but the less objective and therefore the less reliable (Gardos *et*

TABLE I
Some requirements for a therapeutic trial in tardive dyskinesia

1.   Double-blind design.
2.   Adequate number of sufficiently fit and co-operative patients.
3.   Clear diagnostic and descriptive definitions.
4.   Rating scale which is valid and reliable and which allows detailed recording of distribution as well as severity of movements.
5.   Attention to matching for age, duration and severity of TD, neuroleptic and anti-cholinergic medication.
6.   Standard observing and rating conditions.
7.   Any background medication held constant.
8.   Attention to timing of ratings relative to background medication: N.B. depot preparations.

al, 1977; Fann *et al*, 1977). There exist several objective techniques for measuring the severity of TD such as electromyography, accelerometry and pneumatic pressure transducers (Gardos *et al*, 1977) but these have the drawbacks of inconvenience and lack of established validity. The optimal approach may be to employ a combination of objective techniques and clinical ratings.

Given these practical problems, to which solutions should be possible with care, there are two covert theoretical assumptions which are implicit in most pharmacological trials in TD. Firstly, that dyskinesia is the expression of a neurochemical imbalance rather than structural damage. Evidence exists that structural change may be associated with TD (for review, see Jellinger, 1977) and if such presumably irreversible damage contributes substantially to the clinical picture then the potential for pharmacotherapeutic intervention will be limited. Secondly, a related assumption is that dyskinetic syndromes which look clinically similar are the expression of the same underlying pathology. This may not be true at the neurochemical level and if structural factors play a variable role between individuals then reproducible responses to medication would be unlikely.

Pharmacological strategies

A wide range of pharmacological agents have been used in attempts to alleviate TD. The choice has been shaped by the prevailing hypotheses for the underlying neurochemical pathology. The dopamine (DA) overactivity model (Klawans, 1973) has dominated many approaches and Table II provides a summary of the agents which have been used to treat TD with the purpose of affecting, in one way or another, central DA transmission. The majority have not been properly evaluated and those which have been the subject of controlled trials will be considered in more detail in the next section. The most popular approaches have been to inhibit DA transmission by the use of receptor antagonists (such as phenothiazines and butyrophenones) or presynaptic amine depletors such as α-methyl paratyrosine and reserpine. However it is perhaps theoretically predictable that any amelioration in TD would be temporary and would be reversed by further DA receptor proliferation in response to reduced transmission (Kazamatsuri *et al*, 1973). The newer

TABLE II

Agents affecting dopamine systems which have been used to treat tardive dyskinesia

α-methyl-paratyrosine	Phenothiazines
α-methyl DOPA	Butyrophenones
L-DOPA	Oxiperomide
Fusaric acid	Sulpiride
Reserpine	Pimozide
Tetrabenazine	Apomorphine
Oxypertine	Piribedil
Amantadine	Bromocriptine
Monoamine oxidase inhibitors	Lergotrile

DA antagonists such as pimozide and the substituted benzamides (oxiperomide, sulpiride, tiapride and metoclopramide) have a claim to act selectively at the so-called 'D2' receptors—those DA receptors which are not linked to adenylate cyclase (Kebabian and Calne, 1978). There is some evidence from animal studies that D2 receptors may mediate peri-oral dyskinesias in guinea-pigs (Costall and Naylor, 1978) and there is clinical support for the efficacy of oxiperomide in alleviating L-DOPA-induced and spontaneous dyskinesias (Bedard *et al*, 1978). However, it remains to be seen whether the danger of breakthrough supersensitivity is as great with the D2 antagonists as with the more conventional DA antagonists.

Of interest have been attempts to improve TD by the use of DA potentiators such as L-DOPA apomorphine and the ergolines (bromocriptine, piribedil and lergotrile). The L-DOPA strategy has been advocated by Friedhoff (1977) and aims at desensitizing the postsynaptic neurone by gradually increasing stimulation of the DA receptors. In the case of the ergolines, however, it is becoming clear that they are only partial agonists at striatal DA receptors (Kebabian and Calne, 1978) and at high doses may be acting as simple dopamine antagonists. Apomorphine may act to diminish DA release by stimulation of inhibitory presynaptic DA receptors. However the balance between pre- and postsynaptic actions of apomorphine is sensitively dose-dependent, the presynaptic action being evident only at low doses.

The simple DA overactivity model has been extended to one which views the functional balance between transmitters in the basal ganglia as the important issue rather than absolute DA overactivity. Klawans and his colleagues have developed the idea of a balance between DA and acetylcholine (ACh) with the ratio of DA: ACh transmission being raised in TD (Klawans and Rubovitz, 1974). More recently γ-amino-butyric acid (GABA) has also been implicated in operational models, GABA operating in a similar direction to ACh in the balance with DA. Table III provides a list of drugs used to treat TD which would be expected to increase the activity of ACh or GABA. Most have been assessed in small open studies with variable success.

The purpose of this superficial overview has been to give an impression of the various strategies that have been used in the treatment of TD and the following section will consider in more detail the reports of pharmacotherapeutic trials in TD with special attention being given to blind controlled studies.

TABLE III
Agents affecting ACh and GABA systems which have been used to treat tardive dyskinesia

ACh	Physostigmine
	Choline
	Arecoline
	Deanol (2-dimethyl amino ethanol)
	Lecithin
GABA	Sodium valproate (dipropyl acetic acid: Epilim)
	p-chloro-phenyl GABA (Baclofen)
	γ-acetylenic GABA
	SL–76002
	Muscimol
	Benzodiazepines

Pharmacotherapeutic trials

Dopamine receptor antagonists

The three DA receptor blocking agents which have been investigated to the greatest extent in the treatment of TD have been thiopropazate, haloperidol and pimozide. The effectiveness of each of these has been reported in double blind controlled studies (Table IV). Furthermore, several non-blind studies support this conclusion (Schmidt and Jarcho, 1966; Bourgeois and Herbert, 1970; Fog and Pakkenberg, 1970; Curran, 1973; Carruthers, 1971; Pakkenberg and Fog, 1974; Carroll *et al*, 1977; Gibson, 1977). However, the effect of all of these agents appears to be of limited duration (Kazamatsuri *et al*, 1973; Pakkenberg and Fog, 1974; Kazamatsuri *et al*, 1972c; Freeman, 1979). Recently interest has focused on the use of drugs which specifically block D2 receptor sites (see above) e.g., pimozide, oxiperomide, tiapride and metoclopramide. Of these drugs only pimozide has been studied in TD. However in the treatment of L-DOPA-induced dyskinesia both oxiperomide (Bedard *et al*, 1978) and tiapride (Lees *et al*, 1979) have been reported to be of value but metoclopramide (Tarsy *et al*, 1975) seemed to be without effect. Unfortunately the concern with the use of all dopamine receptor antagonists continues to be that they may augment the underlying biochemical pathology while offering at best only temporary alleviation of the dyskinesia. Finally and paradoxically, while most patients show short-term improvement in TD with DA receptor blockers, some may actually become worse (Lal, 1974; Casey and Denney, 1977).

Dopamine depleting drugs

A number of non-blind studies have reported the following DA depleting agents to be of value in alleviating TD: tetrabenzine (Brandrup, 1961; MacCallum, 1970; Fog and Pakkenberg, 1970; Pakkenberg and Fog, 1974); reserpine (Villeneuve *et al*, 1970a; Villeneuve *et al*, 1970b; Schmidt and Jarcho, 1966; Peters *et al*, 1972; Duvoisin, 1972); α-methyl-DOPA (Villeneuve *et al*, 1970a; Villeneuve *et al*, 1970b); α-methylpara-tyrosine (Gerlach *et al*, 1974) and oxypertine

TABLE IV

Double-blind controlled pharmacotherapeutic trials in tardive dyskinesia

Trial drug	Number of patients	Dose of drug per day	Duration of trial drug treatment (weeks)	Effectiveness of trial drugs	Reference
1. Tetrabenazine*	6	100 mg	1	S	Godwin-Austin and Clark, 1971
2. Tetrabenazine†	24	50–150 mg	6	P<0.0005	Kazamatsuri et al, 1972a
3. Tetrabenazine†	6	100–200 mg	18	S	Kazamatsuri et al 1973
4. Thiopropazate*	23	45 mg	3	P<0.0005	Singer and Cheng, 1971
5. Thiopropazate†	9	10–80 mg	4	P<0.05	Kazamatsuri et al, 1972b
6. Haloperidol†	11	2–16 mg	4	P<0.01	Kazamatsuri et al, 1972b
7. Haloperidol†	6	8–16 mg	18	P<0.01	Kazamatsuri et al, 1973
8. Pimozide†	18	6–28 mg	6	P<0.001	Claveria et al, 1975
9. Apomorphine†	8	0.75–6.0 mg	Single injection	S	Smith et al, 1977
10. Methylphendate*	17	80 mg	6	N.S.	Fann et al, 1973
11. D-Amphetamine*‡	6	15–20 mg	Single injection	S§	Smith et al, 1977
12. Deanol*	10	1200 mg	8	N.S.	Simpson et al, 1977
13. Deanol*	6	500–1250 mg	3	N.S.	Tamminga et al, 1977
14. Choline*	20	150–200 mg/kg	2	S	Growdon et al, 1977
15. Physostigmine*‡	5	Max 2.0 mg	Single injection	S	Tamminga et al, 1977
16. Sodium Valproate*	32	900 mg	2	N.S.	Linnoila et al, 1976
17. Baclofen*	20	70 mg	2	P<0.0005	Korsgaard, 1976
18. Baclofen*	18	20–120 mg	3	N.S.	Gerlach, 1977
19. Baclofen*	10	30–90 mg	3	N.S.	Vasavan-Nair et al, 1978
20. Lithium*	15	0.8–1.2 mM☐	3	P<0.01	Gerlach et al, 1975
21. Lithium*	10	0.6–2 mM☐	6	N.S.	Simpson et al, 1976b
22. Lithium*	11	0.8–1.3 mM☐	5	N.S.	Mackay et al, 1980
23. L-Tryptophan*	4	6 gm	2	S.	Prange, 1972
24. Clozapine*	2	Max dose 425 mg	3–5	N.S.	Caine et al, 1979

Key to Table:

* Double blind cross over studies. Placebo and trial drugs administered orally. Control medication in all cases was placebo.

† Double blind studies. Placebo and trial drugs administered orally. Control medication in all cases was placebo but in studies 5 and 6 an additional control group was haloperidol and thiopropazate respectively and in studies 3 and 7 an additional group was haloperidol and tetrabenazine respectively.

‡ Double blind studies. Placebo and trial drugs administered parenterally. Control medication was sterile saline.

S Trial drug 'significantly' better than control. Statistics not reported.

N.S. No significant difference between trial drug and placebo.

S§ Trial drug significantly worse than placebo. Statistics not reported.

☐ Serum lithium concentrations.

(Eckmann, 1968). Crane (1973) failed to confirm the effect of reserpine in an uncontrolled study and Kazamatsuri *et al* (1972c) failed to confirm the effectiveness of α-methyl DOPA in a single-blind study in which nine patients received 1,000 mg a day over a six-week period. The efficacy of tetrabenazine has, however, been confirmed in double blind studies (Table IV) and therefore, among the various DA depletors, the current weight of evidence favours this drug. Compared with the DA antagonists, the DA depleting agents offer two possible therapeutic advantages: (a) the effectiveness of DA depletors may persist whereas benefit derived from DA blockers appears to be short-lived (see Kazamatsuri *et al*, 1973) and (b) DA depletors only rarely seem to cause TD (Duvoisin, 1972; Degkwitz, 1969).

Dopamine-mimetic drugs

Among this group of drugs current studies point to apomorphine as being the most likely to bring therapeutic benefit, although the need for parenteral administration inevitably limits its practical usefulness. It has proved successful in an open single-case study (Carroll *et al*, 1977) and also in two placebo-controlled studies (Tolosa, 1974; Smith *et al*, 1977). It may also be useful in a variety of other dyskinetic disorders (see Carroll *et al*, 1977). Uncontrolled studies with amantadine have yielded conflicting results (Decker *et al*, 1971; Crane and Naranjo, 1971) and a controlled study with methylphenidate failed to detect any significant effect (Fann *et al*, 1973). Aggravation of TD has been reported with amphetamine in a controlled experiment by Smith *et al* (1977). Worsening has also been reported with L-DOPA in a single blind study with five patients (Gerlach *et al*, 1974) and in uncontrolled studies involving forty patients (Hippius and Logemann, 1970), and one patient (Klawans and McKendall, 1971). However, other authors have reported that L-DOPA may on occasion improve TD (Alpert *et al*, 1976; Friedhoff, 1977; and Carroll *et al*, 1977), although the total number of patients accounted for in these studies amounts to only five. It has been suggested that bromocriptine may be of value in TD (Barnes *et al*, 1978) but this has not been borne out in a recent double-blind study (Chase, 1979).

Finally, Hydergine (a mixture of dihydroergocryptine, dihydroergocrystine and dihydroergocornine), which has been suggested as having both stimulant and inhibitory actions at central DA receptors (Hofman *et al*, 1979; Spano *et al*, 1978), has been reported to improve TD in seven out of ten patients in an uncontrolled study (Gomez, 1977).

It is clear from this resumé that the place of DA agonists in the treatment of TD is very uncertain and that further double blind controlled studies are needed to clarify the picture. Clarification will be made more difficult by the partial agonist properties of many of these agents (e.g. bromocriptine) which means that their synaptic action can vary between stimulation and inhibition according to the drug concentration. Relative agonist/antagonist properties may also vary according to brain area (Kebabian and Calne, 1978).

Cholinergic drugs

The principal drugs used to augment cholinergic activity in TD have been physostigmine, deanol, choline and lecithin. Physostigmine given by intravenous injection has improved TD in a placebo controlled double-blind study (Table IV), and three single blind studies (Klawans and Rubovitz, 1974; Fann and Lake, 1974; Davis and Berger, 1978). However, in two uncontrolled studies, Gerlach *et al* (1974) were unable to detect any effect and Tarsy *et al* (1974) found physostigmine increased dyskinetic movements in four out of seven patients. Five early encouraging but anecdotal reports of deanol (2-dimethyl amino ethanol), involving a total of eight patients, were followed by less encouraging results in three larger uncontrolled studies (see Simpson *et al*, 1977), and, finally by negative results in two later double-blind controlled studies (Table IV). Choline has been reported to be of value in uncontrolled studies (Davis *et al*, 1975; Tamminga *et al*, 1977; Davis and Berger, 1978; and Growdon, 1979), and its effect has been confirmed in a double-blind study (Table IV). Lastly, lecithin (phosphatidylcholine), which is a bound form of choline, has been reported to improve TD in two uncontrolled studies (Growdon, 1978; Growdon, 1979). Of these four drugs lecithin perhaps offers the most promise as a practical therapeutic agent, subject to results from controlled studies, because physostigmine has to be given parenterally, the value of deanol has not been confirmed in controlled studies, and choline has a bitter taste and fishy odour.

Both Crane (1971) and Klawans (1973) have suggested that anticholinergic agents may increase the risk of development of TD. Indeed aggravation of TD occurred in three single blind studies with parenteral scopolamine and oral biperiden (Gerlach *et al*, 1974; Gerlach, 1977; Klawans and Rubovitz, 1974). In another single blind study in which patients were assessed during three treatment blocks, (neuroleptics plus anticholinergic antiparkinsonian drugs; neuroleptics alone; anticholinergic antiparkinsonian drugs alone), dyskinetic movements were at their worst during the period of anticholinergic treatment given alone (Turek *et al*, 1972). Furthermore it has been reported that anticholinergics given alone, without neuroleptics, can actually induce TD (Birket-Smith, 1974). Conversely some authors have reported that some patients with TD may improve on anticholinergics (Uhrbrand and Faurbye, 1960; Granacher *et al*, 1975) and the 'rabbit syndrome' appears to respond specifically to anticholinergic therapy (Jus *et al*, 1972; Sovner *et al*, 1977).

Gabacidic drugs

Attempts have been made to correct a postulated imbalance between DA and GABA systems in TD by using drugs to try to increase the activity of the inhibitory neurotransmitter GABA. Baclofen and sodium valproate, both putative GABA potentiators, are the principal drugs that have been used in this group. The effectiveness of baclofen has been confirmed in two controlled studies but another controlled study was unable to detect any significant effect (Table IV). A controlled study claimed that sodium valproate was of value in TD (Linnoila *et al*, 1976), but scrutiny of the results showed that there was no statistically significant difference between placebo and sodium valproate in their effect on oral-buccal dyskinesia. Gibson (1977), in an open study involving twenty-six patients, was also unable to detect any effect of sodium valproate in TD. Furthermore, in L-DOPA-induced dyskinesia sodium valproate proved to have only minimal effect (Price *et al*, 1978) and in three patients with Huntington's Chorea it was without benefit (Symington *et al*, 1978). There is increasing evidence that benzodiazepines can potentiate GABA transmission (Haefely, 1978) and, therefore, it is of some interest to know whether they might be of benefit in TD. However, studies in this area are preliminary and uncontrolled; Singh (1976) found diazepam beneficial in three patients and O'Flanagan (1975) described forty-two patients with clomipramine-induced dyskinesia who responded to clonazepam. Further developments in this GABAcidic approach to TD may depend upon the introduction of more potent and specific potentiators of GABA transmission.

Miscellaneous drugs

A large number of miscellaneous drugs have been investigated as treatments for TD; lithium, papaverine, pyridoxine, barbiturates, oestrogens, progestogens, clozapine, imipramine, isocarboxazid, L-tryptophan, disulfiram, fusaric acid, propranolol, cyproheptadine and manganese. The majority of these drugs have been reported to be successful in the treatment of TD and yet, with the possible exception of lithium, none of them has been properly evaluated. In the case of lithium, the numerous early encouraging reports were not confirmed when the drug was subjected to the discipline of later double-blind controlled studies. In two such studies (Simpson *et al*, 1976b; and Mackay *et al*, 1980), it proved to have no significant effect and in another study (Gerlach *et al*, 1975) it caused only a slight improvement. No doubt this progression from enthusiasm to pessimism would be repeated all too often should other drugs from this miscellaneous group be the subject of controlled studies.

Future strategies

A theme which runs through the published literature on therapeutic trials in TD is the wide variability in response to any particular agent. Some patients improve while others either show no response or get markedly worse. The reason for this variability may lie partly in the inadequacy of trial design but there is already evidence for the existence of distinct pharmacological subtypes within the gross clinical syndrome of TD (Gerlach *et al*, 1974; Casey and Denney, 1977). For example, one putative subgroup respond pharmacologically as if their underlying biochemical pathology was a relative excess of dopaminergic activity over cholinergic activity whereas another subgroup respond pharmacologically as if they had a relative excess of cholinergic activity over dopaminergic activity (Casey and Denney, 1977). These observations could of course explain some of the paradoxial findings with cholinergic and dopaminergic therapy which have already been mentioned.

If pharmacological subtypes have a basis in reality then their definition could be of crucial importance in defining the appropriate treatment for individual patients. The strategy of acute drug challenge as a way of predicting 'who-will-respond-to-what' was suggested by Kobayashi (1977) and has been applied in detail by Casey and Denney (1977). The definition of a *pharmacological signature* for each patient in an acute dose-response design seems to offer the most sensible and economical therapeutic approach to TD at the present time. Correlation of pharmacological response with careful clinical classification may lead to the identification of clinical predictors and even to a better understanding of the underlying neurological disorder(s).

Even if TD does reflect neurochemical imbalance rather than irreversible structural damage, it must be emphasized that until more is known about the mechanisms governing receptor stability then we will remain in a weak therapeutic position. The possibility must be explored of developing drugs which can be used chronically without inducing reactive imbalances in neuronal systems. Until this is possible it seems unlikely that pharmacological treatments for TD will offer anything more than temporary amelioration.

References

AIMS (1976) In *ECDEU Assessment Manual* (ed. W. Guy). Pp 534–537. U.S. Department of Health Education and Welfare, NIMH, Rockville, Maryland.

ALPERT, M., DIAMOND, F. & FRIEDHOFF, A. (1976) Tremographic studies in tardive dyskinesia. *Psychopharmacology*, **12**, 5–7.

BARNES, T., KIDGER, T. & TAYLOR, P. (1978) On the use of dopamine agonists in tardive dyskinesia. *American Journal of Psychiatry*, **135** (1), 132–133.

—— (1979) The concept of tardive dyskinesia. *Trends in Neurosciences*, **2**, 135–136.

BEDARD, P., PARKES, J. & MARSDEN, C. (1978) Effect of new dopamine-blocking agent (Oxiperomide) on drug induced dyskinesias in Parkinson's disease and spontaneous dyskinesias. *British Medical Journal*, i, 954–956.

BIRKET-SMITH, E. (1974) Abnormal involuntary movements induced by anticholinergic therapy. *Acta Neurologica Scandinavia*, **50**, 801–811.

BOURGEOIS, M. & HERBERT, A. (1970) Les dyskinesies tardives des neuroleptiques. *Bordeaux Medical*, **3**, 345–352.

BRANDRUP, E. (1961) Tetrabenazine treatment in persisting dyskinesia caused by psychopharmacea. *American Journal of Psychiatry*, **118**, 551–552.

CAINE, E. D., POLINSKY, R. J., KARTIZINER, R. & EBERT, M. H. (1979) The trial use of clozapine for abnormal involuntary movement disorders. *American Journal of Psychiatry*, **136** (3), 317–320.

CARROLL, B., CURITS, G. & KOKMEN, E. (1977) Paradoxical response to dopamine agonists in tardive dyskinesia. *American Journal of Psychiatry*, **134** (7), 785–789.

CARRUTHERS, S. (1971) Persistent tardive dyskinesia. *British Medical Journal*, iii, 572.

CASEY, D. & DENNEY, D. (1977) Pharmacological characterization of tardive dyskinesia. *Psychopharmacology*, **54**, 1–8.

CHASE, T. N. (1979) Dopamine and GABA syndrome dysfunction and the pathogenises of tardive dyskinesia. Proceedings of the International Symposium on Long Term Effects of Neuroleptics. *Advances in Psychopharmacology*. New York: Raven Press.

CLAVERIA, L., TEYCHENNE, P., CALNE, D., HASKAYNE, L., PETRIE, A., PALLIS, C. & LODGE-PATCH, I. (1975) Tardive dyskinesia treated with pimozide. *Journal of the Neurological Sciences*, **24**, 393–401.

COSTALL, B. & NAYLOR, R. J. (1978) Experimental studies of dopamine function in movement disorders. In *Neurotransmitter Systems and their Clinical Disorders* (ed. N. J. Legg). Pp 129–142. London: Academic Press.

CRANE, G. (1971) Neuroleptics and proneness to motor disorders. Read at 124th Annual Meeting of the American Psychiatric Association, Washington, DC. May 3–7.

—— & NARANJO, E. (1971) Motor disorders induced by neuroleptics. *Archives of General Psychiatry*, **24**, 179–184.

—— (1973) Mediocre effects of reserpine on tardive dyskinesia. *New England Journal of Medicine*, **288** (2), 104–105.

—— (1978) Tardive dyskinesia and related neurologic disorders. In *Handbook of Psychopharmacology, Vol. 10, Neuroleptics and Schizophrenia* (eds. L. L. Iversen, S. D. Iversen and S. H. Snyder). Pp 165–196. New York: Plenum Press.

CURRAN, J. (1973) Management of tardive dyskinesia with thiopropazate. *The American Journal of Psychiatry*, **130**, (8), 925–927.

DAVIS, K., BERGER, P. & HOLLISTER, L. (1975) Choline for tardive dyskinesia. *The New England Journal of Medicine*, **293**, 152.

—— —— (1978) Pharmacological investigations of the cholinergic imbalance hypotheses of movement disorders and psychosis. *Biological Psychiatry*, **13** (1), 23–49.

DECKER, B., DAVIS, J. & JANOWSKY, D. (1971) Amantadine hydrochloride treatment of tardive dyskinesia. *New England Journal of Medicine*, **285**, 1150–1151.

DEGKWITZ, R. (1969) Extrapyramidal motor disorders following long-term treatment with neuroleptic drugs. *Psychotropic Drugs and Dysfunctions of the Basal Ganglion* (P.H.S. Publication No. 1838). Edited by G. E. Crane and R. Gardener. Government Printing Office, Washington, D.C. p. 29.

DUVOISIN, R. (1972) Reserpine for tardive dyskinesia (contd.). *New England Journal of Medicine*, **286**, 611.

ECKMANN, F. (1968) Zur problematik von dauerschaden nach neuroleptischler langzeitbehandelling. *Therapie der Gegenwart*, **107**, 316–323.

FANN, W., DAVIS, J. & WILSON, I. (1973) Methylphenidate in tardive dyskinesia. *The American Journal of Psychiatry*, **130** (8), 922–924.

—— & LAKE, C. K. (1974) Cholinergic suppression of tardive dyskinesia (Gerber, C., McKenzie, G.). *Psychopharmacologia (Berlin)*, **37**, 101–107.

—— STAFFORD, J. R., MALONE, R. L., FROST, J. D. & RICHMAN, B. W. (1977) Clinical research techniques in tardive dyskinesia. *American Journal of Psychiatry*, **134**, 759–762.

FOG, R. & PAKKENBERG, H. (1970) Combined Nitomanpimozide treatment of Huntingdon's Chorea and other hyperkinetic syndromes. *Acta Neurologica Scandinavica*, **46**, 249–251.

FREEMAN, H. (1979) Pimozide as a neuroleptic. *British Journal of Psychiatry*, **135**, 82–83.

FRIEDHOFF, A. (1977) Receptor sensitivity modification (RSM)—a new paradigm for the potential treatment of some hormonal and transmitter disturbances. *Comprehensive Psychiatry*, **18** (4), 309–317.

GARDOS, G., COLE, J. & LABRIE, R. (1977) The assessment of tardive dyskinesia. *Archives of General Psychiatry*, **34**, 1206–1212.

GERLACH, J., REISBY, N. & RANDRUP, A. (1974) Dopaminergic hyposensitivity and cholinergic hypofunction in the patho-physiology of tardive dyskinesia. *Psychopharmacologia (Berlin)*, **34**, 21–35.

—— THORSEN, K. & MUNKVAD, I. (1975) Effect of lithium on neuroleptic-induced tardive dyskinesia compared with placebo in a double-blind cross-over trial. *Pharmacopsychiatrica*, **8**, 51–56.

—— (1977) The relationship between Parkinsonism and tardive dyskinesia. *American Journal of Psychiatry*, **134** (7), 781–784.

GIBSON, A. C. (1977) Tardive dyskinesia and Pimozide. *Proceedings of the Royal Society of Medicine*, **20**, (Suppl. 10), 34–37.

GODWIN-AUSTIN, R. & CLARK, T. (1971) Persistent phenothiazine dyskinesia treated with tetrabenazine. *British Medical Journal*, iv, 25–26.

GOMEZ, E. (1977) Clinical observations in the treatment of tardive dyskinesia with dihydrogenated ergot alkaloids (hydergine), preliminary findings. *Psychiatric Journal of University Ottawa*, **2**, 67–71.

GRANACHER, R., BALDESSARINI, R. & COLE, J. (1975) Deanol for tardive dyskinesia (cont.). *New England Journal of Medicine*, **292**, 926–927.

GROWDON, J., HIRSCH, M., WURTMAN, R. & WIENER, W. (1977) Oral choline administration to patients with tardive dyskinesia. *The New England Journal of Medicine*, **297**, 524–527.

—— (1978) Lecithin can suppress tardive dyskinesia. *The New England Journal of Medicine*, **298** (18), 1029.

—— (1979) Choline and lecithin administration to patients with tardive dyskinesia. *The Canadian Journal of Neurological Science*, **6** (1), 80.

HAEFELY, W. E. (1978) Central actions of benzodiazepines: general introduction. *British Journal of Psychiatry*, **133**, 231–239.

HIPPIUS, H. & LOGEMANN, G. (1970) Zur wirkung von dioxyphenylalanin (L-dopa) auf extrapyramidal motorische hyperkinesen nach langfristiger neruoleptische therapie. *Arzneimittel Forschung*, **20**, 894–896.

HOFMANN, M., TONON, G., SPANO, P. & TRABUCCHI, M. (1979) Mechanisms of dihydroegotoxines effect on prolactin release. *Journal of Pharmacy and Pharmacology*, **31**, 42–44.

JELLINGER, K. (1977) Neuropathologic findings after neuroleptic long-term therapy. *Neurotoxicology* (eds. L. Roizin, M. Shiraka and N. Grcevic), 25–42. New York: Raven Press.

JUS, K., VILLENEUVE, A. & JUS, A. (1972) Tardive dyskinesia and the rabbit syndrome during wakefulness and sleep. *American Journal of Psychiatry*, **129**, 765.

KAZAMATSURI, H., CHIEN, C. & COLE, J. (1972a) Treatment of tardive dyskinesia: clinical efficacy of a dopamine-depletion agent, tetrabenazine. *Archives of General Psychiatry*, **27**, 95–99.

—— —— —— (1972b) Treatment of tardive dyskinesia; short term efficacy of dopamine blocking agents haloperidol and thiopropazate. *Archives of General Psychiatry*, **27** (1), 100–106.

—— —— —— (1972c) Treatment of tardive dyskinesia. *Archives of General Psychiatry*, **27**, 824–827.

—— —— —— (1973) Long-term treatment of tardive dyskinesia with haloperidol and tetra-benazine. *American Journal of Psychiatry*, **130** (4), 479–483.

KEBABIAN, J. W. & CALNE, D. B. (1978) Multiple receptors for dopamine. *Nature*, **277**, 93–96.

KENNEDY, P., HERSHON, H. & McGUIRE, R. (1971) Extrapyramidal disorders after prolonged phenothiazine therapy. *British Journal of Psychiatry*, **118**, 509–518.

KLAWANS, H. & McKENDALL, R. (1971) Observations on the effect of L-dopa on tardive lingual-facial-buccal dyskinesia. *Journal of Neurological Sciences*, **14**, 189–192.

—— (1973) The pharmacology of tardive dyskinesias. *American Journal of Psychiatry*, **130**, 82–86.

—— & RUBOVITZ, R. (1974) Effect of cholinergic and anticholinergic agents on tardive dyskinesia. *Journal of Neurology, Neurosurgery and Psychiatry*, **27**, 941–947.

KOBAYASHI, R. M. (1977) Drug therapy of tardive dyskinesia. *New England Journal of Medicine*, **296** (5), 257–260.

KORSGAARD, S. (1976) Baclofen (Lioresal) in the treatment of neuroleptic-induced tardive dyskinesia. *Acta Psychiatrica Scandinavica*, **54**, 17–24.

LAL, S. (1974) Comparison of thiopropazate and trifluoperazine on oral dyskinesia: a double-blind study. *Current Therapeutic Research*, **16**, 990–997.

LEES, A., LANDER, C. & STERN, G. (1979) Tiapride in Levodopa-induced involuntary movements. *Journal of Neurology, Neurosurgery and Psychiatry*, **4**, 380–383.

LINNOILA, M., VIUKARI, M. & HIETALA, O. (1976) Effects of Sodium Valproate on tardive dyskinesia. *British Journal of Psychiatry*, **129**, 114–119.

MACKAY, A. V. P., SHEPPARD, G., SAHA, B. K., MOTLEY, B. & MARSDEN, C. D. (1980) Failure of lithium treatment in established tardive dyskinesia. *Psychological Medicine*, **10**, 583–587.

MACCALLUM, W. A. G. (1970) Tetrabenazine for extra-pyramidal motor disorders. *British Medical Journal*, i, 760.

O'FLANAGAN, P. M. (1975) Clonazepam in the treatment of drug-induced dyskinesia. *British Medical Journal*, i, 269–270.

PAKKENBERG, H. & FOG, R. (1974) Spontaneous oral dyskinesia: results of tetrabenazine, pimozide, or both. *Archives of Neurology*, **31**, 352–353.

PETERS, H. A., DALY, R. F. & SATO, S. (1972) Reserpine for tardive dyskinesia. *New England Journal of Medicine*, **286**, 106.

PRICE, P., PARICES, J. & MARSDEN, C. (1978) Sodium valproate in the treatment of levodopa-induced dyskinesia. *Journal of Neurology, Neurosurgery and Psychiatry*, **41**, 702–706.

SCHMIDT, W. R. & JARCHO, L. W. (1966) Persistent dyskinesia following phenothiazine therapy. *Archives of Neurology*, **14**, 369–377.

SCHONECKER, M. (1957) Ein eigentumliches syndrom im oralen bereich bei megaphen applikation. *Nervenarzt*, **28**, 35.

SIMPSON, G. M., ZOUBOK, B. & LEE, H. J. (1976a) An early clinical and toxicity trial of Ex. 11-582A in chronic schizophrenia. *Current Therapeutic Research*, **19**, 87–93.

—— BRANCHAY, M., LEE, J., VOITASHEVSKY, A. & ZOUBOK, B. (1976b) Lithium in tardive dyskinesia. *Pharmakopsychiatrica*, **9**, 76–80.

—— VOITASHEVSKY, A., YOUNG, M. & LEE, J. (1977) Deanol in the treatment of tardive dyskinesia. *Psychopharmacology*, **52**, 257–261.

—— LEE, J. H., ZOUBOK, B. & GARDOS, G. (1979) A rating scale for tardive dyskinesia. *Psychopharmacology*, **64**, 171–179.

SINGER, K. & CHENG, M. (1971) Thiopropazate hydrochloride in persistent dyskinesia. *British Medical Journal*, iv, 22–25.

SINGH, M. M. (1976) Diazepam in the treatment of tardive dyskinesia: preliminary observations. *International Pharmacopsychiatry*, **11** (4), 232–234.

SMITH, R., TAMMINGA, C., HARASZJI, J., PANDEY, G. & DAVIS, J. (1977) Effects of dopamine agonists in tardive dyskinesia. *American Journal of Psychiatry*, **134** (7), 765–768.

SOVNER, R. & DIMASCIO, A. (1977) The effects of benztrophine mesylate in the rabbit syndrome and tardive dyskinesia. *American Journal of Psychiatry*, **11**, 1301–1302.

SPANO, P. F. & TRABUCCHI, M. (1978) Interaction of ergot alkaloids with dopaminergic receptors in the rat striatum and nucleus accumbens. *Gerontology*, **24**, Suppl. 1, 106–114.

SYMINGTON, G., LEONARD, D., SHANNON, P. & VAJDA, F. (1978) Sodium valproate in Huntington's disease. *American Journal of Psychiatry*, **135** (3), 352–354.

TAMMINGA, C., SMITH, R., GRICKSEN, S., CHANG, S. & DAVIS, J. (1977) Cholingergic influences in tardive dyskinesia. *American Journal of Psychiatry*, **134** (7), 769–774.

TARSY, D., LEOPOLD, N. & SAX, D. (1974) Physostigmine in choreiform movement disorder. *Neurology*, **24**, 28–33.

—— PARKES, J. & MARSDEN, C. (1975) Metoclopramide and pimozide in Parkinson's disease and levodopa induced dyskinesia. *Journal of Neurology, Neurosurgery and Psychiatry*, **38**, 331–335.

TOLOSA, E. (1974) Paradoxical suppression of chorea by apomorphine. *Journal of the American Medical Association*, **229** (12), 1579–1580.

TUREK, I., KURLAND, A., HANLON, T. & BOHM, M. (1972) Tardive dyskinesia: its relation to neuroleptic and antiparkinson drugs. *British Journal of Psychiatry*, **121**, 605–612.

UHRBRAND, L. & FAURBYE, A. (1960) Reversible and irreversible dyskinesia after treatment with Perphenazine, Chlorpromazine, Reserpine and electroconvulsive therapy. *Psychopharmacologia*, **1**, 408–418.

VASAVAN-NAIR, N. P., YASSA, R., RUIS-NAVARRO, J. & SCHWARTZ, G. (1978) Baclofen in the treatment of tardive dyskinesia. *American Journal of Psychiatry*, **135** (12), 1562–1563.

VILLENEUVE, A., BOSZOMENYI, Z. & DECHAMBAULT, M. (1970a) Tentative De Traitment de dyskinesia post neuroleptiques de type permanent. *Laval Medicine*, **41**, 923–933.

—— & BOSZOMENYI, Z. (1970b) Treatment of drug-induced dyskinesia. *Lancet*, i, 353–354.

WEINER, W. J., CARVEY, P., NAUSIEDA, A. & KLAWANS, H. L. (1978) Diurnal alterations in striatal dopaminergic sensitivity. *Neurology*, **28**, 344.

41 Token economies and schizophrenia: A review

JOHN HALL and ROGER BAKER

Our paper published in 1977 (Baker *et al*, 1977) appeared at a time which represented, in retrospect, the high point of token economy work with chronic institutionalized patients in Britain. In that year two major American books dealing with token economies were published. Paul and Lentz (1977) published a detailed account of their comparison of token economy and milieu therapy programmes with chronic patients. Kazdin's review (1977) volume examined the application of token economy methods to a range of clinical problems, chapter four specifically being concerned with applications to chronic psychiatric patients. Although there have been a number of subsequent useful reviews in journals, some concerning behaviour modification techniques with chronic patients (Matson, 1980) and some covering token economy methods generally (Kazdin, 1982), the use of token methods with chronic patients in Britain has declined. This is illustrated by comparing the survey studies of Hall (1973), and Baker and Rizvi (1984). The former study reviewed 27 working token economies which existed in 1972 in Britain, and was known to have missed some working programmes; the latter study carried out a review of Scottish psychiatric rehabilitation facilities and found only one functioning token economy. What, then, is the present status of the token economy in work with chronic schizophrenic patients?

It is necessary to clarify the use of the term 'chronic patient' in this review. In our own study all patients had been given a clear diagnosis of schizophrenia, checked by the research psychiatrist of the team, and patients who were mentally handicapped or had an organic condition were specifically excluded. Most British token economy studies have used exclusively schizophrenic patients (Woods *et al*, 1984) or groups which were mostly schizophrenic—34 out of the 45 patients in Presly *et al*'s study (1976). In the American studies most patients are schizophrenic, confirmed by phrases such as '76 per cent psychotic' or a detailed diagnostic listing giving, for example, 47 out of 52 patients a diagnosis of schizophrenia. Length of stay criteria or age criteria may vary markedly, but the great majority of studies refer to patient groups which are certainly 75 per cent or more schizophrenic, by diagnostic criteria which vary in their precision. This level of clarity in diagnosis and definition of subjects used is certainly no worse than practice in other areas of published work with chronic patients (Hall, 1979).

Our 1977 paper, together with a related paper (Hall *et al*, 1977a) and an extensive final research report (Hall *et al*, 1977b), reported the main findings of a project undertaken at Stanley Royd Hospital, Wakefield, over a period of six years. When the project was being planned in 1970, treatment of the institutionalized patient was dominated by social therapy and occupational models of treatment. The book *Institutionalism and Schizophrenia*, by Wing and Brown (1970), made no mention of behavioural approaches to treatment. However, Ayllon and Azrin (1968) had already published their book *The Token Economy* and a few other American experimental studies, such as that of Schaefer and Martin (1966), were available to us. The method was thus essentially unknown in British clinical practice, apart from a handful of trial projects, such as the ward developed by David Peck at Lancaster Moor Hospital (Peck and Thorpe, 1971). It was far from clear how much improvement could be expected, and equally unclear what therapeutic factors were central to the apparent success of the early American studies.

As illustrated by the survey of Hall (1973), the project at Wakefield was undertaken at a time of growing interest in the application of behavioural methods to chronic conditions. A community of psychologists and psychiatrists grew up in Britain, in regular contact with each other both informally and through the agency of a number of specialized conferences, such as those organized by the Behavioural Engineering Association in Ireland. It was an exciting time, and the penetration of behavioural methods into professional training syllabuses—for example, the development of the then Joint Board of Clinical Nursing Studies syllabuses in behavioural psychotherapy—resulted in a demand for information about the project and similar projects elsewhere. There were a number of other research based token economy programmes developing at the same time, notably those at Aberdeen, Dundee and Dublin. Stoffelmayr *et al* (1973, 1979) published the results of a multicentre trial conducted in Aberdeen which compared token economy methods with social therapy techniques. Fraser (1978, 1983) conducted a number of studies at Dundee of the main determinants of change in token economies, such as the role of instructions, feedback and response costs. Fernandez (1974) investigated the function of a number of variables, largely by the use of sequential designs, whereby a specified variable was introduced and allowed to exert its effect before the next variable was introduced. Our own distinctive contribution, following the conduct of a pilot study (Baker and Hutchinson, 1974), was to design a study specifically identifying the function of contingent token reinforcement (Baker *et al*, 1977).

Symptom change in token economies

In a review of token economy work with schizophrenic patients, the impact on schizophrenic symptomatology is central, yet the early American studies had made little serious attempt to measure symptom change. This was in part due to the clash between the behavioural and the conventional psychiatric paradigms. From a radical behavioural viewpoint, delusional verbiage was a behaviour much like cleaning your shoes: both may be considered to be shaped and reshapeable by the environment. Our own study showed that symptomatic behaviour, as assessed by a psychiatrist using three standard measures, did not change in the main study. However, there is a body of research using behavioural methods with florid symptoms, largely consisting of single case studies with behavioural methods other than token economies. These studies have been reviewed by Baker (1975) and Gomes-Schwartz (1979) and present fairly clear evidence that it is possible to modify almost any schizophrenic symptom, including the experience and behavioural concomitants of auditory hallucinations. However, the degree of modification found from one patient to another is extremely variable. In the study by Wincze *et al* (1972), seven of ten chronic paranoid schizophrenic patients showed decreases of at least 20 per cent in delusional speech in response to token contingencies, one of the seven showing complete suppression of delusions and another near complete. As with many studies, there was little spontaneous generalization of improvement outside the ward setting, although subsequent special generalization training with eight of the patients effectively reduced delusional speech in four patients. A handful of studies have reported the appearance of aberrant behaviours following modification of symptoms (*inter alia*, Slade, 1972; Lambley, 1973), but florid symptoms such as hallucinations have been totally eradicated without any apparent 'symptom substitution' (*inter alia*, Alumbaugh, 1971). Some studies have reported suppression of all the major symptoms demonstrated by an individual (*inter alia*, Nydegger, 1972; Smith and Carlin, 1972). While it has often been said that such patients have simply been trained to talk less about their symptoms, others (*inter alia*, Saslow, 1967) see no reason why the modification of behaviour should not affect subjective states.

Florid symptoms are only one aspect of schizophrenia. There has been renewed interest in the negative and positive symptoms of schizophrenia (Crow, 1980). The assessment of negative symptoms, such as social withdrawal and apathy, does pose problems (Lewine *et al*, 1983), but the 'social withdrawal' and 'socially embarrassing' factors of the Wing Ward Behaviour Rating Scale (Wing, 1961) are measures of some validity. Five separate British studies of chronic schizophrenic patients (Baker *et al*, 1974; Baker *et al*, 1977; Elliott *et al*, 1979; Fraser, 1978; Presly *et al*, 1976) showed that token economy programmes improve the 'social withdrawal' factor. This includes behaviour such as self-care, speed of movement, and speech. Changes in socially embarrassing behaviour in the five studies were more variable, as would be predicted from Baker *et al* (1977). There is a wealth of other evidence, using a range of assessment methods, that different aspects of social withdrawal can be modified (Hersen, 1979; Matson, 1980). A consistent finding has also been that behaviour change has failed to generalize outside the treatment setting in which it has developed (Shepherd, 1980). This may be overcome by special generalization training (Kazdin, 1977), by moving the token economy into the community (Henderson and Scholes, 1970), or by implementing behaviour modification programmes in the homes of chronic schizophrenic patients by their families (Hudson, 1978).

Other factors in token economies

Although there has been increasing concern to assess symptomatic change in token economies, a number of other aspects of token economy programmes have been investigated, such as individual variations in response to token programmes. Since most token programmes have been carried out with patients who all suffer from chronic schizophrenia, it is not possible to establish diagnosis-specific response rates, although interestingly a careful examination of the appendix of Ayllon and Azrin's book (1968) suggests that the mentally handicapped patients did better than the chronic psychiatric patients. Our colleague, Richard Butler (1979), analysed 51 individual treatment programmes carried out on a token ward, and found that the less withdrawn patients did best on the programme, and the non-responsiveness to token programmes was reduced by individualizing programmes very carefully. Woods *et al* (1984) examined data from six patients exposed to a token programme for five years, suggesting that the programme had a specific therapeutic effect for only three of the patients: this paper also has a useful and detailed discussion of the relative merits of ratings and direct observational techniques in evaluating this type of treatment.

Since changes in behaviour with chronic psychiatric patients are typically slow (Woods and Cullen, 1983) and limited in extent, the question of how best to evaluate token economy programmes is important. Paul and Lentz (1977) directed a considerable part of their own book to describe the several measures they developed in their project. In our own study we encountered the need to improve assessment techniques and carried out a number of studies of staff opinions of behaviour of patients (Hall, 1977) and of the design and use of rating procedures with chronic patients (Hall, 1979; 1980). These led to the publication of REHAB (Baker and Hall, 1983), a new behaviour rating scale for use with chronic psychiatric patients. Similarly, the need to train direct care staff in the use of behavioural methods also became apparent. Two of our colleagues developed a training programme for use with psychiatric nurses, and this led to the publication of a book summarizing the content of the programme (Butler and Rosenthall, 1978). More recently a series of papers by Milne (1982; 1984) have illustrated both the design of training programmes for staff and how to ensure that the results of training generalize to the ward setting.

Why do token economies work?

In 1977 Paul and Lentz were able to state confidently that: 'The overall comparative results on the relative effectiveness of the programs in the current project could not be clearer. The social learning (token) program was significantly more effective than either the milieu program or the traditional hospital program. Its greater effectiveness was consistent across all classes of functioning in the intramural setting.' However, this statement does not indicate *why* token economy programmes are effective. In the years since our 1977 paper was published, considerable doubt has arisen as to whether contingent token reinforcement is the main therapeutic ingredient in a token economy. A token programme involves the introduction of a systematic goal-setting and monitoring system, as well as the use of verbal reinforcement and informational feedback, so the contribution of these factors may outweigh the effect of any material reinforcement available via the tokens. Since the tokens presumably acquire their value to patients by systematic linking to the availability of desired back-up or primary reinforcers, it should be demonstrable that the back-up reinforcers alone can produce systematic change. In none of the quoted studies has this been demonstrated for the group of patients used in the main experimental study. Many of the chronic patients used in token programmes display high levels of anhedonia, i.e. low levels of motivation to experience pleasure. Coupled with the very low cash purchasing power of most token schemes, the incentive to earn tokens is not high, so the level of anhedonia of patients and its relationship to symptom patterns, may be a characteristic on which patients should be selected for token economies (Cook and Simukanda, 1981). For all of these reasons, there have been a number of changes in the way in which token economy programmes are now designed and in the way in which they are conceptualized.

One major change is that the ward-wide standard token packages have been superseded in Britain by more differentiated behavioural regimes, within which tokens may be used for some, but not for all patients (see Matson, 1980; Woods, *et al*, 1984). This change has been stimulated partly because of the evidence of the studies already quoted, but partly because of the continuing reduction in size of the large psychiatric hospitals by the discharge of the least handicapped patients. The wards, formerly full of patients who were relatively similar to each other, are now half empty and contain a more varied and usually more actively disturbed group of patients, less suitable for 'package' programmes. Other treatment approaches have been introduced, such as social skills training (Spencer *et al*, 1983) and problem-solving techniques (D'Zurilla and Goldfried, 1971), and their use in combination with other behavioural techniques means that a 'pure' token economy is now hard to find. Indeed, it is now difficult to imagine that a ward-wide token programme, with tokens as the main therapeutic element for all patients, would be a regime of choice in most psychiatric hospitals in Britain.

Alongside changes in technique have come changes in interpretation. As long ago as 1973 Stoffelmayr found that a token regime was superior to social therapy on all accounts, but noted that nurses on the token economy interacted more frequently with patients and prompted and ordered patients less often than nurses in the control social therapy regime. This might suggest that the nature of staff-patient interaction is the main therapeutic factor. Studies by Fraser (1983) have drawn attention to the role of instructions as the most potent variable in training long-stay patients. This view has also been taken by Lowe and Higson (1983), who point out how verbal self-control methods have been explored relatively little with chronic patients. In our 1977 paper the control group improved significantly more than the experimental group on social withdrawal. Attribution theory could explain this finding. Work with nursery school children has shown that a group previously non-rewarded for drawing drew more than a previously rewarded group, when put in a non-specific situation with drawing materials. Nisbett and Valins (1972) comment that: 'it is possible, at a very tender age, to undermine intrinsic motivation by extrinsic rewards', and this undermining may be displayed with chronic patients. Since the attributional models predicts different results to the behavioural, it merits further investigation.

Another way of conceptualizing some of the information derived from token programmes involves the application of environmental psychology, or 'ward ecology'. Careful examination of the behaviour of chronic patients suggests that their behaviour can be greatly affected by the physical environment within which they live. Studies such as that of Polsky and Chance (1980), examining the patterns of use of space by chronic patients in a ward setting, or of Holahan (1979), looking at the effects of seating arrangements on communication between psychiatric patients, illustrate this trend. The architectural and organizational implications of 'normalization' theory for the care of the mentally handicapped are radical and can equally be applied to the care of the psychiatrically handicapped. Not only the physical environment, but the social environment of a ward can affect patients. The work of Leff and his colleagues (1982) identifies the role of 'expressed emotion' (EE) in the relapse of patients within their families. This work is reviewed in Barrowclough and Tarrier (1984), and certainly it is possible to envisage staff and patients being high on EE with similar potential consequences for vulnerable patients in high contact with them.

One must still ask precisely *what* variable is responsible for the improvements that have resulted from token economies. Our own studies led us to conclude that contingent token reinforcement was *not* responsible, speaking of the token economy as a total environment, rather than as a technique for individual patients or programmes. The work of Fernandez (1974) and Fraser (1978), already referred to, attempted to address this question. Fernandez indicated that some target behaviours show greatest change when instructions and prompting are combined with verbal reinforcement, and that some behaviours can be changed using instruction alone. Fraser used an impressive multiple baseline design, and suggested that instructions about expected behaviour made the most significant contribution to behaviour change. Unfortunately, both these sets of studies used very short experimental phases (two to six weeks), whereas our own, using a 12-month experimental phase, shows that the long-term effectiveness of a Token Economy Programme is confused by the immediate but short-lived effects of contingent token reinforcement (Hall *et al*, 1977a). Nonetheless, the evidence that instructions are perhaps the main therapeutic factor is strong. Fraser clearly thinks so: 'The token economy is therefore seen to achieve its effects solely through the elaborate social information system which is embodied in its application and the conditioning theory of its operation must, as a result, surrender to Occam's razor since there has been no reliable evidence to-date that contingent token presentation is a critical therapeutic variable.' This view has considerable practical implications, since, if comparable results can be achieved without exchangeable tokens, it is no longer necessary to bother to exchange tokens for goods, nor indeed ethically defensible to restrict access to rights and privileges. There would still remain the need to retain a complex goal-setting and monitoring system, together with the information about what behaviour is acceptable, as implied by the elaborate social information system view.

Wing (1977) has advocated on many occasions a three-fold classification of the causation of chronic handicap in schizophrenic patients. He conceives of (a) primary handicaps, arising directly from the psychiatric condition; (b) secondary handicaps relating to the changed reaction or attitude of the patient and relatives to the patient himself; and (c) premorbid handicaps. Only since it has been possible to study schizophrenic patients at home in their family (Creer and Wing, 1974) has it been possible to identify more carefully those handicaps due solely to institutional living. Recent studies have also pointed to the high proportion of patients with a physical disability or untreated medical condition, which further complicates their treatment. This type of analysis suggests that intervention at several different levels is required to meet the full range of needs of the chronic schizophrenic patient. Quite apart from the contingencies which operate in a ward, for example, the appropriate level of social and environmental stimulation still needs to be determined.

Perhaps one test of the influence of token economy methods is to compare the state of the art of psychiatric rehabilitation before the advent of token economies with the present time. General professional views of rehabilitation and the nature of the identified clinical problems, have changed considerably over those 15 years. In 1970 continued discharge of chronic patients was accepted relatively uncritically and most large psychiatric hospitals contained perhaps hundreds of patients who could not immediately be discharged, but for whom a goal-directed social learning regime seemed appropriate. In 1985 the deinstitutionalization movement is proceeding much more cautiously (Bachrach, 1980), and those chronic patients remaining within hospital present a much more differentiated and in general more severe range of problems. One of the requirements of token economy methods is that they need a degree of staff control over patients which is incompatible with the general service move towards greater patient freedom and community alternatives to psychiatric hospitals (Stein and Test, 1978; Wing and Olsen, 1979).

It may seem paradoxical that only as the numbers of chronic patients in hospital have fallen, have important British books on psychiatric rehabilitation been published. Wing and Morris's 1981 volume arose from a working party of the Royal College of Psychiatrists (1980); Watts and Bennett (1983) have produced a comprehensive textbook. The volume edited by McCreadie (1982) contains a chapter specifically on the rehabilitation of schizophrenia, containing a section on behaviour modification methods. A careful reading of these books indicates the major contribution of behavioural methods to present day psychiatric rehabilitation, in four respects. Firstly, an increased emphasis on careful and comprehensive assessment of the patient and his environment, using behavioural methods and relating to regular monitoring procedures. Secondly, a broadening range of behavioural treatment procedures which *may* use individual or group token programmes. Thirdly, a clearer formation of the significance of patient–staff and patient–patient interaction for ward milieux. Fourthly, better guidance on the design of both patient treatment programmes and staff training programmes so that positive results of the programme generalize to the real world. All four of these developments owe much to the token economy practice and research of the last fifteen years, although the token economy itself, in its original 'pure' form, has fallen into abeyance.

References

ALUMBAUGH, R. V. (1971) Use of behaviour modification techniques towards reduction of hallucinatory behaviour: a case study. *Psychological Records*, **21**, 415–417.
AYLLON, T. & AZRIN, N. (1968) *The Token Economy*. New York: Appleton Century Crofts.

BACHRACH, L. L. (1980) Is the least restrictive environment always the best?: Sociological and semantic implications. *Hospital and Community Psychiatry*, **31**, 97–103.

BAKER, R. D. (1975) Behavioural techniques in the treatment of schizophrenia. In *Handbook of Schizophrenia* (eds. A. Forrest and J. Affleck). Edinburgh: Churchill Livingstone.

—— & HALL, J. N. (1983) *REHAB: Rehabilitation Evaluation of Hall and Baker*. Aberdeen: Vine Publishing.

—— —— & HUTCHINSON, K. (1974) A token economy project with chronic schizophrenic patients. *British Journal of Psychiatry*, **124**, 367–384.

—— —— —— & BRIDGE, G. W. K. (1977) Symptom changes in chronic schizophrenic patients on a token economy: a controlled experiment. *British Journal of Psychiatry*, **131**, 381–393.

—— & RIZVI, W. S. (1984) Psychiatric rehabilitation in Scotland: a survey. *Health Bulletin of the Scottish Home and Health Department*, **42**, 187–198.

BARROWCLOUGH, C. & TARRIER, N. (1984) 'Psychosocial' interventions with families and their effects on the course of schizophrenia: a review. *Psychological Medicine*, **14**, 629–642.

BUTLER, R. J. (1979) An analysis of individual treatment on a token economy for chronic schizophrenic patients. *British Journal of Medical Psychology*, **52**, 235–243.

—— & ROSENTHALL, G. (1978). *Behaviour and Rehabilitation*. Bristol: John Wright.

COOK, M. & SIMUKONDA, F. (1981) Anhedonia and schizophrenia. *British Journal of Psychiatry*, **139**, 523–525.

CREER, C. & WING, J. K. (1974) *Schizophrenia At Home*. National Schizophrenia Fellowship, Surbiton.

CROW, T. (1980) Molecular pathology of schizophrenia: more than one disease process? *British Medical Journal*, **280**, 66–68.

D'ZURILLA, T. J. & GOLDFRIED, M. E. (1971) Problem solving and behaviour modification. *Journal of Abnormal Psychology*, **78**, 107–126.

ELLIOTT, P. A., BARLOW, F., HOOPER, A. & KINGERLEE, P. (1979) Maintaining patient improvements in a token economy. *Behaviour Research and Therapy*, **17**, 355–367.

FERNANDEZ, J. (1974) Variables which contribute towards the behavioural improvement shown by subjects in token programmes. Paper presented at the 4th Annual Conference of European Association for Behaviour Therapy, London.

FRASER, D. (1978) *Determinants of Change in Token Economy Programmes*. Report available from the Department of Psychology, Royal Dundee Liff Hospital.

—— (1983) From token economy to social information system: the emergence of critical variables. In *Current Issues in Clinical Psychology, Vol. 1.* (ed. E. Karas). New York: Plenum Press.

GOMES-SCHWARTZ, B. (1979) The modification of schizophrenic behaviour. *Behaviour Modification*, **3**, 439–468.

HALL, J. N. (1973) Ward behaviour modification projects in Great Britain. *Bulletin of British Psychological Society*, **26**, 199–201.

—— (1977) The content of ward rating scales for long-stay patients. *British Journal of Psychiatry*, **130**, 287–293.

—— (1979) Assessment procedures used in studies on long-stay patients: a survey of papers published in the *British Journal of Psychiatry*. *British Journal of Psychiatry*, **135**, 330–335.

—— (1980) Ward rating scales for long-stay patients: a review. *Psychological Medicine*, **10**, 277–288.

—— BAKER, R. D. & HUTCHINSON, K. (1977a) A controlled evaluation of the economy procedures with chronic schizophrenic patients. *Behaviour Research and Therapy*, **15**, 261–283.

—— —— BUTLER, R. J. GWYNNE-JONES, H. & HAMILTON, M. (1977b) *Clinical Applications of Behaviour Modification Techniques with Long-Stay Psychiatric Patients—Final Project Report*. Department of Psychology and Psychiatry, University of Leeds.

HENDERSON, J. D. & SCHOLES, P. E. (1970) Conditioning techniques in a community-based operant environment for psychotic men. *Behaviour Therapy*, **1**, 245–251.

HERSEN, M. (1979) Modification of skills deficits in psychiatric patients. In *Research and Practice in Social Skills Training*. (eds. A. S. Bellack and M. Hersen). New York: Plenum Press.

HOLAHAN, C. J. (1979) Environmental psychology in psychiatric hospital settings. In *Designing for Therapeutic Environments*. (eds. D. Cantor and S. Cantour). Chichester: Wiley.

HUDSON, B. L. (1978) Behavioural social work with schizophrenic patients in the community. *British Journal of Social Work*, **8**, 159–170.

KAZDIN, A. E. (1977) *The Token Economy: a Review and Evaluation*. New York: Plenum.

—— (1982) The token economy: a decade later. *Journal of Applied Behaviour Analysis*, **15**, 431–445.

LAMBLEY, P. (1973) Behaviour modification and the treatment of psychosis: a critique of Alumbaugh. *Psychological Record*, **23**, 93–97.

LEFF, J., KUIPERS, L., BERKOWITZ, R., EBERLEIN-VRIES, R. & STURGEON, D. (1982) A controlled trial of social intervention in the families of schizophrenic patients. *British Journal of Psychiatry*, **141**, 121–134.

LEWINE, R. R. J., FOGG, L. & MELTZER, H. Y. (1983) Assessment of negative and positive symptoms in schizophrenia. *Schizophrenia Bulletin,* **9,** 368–376.

LOWE, C. F. & HIGSON, P. J. (1983) Is all behaviour modification 'cognitive'?. In *Current Issues in Clinical Psychology. Vol. 1.* (ed. E. Karas). New York: Plenum Publishing.

MCCREADIE, R. G. (1982) Schizophrenia. In *Rehabilitation in Psychiatric Practice* (ed. R. G. McCreadie). London: Pitman.

MATSON, J. L. (1980) Behaviour modification procedures for training chronically institutionalized schizophrenics. In *Progress in Behaviour Modification,* **9,** London: Academic Press.

MILNE, D. L. (1982) A comparison of two methods of teaching behaviour modification to mental handicap nurses. *Behavioural Psychotherapy,* **10,** 54–64.

—— (1984) Skill evaluations of nurse-training in behaviour therapy. *Behavioural Psychotherapy,* **12,** 142–150.

NISBETT, R. E. & VALINS, S. (1972) Perceiving the causes of one's own behaviour. In *Attribution: Perceiving the Causes of Behaviour* (eds. E. E. Jones, D. E. Kahouse, H. H. Kelley *et al*). Morristown, N.J.: General Learning Press.

NYDEGGER, R. V. (1972) The elimination of hallucinatory and delusional material by verbal conditioning and assertive training: a case study. *Journal of Behaviour Therapy and Experimental Psychiatry,* **3,** 225–227.

PAUL, G. L. & LENTZ, R. J. (1977) *Psychosocial Treatment of Chronic Mental Patients.* Cambridge, Mass.: Harvard University Press.

PECK, D. F. & THORPE, G. L. (1971) Experimental foundations of token economics: a critique. Paper presented at the 2nd Behavioural Engineering Conference, Wexford.

POLSKY, R. H. & CHANCE, M. R. A. (1980) Social interaction and the use of space on a ward of long-term psychiatric patients. *Journal of Nervous and Mental Disease,* **168,** 550–555.

PRESLY, A. S., BLACK, D., GRAY, A., HARTIE, A. & SEYMOUR, E. (1976) The token economy in the National Health Service: possibilities and limitations. *Acta Psychiatrica Scandinavica,* **53,** 258–270.

ROYAL COLLEGE OF PSYCHIATRISTS (1980) *Psychiatric Rehabilitation in the 1980s.* Royal College of Psychiatrists, London.

SASLOW, G. (1967) A case history of attempted behaviour modification in a psychiatric ward. In *Research in Behaviour Modification* (eds. L. Krasner and L. P. Ullmann). New York: Holt, Rhinehart & Winston.

SCHAEFER, H. H. & MARTIN, P. L. (1966) Behavioural therapy for 'apathy' of hospitalized schizophrenics. *Psychological Reports,* **19,** 1147–1158.

SHEPHERD, G. (1980) The treatment of social difficulties in special environments. In *The Social Psychology of Psychological Problems* (eds. P. Feldman and J. Orford). Chichester: Wiley.

SLADE, P. D. (1972) The effects of systematic desensitization on auditory hallucinations. *Behaviour Research and Therapy,* **10,** 85–91.

SMITH, R. C. & CARLIN, J. (1972) Behaviour modification using interlocking reinforcement on a short-term psychiatric ward. *Archives of General Psychiatry,* **27,** 386–389.

SPENCER, P. G., GILLESPIE, C. R. & EKISA, E. G. (1983) A controlled comparison of the effect of social skills training and remedial drama on the conversational skills of chronic schizophrenic in-patients. *British Journal of Psychiatry,* **143,** 165–172.

STEIN, L. I. & TEST, M. A. (1978) *Alternatives to Mental Hospital Treatment.* New York: Plenum Press.

STOFFELMAYR, B. E., FAULKNER, G. E. & MITCHELL, W. S. (1973) *The Rehabilitation of Chronic Hospitalised Patients—A Comparative Study of Operant Conditioning Methods and Social Therapy Techniques.* Final Report to Scottish Home and Health Department.

—— —— —— (1979) The comparison of token economy and social therapy in the treatment of hard-core schizophrenic patients. *Behavioural Analysis & Modification,* **,** 3–17.

WATTS, F. N. & BENNETT, D. H. (1983) *Theory and Practice of Psychiatric Rehabilitation.* Chichester: Wiley.

WINCZE, J. P., LEITENBERG, H. & AGRAS, W. S. (1972) The effects of token reinforcement and feedback on the delusional verbal behaviour of chronic paranoid schizophrenics. *Journal of Applied Behaviour Analysis,* **5,** 247–262.

WING, J. K. (1961) A simple and reliable subclassification of chronic schizophrenia. *Journal of Mental Science,* **107,** 862–875.

—— (1977) *Schizophrenia and its Management in the Community.* National Schizophrenia Fellowship, Surbition.

—— & BROWN, G. W. (1970) *Institutionalism and Schizophrenia.* Cambridge University Press.

—— & MORRIS, B. (1981). *Handbook of Psychiatric Rehabilitation Practice.* Oxford University Press.

—— & OLSEN, R. (1979) *Community Care for the Mentally Disabled.* Oxford University Press.

Woods, P. A. & Cullen, C. N. (1983) Determinants of staff behaviour in long-term care. *Behavioural Psychotherapy*, **11,** 4–18.

—— Higson, P. J. & Tannahill, N. M. (1984) Token-economy programmes with chronic psychotic patients: the importance of direct measurement and objective evaluation for long-term maintenance. *Behaviour Research and Therapy*, **22,** 41–51.

42 Rehabilitation

ROBIN G. McCREADIE

'Rehabilitation is the process of identifying and preventing or minimizing [the multiple] causes [of severe disablement] while at the same time helping the individual to develop and use his or her talents and thus to acquire confidence and self esteem through success in social roles ... Rehabilitation, therefore, necessitates a long-term commitment to the individual patient' (Royal College of Psychiatrists, 1980). In short, rehabilitation is the management of the long-term mentally ill—in the context of this review, the chronic schizophrenic. Management includes assessment, and physical, psychological and social therapies. As physical and psychological treatments are considered in more detail in this section, more emphasis is placed on social management.

Necessary resources

Facilities necessary for an adequate rehabilitation programme for chronic schizophrenics are of four main types: staffing, accommodation, occupational and social therapies, and support services. A list of 52 services belonging to one or other of the four main types is given in the Appendix. It can be seen that in all four areas both the National Health Service and local authorities contribute to the necessary resources. Levels towards which rehabilitation services should aim have been suggested by the DHSS (DHSS, 1975); for example, local authorities should provide 4–6 hostel places per 100,000 of the general population for short-term care and rehabilitation and 15 to 24 places for long-stay accommodation to include staffed homes, unstaffed accommodation and supervised lodgings.

The degree to which services are present in any given psychiatric hospital and its catchment area vary widely. When the check list described in the Appendix was applied to 18 Scottish psychiatric hospitals serving two-thirds of the Scottish population (McCreadie *et al*, 1985a), the group mean number of services was 50 per cent of the total possible; the hospital with most services (79 per cent of the total possible) had three times as many as the hospital with fewest (23 per cent). The areas in which there were serious deficiencies (for example, staffed hospitals, sheltered workshops and day centres) were those primarily the responsibility of local authorities. In the future the impetus for the development of such services may have to come from the National Health Service—for example, hospital hostels (Affleck, 1981; Wykes, 1982).

If development has not taken place within a hospital's catchment area then the current fashion to transfer patients from hospital to community is a grave disservice to chronic schizophrenics as many become homeless or end up in prison (for an impassioned review, see Weller, 1984).

Assessment

If rehabilitation works (see below), then it must be possible to assess, firstly, the adequacy of a hospital's rehabilitation facilities and, secondly, an individual patient's progress. Which assessments are appropriate for an individual at any given time will depend on the reason for using them. At one extreme, a simple, easy to administer, global assessment of progress may be useful in a busy NHS setting; at the other extreme, a detailed assessment of many individual areas of functioning may be necessary in a research project. What follows is by no means exhaustive but includes assessments mainly originating in the United Kingdom. It must be remembered, however, that no rating scale can supplant the clinician's intimate knowledge of a patient's daily life.

Hospital assessment

It has long been suggested (Bowen, 1965) that a method is needed to assess a hospital's rehabilitation services. Much information about individual hospitals is of course obtained by the Royal College of Psychiatrist's Approval Panels and by visits of the Health Advisory Service. However, a more objective assessment is desirable and is now available (McCreadie *et al*, 1985a). In a study of rehabilitation facilities in 18 Scottish psychiatric hospitals, a straightforward count of the number of facilities provided by each hospital correlated highly with a more detailed assessment of each hospital; hospitals which had better rehabilitation facilities had quite simply more of them. The method of assessment, using a straightforward count (see Appendix), was shown to have some validity as there was a correlation between the range of services provided in a hospital's catchment area and the numbers of misplaced 'new chronic' in-patients within that hospital, a misplaced patient being one who did not in the consultant's opinion need to be in a hospital but could be elsewhere if there were adequate facilities.

Patient assessment

(i) Global assessment

A short simple assessment suitable for use in everyday clinical practice is the Morningside Rehabilitation Status Scale (MRSS) (Affleck and MacGuire, 1984). It examines four main areas—dependency, inactivity, integration and symptoms. Each of the four subscales has eight levels, but a total score can also be obtained giving an overall assessment. Progress through Scottish rehabilitation facilities is associated with an improvement in MRSS scores (McCreadie *et al*, 1985b).

Another recently published global assessment is REHAB (Baker, 1983). In its development it was used mainly with long-stay in-patients. It assesses deviant and general behaviour and five factors—social activity, speech skills, disturbed speech, self-care and community skills. Its value in non-in-patients is yet to be determined.

(ii) Specific assessments

(a) *Symptomatology:* A useful and now widely used rating of chronic schizophrenic symptoms is the Krawiecka Scale (Krawiecka *et al*, 1977). It can be used for both in- and non-in-patients and examines nine areas: positive schizophrenic symptoms—incoherence, delusions, hallucinations, and inappropriate affect (affect has been divided into inappropriate and blunt by Johnstone *et al*, 1978), negative symptoms—blunting of affect and poverty of thought, and non-schizophrenic symptoms—depression, retardation and anxiety.

(b) *Behaviour:* There are many nurse rating scales of ward behaviour (reviewed by Hall, 1980). The Wing Ward Behaviour Scale which examines both socially embarrassing behaviour and social withdrawal (Wing, 1961) is still widely used but is really most appropriate for deteriorated schizophrenic in-patients. The Nurses Observation Scale for In-patient Evaluation (NOSIE) (Honigfeld and Klett, 1965) is an American scale which has been used successfully in the United Kingdom (Philip, 1979) but some Americanisms jar. It gives a total score and has six subscales: social competence, social interest, personal neatness, irritability, manifest psychosis, and retardation. A sensitive instrument for use outside hospital is now needed.

(c) *Occupation:* Industrial therapy has long been an important aspect of the rehabilitation process. Ability to work in such a unit has been measured by several scales, the best established of which is the Griffiths (Griffiths, 1973), in itself an adaptation of an older assessment (Cheadle *et al*, 1967). It assesses task competence, response to supervision, social relationships and enthusiasm. Ability of ratings on this scale to predict resettlement at work has been confirmed (Watts, 1978). Unfortunately, the current economic climate is such that for the foreseeable future chronic schizophrenics are likely to be at the back of the queue when it comes to employment. Thus ratings of ability to work in open employment are for the moment less necessary. More important are measurements of patient's ability to participate in activities of daily living, including self-care, budgeting, cooking and housekeeping. This is the province of occupational therapy but there does not seem to be a widely accepted rating scale for such activities—each unit usually devises its own (e.g. Campbell and McCreadie, 1983).

(d) *Social assessment:* How well chronic schizophrenics get on with others can mean the difference between success and failure in rehabilitation. A lengthy assessment of social adjustment is the Social Behaviour Assessment Scale (SBAS) (Platt *et al*, 1980) but this is too cumbersome for anything but research projects.

More use to clinicians is the Social Adjustment Scale Self-Report (Weissman and Bothwell, 1976). This is a modification of the original scale used by trained interviewers (Weissman and Paykel, 1974). This is a 54-item questionnaire which yields an overall score and a rating of six role areas; work as a worker, housewife or student; social and leisure activities; relationships with extended family; and marital roles as a spouse, parent and member of the family unit. It can be completed in 10–15 minutes by a relative to describe a patient or by a patient to describe himself. A recent study has shown that chronic schizophrenics can accurately describe their social adjustment (McCreadie and Barron, 1984).

Does rehabilitation work?

Does the rehabilitation process affect the chronic schizophrenic? Can it make any impact on the lives of such patients or are organic factors of the disease (Crow, 1982) such that there is an irreversible decline in function?

The principal treatment methods in rehabilitation are medication, psychological therapy and social therapy.

Medication

Medication is 'the ground on which the rehabilitation structure is built' (Royal College of Psychiatrists, 1980). Scottish psychiatrists certainly believe this. A recent survey of 14 Scottish psychiatric hospitals serving more than half of the Scottish population identified 'new chronic' in-patients, defined as patients aged 18–64 years in hospital more than one but less than six years; the biggest single diagnostic category was schizophrenia (McCreadie *et al*, 1983). Only 9 per cent of patients were receiving no medication. Sixty-nine per cent were receiving oral, intramuscular, or both oral and intramuscular antipsychotics, and of these 44 per cent were also receiving antiparkinsonian drugs. In a similar survey of chronic day patients (McCreadie *et al*, 1984), more than half of whom were schizophrenic, 17 per cent were on no medication, 65 per cent were receiving antipsychotic drugs and 30 per cent of the latter group were receiving, in addition, antiparkinsonian medication.

Antipsychotic drugs are effective in postponing relapse. In out-patients recently recovered from an acute schizophrenic episode, oral medication such as trifluoperazine or chlorpromazine was more effective than placebo in preventing relapse over a 12-month period (Leff and Wing, 1971). Also, relapse rates over nine months in chronic schizophrenic out-patients previously well maintained on intramuscular fluphenazine decanoate were much higher in patients switched to placebo injections (66 per cent) when compared with those continuing on active medication (8 per cent) (Hirsch *et al*, 1973). These two studies, however, examined schizophrenics of an 'intermediate' prognosis (Leff, 1973). The role of medication in refractory schizophrenics is less clear. Very high dose therapy may bring modest benefits to some patients (McClelland *et al*, 1976; McCreadie and McDonald, 1977; McCreadie *et al*, 1979), but side-effects such as sedation and liver impairment may occur. At the other extreme, there is little evidence that very low doses of neuroleptics have a protective effect as maintenance therapy in out-patient schizophrenics (Kane *et al*, 1983). Althaough there is considerable interest in the relationship between plasma neuroleptic levels and acute schizophrenia (e.g. Cohen *et al*, 1980), there is as yet no clear cut relationship between such levels and risk of relapse in chronic schizophrenics.

Antipsychotic medication is inevitably associated with side-effects of which the two most troublesome are parkinsonism and tardive dyskinesia. In a review of all known schizophrenics from a discrete geographical area (McCreadie, 1982) more than 30 per cent of patients had one or other side-effect. The value of antiparkinsonian drugs in drug-induced parkinsonism has long been questioned (Mindham *et al*, 1972) and there is no satisfactory treatment for tardive dyskinesia (**Mackay and Sheppard, 1979**). The only option is to reduce the dose with the inherent risk of relapse. Side-effects, especially parkinsonism, are also associated with poor drug compliance (Van Putten, 1974).

Drugs and social measures interact in the rehabilitation process. The relationship between medication and family life is dealt with in detail elsewhere in this book (see **Leff**'s review in the section on 'Social Aspects'), but briefly it appears that antipsychotic medication has a protective effect when schizophrenic patients return home to relatives with high 'expressed emotion' (Vaughn and Leff, 1976). Medication is also of benefit in patients not living with such relatives but who may be exposed to stressful life events (Leff and Vaughn, 1981).

Psychological therapy

Clinical psychologists spend very little time with chronic schizophrenics (McCreadie *et al*, 1985a), their main interest with such patients is in the field of behaviour modification. Controlled studies with chronic schizophrenics on *social skills training* which use techniques such as modelling, role play and feedback through playback of video tapes are few (reviewed by Hersen and Bellack, 1976). One recent controlled study (Shephard, 1978) suggested a clear improvement in social function for the treated group, an improvement which generalized from the immediate treatment situation to the rest of the patients' activities in a day hospital. However, there is still little evidence that learned social skills generalize or are maintained over lengthy periods of time. *Operant conditioning* has been used to improve self care, and social interaction, positive psychotic symptoms and aggressive behaviour. Any improvements are usually transitory, (e.g. Davis *et al*, 1976) and in the case of aggression, negative reinforcement such as time out and fines may increase unwanted behaviour (reviewed by Gomez-Schwartz, 1979).

The usefulness of *token economy* is reviewed in detail elsewhere in this section (**Hall and Baker**). Such programmes can produce improvement but whether contingent tokens are necessary is doubtful (Hall *et al*, 1977). Social reinforcement, feedback of information and suggestions and instructions to nurses may be important factors. However, token economies tend either to become part of the institutional process or break down (Hall and Baker, 1973); also, improvements may not carry over when schizophrenic patients are discharged (reviewed by Hersen, 1976).

Social therapy

General principles

Within the hospital, the life of the chronic schizophrenic has been studied in detail by the Medical Research Council Social Psychiatry Unit (Wing and Brown, 1970). In three psychiatric hospitals there was a clear relationship between the type of environment in which the chronic schizophrenic lived and the severity of symptoms. If the environment was impoverished, e.g. if the patient had few personal possessions and had little contact with the outside world, then the negative symptoms of schizophrenia such as loss of volition and blunting of affect were more severe. The first series of studies showed only a relationship between 'social poverty' and 'clinical poverty' syndromes; they could not demonstrate which was causal. After the initial survey, however, changes were introduced into the hospitals studied with the result that the environment for many patients became more stimulating. Where this happened, it was found that the negative symptoms of schizophrenia lessened; thus it was suggested that the environment could influence the course of the schizophrenic illness. These studies suggest deterioration in the patient's mental state and behaviour can be modified by manipulation of the hospital environment. Encouraging a patient to have personal possessions, welcoming his contact with the outside world and lessening ward restrictions may diminish the negative symptoms of schizophrenia.

A course must be steered, however, between under- and over-stimulating a chronic schizophrenic in-patient. Too much pressure can precipitate an exacerbation of positive schizophrenic symptoms (Wing *et al*, 1964).

Specific measures

(i) Occupational therapy

Although occupational therapists in Scotland are the most committed group to rehabilitation units in psychiatric hospitals (McCreadie *et al*, 1985a) the value of their work has rarely been studied systematically. For in-patients, industrial work rather than occupational therapy may be more successful in improving a patient's willingness and ability to work (Miles, 1971) but improvements can occur in patients attending occupational therapy as well. In occupational therapy, female middle-class patients improved most. In view of the current economic climate, schizophrenics find it difficult to obtain and hold open employment; emphasis on rehabilitation is, therefore, moving away from work towards occupational and social activities. Occupational therapists are becoming increasingly aware of patients in the community (Durham, 1982) and a small but controlled survey of chronic day patient schizophrenics (Campbell and McCreadie, 1983) found brief but intensive occupational therapy was effective in improving patients' skills in such areas as work in the kitchen, shopping, budgeting, laundry and clothes care and general household duties.

(ii) Industrial therapy

Although United Kingdom unemployment rates are high, for most people work is still the main event of the day. Most schizophrenics, however, are unemployed (Freeman *et al*, 1979; McCreadie, 1982). For many years, psychiatric hospital industrial therapy units have given valuable work experience but they tend to attract little non-manual work. As stated above, the ability to work and to develop satisfactory relationships in such units are useful pointers to the schizophrenic's ability to hold down a job in open employment (Watts, 1978). However, very few schizophrenics now progress from hospital-based industrial therapy units to local authority sheltered workshops, employment rehabilitation centres or open employment. Industrial therapy has become for many schizophrenics, especially long-stay in-patients, an end in itself. This is not necessarily an unwelcome development as the single most important factor contributing to the clinical poverty syndrome (Wing and Brown, 1970) was the amount of time spent doing nothing.

(iii) Social work

Chronic schizophrenics living in the community have poor social adjustment (McCreadie and Barron, 1984); compared to a normal community sample, they are less effective at work, in social and leisure activities, and in relationships with close and more distant relatives. The principal series of studies which has examined the effectiveness of social work intervention in discharged schizophrenics is that of Hogarty and co-workers (Hogarty *et al*, 1973, 1974a, 1974b, 1979; Goldberg *et al*, 1977). Social therapy consisted of intensive individual and family social case-work provided by an experienced social worker. Practical problems including situational crises were tackled. It was found on average social therapy was no more effective than placebo in preventing relapse. In patients with few symptoms, however, relapse rates were less over a two-year period when compared with patients who did not receive social therapy. Conversely, patients who still had symptoms such as disorganized overactivity had a greater chance of relapse if given social therapy. It is probable that such patients were over-stimulated and thus relapsed (see above, Wing *et al*, 1964). When the effects of social therapy on the adjustment of non-relapsed patients were studied over a two-year period following hospital discharge, patients treated with combined drug and social therapy adjusted better than those taking the drug alone. Maximum benefits required both maintenance drug and social treatments to continue for more than a year. These conclusions are tentative and methodological weaknesses such as diagnostic procedures in this series of studies have recently been criticized (Barrowclough and Tarrier, 1984).

(iv) Family therapy

At any given time probably three-quarters of known schizophrenics are now living out of hospital and of these, half are with first degree relatives (McCreadie, 1982). The schizophrenic's family assumes considerable importance therefore in the rehabilitation process. The influence of the patient's family is reviewed in more detail elsewhere (**Leff**'s review in section on 'Social Aspects'), but briefly the course of the schizophrenic illness may be affected by the amount of emotion expressed by key relatives towards the patient. If chronic schizophrenics recovered from an acute episode return to hostile, critical relatives, the chances of relapse are increased (Brown *et al*, 1972; Vaughn and Leff, 1976). The significance of high 'expressed emotion' is less clear in the earlier stages of the illness (McMillan *et al*, 1984).

The rehabilitation process should therefore try to modify the attitudes of such relatives. A treatment package including education, a group for relatives and family sessions for relatives and patients has produced a significant reduction in relapse rates (Leff *et al*, 1982). Broadly similar results using a more behavioural approach to family therapy have been found in Californian schizophrenics (Falloon *et al*, 1982). Which aspects of the package are most useful remains to be determined.

Both studies used a detailed assessment of relatives' emotion (the Camberwell Family Index). This instrument is impractical for everyday use in a busy community psychiatric practice; highly critical relatives are probably known to an experienced clinician but others may not be so readily recognized. A relatively quick and accurate estimate of hostility is necessary; work is currently underway comparing the use of a brief scale (Kreisman *et al*, 1979) with the more detailed Camberwell assessment (D. Kreisman, personal communication).

In conclusion, social, psychological and drug therapies can influence the course of a chronic schizophrenic illness. The rehabilitation team should have access to a range of techniques. Which aspect of the rehabilitation process is suitable for any individual patient is decided by thorough assessment of that patient.

Appendix

Range of rehabilitation and support services*

Listed below are 52 different services, widely accepted as important in rehabilitation.

I. Staffing—Rehabilitation unit (n = 18)

Consultant with special interest in rehabilitation; other medical staff; nursing staff; trained occupational therapist; occupational therapy aides or technicians; clinical psychologist; social worker; industrial therapy staff; social therapy staff; voluntary services organizer; physiotherapist; speech therapist; entertainment or recreation officer; art therapist; music therapist; dance therapist; education therapist; horticultural therapist.

II. Staffing—Day hospital (n = 7)

Consultant; other medical staff; nursing staff; trained occupational therapist; occupational therapy aide or technician; clinical psychologist; social worker.

III. Accommodation (n = 8)

Rehabilitation unit; training unit; self-care unit; group home; housing association accommodation; local authority hostel; voluntary agency hostel; other (e.g. supervised lodging).

IV. Occupational and social facilities (n = 10)

Occupational therapy; industrial therapy (repetitive work); industrial therapy (clerical); industrial therapy (woodwork); industrial therapy (machinery); industrial therapy (other); disablement

*Taken from McCreadie *et al* (1985a)

resettlement officer; employment rehabilitation centre; sheltered employment; social club (in-patients).

V. Support services (n = 9)

Day hospital (hospital based); day hospital (ward attendance); day hospital (community based); industrial therapy for day patients; social therapy for day patients; out-patient social club; local authority centre; voluntary agency centre; community psychiatric nurse.

References

AFFLECK, J. W. (1981) The Edinburgh progressive care system. In *Handbook of Psychiatric Rehabilitation Practice* (eds. J. K. Wing and B. Morris). Oxford: Oxford Medical Publications.

—— & MacGUIRE, R. (1984) The measurement of psychiatric rehabilitation status: A review of the needs and a new scale. *British Journal of Psychiatry*, **145**, 517–525.

BAKER, R. (1983) *REHAB: A Multi-Purpose Assessment Instrument for Long-Stay Psychiatric Patients.* Aberdeen, Scotland: Vine Publishing Limited.

BARROWCLOUGH, C. & TARRIER, N. (1984) 'Psychosocial' intervention with families and their effects on the course of schizophrenia: a review. *Psychological Medicine*, **14**, 629–642.

BOWEN, W. A. L. (1965) Need for inspection (or survey) of psychiatric hospital services. In *Psychiatric Hospital Care* (ed. H. Freeman). London: Ballière, Tindall and Cassall.

BROWN, G. W., BIRLEY, J. L. T. & WING, J. K. (1972) Influence of family life on the course of schizophrenic disorders: a replication. *British Journal of Psychiatry*, **121**, 241–258.

CAMPBELL, A. & McCREADIE, R. G. (1983) Occupational therapy is effective for chronic schizophrenic day patients. *British Journal of Occupational Therapy*, **46**, 327–328.

CHEADLE, A. J., CUSHING, D., DREW, C. D. A. & MORGAN, R. (1967) The measurement of the work performance of psychiatric patients. *British Journal of Psychiatry*, **113**, 841–846.

COHEN, B. M., LIPINSKI, J. F., POPE, H. G., HARRIS, P. Q. & ALTESMAN, R. I. (1980) Neuroleptic blood levels and therapeutic effect. *Psychopharmacology*, **70**, 191–193.

CROW, T. J. (1982) Molecular pathology of schizophrenia: more than one disease process. *British Medical Journal*, i, 66–68.

DAVIS, J. R., WALLACE, C. J., LIBERMAN, R. P. & FINCH, B. E. (1976) The use of brief isolation to suppress delusional and hallucinatory speech. *Journal of Behaviour Therapy and Experimental Psychiatry*, **7**, 267–275.

DEPARTMENT OF HEALTH AND SOCIAL SECURITY (1975) *Better Services for the Mentally Ill.* London: HMSO.

DURHAM, T. M. (1982) Community living skills training in psychiatric rehabilitation. *British Journal of Occupational Therapy*, **45**, 233–235.

FALLOON, I. R. H., BOYD, J. L., McGILL, C. W., RAZANI, J., MOSS, H. & CILERMAN, N. (1982) Family man-gement in the prevention of exacerbations of schizophrenia. *New England Journal of Medicine*, 5 J6, 1437–1440.

FREEMAN, H., CHEADLE, A. J. & KORER, J. R. (1979) A method for monitoring the treatment of schizophrenics in the community. *British Journal of Psychiatry*, **134**, 412–416.

GOMEZ-SCHWARTZ, B. (1979) The modification of schizophrenic behaviour. *Behaviour Modification*, **3**, 439–468.

GOLDBERG, S. C., SCHOOLER, N. R., HOGARTY, G. E. & ROPER, M. (1977) Prediction of relapse in schizophrenic out-patients treated by drug and sociotherapy. *Archives of General Psychiatry*, **34**, 171–184.

GRIFFITHS, R. D. P. (1973) A standardized assessment of the work behaviour of psychiatric patients. *British Journal of Psychiatry*, **123**, 403–408.

HALL, J. N. (1980) Ward rating scales for long stay patients: a review. *Psychological Medicine*, **10**, 277–288.

—— & BAKER, R. (1973) Token economy systems: breakdown and control. *Behaviour Research and Therapy*, **11**, 253–263.

—— —— & HUTCHISON, K. (1977) A controlled evaluation of token economy procedures with chronic schizophrenic patients. *Behaviour Research and Therapy*, **15**, 261–283.

HERSEN, M. (1976) Token economies in institutional settings. *Journal of Nervous and Mental Disease*, **162**, 205–211.

—— & BELLACK, A. S. (1976) Social skills training for chronic psychiatric patients: rationale, research findings, and future directions. *Comprehensive Psychiatry*, **17**, 559–580.

HIRSCH, S. R., GAIND, R., RHODE, P. D., STEVENS, B. C. & WING, J. K. (1973) Out-patient maintenance of chronic schizophrenic patients with long-acting fluphenazine: double-blind placebo trial. *British Medical Journal, i,* 633–637.

HOGARTY, G. E., GOLDBERG, S. C. & COLLABORATIVE STUDY GROUP (1973) Drug and sociotherapy in the aftercare of schizophrenic patients: I. One year relapse rates. *Archives of General Psychiatry,* **28,** 54–64.

—— —— SCHOOLER, N. R. & ULRICH, R. F. (1974a) Drug and sociotherapy in the aftercare of schizophrenic patients: II. Two year relapse rates. *Archives of General Psychiatry,* **31,** 603–608.

—— —— —— (1974b) Drug and sociotherapy in the aftercare of schizophrenic patients. III Adjustment of non-relapsed patients. *Archives of General Psychiatry,* **31,** 609–618.

—— SCHOOLER, N. R., ULRICH, R., MUSSARE, F., FERRO, P. & HERRON, E. (1979) Fluphenazine and social therapy in the aftercare of schizophrenic patients. *Archives of General Psychiatry,* **36,** 1283–1294.

HONIGFELD, G. & KLETT, C. J. (1965) The nurses' observation scale for inpatient evaluation. *Journal of Clinical Psychology,* **21,** 65–71.

JOHNSTONE, E. C., CROW, T. J., FRITH, C. D., CARNEY, M. W. P. & PRICE, J. S. (1978) Mechanism of the anti-psychotic effect in the treatment of acute schizophrenia. *Lancet, i,* 848–850.

KANE, J. M., RIFKIN, A., WOERNER, W., REARDON, G., SARANTAKOS, S., SCHIEBEL, D. & RAMOS-LORENZI, J. (1983) Low dose neuroleptic treatment of out-patient schizophrenics. I Preliminary results for relapse rates. *Archives of General Psychiatry,* **40,** 893–896.

KRAWIECKA, M., GOLDBERG, D. & VAUGHAN, M. (1977) A standardised psychiatric assessment scale for rating chronic psychotic patients. *Acta Psychiatrica Scandinavica,* **55,** 299—308.

KREISMAN, D. E., SIMMENS, S. J. & JOY, V. W. (1979) Rejecting the patient: preliminary validation of a self-report scale. *Schizophrenia Bulletin,* **5,** 220–222.

LEFF, J. P. (1973) Influence of selection of patients on results of clinical trials. *British Medical Journal, iv,* 156–158.

—— KUIPERS, L., BERKOWITZ, R., EBERLEIN-VRIES, R. & STURGEON, D. (1982) A controlled trial of social intervention in the families of schizophrenic patients. *British Journal of Psychiatry,* **141,** 121–134.

—— & VAUGHN, C. (1981) The role of maintenance therapy and relatives' expressed emotion in relapse of schizophrenia: a two-year follow-up. *British Journal of Psychiatry,* **139,** 102–104.

—— & WING, J. K. (1971) Trial of maintenance therapy in schizophrenia. *British Medical Journal, iii,* 559–604.

McCREADIE, R. G. (1982) The Nithsdale Schizophrenia Survey. I Psychiatric and social handicaps. *British Journal of Psychiatry,* **140,** 582–586.

—— AFFLECK, J. W. & ROBINSON, A. D. T. (1985a) The Scottish survey of psychiatric rehabilitation and support services. *British Journal of Psychiatry,* **147,** 289–294.

—— & BARRON, E. T. (1984) The Nithsdale schizophrenia survey: IV. Social adjustment. *British Journal of Psychiatry,* **144,** 547–550.

—— —— & WINSLOW, G. (1982) The Nithsdale schizophrenia survey: II. Abnormal movements. *British Journal of Psychiatry,* **140,** 587–590.

—— BURTON, L. L. & WILSON, A. O. A. (1983) The Scottish survey of 'new chronic' in-patients. *British Journal of Psychiatry,* **143,** 564–571.

—— & McDONALD, I. M. (1977) High dosage haloperidol in chronic schizophrenia. *British Journal of Psychiatry,* **131,** 310–316.

—— FLANAGAN, W. L., McKNIGHT, J. & JORGENSEN, A. (1979) High dosage flupenthixol decanoate in chronic schizophrenia. *British Journal of Psychiatry,* **135,** 175–179.

—— ROBINSON, A. D. T. & WILSON, A. O. A. (1984) The Scottish survey of chronic day patients. *British Journal of Psychiatry,* **145,** 626–630.

—— —— —— (1985b) The Scottish survey of 'new chronic' in-patients: two year follow-up. *British Journal of Psychiatry,* in press.

MACKAY, A. V. P. & SHEPPARD, G. P. (1979) Pharmacotherapeutic trials in tardive dyskinesia. *British Journal of Psychiatry,* **135,** 489–499.

McCLELLAND, H. A., FARQUHARSON, R. G., LEYBURN, P., FURNESS, J. A. & SCHIFF, A. A. (1976) Very high dose fluphenazine decanoate. *Archives of General Psychiatry,* **33,** 1435–1439.

MacMILLAN, J. F., GOLD, A., JOHNSTONE, E. C., CROW, T. J. & JOHNSON, A. L. (1984) Expressed emotion in early schizophrenia. *Proceedings of the 14th CINP Congress,* p. 53.

MILES, A. (1971) Long-stay schizophrenic patients in hospital workshops: a comparative study of an industrial unit and an occupational therapy department. *British Journal of Psychiatry,* **119,** 611–620.

MINDHAM, R. H. J., GAIND, R., ANSTEE, B. H. & RIMMER, L. (1972) Comparison of amantidine, orphenadrine and placebo on the control of phenothiazine induced parkinsonism. *Psychological Medicine*, **2,** 406–413.

PHILIP, A. E. (1979) Prediction of successful rehabilitation by nurse rating scale. *British Journal of Psychiatry*, **134,** 422–426.

PLATT, S. D., WEYMAN, A. J., HIRSCH, S. R. & HEWETT, S. (1980) The Social Behaviour Assessment Schedule (SBAS): rationale, contents, scoring and reliability of a new interview schedule. *Social Psychiatry*, **15,** 43–55.

ROYAL COLLEGE OF PSYCHIATRISTS (1980) *Psychiatric Rehabilitation in the 1980s.* Report of the Working Party on Rehabilitation of the Social and Community Psychiatry Section. London: Royal College of Psychiatrists.

SHEPHARD, G. (1978) Social skills training: the generalization problem—some further data. *Behaviour Research and Therapy*, **16,** 287–288.

VAN PUTTEN, T. (1974) Why do schizophrenic patients refuse to take their drugs? *Archives of General Psychiatry*, **31,** 67–72.

VAUGHN, C. E. & LEFF, J. P. (1976) The influence of family and social factors on the course of psychiatric illness: a comparison of schizophrenic and neurotic patients. *British Journal of Psychiatry*, **129,** 125–137.

WATTS, F. N. (1978) A study of work behaviour in a psychiatric rehabilitation unit. *British Journal of Social and Clinical Psychiatry*, **17,** 85–92.

WEISSMAN, M. & PAYKEL, E. S. (1974) *The Depressed Woman: A Study of Social Relationships.* Chicago: Chicago University Press.

—— & BOTHWELL, S. (1976) Assessment of social adjustment by patient self-report. *Archives of General Psychiatry*, **33,** 1111–1115.

WELLER, M. (1984) So-called care in the so-called community. *World Medicine*, **19,** No. 23, 29–31.

WING, J. K. (1961) A simple and reliable subclassification of schizophrenia. *Journal of Mental Science*, **107**, 862–875.

—— & BROWN, G. W. (1970) *Institutionalism and Schizophrenia.* Cambridge University Press.

—— BENNET, D. H. & DENHAM, J. (1964) *The Industrial Rehabilitation of Long-stay Schizophrenic Patients.* Medical Research Council Memo No. 42. London: HMSO.

WYKES, T. (1982) A hostel ward for new long-stay patients: an evaluative study of a 'ward in a house'. *Psychological Medicine*, Monograph Supplement 2, 59–97.

VII.   Outcome

43 Outcome of schizophrenia: Overview

JOHN CUTTING

Historical trends

The literature on the outcome of schizophrenia is extensive. It is probably one of the most researched aspects of the condition. This can be explained by the fact that Kraepelin regarded its characteristic outcome as a defining criterion and certainly a way of discriminating it from manic-depressive psychosis. One of the few definite facts about schizophrenia came to be its poor outcome. In the 90 years since he laid down these rules, however, Kraepelin's pessimism has been challenged. In order to appreciate current views on outcome, it is necessary to trace the main developments this century.

The first change was brought in by Bleuler when he altered the name of the condition from 'dementia praecox' to 'schizophrenia'. The purpose of this was to emphasize the difference between the psychological impairment in schizophrenia and that seen in dementia of undoubted organic origin, such as Alzheimer's disease. He believed that schizophrenia led to an impairment of mental functions through a particular sort of emotional disturbance, an 'affective dementia', whereas Alzheimer's disease produced a genuine 'intellectual dementia'. Whatever the truth of this, his views encouraged the idea that an 'affective dementia' was potentially reversible, whereas an 'intellectual dementia' was not.

North American psychologists and psychiatrists took this further in the 1920s, 1930s and 1940s and objected strongly to the term dementia being attached to the condition. They were influenced by psychoanalysis, social notions of mental disorder and, later, behaviourism, and regarded schizophrenia as a learned reaction to adverse social or emotional events in early life. They replaced the word dementia by the terms 'psychological deficit' or 'psychological deterioration'. The advantage of this reformulation was that schizophrenia became potentially treatable by psychological and social means, although as it later became clear, the North Americans widened the diagnostic criteria to fit their new views.

In Britain during the 1960s, the social revolution in psychiatry led to a modified version of these ideas. Schizophrenics remained in the back wards of mental hospitals, it was claimed, not primarily because of their condition, but because they were institutionalized. If they had been given sufficient stimulation and encouragement, it was argued, they would not now be showing such 'symptoms' as poverty of speech or flattening of affect. This idea, that much if not all of the social deterioration stemmed from neglect, prevailed until the late 1970s. It was regarded as an iatrogenic effect, and one that all psychiatrists should be ashamed of. An active discharge policy was then initiated and when the wards did not fill up again, this was regarded as proof of the social origin of schizophrenic deterioration.

The truth was more complex, however, because a number of other changes were taking place in the early 1960s. First and foremost, neuroleptics were introduced, which undoubtedly had a radical effect on outcome. Secondly, clinical psychologists were setting up behavioural programmes—token economies, rehabilitation workshops—in the big mental hospitals with the aim of strengthening relatively intact mental functions and discouraging asocial behaviour. Thirdly, the successful discharge from hospital of many chronic schizophrenics and the reduction to a minimum of new long-stay patients did not mean that deterioration had necessarily been reversed or prevented. Part of what was happening was that the alternative facilities which were being set up—day hospitals, hostels, sheltered accommodation—began to fill up with deteriorated schizophrenics. Superficially, social outcome appeared to have improved, in the sense that the majority of schizophrenics were 'hanging on' in the community, but careful clinical and psychological assessment of such people (see below) revealed considerable residual psychopathology and psychological impairment.

The final development in furthering our understanding of the outcome of schizophrenia was the introduction of CT scanning in the late 1970s. Radiological examination of chronic schizophrenics revealed that a sizeable proportion had enlarged cerebral ventricles, indistinguishable from that seen in patients with mild or moderate Alzheimer's disease. This led several investigators to resurrect Kraepelin's notion of dementia praecox. Opinions on the outcome of schizophrenia seemed to have come full circle back to Kraepelin.

Before putting these trends in perspective and trying to tie up the psychological, organic and social strands, it is necessary to look at the main studies on *general outcome*, examine the possible *specific outcomes* and assess the importance of the numerous *factors* which have been claimed to affect *prognosis*.

General outcome

About 10 first-class studies on general outcome have been carried out during the century: by Kraepelin in Munich in 1913, Langfeldt in Norway in 1937, Harris *et al* in London in 1956, Holmboe and Astrup in Norway in 1957, Brown *et al* in London in 1966, Manfred Bleuler in Zurich in 1972, Bland and Orn in Canada in 1978, Brockington in London in 1978, the WHO collaborative study in 10 countries in 1979, and Huber *et al* in Bonn in 1979. They are summarized in Table I.

The most useful figures to emerge concern the extremes of good and bad outcome. These are defined differently in each study, but for purposes of comparison good outcome in the Table is regarded as discharge from hospital without re-admission at any time, and bad outcome as continuous stay in hospital throughout follow-up or moderate to severe intellectual or social impairment at last follow-up.

TABLE I

Outcome in schizophrenia: analysis of best follow-up studies

Investigator	Year	Length of follow-up	Number of patients	Outcome		
				Good* %	Intermediate %	Bad* %
Unspecified admissions:						
Kraepelin	1913	10 years	1,054	4	13	83
Langfeldt	1937	10 years	100	17	23	60
Harris *et al*	1956	5 years	123	14	43	43
Brown *et al*	1966	5 years	339	17	42	41
Bleuler	1972	20 years	208	10	61	29
IPSS	1979	2 years	811	27	47	26
Huber *et al*	1979	22 years	502	10	43	35
Mean				13	42	45
First admissions:						
Holmboe & Astrup	1957	6 years	255	29	38	33
Brown *et al*	1966	5 years	111	35	37	28
Bleuler	1972	20 years	66	32	45	23
Bland & Orn	1978	13 years	45	21	42	37
Mean				29	41	30

* Good—no further readmissions; bad—continuous in-patient or severe or moderate social or intellectual impairment at last follow-up.
(Reprinted from the Psychology of Schizophrenia, Cutting, 1985, Churchill Livingstone)

Two main points emerge from the Table. First, there is a marked difference in outcome after a first admission (good—29 per cent; bad—30 per cent) compared with subsequent admissions (good—13 per cent; bad—45 per cent). Secondly, there has been a slight overall improvement in outcome over the century, mainly involving the proportion with a bad outcome (83 per cent in the 1900s; 60 per cent in the 1930s; 43 per cent in the 1950s and 26 per cent in the 1970s). Some commentators have seen in these figures a trend for schizophrenia to have become milder in nature, as the apparent improvement preceded the neuroleptic era. In my view, this is a doubtful conclusion because of the different attitudes to admission and discharge that must have prevailed, attitudes which are largely independent of the severity of the condition.

In general, about one-quarter of patients after a first admission nowadays do very well (complete recovery), about one-quarter do badly (chronic social and intellectual impairment requiring frequent admissions and much community support) and about one-half do moderately well (occasional subsequent admissions, some neurotic symptoms, and some social impairment manifest as difficulty in interpersonal relationships).

Specific outcomes

Specific outcome is usually described in terms of the frequency and length of admissions, the severity of psychotic and neurotic symptoms, the degree of psychological impairment and the level of social functioning.

Death: Schizophrenics have a higher mortality than the general population. In the early decades of the century this was mainly accounted for by an increase in intercurrent infections amongst institutionalized patients, but is now attributable to a higher suicide rate (about three times that in the general population and about 5 per cent of all schizophrenics).

Institutionalization: Continuous stay in hospital is very rare these days. There is a small accumulation of what are known as the 'new long-stay patients', but in general the more severely affected patients are accommodated in day hospitals and hostels, although these, of course, possess many of the malign characteristics of an institution.

Remittent course: The most common outcome is, according to Wing (1982), who has studied the matter more than anyone: 'to alternate for decades between acute psychotic phases and phases of improvement or recovery'.

In some patients, a remitting course is particularly striking, so much so that the original diagnosis of schizophrenia has been questioned and diagnoses such as 'cycloid psychosis' substituted. Some such patients may have a separate condition, but this decision should be made on the basis of psychopathological and psychological differences and not course alone.

Persistent psychopathology: This is surprisingly high in all the studies which have looked for it. About 15 per cent of discharged schizophrenics are deluded or hallucinated at any point in time, about 30 per cent have what are now known as negative symptoms—affective flattening, attentional impairment, poverty of speech, impoverishment of motivation and inability to feel intimate—and as many as 70 per cent have neurotic symptoms, particularly depression.

Psychological deficit: Cognitive impairment severe enough to be picked up on tests for organic impairment (e.g. Hinton and Withers' battery) is found in 65 per cent of chronic in-patients and about 20 per cent of out-patients. In such cases orientation, attention and memory are all affected, and patients resemble moderately severe cases of Alzheimer's disease in this respect. Some investigators, notably Huber, have claimed to have identified a more subtle psychological deficit in as many as 80 per cent of schizophrenics, but the manifestations of this—e.g. decreased initiative, reduced capacity for adaptation—are so widespread in other psychological conditions and even in normal people that the validity of the claim must be in doubt at the moment.

Social impairment: About one half of schizophrenics in the community are functioning at a lower social level than the general population. This is obviously a difficult issue to be sure about. In the days of virtual full employment, unemployment was a relatively good measure of impaired social functioning, whereas nowadays it is not. Social isolation, identified in 58 per cent of schizophrenics in Brockington's study in the 1970s, is a loose measure, but in view of the evidence that overinvolved and overcritical relatives contribute to relapse, a schizophrenic who chooses to live in relative social isolation could be regarded as quite sensible.

Recovery: Although Kraepelin regarded this as rare, it is one of the few points, in my view, where he was wrong. Some investigators, earlier this century, were inclined to change the diagnosis retrospectively if a patient had clearly recovered, and this was partly responsible for the gloomy prognosis which became attached to the condition. The whole issue of outcome and recovery in schizophrenia is inextricably linked with the diagnostic criteria used. The increasing acceptance of DSM-III criteria, which require the condition to have lasted at least six months, means that patients with a poor prognosis are over-represented in DSM-III schizophrenia, whilst patients who recover rapidly are excluded. The issue, and it is a central issue in schizophrenia, is whether poor outcome should be made an integral part of the defining criteria. In my view, this is wrong, as outcome in any illness, physical or mental, is usually governed by factors extrinsic to the actual condition itself. This theme will be elaborated in the next two sections.

Factors influencing outcome

A large number of factors have been reported to affect outcome. They can be divided into premorbid (sex, body build, family history, early life experiences, personality, recent life experiences, cerebral dysfunction); previous psychiatric illness; nature of the current episode (diagnostic criteria, particular phenomena, psychological aspects, mode of onset); and subsequent factors (culture, life situation, family atmosphere, treatment, personal attitude towards the condition).

The best evaluation is undoubtedly the International Pilot Study of Schizophrenia, sponsored by the WHO, in which psychiatrists in 10 countries co-operated and used the same interviewing technique and diagnostic criteria (PSE, CATEGO). In this study 47 potential predictors were ranked according to how much of the variance they accounted for. They were grouped into three sets—socio-demographic, past history and current episode—thus allowing a more balanced perspective than is possible in smaller studies, some of whose claims fade into insignificance by comparison.

Several major points emerged from this study. First, the five most powerful overall predictors of poor outcome were social isolation, long duration of the episode, a history of past psychiatric treatment, being unmarried and a history of behavioural symptoms in childhood (e.g. truancy, tantrums). Secondly, all 47 potential predictors only accounted for 38 per cent of the variance, and each of the three sets was roughly equal in its predictive power. Thirdly, different sets of factors predict different measures of outcome. Premorbid social maladjustment, as one might expect, is a good predictor of poor social outcome. Rather surprisingly, however, the form of the current illness was an unreliable predictor of any sort of outcome. Fourthly, the outcome was quite markedly different in the various countries, in general being better in the *less* developed countries (e.g. Nigeria, Colombia) than in the more developed countries (e.g. Soviet Union, Denmark). In the five-year follow-up, not yet published, differences between countries are not so striking for typical schizophrenia and the apparent differences in the two-year follow-up can be accounted for by a higher rate in underdeveloped countries of atypical presentations with a good prognosis but still within the CATEGO diagnostic category (Wing, personal communication).

What of the other factors mentioned at the beginning of this section? In general a poor premorbid social and sexual adjustment is the most powerful predictor of poor outcome, but flattening of affect, absence of depression or elation and long duration of the current episode are further predictors of poor outcome; and the most important subsequent events are whether neuroleptics are regularly given and the quality of the family atmosphere to which a patient is discharged. The efficacy of neuroleptics is undoubted in the short and medium term (up to five years), whereas Manfred Bleuler has questioned whether they affect the long-term outcome (10–20 years). There is some recent evidence from Crow and his colleagues in North London that early treatment with neuroleptics does affect the relapse rate in the short-term and I suspect that Manfred Bleuler is wrong to question their long-term efficacy. The adverse effect of living with overinvolved and critical relatives is in doubt at the moment, as two competent investigators (Crow—against, Leff—in favour) have come to different conclusions on the matter. It is probable, in my view, that some aspect of a patient's subsequent life situation does predispose to relapse, but what it is (overinvolved relative? critical relative? life events?) is still not clear, nor whether neuroleptics merely prevent florid relapses of delusions and hallucinations or prevent the emergence of negative symptoms, psychological deficit and social impairment.

Conclusions

The outcome of schizophrenia, despite extensive studies of the matter and despite its apparent ease of measurement, is still a puzzle. In one sense Kraepelin was right to emphasize its gloomy prognosis, as schizophrenia disrupts the quality of life more than any other psychiatric disorder with the exception of Alzheimer's disease and other organic dementias, and even they generally only affect the pattern of life in the '60s and beyond. In another sense he was wrong to dismiss the possibility of recovery or a restricted life in the community.

Two issues are chiefly responsible for the uncertainty which surrounds the problem of outcome. The first is the continuing debate concerning the most appropriate diagnostic criteria. In the last decade, over a dozen operational criteria have been suggested. Their reliability, in the sense that two or more observers, even hastily trained lay people, will readily agree on the same diagnosis in the same patient, is extremely high. Their validity, however, is completely unknown. In fact, outcome is the most frequently used measure of their validity, and it is therefore almost meaningless to ask, 'what is the outcome of schizophrenia?' when the condition is defined as having a particular outcome. Moreover, outcome is largely determined by the level of premorbid adaption to life, and is not a valid criterion of any condition, whether physical or mental.

This links with the second issue, the problem of distinguishing between pathogenic (causal) and pathoplastic (modifying) factors. For example, schizophrenia is more common in those whose premorbid personality was schizoid in nature and yet the presence of a schizoid personality ensures a worse prognosis to an established schizophrenia. It would appear that a schizoid personality is both cause and modifier of outcome, but it might be, as some have argued, that a schizoid personality and schizophrenia are both manifestations of the same genotype and psychological make-up. If this is the case, then it becomes impossible to identify separate prognostic factors as they are merely manifestations of the same condition. This is particularly true of the recent finding of enlarged ventricles on CT scanning. Are they a pointer to a genuine cause in some schizophrenics or a modifying influence in all schizophrenics? In my view, they are probably both, which makes the issue of a characteristic outcome all the more complex.

There is some evidence that the unitary concept of schizophrenia is breaking down, more than at any point this century. There is a tendency to emphasize the subtype, paranoid versus hebephrenic, Type I versus Type II, and to identify their separate causes and outcomes. I am in favour of this, as it seems to me that much of the literature on outcome of schizophrenia in general only underlines the heterogeneous nature of the condition.

The most definite points that one can make about the outcome of schizophrenia are as follows: (1) The longer the condition has lasted, up to a cut-off point of about five years, the worse is the outcome. (2) The sooner neuroleptics are begun, the better is the prognosis, with some doubt remaining about the very long-term outcome. (3) The more premorbid abnormalities that exist (whether social, personality or organic) and the worse the eventual life situation (in terms of adverse social or emotional events) the worse is the prognosis. (4) Some subtypes, which may indeed be better regarded as separate conditions, have different outcomes. (5) The nature of the care which a schizophrenic receives, whether organic (neuroleptics), social (where they live, what they do) or psychological (behavioural manipulation, rehabilitation), is a powerful factor in influencing outcome, but not all of their eventual psychopathology, psychological deficit or social maladroitness can be attributed to it. A significant element in the outcome is the intrinsic nature of the condition, though so far this eludes definition and measurement.

References

BLAND, R. C. & ORN, H. (1978) 14 year outcome in early schizophrenia. *Acta Psychiatrica Scandinavica*, **58,** 327–338.

BLEULER, M. (1972) *The Schizophrenic Disorders.* Translated in 1978. New Haven: Yale University Press.

BROCKINGTON, I. F., KENDELL, R. E. & LEFF, J. (1978) Definitions of schizophrenia: Concordance and prediction of outcome. *Psychological Medicine*, **8,** 387–398.

BROWN, G. W., BONE, M., DALISON, B. & WING, J. K. (1966) *Schizophrenia and Social Care.* Institute of Psychiatry, Maudsley Monographs No. 17. Oxford University Press.

HARRIS, A., LINKER, I., NORRIS, V. & SHEPHER, M. (1956) Schizophrenia: a social and prognostic study. *British Journal of Preventive and Social Medicine*, **10,** 107–114.

HOLMBOE, R. & ASTRUP, C. (1957) A follow-up study of 255 patients with acute schizophrenia and schizophreniform psychoses. *Acta Psychiatrica et Neurologica Scandinavica*, Suppl. 115.

HUBER, G., GROSS, G. & SCHEUTTLER, R. (1979) *Schizophrenie. Eine verlaufs- und sozial-psychiatrische Langzeitstudie.* Berlin: Springer.

KRAEPELIN, E. (1913) *Dementia Praecox and Paraphrenia.* Translated from Eighth Edition of *Psychiatrie, Vol. III,* Part 2 in 1919. Edinburgh: E. & S. Livingstone.

LANGFELDT, G. (1937) *The Prognosis in Schizophrenia and the Factors Influencing the Course of the Disease.* Copenhagen: Levin & Munksgaard.

WING, J. K. (1982) Course and prognosis of schizophrenia. In *Handbook of Psychiatry, Vol. 3* (eds. J. K. Wing and L. Wing). Cambridge University Press.

WORLD HEALTH ORGANIZATION (1979) *Schizophrenia: An International Follow-up Study.* Chichester: John Wiley.

44 Schizophrenic deterioration: A discussion

1. Manfred Bleuler

In this article the concept 'schizophrenic psychosis' is to be understood as in DSM-II. 'Deteriorated schizophrenic psychosis' means a chronic schizophrenic psychosis in which not only single symptoms (e.g. delusions) continue to exist in the long term but also an altered cognitive and affective life.

The experience on which my findings are based is the everyday experience of 50 years, since I lived so many years under the same roof as schizophrenics. It is also based on many years of systematic investigation of the course of the disease, involving 556 selected schizophrenics and about 11,806 of their relatives. These investigations also enabled me to compare the course of the disease in 591 schizophrenic relatives.

The incidence of deterioration

About 10 per cent of schizophrenics sink into such a severe state of deterioration that they need permanent nursing care. About 35 per cent show long-lasting mild psychotic signs and live at home, in hostels or in open hospital wards. However, only about half of these chronic mild cases are deteriorated. The others show mainly single psychological signs or symptoms (e.g. passivity or delusions). About 35 per cent of the patients appear cured and almost cured for long periods but are threatened by new acute psychotic phases. About 20 per cent are stable and cured over many years.

The factors which influence deterioration

(1) *Decade of onset:* The above figures are only valid for patients admitted after the 1940s. Schizophrenia in the first decades of this century was, on average, more severe, yet the numbers of the severely deteriorated and of the permanently cured remained the same.

(2) *Family history:* Although schizophrenic psychoses of siblings and other blood relatives often run quite a different course, the course and result of schizophrenias of blood relatives are more alike than those of non-related patients.

(3) *Phase of illness:* Of the illnesses which result in deterioration approximately one half occur after acute phases of the disease and the other half after a chronic course. Improvement and cures are not at all rare in cases in whom acute phases preceded the deterioration, but this can hardly be expected when the development has been purely chronic.

(4) *Early upbringing:* In the history of schizophrenics one does not find broken homes or adverse conditions in childhood more frequently than in the history

of addicts or many personality disorders. However, there exists a statistically significant correlation between adverse childhood conditions and schizoid personality in the history of schizophrenics.

Conclusions

The approximate figures which I quoted regarding the long-term development and final result of schizophrenic psychoses have general validity in the countries with western culture and in the second half of our century. At other times and in different settings the course of the schizophrenic disease is not the same. International experience has been that, in many African and some Asian countries, there is a more benign and phasic course. This might be due to a higher mortality of the severely ill in these countries.

It seems probable that the improvement in prognosis which has taken place since the middle of this century has something to do with the improvement of treatment, nursing care and efforts at rehabilitation. Yet it must be noted that even with modern treatment with neuroleptics the number of permanently cured individuals has not increased. According to my own statistics not one of the permanently cured patients has, during the last few years, been under continuous medication. Although modern treatment has caused the disappearance of severe permanent states immediately following a first acute attack it has not succeeded in reducing the number of severely deteriorated cases from the level of 10 per cent.

The symptomatology of patients who later recover can for a long period not always be distinguished from the symptomatology of those patients who remain permanently deteriorated. Benign and malignant cases often occur in the same family. Therefore, the concept of 'schizophrenic psychoses', covering both cases with and without permanent deterioration, is still justified. Clinical experience shows that it is not possible to contrast the 'real' or malignant schizophrenia as a sharply defined disease entity from benign schizophrenia as another disease entity. Why do certain psychiatrists try to restrict the term schizophrenia or dementia praecox to that of a completely incurable disease, and exclude benign schizophrenias? The chief reason is probably the suggestive influence of the concept of 'disease entity'. This supposes the existence of diseases with uniform cause, uniform symptomatology and uniform development. It is impossible in many medical conditions, and even more so in psychiatric conditions, to carve out such clearly circumscribed disease entities.

According to the findings mentioned above there are two different family influences on schizophrenic events. One influence is the disposition to a schizophrenic illness, the other a disposition to the course of the illness. In neither of the two cases is the family influence decisive, nor is the family influence purely an inherited trait. The inherited tendency to personality development is closely linked with the family's effect on a subject's environment.

While adverse conditions in childhood cannot have a statistically visible influence on the onset of schizophrenia they can determine whether the prepsychotic personality is schizoid or not, and thereby increase the likelihood of chronicity and deterioration.

2. *David Abrahamson*

The image of progressive deterioration that has for so long dominated thinking about chronic schizophrenia owes a great deal to the profound impact made by long-stay patients. The silent, immobile figures that form the nucleus of mental hospital populations produce an indelible impression of a state which it is feared other patients may recreate given sufficient time. Debate about its aetiology has diverted attention away from a re-examination of whether such patients do deteriorate progressively or not.

Relationship between individual and group deterioration

Studies in which groups of long-stay patients have been compared according to length of hospital stay have demonstrated statistically significant associations between time in hospital and the severity of negative handicaps such as poverty of affect and speech, underactivity and social withdrawal. A survey of almost 300 long-stay schizophrenic patients at Goodmayes, a typical catchment area hospital, produced the expected highly significant correlation between the length of stay and social withdrawal. The pattern throughout mirrored the one demonstrated by Wing and Brown in their classic study of three hospitals.

One need not suppose that such group patterns result from a homogeneous patient population. It might be that over a period of 50 years, different cohorts of patients will have had different degrees of initial deterioration. This would, in retrospect, produce a misleading impression of gradual *individual* deterioration.

Longitudinal course

The usual practice in assessing outcome is to group patients according to length of stay in hospital. This length of stay is divided into five-year stretches. When I examined the social withdrawal scales when length of stay was divided into year stretches, I found much greater variation than expected, with no sustained worsening from year to year in the earlier decades. It was not until the end of the third decade that scores increased markedly and persistently to establish the overall correlation between length of stay and social withdrawal. This is inconsistent with individual deterioration, unless there was a cumulative effect which only manifested itself when a late threshold was reached.

However, the case notes of three samples of patients, with the most, an intermediate degree and minimal disability, disclosed courses with a surprising degree of long-term consistency. Levels of disability at the time of survey were strikingly similar to those recorded at or shortly after the index admission, even when this had taken place four or five decades earlier. In less than 10 per cent was the final state worse than the initial, and even here, the deterioration had been almost entirely confined to the first third of their admission. Improvement, which occurred in about 25 per cent of patients, had in contrast developed predominantly in the middle or last third of their admission. The pattern was thus the reverse of that predicted by either a progressive or threshold deterioration model.

These were particularly surprising findings. Patients with the greatest amount of disability accounted for the 'back-ward' stereotype, and were largely responsible for the statistical correlation between length of stay and social withdrawal in the population as a whole. Other studies have shown that such patients have disabilities which are maximal on admission or relatively soon afterwards, and the correlation appears to reflect the paucity of similar patients in the shorter stay groups, due to changes in the pattern of schizophrenia. In essence they appear to have been *selected* rather than *formed* by the institution.

The overall picture that emerged was remarkably similar to that described by Manfred Bleuler—whose findings were not known to me at that time. His thesis is that there is an approximate equilibrium over long periods, without precluding improvement even after decades. Such equilibrium he conceives as a plateau.

Discussion

One of the most striking features of schizophrenic 'deterioration' is that patients were frequently described as demented or institutionalized, according to the period, despite comments in the case notes that belied the terms. The misuse of these terms probably stemmed from the second class status of chronic patients. As the general feeling is that deterioration worsens with time, resources were concentrated on early cases.

This was particularly unfortunate in institutions that might have been well placed to develop long-term strategies to take advantage of stable plateaus and promote improvements, however late in the course.

Outside hospital the same misconception leads to continuing neglect of the rhythm of rehabilitation. Interventions are more commonly timed according to the short-term availability of resources or enthusiasm, than tuned to the needs of the individual for as long as handicaps persist.

More is known about the determinants of acute relapse than of the plateaus that form the major part of most outcomes. Still less has been established about the relationship between plateaus and phases of change, or the varying effects of social and other influences at different stages.

Most fundamentally, attempts to explain chronic schizophrenia have been based on misconceptions about its course. The concept of institutionalization depended on the assumption of fundamental differences between hospital and community courses. The disease process theory, derived from the work of Crow and colleagues, is again asserting itself over the psychosocial model, but I am concerned that it should not contain the same misconception about progression as Kraepelin's model did.

45   The natural history of schizophrenia in the long term

LUC CIOMPI

It is well known that in some small European countries there exist especially favourable conditions for certain types of research which elsewhere meet enormous difficulties. This is exemplified in Denmark and other Scandinavian countries by the famous studies on the influence of genetic and environmental factors in schizophrenia, which were made possible by the exceptional availability of well organized national registers on twins, adoptees and psychotics.

Some time ago we realized that similar favourable conditions exist in Switzerland for long-term follow-up research. It possesses the advantages of being a small and well ordered country without wars and major troubles during the last 100 years, leading to intact and meticulously well kept records of population movements, combined with an exceedingly low social mobility within a very limited geographic area. These features made it possible to trace and find within a short period over 96 per cent of all former patients, even after many changes of address through several decades. Another advantage is the division of the country into 23 political districts or 'cantons', each one with its own hospitals and health care organizations, which have provided for many decades clearly delimited catchment areas, forming an ideal basis for epidemiological research.

These favourable conditions led at the beginning of the sixties to the mounting in one of these districts of the so-called 'Enquête de Lausanne', an extended follow-up research programme on the long-term evolution of mental illnesses of all kinds. The programme was initiated by C. Müller and carried out by L. Ciompi and collaborators over more than ten years. About 50 papers dealing with the long-term evolution of various psychiatric conditions have been published within the framework of this project; a final synthesis is currently in elaboration. The findings concerning schizophrenia have been published in the form of a monograph (Ciompi and Müller, 1976). In the following, some of the most important findings of this study are briefly summarized, with particular reference to the problems of treatment.

The general framework of the schizophrenia study

The 5,661 former patients of the Psychiatric University Hospital of Lausanne, included in the 'Enquête de Lausanne', represent all the psychiatric patients born between 1873 and 1897, hospitalized from the beginning of the century until 1962 in a catchment area with about 500,000 inhabitants today. Age criteria were chosen in order to obtain from all the survivors virtually life-long follow-ups until at least the age of 65 years. Systematic additional cause-of-death and mortality studies provided precise information about the most important selection factors operating in the samples that were finally examined, since attrition was mainly due to death.

One thousand, six hundred and forty-two patients (29 per cent) were diagnosed as schizophrenic at first admission, according to strict Bleulerian criteria, which do not include a bad outcome as obligatory. Heavy mortality during the follow-up period and some other minor factors, probably introducing a slightly favourable bias in the course of the illness, reduced the initial sample to 289 patients. These were personally re-examined by an experienced psychiatrist in their homes, using a semi-structured interview of about two hours duration. Additional information was systematically collected from hospital files, family members, authorities etc.

The average duration of follow-up from first admission to re-examination was 36.9 years. The longest catamnesis was 65 years and about 50 per cent of the cases had a catamnesis of more than 40 years. To our knowledge, based on a synopsis of papers published in 1970 by Stephens and augmented by ourselves, these are the longest known follow-ups of such a large number of schizophrenics in world literature. The follow-up observations were classified under 6 main headings (which could be viewed, according to a concept recently introduced by Strauss and Carpenter (1977), as 'linked-open systems') namely: (a) the end-states at follow-up; (b) the development of schizophrenic symptoms and syndromes; (c) the development of additional, not specifically schizophrenic, symptoms (for instance depression, anxiety, etc.); (d) the development of organic brain syndromes; (e) the development of social adaptation; and (f) the overall course (combined measure of the preceeding evolving aspects).

In order to identify some of the main factors influencing the long-term course, every aspect of outcome was statistically related to a set of more than 20 general, anamnestic, psychopathological and situational variables.

Overall outcome

From the many aspects of outcome studied, we will briefly report here the following four: admission to hospital, types of course, global outcome of schizophrenia, social outcome.

Regarding *admission to hospital*, it is interesting to note that the total duration was less than one year for about half of the probands. On the other hand, about one-quarter spent more than 20 years in hospitals. A very similar picture is obtained when the duration of admission to hospital is related to the total follow-up period. Most patients spent less than 10 per cent of the whole follow-up period in hospital, but about one-quarter of the probands remained there nearly all of the time.

By combining the type of onset, the form of development and the end-state reached (in the sense of M. Bleuler), a great variety of *types of course* were observed. It is noteworthy that an acute onset combined with a phasic course and a favourable outcome was exhibited by 25 per cent of the sample and was the most frequent and also the most favourable type. The most unfavourable one (Bleuler's so-called 'catastrophic schizophrenia'), beginning with an acute onset and leading directly to a severe end-state, affected 6 per cent of the sample and was sixth in order of frequency.

The *global outcome* of schizophrenia, as measured by the end-states reached was favourable in 49 per cent of the cases, 27 per cent complete remissions and 22 per cent minor residuals, compared to 42 per cent with unfavourable outcomes of intermediate or severe degree. In comparison with the situation at first admission, mental health was completely or partially improved in about two-thirds of the cases.

Concerning *social outcome* at follow-up, we found about two-fifths of the patients living with their family or by themselves, one-fifth in community institutions, and the rest in hospitals. Although the mean age of our probands was 74 years at follow-up, more than half (51 per cent) were still working; about two-thirds of them in part-time and one-third in a full-time occupation. The final social adaptation was assessed from a combination of social dependency and from quality and quantity of social contacts. Combined in a global score, the overall social adaptation appeared as good or fair in only about one-third of the cases, whereas it was intermediate or bad in two-thirds. This showed that the main residuals or consequence of the illness were not in the field of persisting schizophrenic psychopathology, but of impaired social functioning.

Relations between outcome, treatment and other variables

Concerning the relations of outcome with treatment, as well as with some other important variables, the study provides the probably unique opportunity to compare the course and outcome of first admissions from the beginning of the century until the sixties. In order to examine the possible influence of the introduction of new treatment methods, we divided our sample into six decades according to first admission, and also into three main groups: first the patients admitted before the beginning of the active shock treatment era in 1933 (61 per cent), second the patients first admitted between 1933 and the introduction of neuroleptics in 1953 (35 per cent), and third the patients first admitted after 1953. The last group with only 4 per cent was, however, too small for valid statistical comparisons. The surprising and disappointing finding was that no statistically significant difference could be found between the outcomes of first admissions during this whole, very extended period of observation. In other words, the schizophrenic patients first admitted in the forties or fifties had no better long-term course than those first admitted at the beginning and during the three first decades of the century!

This seems to show that the apparent improvements in treatment methods, hospital conditions, psychological understanding, etc., from the beginning of the century until at least the fifties, with the possible exclusion of the neuroleptics because the last subgroup was too small, made no difference at all to the course of the illness. Closer examination reveals, however, several selective sampling factors, partly related to mortality. Among them an increasing proportion of prognostically more unfavourable schizophrenics with late onset during the later decades could conceal more favourable courses in recent years. But such possibly hidden improvements were not overwhelming enough to counterbalance the sampling effects mentioned.

A second important finding, which points in the same direction, is the relationship between the outcome on one hand and various methods of treatment on the other, such as electroshock (given to 6.5 per cent of patients), insulin (12.5 per cent), pre-neuroleptic drugs (31 per cent), or complete lack of any particular therapy (50 per cent). Here also, no significant differences of outcome could be found between all these different approaches.

Again these results should be interpreted with great care. Various treatments could have been effective for a short time without, however, improving the final outcome. Furthermore, there is no guarantee that the different groups of patients and treatments are really comparable. It might well be, for instance, that only the most unfavourable cases received electroshock and insulin, which in contrast were given very seldom or not at all to the most favourable cases. The only thing that once more can be safely said is that any possible favourable effects of the treatments mentioned were certainly not overwhelming enough to counterbalance the likely biases.

Continuing in the same line, some other negative findings may be of particular interest. Contrary to common beliefs and information in the literature, no specific relations at all were found between the different aspects of outcome and sex, constitution, heredity (schizophrenia or other mental illnesses), intelligence, school education, and age of onset.

Except for the obviously circular relations between outcome and several aspects of the current situation such as housing, employment and perhaps physical health, it seemed that three general factors emerged, which were determinants for the overall outcome, namely:

1. A *personality factor:* the better adapted and the more harmonious the premorbid personality was, the more probable statistically was a favourable course of illness.
2. An *illness-Gestalt-factor* (which is perhaps related to or even identical with the personality factor): the more florid and transient certain main characteristics of the illness were (such as type of onset, productivity and acuteness of the initial symptomatology, developing form), the more probable statistically was a favourable course of illness.
3. An *age factor:* it was found that the latter half of life often exerts a levelling, smoothing and calming influence on schizophrenia. The further the person advanced into old age, the more probable statistically was a favourable course of illness.

Comment

During recent years, not only our own, but also two other major long-term studies on schizophrenia have been published in German, providing together a view of the course of about 1,000 cases over several decades. In 1972, also from Switzerland, came Manfred Bleuler's book, which has just been translated into English, on a very careful 22 year follow-up investigation of 208 schizophrenics in Zurich, and in 1979 appeared the important study by Gerd Huber and co-workers from Bonn on 502 schizophrenics followed-up after an average of 21.4 years. These three studies, closely comparable in their methodology and framework, in spite of a quite different theoretical approach by Huber, were undertaken completely independently of each other. The concordance of the results in general, as well as in many details, is striking.

Thus, favourable end-states were found in 53 per cent of cases by Bleuler, 49 per cent by us in an identical evaluation, and 57 per cent by Huber and collaborators. In all three studies, a great variety of developing types was found by combining various aspects (Huber for instance identified initially 72 types of development which he condensed to 12, as compared to the eight types reported, with very similar frequencies, by Bleuler and ourselves).

Many findings are very similar concerning the variables related to favourable or unfavourable outcome, such as for instance the premorbid personality and social adaptation, the type of onset, the form of development, and to some extent also the initial symptomatology. A common finding, with some minor variations, was also the lack of correlation between course and outcome on one hand and genetic factors on the other (as assessed by schizophrenia or other mental illnesses among family members).

Concerning the influence of treatment, however, the findings are somewhat different. Bleuler avoided statistical calculations because of the enormous inherent methodological uncertainties. Huber on the other hand, whose cases were examined between 1945 and '59, identified some possible, but questionable, indications of a positive long-term effect of neuroleptics as well as of electroshock treatment, especially when they were given shortly after the onset of the illness. This points to a possible bias, as the cases with chronic onset have a worse prognosis.

Our own stand is, as mentioned, intermediate. We would certainly fully agree with Bleuler's (1972) very thoughtful general reflections on the effective factors in the treatment of schizophrenia. He considers that three principles are vitally important in every one of the many old and new therapeutic approaches. The first consists in therapists relating constantly and actively to the healthy aspects of the psychotic patient. The second concerns the therapeutic effect of sudden and surprising changes in general, social and somatic conditions, often leading to a mobilization of hidden resources. The third consists in calming actions and influences which can be introduced in many ways, the best of them being talking and togetherness, and another being neuroleptic drugs. Bleuler is, however, against a regular, heavy and prolonged use of such drugs, giving many convincing arguments on the basis of his long-term observations. It is striking, and emphasized by Bleuler himself, how these three general therapeutic principles can be seen at work in nearly all treatment methods in schizophrenia, as in many other mental conditions and even in normal growth and creativity. Bleuler is convinced that a 'specific treatment of schizophrenia' does not exist.

On the same lines is the following general conclusion we can draw from our own recent long-term investigations and those of the authors mentioned. For everyone who does not link the concept of schizophrenia itself to an obligatory bad outcome, the enormous variety of possible evolutions shows that *there is no such thing as a specific course of schizophrenia*. Doubtless, the potential for improvement of schizophrenia has for a long time been grossly underestimated. In the light of long-term investigations, what is called 'the course of schizophrenia' more closely resembles a life process open to a great variety of influences of all kinds than an illness with a given course. Just as in normal life processes, here what we call illness may represent the complex and variable reaction to an equally complex global situation of a given person, with his particular sensibilities and idiosyncracies, personality structure, behaviour and communication patterns, and past and present experiences. Several important environmental influences on the course have already clearly been identified, among them family attitudes and stressful life-events according to investigations by Brown *et al* (1968; 1972) and Vaughn and Leff (1976), as well as the expectations of the patient himself, his family and surrounding persons which, according to our own recent research, seem often to act strongly as self-fulfilling prophecies (Ciompi *et al*, 1979).

Such a conclusion may be both bewildering and encouraging at the same time. Practically none of the old and seemingly secure dogmas about this illness hold when we look at them closely and long enough. But also no approach which takes the person into account more than the illness, and is hence 'psychotherapeutic' in a wider or narrower sense, has to be *a priori* discarded. Viewing schizophrenia as closer to a life process than to an illness might not be a less useful concept for therapeutic purposes than any other. Anyhow it inspires hope as well as modesty in dealing and communicating with our fellow men hidden by the fascinating and as yet unsolved enigma of psychotic alienation.

References

BLEULER, M. (1978) Die Schizophrenen Geistesstörungen im Lichte langjähriger Kranken- und Familiengeschichten. Thieme, Suttgart 1972. *The Schizophrenic Disorders: Long-term Patient and Family Studies*, translated by S. M. Clemens. Yale University Press, Newhaven and London.

BROWN, G. W. & BIRLEY, J. L. T. (1968) Crises and life changes and the onset of schizophrenia. *Journal of Health and Social Behaviour*, **9**, 203–214.

——— ——— & WING, J. K. (1972) The influence of family life on the course of schizophrenic disorders; a replication. *British Journal of Psychiatry*, **121**, 241–258.

CIOMPI, L., DAUWALDER, H. P. & AGUE, C. (1979) Ein Forschungsprogram zur Rehabilitation psychisch Kranker: III. Längsschnittuntersuchung zum Rehabilitationserfolg und zur Prognostik. *Nervenarzt*, **50**, 366–378.

——— & MULLER, C. H. (1976) *Lebensweg und Alter der Schizophrenen*. Eine katamnestische Langzeit-studie bis ins Senium. Springer, Berlin-Heidelberg-New York.

HUBER, G., GROSS, G. & SCHEUTTLER, R. (1979) *Schizophrenie. Eine verlaufs- und sozial-psychia-trische Langzeitstudie*. Springer, Berlin-Heidelberg-New York.

STEPHENS, J. H. (1970) Long-term courses and prognosis in schizophrenia. *Seminars in Psychiatry*, **2**, 464–485.

STRAUSS, J. S. & CARPENTER, W. T., JR. (1977) The prediction of outcome in schizophrenia. III. Five-year outcome and its predictors. *Archives of General Psychiatry*, **34**, 159–163.

VAUGHN, C. & LEFF, J. (1976) The measurement of expressed emotion in the families of psychiatric patients. *British Journal of Social and Clinical Psychology*, **15**, 157–165.

46 Depressive symptoms in schizophrenia: Some observations on the frequency, morbidity and possible causes

D. A. W. JOHNSON

The presence of depressive mood disorders in schizophrenia has been recognized since the days of Kraepelin and Bleuler. In particular, it has been suggested that patients may manifest a depressive syndrome when their psychosis has aborted. Mayer-Gross (1920) first suggested the syndrome of post-psychotic depression when he described denial of the future or despair as a mode of reacting to a psychotic experience. Further observations were made by Claude *et al* (1924) and Claude (1930), but Eissler (1951) presented the first extensive description of the syndrome. He noted two phases of the schizophrenic breakdown: an initial phase of acute symptoms and a subsequent phase of relative clinical muteness.

Semrad (1966), describing the recovery from an acute schizophrenic episode, identified an initial three to four months regression followed by a longer period when he functions as a 'depressed' patient. He claimed it is during this latter period that the patient works to establish his relationships. The onset of depression heralds progress, represents a good prognostic sign and presents new opportunities for therapeutic intervention, according to the description offered. Other authors have also suggested that the development of post-psychotic depression may be a favourable prognostic sign (Phillips, 1953; Schofield *et al*, 1954; Huston and Pepernik, 1958; Vaillant, 1962; 1964), and that it indicates an improved possibility of good psychosocial adjustment (Wildroe, 1966; Hoedmaker, 1970; Roth, 1970; Kayton, 1973), of these reports the only systematic research was Kayton's retrospective study. A more recent prospective study by McGlashan and Carpenter (1976b) failed to show any association between outcome and post-psychotic depression. In contrast Mandel *et al* (1982) found that depressed schizophrenic patients had a more chronic psychiatric history and they were more likely to experience a future relapse. The value of depression as a prognostic index is unclear and needs further clarification. The literature on the frequency of post-psychotic depression was reviewed by McGlashan and Carpenter (1976a), who failed to find an agreement concerning either the definition or the symptoms of the condition (Steinberg *et al*, 1967; Stern *et al*, 1972; Donlon and Blacker, 1973; Rada and Donlon, 1975). They reported that only four studies were identified and each had serious methodological problems but, on the basis of these reports, they estimated the frequency at 25 per cent. Their own prospective study suggested a higher frequency of 50 per cent (McGlashan and Carpenter, 1976b). A more recent survey Mandel *et al*, 1982) agrees with the earlier assessment, with 25 per cent of these patients developing depression within five months of discharge from hospital.

Although most research has been concerned with depression following the psychotic disorder, depression may develop at other times in the life of a schizophrenic patient. It is clear from studies which include patients who have been established on maintenance treatment that the frequency of depression may be high even after long periods in remission (Leff and Wing, 1971; Hirsch *et al*, 1973; Knights *et al*, 1979). Random interviews have suggested that neurotic symptoms, many of a depressive type (worrying, simple depression, loss of energy, loss of interest) are the principal symptoms causing distress to the chronic schizophrenic patient in the community (Cheadle *et al*, 1978) and this confirmed an earlier observation by Leff (1976). A prospective survey suggested that for chronic schizophrenic patients on regular neuroleptic medication the risk for an episode of depression was over three times the risk of an acute schizophrenic relapse, and that over a two-year period the total duration of morbidity from depression was more than twice the duration of morbidity from acute schizophrenic symptoms (Johnson, 1981a). Conrad (1958) claimed that some patients experience a prodromal phase of mood disturbance before treatment had been prescribed, which may be indistinguishable from endogenous depression. A retrospective analysis of symptoms by Herz and Melville (1980) showed that an acute schizophrenic relapse may be preceded by a non-psychotic prodromal mood disorder. In addition, depressive symptoms have been shown to be present at the time of an acute schizophrenic relapse (McGlashan and Carpenter, 1976b; Knights *et al*, 1979). A recent prospective double blind controlled study goes some way to confirm both these observations: Johnson *et al* (1983) found that about 20 per cent of patients had a definite rise in affective symptoms before an overt schizophrenic relapse and that the acute schizophrenic symptoms were associated with a rise of depressive symptoms on the Hamilton Depression Rating Scale in 40 per cent of patients. These results were the same for drug treated and drug free patients.

Considerations of the aetiology of depressive symptoms have only recently been extended beyond the psychodynamic theories of post-psychotic depression. The neuroleptic drugs have been alleged to have a depressant effect in some patients, particularly certain depot preparations (d'Alarcon and Carney, 1969; Falloon *et al*, 1978), but this is unlikely to be a simple relationship since in some double blind controlled trials the placebo group has experienced a similar frequency of depressive symptoms as the active drug recipients (Leff and Wing, 1971; Hirsch *et al*, 1973). Johnson (1981a) found a high prevalence of depression in untreated first illness patients and drug free relapsed chronic schizophrenic patients. A double blind controlled trial also failed to show any difference in the frequency of depression in patients treated with oral or depot forms of a drug (Schooler *et al*, 1980). Galdi *et al* (1981) have suggested that certain genetic subtypes with a strong familial history of depression may be predisposed to respond to neuroleptics with a pharmacogenic depression. **Hirsch (1983)** replied to this suggestion by claiming that, since depressive symptoms are more frequent during an acute exacerbation of schizophrenia and less once treatment has been started, this is incompatible with pharmacogenic depression. His own explanation is that depressive symptoms resolve less quickly than schizophrenic symptoms—a concept of 'revealed' depression

(**Hirsch, 1982**). To cloud the debate further a number of trials have suggested that some oral (Brockington *et al*, 1978; Johnson, 1979) and depot neuroleptics (Young *et al*, 1976) may have an antidepressant effect in non-schizophrenic patients, and that flupenthixol decanoate may have an antidepressant or mood elevating effect in acute schizophrenia (Johnson and Malik, 1975; Hamilton *et al*, 1979). Any effect on mood may be dose related since most studies suggesting an antidepressant effect have used quite small doses and Johnson (1981a) found that depression was more frequent with the highest dose ranges. The possible contribution of drugs to mood disorders in schizophrenia is complicated even further by the existence of an extrapyramidal syndrome (akinetic depression) which resembles depressive illness, but is in fact a form of drug-induced parkinsonism and responds to the prescription of anticholinergic drugs. A number of authors (Klein and Davis, 1969; Rifkin *et al*, 1975; van Putten and May, 1978) have drawn attention to this frequently overlooked syndrome. Johnson (1981a) estimated that it is responsible for 10 to 15 per cent of depressive type symptoms. Ayd (1975) speculated that such depressions are an affective manifestation of an extrapyramidal reaction.

The schizophrenic illness carries with it an increased risk of suicide. Miles (1977) reviewed all the available studies and estimated that 10 per cent of schizophrenics died by suicide. Markowe *et al* (1967) estimated that in the United Kingdom the risk of suicide in schizophrenia is fifty times that of the normal population. In the United States of America, Pokorny (1964) calculated the suicide rate for the male schizophrenic was 167 per 100,000 per year, compared to the national rate of 10 per 100,000 per year; Miles (1977) estimated that approximately 3,800 schizophrenics per year committed suicide in the United States. Roy (1982), in a matched controlled study, found 50 per cent committed suicide within three months of discharge from in-patient care, and significantly more suicides had a previous history of depression (57 per cent), were depressed in their last episode of contact (53 per cent) and had their last admission for depression or suicidal ideation (55 per cent). Studies have failed to show any direct causal relationship between neuroleptic medication and suicide in schizophrenia (Farberow *et al*, 1961; Cohen *et al*, 1964; Warnes, 1968; Roy, 1982). In one series some suicides occurred shortly after the phenothiazines had been stopped (Cohen *et al*, 1964). In a recent blind prospective follow-up of chronic schizophrenic patients, significantly more patients attempted to harm themselves in the no-treatment group than those who remained on regular neuroleptic medication. In each case the act was associated with a deterioration of mental state, which included a rise in depression as measured by the Hamilton Depression Scale in half the episodes (Johnson *et al*, 1983).

Despite the frequency and complexity of the depressive syndromes in schizophrenia (Knights *et al*, 1979; Galdi *et al*, 1981; **Hirsch, 1982**), it is a subject which, until very recently, had received little systematic or prospective study, particularly in patients on regular medication. Until the aetiology of these syndromes is more clearly understood the treatment must remain empirical and imprecise. One common strategy is to prescribe antidepressant medication although the efficacy of using tricyclic antidepressants is relatively unexplored. Michel and Kolakowska (1981) identified 14 per cent of in-patients or day patients receiving a combination of neuroleptic and antidepressant drugs. Johnson (1983) found that 28 per cent of schizophrenics treated as out-patients had been prescribed antidepressants in addition to neuroleptics during a single year. Yet only two double blind trials have attempted to investigate the effect of tricyclic drugs on new episodes of depression in schizophrenic patients maintained on neuroleptic drugs. Johnson (1981a) failed to show any overall significant advantage for nortriptyline although a trend existed for the 'good improvement' group on active drug. Rifkin and Siris (1984) in a small group of post-psychotic depressions, who had previously failed to respond to anticholinergic drugs to exclude akinetic depression, demonstrated a response to tricyclic antidepressants. Prusoff *et al* (1979) showed some advantage for a combination of amitriptyline with perphenazine in maintenance therapy of depressed schizophrenic out-patients, but only after four months' treatment. Unfortunately the addition of amitriptyline significantly increased the amount of thought disorder with a consequent failure of more than 50 per cent of the patients to complete more than one month on the combination treatment. Despite the improvement in depressive symptoms the final analysis showed no overall advantage for either treatment. Neither Johnson (1981a) nor Rifkin and Siris (1984) confirmed the worsening of psychotic symptoms with the addition of a tricyclic antidepressant, but Johnson reported a significant increase in side-effects with the combination therapy.

The literature on depression in schizophrenia has consistently stressed the frequency and clinical importance of this syndrome. However, it is clear that as yet there is no consensus view on causation and this probably reflects the complex aetiology (Johnson, 1982). Much emphasis has been placed on post-psychotic depression and a possible depressogenic effect of neuroleptic medication, and this has led to a neglect of certain other potentially important areas. As a consequence it remains difficult for the clinician to put the problem in perspective and there is little guidance on management. The author would suggest that the following topics require further research and clarification.

Personality: It is well recognized that the development of depression in a non-schizophrenic is influenced by the personality of the patient. Certain experiences, such as an early parental loss may increase this vulnerability. In schizophrenia it is not only important to consider the premorbid personality, but in many patients the influence of the illness upon personality development. The illness may alter maturation either by a biological influence or by exposing the developing personality to a range of abnormal learning experiences. So far only Roy *et al* (1983) has studied personality vulnerability in the causation of depression in schizophrenia.

Life events: The presence of an excess of life events three to six months before the onset of depression has been repeatedly demonstrated. A recent review (Paykel *et al*, 1984) concluded that neurotic and endogenous depression were very similar in this respect. It has also been shown that life events can precipitate acute episodes of schizophrenia (Brown and Birley, 1968; Birley and Brown, 1970; Hogarty, 1984; Leff *et al*, 1984). It is, therefore, possible that life events may be associated with depression in schizophrenia either by activating the schizophrenic process or by independently precipitating a mood change. The implications for treatment might be considerable.

Post-psychotic depression: Recent research increasingly suggests that 'revealed' depression is a major cause of this syndrome. Despite early claims and considerable interest, no prospective study has been undertaken to examine the psychodynamic theories. Mandel *et al* (1982) have suggested that this syndrome may be associated with a poor prognosis in terms of risk for a further episode of acute schizophrenia, but the full implications for future social or work function remain unexplained. The potential of this syndrome as an index for outcome either of the acute episode or of the long-term prognosis remains relatively unexplored.

Akinetic depression: It seems certain that some patients who present with the symptom of depression, or are diagnosed as depressed, are suffering from this extrapyramidal syndrome which responds rapidly to antiparkinsonian drugs. It is recognized that it may be difficult to separate the two syndromes, but no attempt has been made to establish the profile of symptoms present or whether the condition represents a true depressed state. The risks to the patient, the relevance to neuroleptic response, and the possibility that anticholinergic drugs may be influencing the mental state by other pathways remains unexplored.

Pharmacogenic depression: A direct depressogenic effect by the neuroleptic drugs remains uncertain and if present it is likely to be only a small contributory cause. However, this action could be of considerable importance since it may be related to particular drugs or dose range. Current research is directed at very low dose maintenance therapies. It has been suggested that although a reduced dose may increase the risk of a relapse this may be compensated by other factors such as reduced risk of side-effects and an improved quality of life.

Natural history of schizophrenia: Depressive symptoms may be an integral part of schizophrenia. Research results suggest that their presence may be an early warning of relapse, an indication that an acute episode is responding to treatment with the acute symptoms resolving, and more specifically that the postpsychotic syndrome may indicate a poor prognosis. The frequency of depressive symptoms at all stages of treated and untreated schizophrenia must suggest a relationship with the illness process. A clearer understanding of this relationship has important implications both for the immediate treatment of symptoms and the long-term management of schizophrenia.

Diagnostic dilemma: schizophrenia v. schizoaffective illness: The possibility of a separate diagnostic category has been suggested. However, the present use of the term schizoaffective has little clinical significance since the term is not used in any consistent way. Brockington and Leff (1979) demonstrated a very low concordance between the eight definitions of schizoaffective illness currently in use, and these were much lower than the concordance found for diagnostic categories such as schizophrenia and mania. In an analysis of treatment response schizodepressive patients showed a trend to a better response to chlorpromazine, but the overall response to drugs was poor (Brockington *et al*, 1978). At the present time the data available do not allow any firm conclusion on the presence or absence of the schizoaffective concept (Brockington *et al*, 1979).

References

D'Alarcon, R. & Carney, M. W. P. (1969) Severe depressive mood changes following slow release intramuscular fluphenazine injection. *British Medical Journal, i*, 564–567.

AYD, F. J. (1975) The depot fluphenazines: A reappraisal after ten years' clinical experience. *American Journal of Psychiatry*, **132,** 491–500.

BIRLEY, J. L. T. & BROWN, G. W. (1970) Crisis and life changes preceding the onset of schizophrenia. *British Journal of Psychiatry*, **116,** 327–333.

BROCKINGTON, I. F., KENDELL, R. E., KELLETT, J. M., CURRY, S. H. & WAINWRIGHT, S. (1978) Trials of lithium, chlorpromazine and amitriptyline in schizoaffective patients. *British Journal of Psychiatry*, **133,** 162–168.

—— & LEFF, J. P. (1979) Schizoaffective psychosis: definitions and incidence. *Psychological Medicine*, **9,** 91–99.

—— KENDELL, R. E., WAINWRIGHT, S., HILLIER, V. F. & WALKER, J. (1979) The distinction between the affective psychoses and schizophrenia. *British Journal of Psychiatry*, **135,** 243–248.

BROWN, G. W. & BIRLEY, J. L. T. (1968) Crises and life changes and the onset of schizophrenia. *Journal of Health and Social Behaviour*, **9,** 203–214.

CHEADLE, A. J., FREEMAN, H. L. & KORER, J. (1978) Chronic schizophrenia patients in the community. *British Journal of Psychiatry*, **133,** 211–227.

CLAUDE, H. (1930) Schizomania à forme imaginative. *L'Encéphale*, **25,** 10.

—— BOREL, S. & ROBIN, G. (1924) Démence precoce, schizomanie et schizophrénie. *L'Encéphale*, **19,** 45.

COHEN, S., LEONARD, C. V., FARBEROW, N. L. & SCHNEIDMAN, E. S. (1964) Tranquillizers and suicide in the schizophrenic patient. *Archives of General Psychiatry*, **11,** 312–321.

CONRAD, K. (1958) Die Beginnende Schizophrenia: Versuch Einer Gestaltanalyse Des Wahns. Stuttgart: Thieme.

DONLON, P. T. & BLACKER, K. H. (1973) Stages of schizophrenia decompensation and reintegration. *Journal of Nervous and Mental Disease*, **157,** 200–208.

EISSLER, K. R. (1951) Remarks on the psycho-analysis of schizophrenia. *International Journal of Psychoanalysis*, **32,** 139–156.

FALLOON, I., WATT, D. C. SHEPHERD, M. (1978) A comparative controlled trial of pimozide and fluphenazine decanoate in the continuation therapy of schizophrenia. *Psychological Medicine*, **8,** 59–70.

FARBEROW, N. L., SCHNEIDMAN, E. S. & CALISTA, L. (1961) Suicide amongst schizophrenic mental hospital patients. In *The Cry for Help* (eds. Farberow and Schneidman). New York: McGraw-Hill.

GALDI, J., RIEDER, R. O., SILBER, D. & BONATO, R. R. (1981) Genetic factors in the response to neuroleptics in schizophrenia: a psychopharmacogenetic study. *Psychological Medicine*, **11,** 713–728.

HAMILTON, M., CARD, I. R., WALLIS, G. G. & MAHMOUD, M. R. (1979) A comparative trial of the decanoates of flupenthixol and fluphenazine. *Psychopharmacology*, **64,** 225–229.

HERZ, M. I. & MELVILLE, C. (1980) Relapse in schizophrenia. *American Journal of Psychiatry*, **137,** 801–805.

HIRSCH, S. R. (1982) Depression 'revealed' in schizophrenia. *British Journal of Psychiatry*, **140,** 421–424.

—— (1983) The causality of depression in schizophrenia. *British Journal of Psychiatry*, **142,** 624–625.

—— GAIND, R., ROHDE, P. D., STEVENS, B. C. & WING, J. K. (1973) Outpatient maintenance of chronic schizophrenic patients with long-acting fluphenazine: double blind placebo trial. *British Medical Journal*, i, 633–637.

HOEDEMAKER, F. S. (1970) Psychotic episodes and postpsychotic depression in young adults. *American Journal of Psychiatry*, **127,** 606–610.

HOGARTY, G. E. (1984) Depot neuroleptics: the relevance of psychosocial factors—A United States perspective. *Journal of Clinical Psychiatry*, **45,** 36–42.

HUSTON, P. E. & PEPERNIK, M. C. (1958) Prognosis in schizophrenia. In *Schizophrenia: A Review of the Syndrome* (ed. L. Bellack). New York: Logos Press.

JOHNSON, D. A. W. (1979) A double-blind comparison of flupenthixol, nortriptyline and diazepam in neurotic depression. *Acta Psychiatrica Scandinavica*, **59,** 1–8.

—— (1981a) Studies of depressive symptoms in schizophrenia: I. Prevalence of depression and its possible causes; II. A two year longitudinal study of symptoms; III. A double blind trial of orphenadrine against placebo; IV. A double blind trial of nortriptyline for depression in chronic schizophrenia. *British Journal of Psychiatry*, **139,** 89–101.

—— (1981b) Epidemiological evaluation of maintenance antipsychotic treatment. In *Epidemiological Impact of Psychotropic Drugs* (eds. G. Tognoni, C. Bellantuono, and M. Lader). North Holland: Elsevier.

—— (1982) The long-acting depot neuroleptics. In *Recent Advances in Clinical Psychiatry* (ed. K. Granville-Grossman). Edinburgh: Churchill Livingstone.

—— (1983) Is additional medication required in the maintenance treatment of schizophrenia? In *Modern Trends in the Chemotherapy of Schizophrenia* (ed. P. Hall). VII World Congress of Psychiatry, Vienna.

—— & MALIK, N. A. (1975) A double blind comparison of flupenthixol decanoate and fluphenazine decanoate in the treatment of acute schizophrenia. *Acta Psychiatrica Scandinavica*, **51**, 257–267.

—— PASTERSKI, G., LUDLOW, J. M., STREET, K. & TAYLOR, R. D. W. (1983) The discontinuance of maintenance neuroleptic therapy in chronic schizophrenia patients: drug and social consequences. *Acta Psychiatrica Scandinavica*, **67**, 339–352.

KAYTON, L. (1973) Good outcome in young adult schizophrenia. *Archives of General Psychiatry*, **29**, 103–110.

KLEIN, D. F. & DAVIS, J. M. (1969) *Diagnosis and Drug Treatment of Psychiatric Disorders*. Baltimore: Williams and Wilkins.

KNIGHTS, A., OKASHA, M. S., SALIH, M. A. & HIRSCH, S. R. (1979) Depressive and extrapyramidal symptoms and clinical effects: A trial of fluphenazine versus flupenthixol in maintenance of schizophrenic outpatients. *British Journal of Psychiatry*, **135**, 515–523.

—— & HIRSCH, S. R. (1981) Revealed depression and drug treatment for schizophrenia. *Archives of General Psychiatry*, **38**, 806–811.

LEFF, J. (1976) The assessment of psychiatric and social state. *British Journal of Clinical Pharmacology*, **3**, Supplement 2, 385–390.

—— & WING, J. K. (1971) Trial of maintenance therapy in schizophrenia. *British Medical Journal*, iii, 559–604.

—— KUIPERS, L. & BERKOWITZ, R. (1984) Psychosocial relevance and benefit of neuroleptic maintenance: experience in the United Kingdom. *Journal of Clinical Psychiatry*, **45**, 43–49.

MANDEL, M. R., SEVERE, J. B., SCHOOLER, N. R., GELENBERG, A. J. & MIESKE, M. (1982) Development and prediction of postpsychotic depression in neuroleptic-treated schizophrenics. *Archives of General Psychiatry*, **39**, 197–203.

MARKOWE, M., STEINERT, J. & HEYWORTH-DAVIES, F. (1967) Insulin and chlorpromazine in schizophrenia: a ten year comparative study. *British Journal of Psychiatry*, **113**, 1101–1106.

MAYER-GROSS, W. (1920) Über die Stellungsnahme auf abgelaufenen akuten Psychose. *Zeitschrift Für Die Gesamte Neurologie Und Psychiatrie*, **60**, 160–212.

McGLASHAN, T. H. & CARPENTER, W. T. (1976a) Postpsychotic depression in schizophrenia. *Archives of General Psychiatry*, **33**, 231–239.

—— —— (1976b) An investigation of the postpsychotic depressive syndrome. *American Journal of Psychiatry*, **133**, 14–19.

MELLOR, C. S. (1970) First rank symptoms of schizophrenia. *British Journal of Psychiatry*, **117**, 15–23.

MICHEL, K. & KOLAKOWSKA, T. (1981) A survey of prescribing psychotropic drugs in two psychiatric hospitals. *British Journal of Psychiatry*, **138**, 217–221.

MILES, P. (1977) Conditions predisposing to suicide: a review. *Journal of Nervous and Mental Disease*, **164**, 231–246.

PAYKEL, E. S., RAO, B. M. & TAYLOR, C. N. (1984) Life stress and symptom pattern in out-patient depression. *Psychological Medicine*, **14**, 559–568.

PHILLIPS, L. (1953) Case history data and prognosis in schizophrenia. *Journal of Nervous and Mental Disease*, **117**, 515–535.

POKORNY, A. (1964) Suicide rates in various psychiatric disorders. *Journal of Nervous and Mental Disease*, **139**, 499–506.

PRUSOFF, B. A., WILLIAMS, D. H., WEISSMAN, M. M. & ASREACHAN, B. M. (1979) Treatment of secondary depression in schizophrenia. *Archives of General Psychiatry*, **36**, 569–575.

RADA, R. T. & DONLON, P. T. (1975) Depression and the acute schizophrenic process. *Psychosomatics*, **16**, 116–119.

RIFKIN, A., QUITKIN, F. & KLEIN, D. F. (1975) Akinesia, a poorly recognised drug-induced extrapyramidal behaviour disorder. *Archives of General Psychiatry*, **32**, 672–674.

—— & SIRIS, S. (1984) *Double-Blind Trial of a Tricyclic Antidepressant Versus Placebo in Postpsychotic Depression*. Paper presented at Symposium in Seefeld, Austria.

ROTH, S. (1970) The seemingly ubiquitous depression following acute schizophrenic episodes, a neglected area of clinical depression. *American Journal of Psychiatry*, **127**, 91–98.

ROY, A. (1982) Suicide in chronic schizophrenia. *British Journal of Psychiatry*, **141**, 171–177.

—— THOMPSON, R. & KENNEDY, S. (1983) Depression in schizophrenia. *British Journal of Psychiatry*, **142**, 465–470.

SCHOFIELD, W., HATHAWAY, S. R. & HASTINGS, D. W. (1954) Prognostic factors in schizophrenia. *Journal of Consulting Psychology*, **18**, 155–156.

SCHOOLER, N. R., LEVINE, J., SEVERE, J. B., BRAUZER, B., DIMASCIO, A., KLERMAN, G. L. & TUASON, V. B. (1980) Prevention of relapse in schizophrenia: An evaluation of fluphenazine decanoate. *Archives of General Psychiatry*, **37,** 16–24.

SEMRAD, E. V. (1966) Long-term therapy in schizophrenia. In *Psychoneuroses and Schizophrenia* (ed. E. L. Usdin). Philadelphia: J. B. Lippencott.

STEINBERG, H. R., GREEN, R. & DURELL, J. (1967) Depression occurring during the course of recovery from schizophrenic symptoms. *American Journal of Psychiatry*, **124,** 699–702.

STERN, M. J., PILLSBURY, J. A. & SONNENBERG, S. M. (1972) Postpsychotic depression in schizophrenics. *Comprehensive Psychiatry*, **13,** 591–598.

VAILLANT, G. E. (1962) The prediction of recovery in schizophrenia. *Journal of Nervous and Mental Disease*, **135,** 534–543. .

—— (1964) Prospective prediction of schizophrenic remission. *Archives of General Psychiatry*, **11,** 509–518.

VAN PUTTEN, T. & MAY, P. R. A. (1978) Akinetic depression in schizophrenia. *Archives of General Psychiatry*, **35,** 1101–1107.

WARNES, H. (1968) Suicide in schizophrenics. *Diseases of the Nervous System*, **29,** 35–40.

WILDROE, H. J. (1966) Depression following acute schizophrenic psychosis. *Journal of Hillside Hospital, New York*, **15,** 114–122.

YOUNG, J. O., HUGHES, W. C. & LADER, M. (1976) A controlled comparison of flupenthixol and amitriptyline in depressed patients. *British Medical Journal, ii,* 1116–1118.

47 Depression 'revealed' in schizophrenia

1. Steven R. Hirsch

Since Helmchen and Hippius (1967) noted that half a sample of 120 schizophrenics had depressive symptoms at the time of admission, more than 30 papers have appeared associating depressive symptoms in schizophrenics with neuroleptic medication (Ananth and Chadirian, 1980). Many authors and clinicians in fact think that a causal relationship has been proven, and the term 'pharmacogenic depression' and the associated concept 'akinetic depression' have come into use. The assumptions underlying these concepts and the evidence to support them need critical examination. They will be considered with the results of more recent studies which answer some of the outstanding questions, but in turn raise new ones about the relationship of schizophrenia and depression to their underlying pathophysiology.

The concept of *pharmacogenic depression* assumes that depressive symptoms are a side effect of neuroleptic medication. However, reports of the frequency of depression in schizophrenia vary widely according to the method used—for example, in one study we reported that about 15 per cent of chronic schizophrenics in out-patients required antidepressant medication over 9 months whether they were on depot neuroleptics or had been withdrawn (Hirsch *et al*, 1973). In another sample of 37 schizophrenics, followed for 6 months from the time they were discharged from hospital, just over half were found to develop depressive symptoms at some point during this period (Knights *et al*, 1979). Obviously, the results differed because of the methodology. In fact, most reports in the literature fail to provide the basic facts necessary to interpret their results, including: (a) The length of time patients are observed—so one can tell if depression is rare or common during the period of observation. (b) The method of case detection—so one can compare one series of patients with another and know the likelihood of observing depression, if observations were made frequently or only, say, every nine months. (c) The criteria used to identify symptoms or rate their presence.

In order to demonstrate that pharmacogenic depression occurs, one needs to be able to show that depressive symptoms are more common in patients receiving neuroleptics than a comparable group receiving no drugs or placebo. Until recently there were no prospective studies comparing patients with and without medication over the same time period, except one single crude attempt (Hirsch *et al*, 1973).

The concept of *akinetic depression* is a variation on the concept of pharmacogenic depression. It was coined by Van Putten and May (1978) because they noted patients without other symptoms of drug-induced parkinsonism were slow and lethargic as well as seemingly depressed, and rapidly improved when anticholinergics were administered. However, Quitkin *et al* (1978) had made the point that those symptoms which respond to anticholinergics are part of drug-induced parkinsonism. One would need to demonstrate that a depressive syndrome can be reliably differentiated from the parkinsonian syndrome before 'akinetic depression' could be regarded as a separate clinical entity. Möller and von Zerssen (1981) have in fact shown that depressive symptoms are as common in schizophrenics on anticholinergics as in those who are not, and Johnson (1981a; b) has shown that anticholinergics are no more effective than placebo for the treatment of depression in schizophrenics. There is therefore little reason to regard the akinetic syndrome as a form of depression, though the concept has heuristic value to remind us that apparently anergic depressed schizophrenics may have drug-induced parkinsonism.

A third concept, *post-psychotic depression*, refers to the possibility that depression may occur as schizophrenics recover insight into their illness and life situation. From a nosological point of view depression which occurs as a reaction to being ill is no different from any other 'reactive depression' such as that following bereavement or divorce, and we do not speak of 'post-divorce depression'! No one has even shown whether or not the number of such cases is negligible. Depression and schizophrenia could, logically, occur together *merely as a matter of chance*. If so, depression should occur with an equal frequency at any phase in the illness, but reports from Shanfield *et al* (1970), Donlon *et al* (1976) plus recent studies by Knights and Hirsch (1981), Johnson (1981a; b) and Möller and von Zerssen (1981), show that this is not the case.

Finally, depression may be *an integral part of the schizophrenic process*, commonly present, but unnoticed during the acute phase when the florid psychosis is most evident and other symptoms are understandably ignored. In this case we could expect depressive symptoms to be more prevalent in the acute phase when the psychosis is more active and decrease rather than increase with neuroleptic treatment. Recent studies summarized below have shown that this is the case. In fact, it can be hypothesized that if depressive symptoms are caused by neuroleptic medication one could expect them to increase rather than decrease after treatment begins—if they decrease it would not support the hypothesis of pharmacogenic depression.

Three recent studies have done this. A sample including all interviewable schizophrenics admitted from a catchment area over one year, showed that depressive symptoms decreased significantly during the three-month interval from the time of admission (Knights and Hirsch, 1981). Sixty-five per cent of the patients had at least three depressive CATEGO syndromes on the Present State Examination (Wing *et al*, 1974) present on admission, and over 80 per cent had at least one. At the end of three months depressive symptoms were almost as prevalent in schizophrenics as in a comparison group of neurotics and depressives from the same catchment area over the same period of time. Another group of schizophrenics, followed from the time of discharge when they began depot neuroleptics, had a lower prevalence of depressive symptoms when going on the medication, but these also decreased, though not significantly, over the following six months.

Using a different method of assessment, based on the IMP Scale, Möller and von Zerssen (1981) reported a series of 280 schizophrenics, of whom 48 per cent had depressive symptoms on admission and 14 per cent at discharge. Only 14 per cent developed depressive symptoms who did not have depression on admission. Johnson (1981a; b) found a high prevalence of depressive symptoms, as defined by a Hamilton Rating Scale (HRS) or a Beck self-rating inventory (BDI) score of over 15 in first illness acute schizophrenics, acute on chronic relapsed schizophrenics, and chronic schizophrenics in remission. There was no difference in the prevalence of depression in any group, whether they were on medication at the time or had never been treated with drugs. Furthermore, a follow-up of 30 chronic schizophrenics over two years, with monthly assessments from the time they entered the study on relapse, showed that 60 per cent experienced at least one episode of depressive illness (HRS or BDI over 15) at some time during the study. Depression alone was responsible for 70 per cent of the patients' morbidity measured in weeks over the two year period, while only 30 per cent could be ascribed to schizophrenia alone or schizophrenic symptoms plus depression. Neither anticholinergics nor antidepressants proved to be significantly better than placebo in reducing symptoms, which tended to go and come spontaneously in at least half of those affected.

Taken together these results from different centres are incompatible with the hypothesis that neuroleptics are a common cause of depressive symptoms in schizophrenia. Perhaps even more important is the question they raise about our concept of schizophrenia and the distinction between schizophrenia and depression—the old concept of a unitary psychosis springs to mind. Because of the high frequency of depressive symptoms in schizophrenia, occurring whether patients are on neuroleptic medication or not, their tendency to recur, and the fact that they remit rather than increase after treatment has begun, all suggest that depressive symptoms are an integral part of the schizophrenic syndrome and must, therefore, share with schizophrenia common pathophysiological processes. Like the situation in the game of chess called 'revealed check', these symptoms tend to remain hidden from clinicians behind the florid features of psychosis, only to be revealed during the remission phase. This new evidence suggests that re-examination of the underlying relationship between depression and schizophrenia is required.

References

ANANTH, J. & CHADIRIAN, A. M. (1980) Drug induced mood disorder. *International Pharmacopsychiatry*, **15**, 58–73.
DONLON, P. T., RADA, R. T. & ARORA, K. K. (1976) Depression and the reintegration of acute schizophrenia. *American Journal of Psychiatry*, **133**, 1265–1268.
HELMCHEN, H. & HIPPIUS, H. (1967) Depressive Syndrome im Verlauf neuronleptischer Therapie. *Nervenarzt*, **38**, 445.
HIRSCH, S. R., GAIND, R., ROHDE, P. D. *et al* (1973) Out-patient maintenance of chronic schizophrenic patients with long-acting fluphenazine: A double-blind placebo trial. *British Medical Journal*, i, 633–637.
JOHNSON, D. A. W. (1981a) Studies of depressive symptoms in schizophrenia. *British Journal of Psychiatry*, **139**, 89–101.
—— (1981b) Studies of depressive symptoms in schizophrenia: III. A double-blind trial of orphenadrine against placebo. *British Journal of Psychiatry*, **139**, 96–97.
KNIGHTS, A., OKASHA, M. S., SALIH, M. *et al* (1979) Depressive and extrapyramidal symptoms and clinical effects: A trial of fluphenazine versus flupenthixol in maintenance of schizophrenic out-patients. *British Journal of Psychiatry*, **135**, 515–523.
—— & HIRSCH, S. R. (1981) 'Revealed' depression and drug treatment for schizophrenia. *Archives of General Psychiatry*, **38**, 806–811.
MÖLLER, H. J. & VON ZERSSEN, D. (1981) Depressive Symptomatik in stationären Behandlungsverlauf von 280 schizophrenen Patienten. *Pharmacopsychiatria*, **14**, 172–179.

QUITKIN, F., RIFKIN, A., KANE, J. *et al* (1978) Long-acting oral vs injectable antipsychotic drugs in schizophrenics: A one-year double-blind comparison in multiple episode schizophrenics. *Archives of General Psychiatry*, **35,** 889–892.

SHANFIELD, S., TUCHER, G. J., HARROW, M. *et al* (1970) The schizophrenic patient and depressive symptomatology. *Journal of Nervous and Mental Disease*, **151,** 203–210.

VAN PUTTEN, T. & MAY, P. R. A. (1978) 'Akinetic depression' in schizophrenia. *Archives of General Psychiatry*, **35,** 1101–1107.

WING, J. K., COOPER, J. E. & SARTORIUS, N. (1974) *The Measurement and Classification of Psychiatric Symptoms.* London: Cambridge University Press.

2. Joe Galdi

The phenomenon of post-treatment depression in schizophrenia has become the subject of considerable controversy regarding its causality (Ananth and Chadirian, 1980; McGlashan and Carpenter, 1976a). But as the recent commentary by **Hirsch** (**1982**) emphasizes, the most controversial issue is focused on whether this depression is neuroleptic-induced. Hirsch himself refutes neuroleptic induction on the basis of various uncontrolled data which seem ostensibly incompatible with this causality. Results indicating that pre-treatment depressions appear in a high proportion of recently hospitalized schizophrenics, occur in drug free patients, and frequently remit or decrease following neuroleptic therapy are cited as evidence contradicting neuroleptic induction. Hirsch therefore proposes an alternative view: that this post-treatment depression is an integral, 'revealed' aspect of the schizophrenia syndrome which arises from the same pathophysiological process (McGlashan and Carpenter, 1976b).

There are several theoretical and methodological issues not addressed by Hirsch, however, which might render this or any theory concerning the causality of this depression premature if not too all encompassing.

(1) Significant pretreatment depression in a recently hospitalized schizophrenic could signify many things. First, by current American criteria (RDC or DSM-III) such a patient might receive an 'affective' or 'schizoaffective' diagnosis, a trend (especially characteristic of research settings) which attempts to mimic the more stringent diagnostic practices of European psychiatry. Yet one might wonder if such practices were operative in the studies quoted by Hirsch as refuting neuroleptic induction. Knights and Hirsch (1981), for example, indicated the presence of PSE depressive CATEGO syndromes in a sample of acute schizophrenics which were almost as frequent as their presence in a control sample of hospitalized depressives. The comparatively lesser severity of symptoms in the sample as a whole, furthermore, did not exclude the possibility that, in many patients, severity was equivalent to that found in the depressives. Möller and von Zerssen (1982) likewise reported significant depression in a substantial number of recently hospitalized schizophrenics, 60 per cent of whom were first admissions and 44 per cent acutely precipitated. In the samples reported by Johnson (1981), depression (Hamilton Depression Scales >15) on admission was evident in seven, and pre-admission depression (past 2 months) in another 11, of 37 never-treated first illness schizophrenics. A few of these patients, however, had originally been diagnosed for depression, while still others had a history of depresssion for which they may have previously attended hospital. In another sample of relapsed schizophrenics who

had been drug free for at least two months, 24 of 79 met depression criteria on the Hamilton Scale. In addition to the secondary status apparently accorded depression in these patients, the reported use of Schneiderian symptoms as a basis for diagnosing schizophrenia may also be questionable since these symptoms also occur, if less frequently, in manics and psychotic depressives.

Given that many patients in the above studies were initially depressed, findings such as reported by Knights and Hirsch (1981) indicating that initially depressed patients tend to remain depressed after drug therapy, are neither unexpected nor evidence against neuroleptic induction, since neuroleptics might have impaired remission or regression, or ceiling effects on ratings might have limited the ability to determine psychometrically whether symptoms had actually worsened in some patients (see below).

Secondly, since depression is frequently observed as the first sign of relapse in out-patient schizophrenics maintained on neuroleptics (Floru *et al*, 1975; Hertz and Melville, 1981; Hogarty *et al*, 1979; Mandel *et al*, 1982), it would not be unusual to find that relapsed patients are frequently depressed when rehospitalized. Some pre-treatment depressions in recently admitted patients could therefore be neuroleptic-induced.

Third, even among relapsing schizophrenics who previously ceased taking neuroleptics for any time (e.g. Johnson, 1981), the neuroleptic induction of depressions observed at time of hospitalization cannot be ruled out. This contention is supported by the Casey *et al* (1960) finding that neuroleptics can have long-lasting residual effects which may be depressogenic. In this study, patients were randomly assigned to chlorpromazine (fixed 400 mgs/day) and placebo (plus other drugs), treated for 3 months, and then randomly *reassigned* to these same treatments for another 3 months. After 6 months, patients who were initially assigned to chlorpromazine but subsequently reassigned to placebo were significantly more depressed than patients who, by sequential randomization, were treated with placebo for the entire period. Such residual depressogenic effects might conceivably be due to biochemical changes attending chronic receptor blockade which persist in spite of drug withdrawal. Similar effects may also be responsible for the long delay of relapse following neuroleptic withdrawal in chronically medicated out-patients.

(2) The causes of post-treatment depression in schizophrenia may be heterogeneous, but a substantial proportion of these depressions are probably *pharmacogenic*. In a recent study (Galdi *et al*, 1981), we reported, in one sample, that schizophrenics who had depressed first-degree relatives were significantly more depressed after 4–6 weeks of neuroleptic therapy than similar patients treated with placebo. Schizophrenics who had schizophrenic first-degree relatives failed to show differences in the effect of neuroleptics and placebo on depression. In a second, uncontrolled sample in which sensitive ratings scales were used, depression increased in patients who had a depressed parent but decreased in patients who had a schizophrenic parent. Yet these subgroups could not be differentiated at pre-treatment on the basis of presenting symptoms including depression, in one sample, while in another, patients who had depressed relatives were slightly more depressed, although this was mainly due to higher anxiety. Although we cannot speak to the rigour of the DSM-II criteria applied in these samples where prior psychiatric history was assessed, 70 per cent of the schizophrenics with depressed relatives were described by

admitting psychiatrists as being chronically ill. This chronicity indirectly confirmed the poor prognostic character of post-treatment depressions reported by others (Mandel *et al*, 1982). A similar finding from the Hogarty *et al* (1979) study of relapsed schizophrenics maintained on depot neuroleptics, furthermore, supports the view that many of the depressions observed in recently hospitalized schizophrenics may also be pharmacogenic. In this study, relapsed patients, whose symptoms frequently revealed a distinct 'affective quality' on hospitalization, were found to have significantly more affective illnesses in first-degree relatives than non-relapsed patients.

(3) Post-treatment depressions in schizophrenics which are pharmacogenic are frequently accompanied by pseudo-parkinsonism and, less often, akathisia. Our findings revealed more severe demonstrations of these extrapyramidal symptoms EPS in schizophrenics who had depressed first-degree relatives (some mild EPS also occurred more frequently but failed to reach significance), and correlations between these EPS and depressive symptoms which, though not well co-ordinated, ranged 0.49–0.79 in these patients. These findings not only implicated neuroleptics in the induction of this depression, but suggested that these more severe EPS may also be pharmacogenic. The genetic selectivity of these drug-induced symptoms also contradicts past tendencies to trivialize them as simply 'drug-induced' or notions that the depression is not a real depression. Our findings instead imply that severe pseudo-parkinsonism (and possibly akathisia) as well as its correlated depression may result from the interaction of neuroleptics with a genetic defect affecting the nigrostriatal dopaminergic system of patients with associated disorders. We applied the terms 'pharmacogenic depression' and 'pharmacogenic pseudo-parkinsonism' to distinguish these responses, emphasizing their potential diagnostic utility. In this sense, we can agree with **Hirsch (1982)** as to the pathophysiological significance of this depression.

(4) Post-treatment depressions of the pharmacogenic (nigrostriatal variety may be responsive to anticholinergic drugs. Although difficulties in co-ordinating data in one sample and obtaining accurate data in another precluded our estimating the effect of anticholinergic drugs on post-treatment depression in our study (Galdi *et al*, 1981), we were able to provide evidence supporting anticholinergic responsiveness in a third sample. This sample consisted of small numbers of genetically subtyped schizophrenics who presented EPS (at early emergence) following routine treatment with neuroleptics. Predictably, seven patients who had depressed first-degree relatives had significantly higher depression, pseudo-parkinsonism, and total EPS scores than four patients who had schizophrenic first-degree relatives when EPS emerged. In both subgroups, EPS responded similarly to benztropine and amantadine (a dopamine agonist), although change appeared more dramatic in patients who had depressed first-degree relatives. In addition, only these latter patients showed evidence of reduced clinical symptomatology including depression after treatment. Similarly, Johnson (1981) reported orphenadrine (albeit only 100 mgs/day) to be more effective than placebo in treating post-treatment depressions, although the difference was not significant and less than half of the patients responded. However, that not all depressions respond fully to anticholinergics is not necessarily contradictory since dopamine-acetylcholine balance may be involved and remission might depend on the relative

potency and bioavailability of drugs antagonizing the system (Snyder *et al*, 1974).

What these preliminary findings also suggest is that difficulties exist in interpreting results from studies such as quoted by Hirsch in which anticholinergics are used in an uncontrolled fashion, and liberally, perhaps prophylactically, prescribed. Since depressions arising during neuroleptic therapy are frequently accompanied by parkinsonian symptoms which are almost reflexively treated with anticholinergics, a reduction of depression in at least some patients would not be unexpected. By contrast, since tricyclic antidepressants may be less potent anticholinergics than the anticholinergic antiparkinson agents, it is doubtful that, in the presence of neuroleptic therapy, they can alleviate depressions which are neuroleptic-induced (Johnson, 1981); van Kammen *et al* (1980) recently suggested that some of these depressions may be responsive to lithium.

(5) Finally, there exist many psychometric problems inherent to measuring direction of symptom change with rating scales that should be considered in judging whether depression has been induced by neuroleptics. Depression in schizophrenics, for example, might appear (via 'halo' effects) more severe during early psychotic phases than during subsequent non-psychotic or less severe phases simply by association with greater severity, all else equal. Second, most linear rating scales are prone to regression toward the mean which could affect the direction of change observed, especially if depressive symptoms were initially rated more severe (high) on the scale. Third, scales vary considerably in their ability to sense change let alone its direction. In our study, for example, the semi-molecular Inpatient Multi-dimensional Psychiatric Scale revealed increased depression in schizophrenics with depressed heredity, while the molar Brief Psychiatric Rating Scale revealed no change or trivial decreases in these same symptoms. This difference occurred in spite of very high interscale correlations and the fact that both scales were reliably completed by the same raters in the same interviews. These selected problems imply that, since scaled ratings may not accurately reflect change in symptoms over time, issues bearing on drug induction are probably best addressed through placebo controls and judgements of relative change. In the absence of such controls, even if neuroleptics worsened depression or impaired its remission, it might still be possible to conclude from the data that the depression just remitted more slowly (McGlashan and Carpenter, 1976b) or that it was simply unmasked (**Hirsch, 1982**).

A further methodological issue suggested by our own studies arises from the probable biologic-genetic heterogeneity of schizophrenia and its relationship to post-treatment depressions. If we had simply grouped all patients together, our findings would have revealed what Knights and Hirsch (1981) and others have reported: slightly decreased depression from pre-treatment levels. The extent of decrease observed in any sample, moreover, might depend on the relative weighting of biologically different subgroups in the sample. The diagnostic criteria used, which might vary these weights, could also have an impact on what is observed.

What these various points seem to indicate is that depression in schizophrenia is a complex phenomenon from both methodological and theoretical perspectives. No single theory may adequately explain all of the data. Our own studies support a concept of 'pharmacogenic depression' which occurs in genetically predisposed patients as one type. In many, if not most patients, this depression is co-mingled with pseudo-parkinsonism, from which it may be indistinguishable. Mild as opposed to severe expressions of this depression, however, particularly if only accompanied by akinesia, may be difficult to discriminate. Preliminary evidence suggests that it is responsive to anti-cholinergics and may be of nigrostriatal origin. Since it may be part of the pathophysiology of the disorder, it must also be assumed that it can occur spontaneously in the absence of neuroleptics. In our opinion, this depression may actually represent an extrapyramidal (motor) component of a dopaminergic-related disorder which often induces a subjective dysphoria that is secondary in nature (cf. Hogarty *et al*, 1979). On the other hand, I have also interviewed schizophrenic patients who are ostensibly depressed in conjunction with a severe pseudo-parkinsonian reaction who persistently deny being depressed.

The significance of pre-treatment depressions, by contrast, in the absence of diagnostic laxity, may be ambiguous. Some of these depressions may be neuroleptic-induced, persisting long after pre-admission drug withdrawal, others may be purely reactive and remit with neuroleptic therapy. Findings such as Möller and von Zerssen's (1982), of initial remission of depression followed by subsequent increases in some patients, may be difficult to explain from any viewpoint. (However, in Casey *et al*, quoted above, chlorpromazine at 400 mgs/day decreased initial depression in spite of subsequent residual effects.) Obviously, additional controlled studies of these depressive phenomena are needed. In this regard, we are struck by growing reports associating depression in schizophrenia with increased risks for tardive dyskinesia. Such studies should therefore probably look prospectively at the long-term effects of neuroleptics in depressed schizophrenics.

Lest it be misunderstood, no findings to date appear to support the notion that schizophrenics predisposed to post-treatment depressions are diagnostically unique (further evaluation is indicated) nor that the use of rigorous diagnostic criteria can circumvent their occurrence (Galdi *et al*, 1981).

References

ANANTH, J. & CHADIRIAN, A. M. (1980) Drug induced mood disorder. *International Pharmacopsychiatry*, **15,** 58–73.

CASEY, J. F., BENNETT, I. F., LINDSEY, C. J. *et al* (1960) Drug therapy of schizophrenia: a controlled study of the relative effectiveness of chlorpromazine, promazine, phenobarbital and placebo. *Archives of General Psychiatry*, **117,** 997–1003.

FLORU, L., HEINRICH, K. & WITTEK, F. (1975) The problem of postpsychotic schizophrenic depression and their pharmacological induction. *International Pharmacopsychiatry*, **10,** 230–239.

GALDI, J., RIEDER, R. O., SILBER, D. & BONATO, R. R. (1981) Genetic factors in the response to neuroleptics in schizophrenia: a psychopharmacogenetic study. *Psychological Medicine*, **11,** 713–728.

HERTZ, M. I. & MELVILLE, C. (1981) Relapse in schizophrenia. *American Journal of Psychiatry*, **137,** 801–805.

HIRSCH, S. R. (1982) Depression 'revealed' in schizophrenia. *British Journal of Psychiatry*, **140,** 421–424.

HOGARTY, G. E., SCHOOLER, N. R., ULRICH, R. *et al* (1979) Fluphenazine and social therapy in the aftercare of schizophrenic patients. *Archives of General Psychiatry*, **36,** 1283–1294.

JOHNSON, D. A. W. (1981) Studies of depressive symptoms in schizophrenia. *British Journal of Psychiatry*, **139,** 89–101.

KNIGHTS, A. & HIRSCH, S. R. (1981) 'Revealed' depression and drug treatment for schizophrenia. *Archives of General Psychiatry*, **38**, 806–811.

MANDEL, M. R., SEVERE, J. B., SCHOOLER, N. R. *et al* (1982) Development and prediction of postpsychotic depression in neuroleptic-treated schizophrenics. *Archives of General Psychiatry*, **39**, 197–203.

McGLASHAN, T. H. & CARPENTER, W. T. (1976a) Postpsychotic depression in schizophrenia. *Archives of General Psychiatry*, **33**, 231–239.

—— —— (1976b) An investigation of the postpsychotic depressive syndrome. *American Journal of Psychiatry*, **133**, 14–19.

MÖLLER, H. J. & VON ZERSSEN, D. (1982) Depressive states occurring during the neuroleptic treatment of schizophrenia. *Schizophrenia Bulletin*, **8**, 109–117.

SNYDER, S., GREENBERG, D. & YAMAMURA, H. I. (1974) Antischizophrenic drugs and brain cholinergic receptors. *Archives of General Psychiatry*, **31**, 58–61.

VAN KAMMEN, D. P., ALEXANDER, P. E. & BUNNEY, W. E. (1980) Lithium treatment in postpsychotic depression. *British Journal of Psychiatry*, **136**, 479–485.

3. Steven R. Hirsch

The strength of the concept of 'revealed' depression in schizophrenia lies in its economy and simplicity. If depressive symptoms are an integral part of the schizophrenic process, these symptoms could be expected to be most frequent when the symptoms of schizophrenia are most severe and be less prevalent as the condition remits. A post-psychotic reactive depression consequent on the return of insight, or depression which is a result of drug treatment, should get worse, not better, after treatment is commenced and not be most extant in the acute untreated phase. Numerous studies quoted by Hirsch (1982) and Galdi *et al* (1981) confirm a high prevalence of depression in acutely admitted schizophrenia, 50 per cent of cases or more. In his critique, Galdi endeavours to show how a number of factors may have contributed to this high rate of depression in acute schizophrenia yet may also be compatible with the concept of a neuroleptic-induced depression. It is important to realize that the apparent conceptual conflict between us may be more one of emphasis than flat disagreement. Our argument can be rephrased; if depressive symptoms can be proved to be most frequent during an acute exacerbation of schizophrenia and decrease after treatment begins, it is incompatible with the concept of pharmacogenic depression as the *main* explanatory hypothesis. This is not to say that the causes are not heterogeneous but only that drug-induced depression is not the main factor.

Galdi builds his argument by introducing a large number of assumptions about other researchers' data, mostly based on conjecture, which would account for a misleading high prevalence rate for depression in schizophrenia apparently independent of a neuroleptic-inducing effect. The first is 'diagnostic laxity'—unlikely, given that all the studies quoted used research criteria which, though differing from centre to centre, produced very similar results. Thus we used the PSE-CATEGO criteria of Wing *et al* (1974), Johnson used the Feighner Criteria and Möller used the IMPS and the DiaSika programme. According to Möller and von Zerssen (1981; 1982) 15–17 per cent of patients developed depression following admission, in addition to the 50 per cent who had depression on admission. These indeed could be drug-induced but they are a minority. In fact Johnson (1981) found a higher rate of depression among first admission untreated schizophrenics, of whom half were depressed, than among patients who had been on neuroleptics previously or at the time of admission, of whom a third were depressed. Thus the drug-induced depression concept cannot explain the higher prevalence rate of depressive symptoms found in the untreated among all acute schizophrenics. Casey *et al*'s (1960) finding that depression occurred in a higher frequency in schizophrenics treated with neuroleptics until six months prior to assessment than patients never treated, and Galdi's finding (1981) that the incidence of persisting depressive symptoms was higher in schizophrenics treated with neuroleptics than those who received placebo, provided that they had a family history of depression, are as yet unreplicated isolated observations, but they would support the existence of a neuroleptic-induced depression in schizophrenia if confirmed.

The strong association between drug-induced extra-pyramidal symptoms, especially hypokinesis, muscular rigidity and loss of movement with depression (0.49–.79, Galdi, 1981) itself raises problems of interpretation. No one has shown that depression can be reliably distinguished from pseudo-parkinsonism with loss of movement but without depression, so the relationship may be spurious and the only drug-induced effect may be parkinsonism, not depression. The apparent responsiveness of the symptoms to anticholinergics does not solve this problem. Johnson's assessment (1981) was based on depressive feelings and distress as well as a high Hamilton score so it would seem that his patients were depressed, in which case it remains to be determined what proportion of the patients recorded as depressed in other studies have depression, drug-induced parkinsonism, or both.

Perhaps Galdi's most telling point about studies based on following up symptoms over time is the tendency for ratings, especially the more extreme ones, to regress to the mean. As he suggests, this can be overcome by comparing drug and placebo-treated groups, blindly rated over a time, to see if the prevalence and rating of depressive symptoms changes at different rates in the two groups. The point is to prove that a decrease noted to occur in affective symptoms over time is not an artefact inherent in repeated ratings.

Depression, as a common syndrome in acute as well as chronic patients with schizophrenia has now been revealed by numerous recent studies. As we postulated (Knights and Hirsch, 1981) causation may well prove to be heterogeneous, but as yet the most economical main hypothesis is a shared pathophysiological mechanism accounting in part for schizophrenic and depressive symptoms, and not a drug-induced one. Only further research, not polemics, can resolve this issue.

References

CASEY, J. F., BENNETT, I. F., LINDLEY, C. J. *et al* (1960) Drug therapy of schizophrenia: a controlled study of the relative effectiveness of chlorpromazine, promazine, phenobarbitol and placebo. *Archives of General Psychiatry*, **117**, 997–1003.
GALDI, J., REIDER, R. O., SILBER, D. & BONATO, R. R. (1981) Genetic factors in the response to neuroleptics in schizophrenia: a psychopharmacogenetic study. *Psychological Medicine*, **11**, 713–728.
HIRSCH, S. R. (1982) Depression 'revealed' in schizophrenia. *British Journal of Psychiatry*, **140**, 421–424.
JOHNSON, D. A. W. (1981) Studies of depressive symptoms in schizophrenia. *British Journal of Psychiatry*, **139**, 89–101.

KNIGHTS, A. & HIRSCH, S. R. (1981) Revealed depression and drug treatment for schizophrenia. *Archives of General Psychiatry*, **38**, 806–811.

MÖLLER, H. J. & VON ZERSSEN, D. (1981) Depressive Symptomatik in Stationären Behandlungsverlauf von 280 schizophrenen Patienten. *Pharmakopsychiatrie*, **14**, 172–179.

—— & VON ZERSSEN, D. (1982) Depressive states occurring during the neuroleptic treatment of schizophrenia. *Schizophrenia Bulletin*, **8**, 109–117.

WING, J. K., COOPER, J. E. & SARTORIUS, N. (1974) *The Measurement and Classification of Psychiatric Symptoms*. London: Cambridge University Press.

Index

Compiled by Stanley Thorley

References in **bold type** indicate complete papers. With the exception of major direct quotations references to the literature have not been included.

PROPERTY OF
RIVERWOOD COMMUNITY MENTAL HEALTH